Medical Spanish
Dictionary pocket

english–spanish
spanish–english

A
B
C
D
E
F
G
H
I
J
K
L
M
N
O
P
Q
R
S
T
U
V
W
X
Y
Z

D1247771

www.media4u.com

Editors: Carla Maute M.D., Stephanie Prinz M.D., Santiago Otero Lopez-Cubero M.D., Jose Miguel Espinosa Saldaña, Ingo Haessler M.D.
Cover Illustration: Franka Krueger
Illustration: Anna Donska, Ilka Barthauer
Printer: Koesel GmbH, 87435 Kempten, Germany, www.koeselbuch.de
Publisher: Börm Bruckmeier Publishing LLC, www.media4u.com

© 2003, by **Börm Bruckmeier Publishing LLC**
63 16th Street, Hermosa Beach, CA 90254
www.media4u.com
First Edition

IMPORTANT NOTICE - PLEASE READ!
This book is based on information from sources believed to be reliable, and every effort has been made to make the book as complete and accurate as possible and to describe generally accepted practices based on information available as of the printing date, but its accuracy and completeness cannot be guaranteed. Despite the best efforts of editors and publisher, the book may contain errors, and the reader should use the book only as a general guide and not as the ultimate source of information about the subject matter.
This book is not intended to reprint all of the information available to the authors or publisher on the subject, but rather to simplify, complement and supplement other available sources. The reader is encouraged to read all available material and other references to learn as much as possible about the subject.
This book is sold without warranties of any kind, expressed or implied, and the publisher and authors disclaim any liability, loss or damage caused by the content of this book.
IF YOU DO NOT WISH TO BE BOUND BY THE FOREGOING CAUTIONS AND CONDITIONS , YOU MAY RETURN THIS BOOK TO THE PUBLISHER FOR A FULL REFUND.

Printed in Germany
ISBN 1-59103-211-3

Preface

Communication is critical in medicine. Language should never be a barrier between medical professionals and patients.

Medical Spanish Dictionary pocket provides you with a handy reference that will enhance your ability to communicate with your Spanish-speaking patients and to understand them with greater ease and precision.

Medical Spanish Dictionary pocket offers accurate translations for almost every health-related term likely to occur in a conversation between a healthcare professional and a Spanish-speaking patient.

Medical Spanish Dictionary pocket is also published as software for PDA. Go to our web site at www.media4u.com for details.

We hope that **Medical Spanish Dictionary pocket** will be helpful to you in your practice! Please write (service@media4u.com) to tell us what we can do to make it even better.

From the editors and the publisher   June 2003

Additional titles in this series:
Differential Diagnosis pocket
Drug pocket 2003
Drug Therapy pocket
ECG pocket
Homeopathy pocket
Medical Abbreviations pocket
Medical Spanish pocket
Medical Spanish pocket plus
Normal Values pocket
Surgery pocket

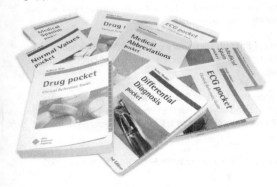

Börm Bruckmeier Publishing LLC on the Internet:
www.media4u.com

Contents

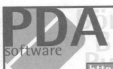

1. Basics

1.1 Spanish Language

Pronunciation

The Spanish alphabet has 30 letters.y

Letter	Name	Pronunciation
A	a	like 'a' in afternoon
B	be	softer than English 'b'
C	ce	like 'k' in 'key' before a, o, u or consonants, before e, i like 'th' in 'then' is the pronunciation in Spain; c like 's' in 'say' in Latin America
CH	che / ce hache	like 'ch' in chest
D	de	softer than English 'd'
E	e	like 'e' in contents
F	efe	same as 'f' in English
G	ge	mostly like 'g' in 'guess' like h before e, i, but ...gui..., ...gue... is spoken as 'g' in 'guess'
H	hache	silent
I	i	like 'i' in 'ski'
J	jota	similar to the 'h' in 'hospital'
K	ka	like 'k' in 'key'
L	ele	like 'l' in 'lemon'
LL	elle / doble ele	like 'y' in 'yellow'
M	eme	same as in English
N	ene	same as in English
Ñ	eñe	like 'ny' in 'canyon'
O	o	like 'o' in 'low'
P	pe	same as in English
Q	cu	like 'k'
R	ere	similar to 'r' in 'interest', stronger than English 'r'
RR	erre	strong spanish 'r', always trilled

Letter	Name	Pronunciation
S	ese	like 'ss' in 'stress'
T	te	between English 't' and 'd'
U	u	like 'u' in 'true'
V	ve / uve	like English 'b'
W	uve doble	similar to 'w' in 'word'
X	equis	like 's', 'ks'
Y	i griega	like 'y' in 'yes'
Z	zeta	like 's'; before e and i like the English 'th' in Spain like 's' in Latin America

How to stress correctly in Spanish

- Stress words ending with a vowel, n or s on the next to the last syllable, e.g. ayudar (to help)
- Stress the last syllable in words ending with consonants other than n or s, e.g. calor (heat)
- Any word that follows a different stress pattern must have an accent on the vowel of the stressed syllable, e.g. corazón (heart)

Articles

- Masculine articles are el, los, and uno, unos.
- Feminine articles are la, las, and una, unas.
- In most cases, nouns ending in -o are masculine, and nouns ending in -a are feminine.
- Exceptions: día (day) is masculine, mano (hand) is feminine. A few other exeptions are the masculine words raticida, insecticida, herbicida, pesticida.
- Words ending in -dad, -ián, -tad, -umbre are feminine.
- Names of days of the week, months, rivers, mountains etc. are always masculine and often end in -o, -e, -u, -y.
- Articles in the following tables are given, if the word doesn't end in -a or -o, or if it is an exception. (ms) stands for masculine

singular, (fs) for feminine singular, (mp) for masculine plural, (fp) for feminine plural.

Plurals
- Words are made plural by adding -s or -es to the end of the word.
- Add -s, if the word ends in an unaccented vowel.
- Add -es, if the word ends in an accented vowel, consonant or -y.

Contractions
- 'to the' is expressed as 'a la', if a feminine noun follows, as 'al', if the following noun is masculine.
- 'of the' is expressed as 'de la', if a feminine noun follows, as 'del', if the following noun is masculine.

Sentence marks
- In Spanish, there are also inverted question and exclamation marks before a question or exclamation, e.g. ¿De dónde es? ¡Qué interessante!

Pre- and Suffixes
- 'des-' at the beginning of a word is used to express the opposite of the original word.
- '-ito', '-ita' at the end of the word is used to express the diminutive.
- 'ísimo, -a' at the end of the word is used to express the augmentative.
- '-tad' or '-dad' are related to the English '-ty' as in quality.
- '-ería' at the end of the word marks up the location where the object is manufactured, sold etc.
- '-mente' at the end of the feminine adjective forms the correspondending adverb.

Common Questions

Common questions	Preguntas comunes
Are there...?	¿Hay...?
Are you...?	¿Está usted (Vd.) ...?
Can I...?	¿Puedo...?
Do you have...?	¿Tiene Vd....?
Do you have...?	¿Tiene Vd....?
Do you remember?	¿Recuerda Vd.?
Do you use...?	¿Usa Vd....?
For how long?	¿Desde cuándo?; ¿Por cuánto tiempo?
Have I seen you before?	¿Lo he visto antes?
Have you had...?	¿Ha tenido Vd.?
How are you?	¿Cómo está Vd.?
How many years ago?	¿Hace cuantos años?
How much?	¿Cuánto?
Is it better / worse?	¿Está mejor / peor?
What did you say?	¿Cómo?; ¿Qué dijo?; ¿Mande?
What do you have?	¿Qué tiene Vd.?
What do you need?	¿Qué necesita Vd.?
What is it?	¿Qué es esto?
What time is / was it?	¿Qué hora es / ¿A qué hora fue?
What?	¿Qué?
What's the matter?	¿Qué pasa?
What's your name?	¿Cómo se llama?
When?	¿Cuándo?
Where do you come from?	¿De dónde es Vd.?
Where is...?	¿Dónde está?
Which side?	¿En qué lado
Which year?	¿En qué año?
Who is this?	¿Quién es este?
Why? / Because...	¿Por qué? / Porque...

1.2   Basic Anatomy

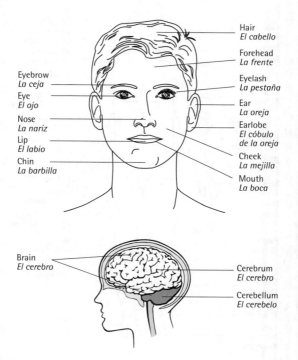

Hair
El cabello

Forehead
La frente

Eyelash
La pestaña

Ear
La oreja

Earlobe
*El cóbulo
de la oreja*

Cheek
La mejilla

Mouth
La boca

Eyebrow
La ceja

Eye
El ojo

Nose
La nariz

Lip
El labio

Chin
La barbilla

Brain
El cerebro

Cerebrum
El cerebro

Cerebellum
El cerebelo

Head / *La cabeza*

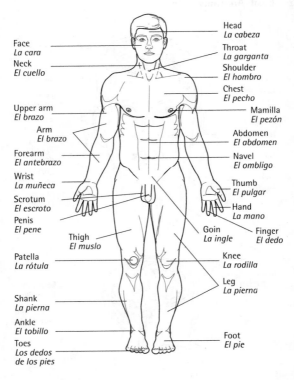

Male body, anterior view / *El cuerpo masculino, vista anterior*

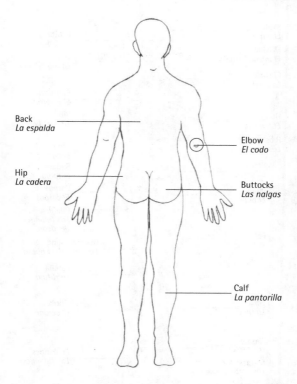

Back
La espalda

Elbow
El codo

Hip
La cadera

Buttocks
Las nalgas

Calf
La pantorrilla

Male body, posterior view / *El cuerpo masculino, vista posterior*

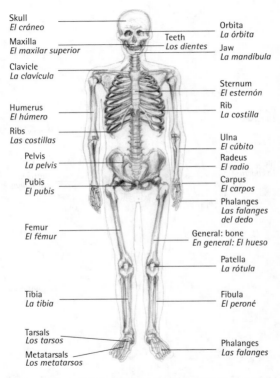

Skull
El cráneo

Maxilla
El maxilar superior

Clavicle
La clavícula

Humerus
El húmero

Ribs
Las costillas

Pelvis
La pelvis

Pubis
El pubis

Femur
El fémur

Tibia
La tibia

Tarsals
Los tarsos

Metatarsals
Los metatarsos

Orbita
La órbita

Teeth
Los dientes

Jaw
La mandíbula

Sternum
El esternón

Rib
La costilla

Ulna
El cúbito

Radeus
El radio

Carpus
El carpos

Phalanges
*Las falanges
del dedo*

General: bone
En general: El hueso

Patella
La rótula

Fibula
El peroné

Phalanges
Las falanges

Skeleton, anterior view / *El esqueleto, vista auterior*

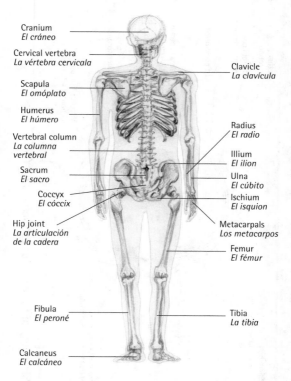

Cranium
El cráneo

Cervical vertebra
La vértebra cervicala

Clavicle
La clavícula

Scapula
El omóplato

Humerus
El húmero

Radius
El radio

Vertebral column
*La columna
vertebral*

Illium
El ilion

Sacrum
El sacro

Ulna
El cúbito

Coccyx
El cóccix

Ischium
El isquion

Hip joint
*La articulación
de la cadera*

Metacarpals
Los metacarpos

Femur
El fémur

Fibula
El peroné

Tibia
La tibia

Calcaneus
El calcáneo

Skeleton, posterior view / El esqueleto, vista posterior

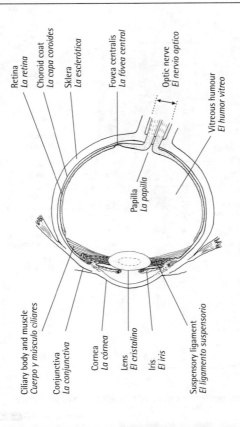

Structures of the eye / *Las estructuras del Ojo*

Retina
La retina

Choroid coat
La capa coroides

Sklera
La esclerótica

Fovea centralis
La fóvea central

Optic nerve
El nervio optico

Vitreous humour
El humor vítreo

Papilla
La papilla

Ciliary body and muscle
Cuerpo y músculo ciliares

Conjunctiva
La conjunctiva

Cornea
La córnea

Lens
El cristalino

Iris
El iris

Suspensory ligament
El ligamento suspensorio

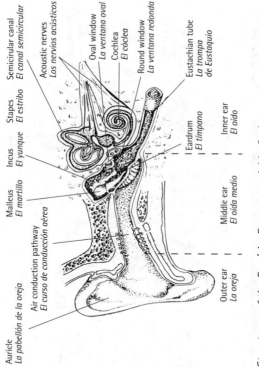

Semicircular canal
El canal semicircular

Acoustic nerves
Los nervios acústicos

Oval window
La ventana oval

Cochlea
El cóclea

Round window
La ventana redonda

Eustachian tube
*La trompa
de Eustaquio*

Stapes
El estribo

Incus
El yunque

Eardrum
El tímpano

Inner ear
El oído

Malleus
El martillo

Air conduction pathway
El curso de conducción aérea

Middle ear
El oída medio

Outer ear
La oreja

Auricle
La pabellón de la oreja

Structures of the Ear / *La Estructura del la Oreja*

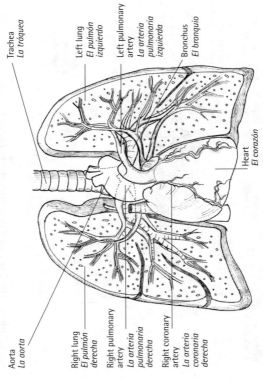

Structures of the lung / La estructura del pulmón

Trachea
La tráquea

Left lung
El pulmón izquierdo

Left pulmonary artery
La arteria pulmonaria izquierda

Bronchus
El bronquio

Heart
El corazón

Aorta
La aorta

Right lung
El pulmón derecha

Right pulmonary artery
La arteria pulmonaria derecha

Right coronary artery
La arteria coronaria derecha

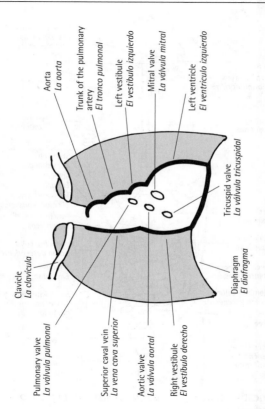

Aorta
La aorta

Trunk of the pulmonary artery
El tronco pulmonal

Left vestibule
El vestibulo izquierdo

Mitral valve
La válvula mitral

Left ventricle
El ventriculo izquierdo

Tricuspid valve
La válvula tricuspidal

Clavicle
La clavicula

Diaphragm
El diafragma

Pulmonary valve
La válvula pulmonal

Superior caval vein
La vena cava superior

Aortic valve
La válvula aortal

Right vestibule
El vestibulo derecho

Silhouette of the heart / La silueta del corazón

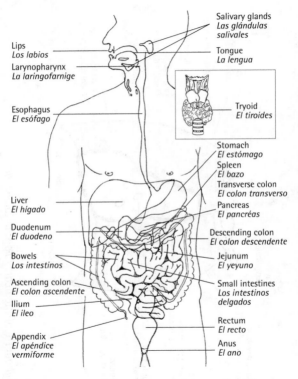

Salivary glands
Las glándulas salivales

Tongue
La lengua

Lips
Los labios

Larynopharynx
La laringofarnige

Esophagus
El esófago

Tryoid
El tiroides

Stomach
El estómago

Spleen
El bazo

Transverse colon
El colon transverso

Pancreas
El pancréas

Liver
El hígado

Duodenum
El duodeno

Descending colon
El colon descendente

Bowels
Los intestinos

Jejunum
El yeyuno

Ascending colon
El colon ascendente

Small intestines
Los intestinos delgados

Ilium
El ileo

Appendix
El apéndice vermiforme

Rectum
El recto

Anus
El ano

Digestive system / *El aparato o sistema digestivo*

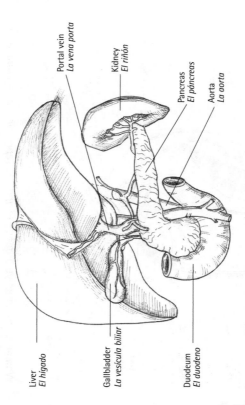

Portal vein
La vena porta

Kidney
El riñón

Pancreas
El páncreas

Aorta
La aorta

Liver
El hígado

Gallbladder
La vesícula biliar

Duodeum
El duodeno

Digestive system / *El aparato o sistema digestivo*

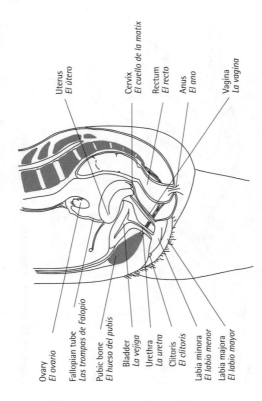

Ovary
El ovario

Fallopian tube
Las trompas de Falopio

Pubic bone
El hueso del pubis

Bladder
La vejiga

Urethra
La uretra

Clitoris
El clitoris

Labia minora
El labio menor

Labia majora
El labio mayor

Uterus
El útero

Cervix
El cuello de la matix

Rectum
El recto

Anus
El ano

Vagina
La vagina

Woman's reproductive organs / *El aparato reproductivo de la mujer*

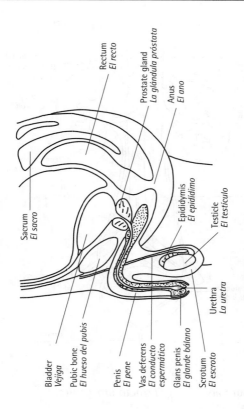

Rectum
El recto

Prostate gland
La glándula próstata

Anus
El ano

Epididymis
El epidídimo

Testicle
El testículo

Urethra
La uretra

Sacrum
El sacro

Bladder
Vejiga

Pubic bone
El hueso del pubis

Penis
El pene

Vas deferens
El conducto espermático

Glans penis
El glande bálano

Scrotum
El escroto

Man´s reproductive organs / *El aparato reproductivo del hombre*

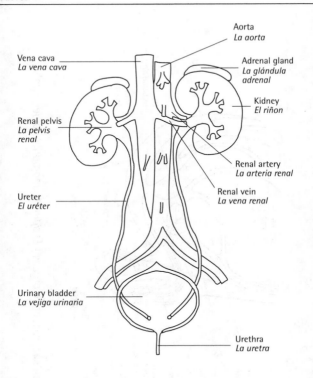

Aorta
La aorta

Vena cava
La vena cava

Adrenal gland
La glándula adrenal

Kidney
El riñon

Renal pelvis
La pelvis renal

Renal artery
La arteria renal

Renal vein
La vena renal

Ureter
El uréter

Urinary bladder
La vejiga urinaria

Urethra
La uretra

Genitourinary Tract / *El tracto uro-genital*

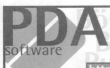

English – Spanish
Dictionary

A

a, an un, una
abdomen abdomen, vientre
abdominal abdominal, del vientre; ~ **aneurysm** aneurisma abdominal; ~ **aponeurosis** aponeurosis abdominal; ~ **bandage** vendaje abdominal, faja; ~ **belt** vendaje abdominal, faja; ~ **bloating** flatulencia, meteorismo, presencia de gas en el vientre o intestino; ~ **breathing** respiración diafragmática; ~ **cavity** cavidad abdominal; ~ **cramp** cólico, espasmo abdominal, retortijón; ~ **fascia** aponeurosis abdominal; ~ **gas** meteorismo, presencia de gas en el vientre o intestino; ~ **pain** dolor abdominal, dolor pélvico; ~ **palpation** palpación del abdomen; ~ **skin reflex** reflejo cutáneo abdominal; ~ **tap** paracentesis; ~ **trauma** traumatismo abdominal
abdominalgia dolor abdominal, dolor pélvico
abdominoplasty abdominoplastia
abducens paralysis parálisis del nervio motor ocular externo
abduction abducción; ~ **fracture** fractura en abducción; ~ **splint** férula de abducción
abductor abductor
aberrant aberrante, anormal, extraño
abetalipoproteinemia abetalipoproteinemia
abiogenesis abiogénesis
abiotic degradation degradación abiótica
abiotrophy abiotrofia
ablation desprendimiento, extirpación, ablación; ~ **of the vitreum** ablación del vítreo
abnormal aberrante, anormal, anómalo; ~ **fibrinogens** fibrinógenos anormales
abnormality anomalía, desviación de la norma, irregularidad, anormalidad
abortifacient medicamento abortivo, substancia abortiva
abortion aborto, interupción del embarazo; ~ **pill** píldora abortiva
about aproximadamente
above arriba, sobre
abrasion abrasión, erosión dentaria, desgaste, raspadura, decorticación; ~ **of the cornea** abrasión corneal, ulceración del epitelio corneal producida por fricción
abreaction abreacción, la catarsis, una liberación emocional
abrupt abrupto, repentino, brusco
abruptio placentae abruptio placentae
abscess absceso
abscisic acid ácido absísico
absence ausencia, pérdida momentánea del conocimiento; ~ **seizure** ausencia, pérdida momentánea del conocimiento
absent-minded distraído, olvidadizo, irritado
absinthe ajenjo
absolute absoluto; ~ **alcohol** alcohol absoluto; ~ **error** error absoluto; ~ **healing index** tasa absoluta de curación; ~ **lethal concentration** concentración letal absoluta
absorbance absorbancia
absorbed concentration concentración absorbida; ~ **dose** dosis absorbida
absorbent cotton algodón hidrófilo
absorbing absorción, captación, retención
absorptance absortancia
absorption absorción, penetración a través de la piel o de las mucosas; ~ **coefficient** coeficiente de absorción; ~ **factor** factor de absorción; ~ **spectrum** espectro de absorción
abstinence abstinencia, privación voluntaria
abstract resumen
abstract thinking pensamiento abstracto
abulia abulia, debilitación de la voluntad
abuse, to lastimar, dañar, abusar
acanthocheilonema microfilaria, forma prelavaria del helminto filariásico
acanthocytosis acantocitosis
acariasis acariasis, enfermedad de los acáridos, de la acarina
acarodermatitis dermatitis por ácaros
acarus scabiei acarus scabiei
acataphasia agramatismo, acatafasia
acathisia acatisia, tasicinesia
accelerated skin aging envejecimiento prematuro de la piel
acceleration aceleración
acceptor site centro aceptor
accessory concomitante, acompañante
accident accidente; ~ **at work** accidente de trabajo
accidental accidental, al azar, sin importancia,

casual, involuntario; ~ **death** muerte por accidente; ~ **irradiation** irradiación accidental; ~ **poisoning** intoxicación accidental

accident-prone propenso a accidentes

acclimatization aclimatación, aclimatización

acclimatized inoculum inóculo aclimatado

accommodation acomodación (f), ajuste (m), adaptación (f); ~ **range** escala de adaptación, grado de acomodación

accreditation acreditación

accretion acrementación, la unión, el crecimiento

accumulation acumulación

accuracy exactitud, fiabilidad, precisión; ~ **of a test** fiabilidad de un instrumento; ~ **of movement** precisión de movimiento

ACE enzima de conversión de la angiotensina, enzima convertidora de angiotensina

Ace bandage venda elástica, apósito contentivo

acephalia acefalia

acephaly acefalia

acetabulae zonas acetabulares

acetabular fossa fosa acetabular

acetabulum acetábulo

acetaminophen paracetamol

acetate kinase acetato-cinasa

acetazolamide acetazolamida

acetoacetato acetoacetato

acetoacetic acid ácido acetoacético

acetone acetona; ~ **bodies** cuerpos cetónicos

acetonemic vomiting vómito acetonémico

acetonuria cetonuria, acetonuria, presencia de cueropos cetónicos en la orina

aceto-phenetidin fenacetina

acetyl cysteine acetil cisteina

acetylation acetilación

acetylcholine acetilcolina; ~ **intoxication** intoxicación por acetilcolina

acetylcholinesterase acetilcolinesterasa, colinesterasa verdadera

acetylcoenzyme A acetilcoenzima A

acetylsalicylic acid aspirina, ácido acetilsalicílico

ACH hormona corticosuprarrenal

achalasia acalasia del esofago

ache dolor constante, la dolencia; ~ , **to** doler

Achilles tendon tendón de Aquiles

aching doloroso, dolorido

achlorhydria aclorhidria, anacidez, anaclorhidria

achondroplasia acondroplasia

achroacyte linfocito

achromatopsia acromatopsia

acid ácido; ~ **-base balace** equilibrio acidobásico; ~ **-fast** ácidorresistente; ~ **phosphatase** fosfatasa ácida; ~ **rebound** acidez reactiva

acidification acidificación

acidified methanol metanol acidificado

acidity acidez

acidocyte leucocito neutrofilo, granulocito acidófilo

acidophil leucocito neutrofilo, granulocito acidófilo

acidophilic cell leucocito neutrofilo, granulocito acidófilo

acidosis acidosis, aumento de la acidez en líquidos y tejidos del cuerpo

acidotic acidótico; ~ **coma** coma acidótico; ~ **dyspnea** disnea acidótica; ~ **respiration** respiración acidótica

aciduria aciduria

acinetobacter acinetobacter

acne acné; ~ **necrotica** acné necrótica; ~ **pustule** pústula de acné, grano, espinilla, granito, barro; ~ **rosacea** acné rosácea, rosácea, eritrosis facial

acoustic acústico; ~ **nerve** nervio coclear, nervio auditivo; ~ **neuroma** neuroma acústico; ~ **trauma** trauma acústico

acquired adquirido; ~ **deafness** sordera adquirida, hipoacusia adquirida, sordera accidental; ~ **hyperostosis syndrome** síndrome de hiperortocitosis; ~ **immunodeficiency syndrome** síndrome de inmunodeficiencia adquirida, el SIDA

acrania acrania

acrocyanosis acrocianosis, coloración rojiazulada de los extremos corporales

acrodynia acrodinia, quiropodalgia

acromegaly acromegalia

acromio-clavicular acromioclavicular

acromioclavicular joint articulación acromioclavicular

acromion acromion

acro-osteolysis acroosteolisis
acroscleroderma esclerodactilia, acrosclerosis
acrosome acrosoma
across a través, al otro lado
ACTH ACTH (hormona), hormona adrenocorticotropa
actin actina; ~ **filaments** microfilamentos
actinic keratosis queratosis senil, queratosis actínicas, lesiones cutáneas escamosas derivadas de la exposición excesiva y crónica al sol
actinodermatitis dermatitis lumínica, actinodermatitis
actinodermatosis dermatitis lumínica, actinodermatitis
actinomyces actinomicetos
actinomycosis actinomicosis
activate, to activar, estimular, acelerar, reactivar
activated activado; ~ **carbon** carbón activado; ~ **charcoal** carbón activado; ~ **host cell** activación de la célula huésped
activated water agua activada
activation activación
activator activador
active activo, en actividad, eficaz; ~ **anaphylaxis** anafilaxis activa; ~ **hyperemia** hiperemia activa, hiperemia arterial; ~ **ingredient** principio activo, sustancia activa; ~ **medication** medicamento activo; ~ **principle** principio activo, sustancia activa; ~ **site** centro activo, sitio activo
activity actividad; ~ **coefficient** coeficiente de actividad
actual real
acuity acuidad, agudeza
acupressure acupresión, digitopuntura
acupuncture acupuntura
acute agudo, súbito y breve, grave; ~ **abdomen** abdomen agudo; ~ **care** cuidados intensivos, medicina intensiva; ~ **glomerulonephritis** glomerulonefritis aguda; ~ **laryngotracheobronchitis** garrotillo, crup laríngeo, crup diftérico, laringotraqueítis, infección vírica aguda del conducto respiratorio; ~ **leukemia** leucemia aguda; ~ **liver failure** insuficiencia hepática aguda; ~ **lymphoblast leukemia** leucemia linfoblástica aguda, leucemia linfocítica,

leucemia linfática, leucemia linfógena, leucemia linfoide; ~ **lymphocytic leukemia** leucemia aguda linfoide; ~ **monoblast leukemia** leucemia monoblástica; ~ **mountain sickness** mal de montaña agudo; ~ **myeloblast leukemia** leucemia mieloblástica; ~ **myeloid leukemia** leucemia aguda mieloide; ~ **otitis media** otitis media aguda; ~ **pain** dolor agudo; ~ **-phase protein** proteína de fase aguda; ~ **pulmonary edema** edema agudo pulmonar; ~ **renal failure** insuficiencia renal crónica; ~ **tonsillitis** angina aguda; ~ **toxicity** toxicidad aguda; ~ **trauma** traumatismo agudo; ~ **tubulo-interstitial nephropathy** nefropatía tubulointersticial
acyclovir aciclovir
acyl dehydrogenase acil-CoA-deshidrogenasa
Adam's apple bocado de Adán, nuez de adán
adaptation adaptación
adaptor DNA, ADN de unión, ADN de enlace; ~ **RNA** tRNA adaptador
add, to añadir, adicionar, agregar
addiction adicción, dependencia de drogas, morfinomanía, tendencia, propensión, adictovicio, habito malo
addictive drug droga adictiva, droga toxicomanígena, droga causante de dependencia
Addis count cuenta de Addis
Addison's disease enfermedad de Addison
additional adicional, añadido, complementario, suplemental
additive aditivo, sustancia añadida a alimentos
add-on aditivo, sustancia añadida a alimentos
address dirección
adduction aducción; ~ **contracture** contractura por aducción; ~ **fracture** fractura por aducción
adductor reflex reflejo de los aductores
adenine adenina
adenitis adenitis, inflamación de las glándulas
adenocystic carcinoma carcinoma adenoide quístico, cilindroma
adenoepithelioma adenoepitelioma, epitelioma glandular
adenofibroma fibroadenoma, adenoma fibroso
adenoma adenoma (m), tumor benigno de estructura glandular

adenomatoid carcinoma adenocarcinoma

adenomatous adenomatoso; ~ **carcinoma** adenoepitelioma, epitelioma glandular; ~ **polyp** pólipo adenomatoso, adenoma polipoide benigno

adenopathy adenopatía

adenosine adenosina; ~ **deaminase** adenosina-desaminasa; ~ **monophosphate** adenosina monofosfato; ~ **triphosphate** trifosfato de adenosina

adenosinetriphosphatase adenosinatrifosfatasa

adenotomy adenotomía, linfadenectomía

adenoviral vector vector adenoviral

adenovirus adenovirus

adenylate kinase adenilato-cinasa

adenylylcyclase adenilato-ciclasa

adequate adecuado, apropiado, propio

adherence assay ensayo de adherencia

adherent pericardium pericarditis adhesiva, pericarditis constrictiva

adhesion adhesión, fijación, unión anormal de tejidos u órganos

adhesive adhesivo; ~ **bandage** vendaje adhesivo, venda adhesiva; ~ **colpitis** vaginitis adhesiva, vaginitis senil; ~ **dressing** vendaje adhesivo, venda adhesiva; ~ **plaster** esparadrapo, curita; ~ **tape** cinta adhesiva

adipoceratous corpse cadáver conservado en cera grasa (en adipocira)

adipose cell célula cebada; ~ **tissue** tejido adiposo, tejido grasoso

adiuretin vasopresina

adjustment acomodación, ajuste, adaptación; ~ **disorder** trastorno de adaptación

adjuvant adyuvante, sustancia que contribuye a la acción de otra, sustancia añadida a una vacuna que refuerza su efecto

administer, to administrar

admission rate tasa de admisiones; ~ **to hospital** admisión en un hospital, hospitalización

Admissions (in the hospital) internación, ingresos

adnexa anexo, anejo

adnexal anexial, de los anejos, del anexo; ~ **carcinoma** carcinoma de los anejos, cáncer del anexo, tumor de los anejos; ~ **mass** tumor de los anejos, masa anexial; ~ **tuberculosis** tuberculosis de los anexos; ~ **tumor** tumor de los anejos, masa anexial

adnexectomy histerosalpingooforectomía

adnexitis enfermedad inflamatoria pélvica, anexitis, adnexitis

adolescent adolescente, joven; ~ **coxa vara** coxa vara adolescente, coxa adducta, la epifisiólisis

adrenal suprarrenal; ~ **cortex** corteza suprarrenal, corteza adrenal; ~ **glands** glándulas adrenales, glándula suprarrenales; ~ **glycosuria** glucosuria adrenal; ~ **insufficiency** insuficiencia suprarrenal; ~ **system** sistema cromafínico

adrenalectomy adrenalectomía

adrenalin(e) epinefrina, adrenalina; ~ ~ **blocking** adrenolítico, sustancia que inhibe la respuesta a la adrenalina; ~ **inhibitor** adrenolítico, sustancia que inhibe la respuesta a la adrenalina

adrenergic adrenérgico, activado por la adrenalina; ~ **antagonist** antagonista adrenérgico, bloqueador adrenérgico, simpaticolítico; ~ **blocker** antagonista adrenérgico, bloqueador adrenérgico, simpaticolítico; ~ **receptor** receptor adrenérgico

adrenocorticotropic hormone coticotropina, hormona ACTH, hormona adrenocorticotropa

adrenodoxin adrenodoxina

adrenogenital adrenogenital; ~ **syndrome** síndrome adrenogenital

adrenolytic adrenolítico, sustancia que inhibe la respuesta a la adrenalina

adrenoreceptor receptor adrenérgico

adriamycin adriamicina, doxorrubicina

adsorption adsorción, fijación a una superficie, cf absorción, penetración a través de la piel o de las mucosas; ~ **chromatography** cromatografía de adsorción; ~ **immobilization** enlace iónico, inmovilización por adsorción

adult adulto; ~ **respiratory distress syndrome** síndrome de insuficiencia respiratoria del adulto

advance directives directivas de adelanto,

procuración
adventitious adventicio; ~ **agent** agente adventicio; ~ **deafness** sordera adquirida, hipoacusia adquirida, sordera accidental
adverse adverso, contrario, desfavorable; ~ **effects** efectos adversos; ~ **reaction** reacción adversa, efecto colateral
adversity revés, contrariedad, fracaso
advice asesoramiento, consejo
adviser asesor
adynamic fever fiebre adinámica
adjuvant chemotherapy quimioterapia adyuvante
aerasthenia aeroastenia, aeroneurosis
aerobic aerobio, que necesita la presencia de oxígeno
aerogenic aerogénico
aero-otitis media barotraumatismo del oído
aerophagy aerofagia, acción de tragar aire, deglución inconsciente de aire
aerosinusitis aerotitis media (en una cavidad en el cráneo)
aerosol aerosol, solución de un producto destinado a ser inhalado; ~ **inhaler** inhalador de epinefrina broncodilatadora
aerospace medicine medicina espacial, aeroespacial
aerotolerant aerotolerante
aesthetic surgery cirugía estética, cirugía plastica
a–fetoprotein a-fetoproteína
affect sentimiento, emoción
affected afectado; ~ **area** lesión, daño, desperfecto, traumatismo, herida, lastimadura
affective afectivo, emocional; ~ **bond** relación afectiva, vinculación afectiva; ~ **climate** clima afectivo, ambiente emocional; ~ **disorder** trastorno afectivo, trastorno de humores; ~ **psychosis** trastorno afectivo mayor, psicosis afectiva, trastorno psicótico afectivo; ~ **rapport** relación afectiva, vinculación afectiva
affinity afinidad, analogía, semejanza, interacción entre un medicamento y el receptor de membrana; ~ **chromatography** cromatografía de afinidad; ~ **constant** constante de afinidad
affliction aflicción

aflatoxin aflatoxina
AFP alfa-fetoproteína, AFP
afebrile apirético, sin fiebre
African trypanosomiasis tripanosomiasis, tripanosomosis
after después de, tras; ~ **care services** cuidados posteriores, fase posterior al tratamiento, servicios de terapia de convalescencia; ~ **childbirth** posparto, después del parto; ~ **dinner** posprandial, que se presenta después de una comida
afterbirth segundo parto, placenta
aftereffect postefecto
afterload (of blood pressure) presión diastólica
afternoon tarde
again de nuevo, otra vez
against contra
agalactia agalactia, falta o disminución de la secreción de leche
agamma–globulinemia agammaglobulinemia, déficit de gammaglobulina en la sangre
agar agar; ~ **diffusion test** prueba de difusión en agar; ~ **gel** gel de agar
agarose agarosa; ~ **gel electrophoresis** electroforesis en gel de agarosa
age edad, generación; ~ **at death** edad de fallecimiento; ~ **-sex pyramid** pirámide de población
agent sustancia, -agente
agglomerate aglomerado
agglomeration glomeración
agglutinating antibody aglutinina
agglutination aglutinación
agglutinin aglutinina
aggravation agravamiento, empeoramiento
aggregation agregación, concentración
aggressive fibromatosis fibromatosis agresiva
aggressiveness agresividad
aging envejecimiento, senscencia
agitated agitado, inquieto, nervioso
agitation agitación, euforia, inquietud y actividad aumentada
agonist agonista, músculo que participa con otro en un mismo movimiento, medicamento que estimula células de manera natural
agony agonía
agoraphobia agorafobia, ansiedad y miedo a los lugares públicos, abiertos o concurridos

agrammatism agramatismo, acatafasia

agranulocytosis agranulocitosis, disminución o ausencia de leucocitos granulados en la sangre

ague escalofríos, fríos

AID inseminación artificial a partir de un donante

aid, to asistir, ayudar, apoyar

AIDS síndrome de inmunodeficiencia adquirida, SIDA; ~ **dementia complex** complejo demencial del SIDA; ~ **patient** enfermo de SIDA

air aire; ~ **embolism** embolia gaseosa; ~ **suction system** dispositivo de aspiración de aire; ~ **swallowing** aerofagia, acción de tragar aire, deglución inconsciente de aire

airborne volando, en el aire; ~ **allergen** alergeno respiratorio, anafilactógeno respiratorio; ~ **favism** favismo por inhalación; ~ **transmission** transmisión aérea

airtight hermético, impenetrable

airway hyperresponsiveness hiperreactividad bronquial; ~ **obstruction** obstrucción aérea

airways vías respiratorias

akathisia acatisia, intranquilidad motora (agitación 2), incapacidad de permanecer sentado con tranquilidad

akinesia acinesia, ausencia de movimiento

alanine alanina; ~ **transaminase** alanina-aminotransferasa, alanina transaminasa, GPT

albendazole albendazol

Albrecht root-canal filling empaste radicular de Albrecht

Albright-McCune-Sternberg syndrome síndrome de Albright, enfermedad de Albright

albumin albúmina, proteína principal en la sangre

albuminuria albuminuria, excreción de albúmina

Alcock canal conducto pudendo, conducto de Alcock

alcohol alcohol; ~ **abuse** abuso de alcohol, alcoholismo; ~ **amnesic disorder** trastorno amnésico alcohólico; ~ **dehydrogenase** alcohol deshidrogenasa; ~ **oxidase** alcohol-oxidasa; ~ **poisoning** intoxicación alcohólica; ~ **test** prueba de alcoholemia, alcotest

alcoholic alcohólico; ~ **delirium** delirio

alcohólico; ~ **dementia** demencia alcohólica; ~ **drink** bebida alcohólica; ~ **encephalopathy** encefalopatía alcohólica; ~ **myocardiopathy** miocardiopatía alcohólica; ~ **polyneuritis** polineuritis alcohólica

alcoholism alcoholismo

alcoholometer alcohómetro, alcoholimetría

aldehyde aldehído; ~ **dehydrogenase** aldehído-deshidrogenasa

aldolase aldolasa

aldosterone aldosterona; ~ **antagonist** antagonista de la aldosterona

alendronate alendronato

alert alerta

alexia alexia

algae algas

algesia algesia

algophobia algofobia

algorithm algoritmo

alienation alienación, despersonalización, sensación de extrañeza personal

alimentary alimentario; ~ **canal** tracto intestinal, tubo digestivo, aparato digestivo

aliquot alícuota

a little poco, un poco

alive vivo

alkaline alcalino, que posee las reacciones de un álcali; ~ **phosphatase** fosfatasa alcalina, fosfatasa ácida

alkaloid alcaloide, sustancia vegetal básica

alkalosis alcalosis, disminución de la acidez de sangre y tejidos

alkaptonuric arthritis artritis alcaptonúrica

alkylate alquilato

alkylating agent agente alquilado, agente alquilante

all cada (uno, -a), todo; ~ **the time** perenne, perpetuo, persistente

ALL leucemia linfoblástica aguda, leucemia linfocítica, leucemia linfática, leucemia linfógena, leucemia linfoide

allantoic alantoideo; ~ **cavity** cavidad alantoidea; ~ **membrane** membrana alantoidea

allele alelo; ~ **displacement** sustitución alélica; ~ **replacement** sustitución alélica

allelotype alelotipo

allergen alergeno, sustancia que provoca

reacciones alérgicas

allergic alérgico; ~ **angiitis** angiitis alérgica, angeítis alérgica, angitis alérgica; ~ **arthritis** artritis alérgica; ~ **contact dermatitis** dermatitis alérgica de contacto; ~ **dermatitis** dermatitis alérgica; ~ **diathesis** diatesis alérgica; ~ **eczema** eczema alérgico; ~ **glomerulonephritis** glomerulonefritis alérgica; ~ **interstitial pneumonitis** alveolitis alérgica extrínseca; ~ **panmyelopathy** panmielopatía alérgica; ~ **reaction** atópico, alérgico, respuesta alérgica; ~ **response** atópico, alérgico, respuesta alérgica; ~ **rhinitis** rinitis alérgica, fiebre de heno; ~ **urticaria** urticaria alérgica

allergist alergista, especialista en alergias, alergólogo

allergology alergología

allergy alergia; ~ **test** análisis de alergia; ~ **to peanuts** hipersensibilidad a los cacahuates

alloantibody aloanticuerpo

allogenic alogénico; ~ **graft** aloinjerto, homoinjerto, donación alogénica, trasplante alogénico; ~ **transplant** aloinjerto, homoinjerto, donación alogénica, trasplante alogénico

allograft aloinjerto, homoinjerto, donación alogénica, trasplante alogénico

allopathy alopatía

allopurinol sodium alopurinol

allosteric enzyme enzima alostérica

allowable maximum imprecision imprecisión máxima tolerable; ~ **maximum inaccuracy** inexactitud máxima tolerable

allozyme aloenzima

almond oil aceite de almendra

alobar holoprosencephaly arinencefalia

aloe vera aloe vera, áloe

alopecia alopecia, caída general o parcial de cabellos o pelos

a lot mucho, bastante

alpha alpha; ~ **-amylase** alpha-amilasa; ~ **1-antitrypsin** alpha1-antitripsina; ~ **2-antiplasmin** alpha2-antiplasmina; ~ **-fetoprtein** alfa-fetoproteína, AFP; ~ **interferon** interferón leucocitario, interferón alfa; ~ **receptor** receptor alfa

alphaadrenergic alfaadrenérgico; ~ **receptor** receptor alfaadrenérgico

altered consciousness alteración de la conciencia

alternate, to alternar, sucederse dos o más acciones o administraciones de medicamentos

alternative alternativo; ~ **medicine** medicina paralela, medicina alternativa; ~ **pathway** vía alternativa

although aunque, bien que

altitude altitud; ~ **alkalosis** alcalosis de altitud; ~ **sickness** mareos, mal de altura, soroche, vértigo

aluminum aluminio

alveolar alveolar; ~ **capillary plexus** red capilar alveolar; ~ **inflammation** alveolitis, inflamación de los alvéolos del pulmón; ~ **macrophage** macrofago alveolar; ~ **phagocyte** macrofago alveolar

alveolitis alveolitis, inflamación de los alvéolos del pulmón

alveolus alvéolo

alymphocytosis alinfocitosis

Alzheimer dementia enfermedad de Alzheimer

Alzheimer disease enfermedad de Alzheimer

amalgam amalgama; ~ **filling** amalgama dental

amanita amanita, oronja

amantidine amantadina

amaurosis amaurosis, ceguera; ~ **fugax** amaurosis fugax

amber codon codón ámbar; ~ **mutation** mutación ámbar

amblyopia ambliopía, visión bizcada, visión reducida

ambulance ambulancia; ~ **service** servicio de ambulancias

ambulant ambulante, ambulatorio

ambulatory ambulante, ambulatorio; ~ **care** centro ambulatorio, clínica ambulatoria, tratamiento ambulatorio, atención ambulatoria, servicio ambulatorio; ~ **ECG monitoring** control ECG ambulatorio; ~ **patient** ambulatorio, paciente externo

ameba amiba, ameba

amebiasis amebiasis

amebic amebiano; ~ **colitis** colitis amebiana, disentería amebiana; ~ **dysentery** colitis amebiana, disentería amebiana; ~ **enteritis** enteritis amebiana; ~ **hepatitis** hepatitis amebiana

amebicide antiamebiano

amelanotic nevus nevus acrómico, nevus despigmentado

amenorrhoea amenorrea, ausencia de la menstruación

American Mountain Fever fiebre (f) de montaña americana

amikacin amikacina

amine amina, compuesto químico relacionado con el amoníaco; ~ **oxidase** amina-oxidasa

amino acid polymer polipéptido; ~ **-aciduria** aminoaciduria

aminoacid aminoácido

aminobutyric acid ácido aminobutírico

aminoglycoside aminoglicósido

aminolevulinic acid ácido aminolevulínico

amitriptyline amitriptilina

AML leucemia aguda mieloide

amlodipine amlodipino

ammonia amoníaco

ammoniac gum goma amoniaca

ammoniacal dermatitis dermatitis del pañal

ammonium amonio; ~ **hydrogen carbonate** carbonato ácido de amonio; ~ **lauryl sulfate** laurilsulfato de amonio; ~ **sulphate** sulfato de amonio

Ammon's horn hipocampo, asta de Ammon

amnesia amnesia, pérdida total o parcial de la memoria

amnesic aphasia afasia sensorial, afasia de Wernicke

amniocentesis amniocéntesis

amnion amnios

amnioscopy amnioscopia

amniotic amniótico; ~ **embolism** embolismo amniótico; ~ **fluid** líquido amniótico; ~ **fluid cells** células de líquido amniótico; ~ **sac** bolsa de aguas, saco amniótico

amniotomy amniotomía

amoeba amiba, ameba

amoebic amebiano; ~ **meningoencephalitis** meningo-encefalitis amebiana; ~ **pericarditis** pericarditis amebiana

amount cantidad; ~ **of substance** cantidad de sustancia

amoxicillin amoxicilina

ampere ampere

amperometry amperimetría

amphetamine anfetamina

amphiarthrosis articulación cartilaginosa, anfiartrosis, juntura cartilaginosa

ampholytic agent anfolito, el coloide anfótero

ampholytoid anfolito, el coloide anfótero

amphoteric anfotérico, anfótero; ~ **ion** ión anfótero, anfoíon, ion dipolar, ion hibrido

amphotericin B anfotericina B

amphoterous anfotérico, anfótero

ampicillin ampicilina

amplification amplificación

amplimer amplímero

amplitude amplitud; ~ **of pelvis** amplitud de la pelvis

ampule ampolla, envase de vidrio o plástico

amputate, to amputar

amputation amputación; ~ **of a finger** amputación de un dedo; ~ **of upper arm** amputación del brazo

amputee amputado; ~ **arm amputee** amputado de un brazo

amygdalase glucosidasa

amygdaline exudate exudado amigdalino

amylase amilasa

amyloid amiloide; ~ **arthritis** artritis amiloidea; ~ **degeneration** amiloidosis, degeneración amiloidea; ~ **deposits** placas seniles, depósitos amiloides; ~ **fibril protein** proteína beta amiloide; ~ **liver** hígado amiloideo, hígado círeo; ~ **nephrosis** nefrosis amiloidea; ~ **peptide** proteína amiloide; ~ **plaques** placas seniles, depósitos amiloides; ~ **protein** proteína amiloide; ~ **spleen** bazo amiloideo

amyloidosis amiloidosis, degeneración amiloidea; ~ **of the conjunctiva** amiloidosis conjuntiva

amyotonia amiotonía; ~ **congenita** enfermedades neuromusculares

amyotrophic amiotrófico; ~ **lateral sclerosis** esclerosis lateral amiotrófica, la enfermedad de Charcot

amyotrophy amiotrofia

anabolic anabolico; ~ **steroid** esteroida anabolica y androgenica

anabolism anabolismo

anachlorhydria anaclorhidria, aclorhidria, anacidez

anacidity anacidez, aclorhidria, anaclorhidria

anacrotic pulse anacrotismo

anacusis anacusia, sordera neuronal, cofosis

anaerobic anaerobio, que no necesita oxígeno; ~ **bacteria** bacterias anaerobias; ~ **chamber** cámara anaerobia; ~ **culture** cultivo para anaerobios; ~ **decay** degradación anaerobia; ~ **digestion** degradación anaerobia; ~ **gram-negative coccus** coco anaerobio gramnegativo; ~ **gram-negative rod** bacilo anaerobio gramnegativo; ~ **gram-positive coccus** coco anaerobio grampositivo; ~ **gram-positive rod** bacilo anaerobio grampositivo; ~ **incubation system** sistema anaeróbico de incubación

anaerogenic anaerogénico

anal anal, relativo o perteneciente al ano; ~ **fissure** fisura anal; ~ **intercourse** coito anal; ~ **itching** prurito anal; ~ **mucus** muco anal; ~ **orifice** ano, sieso, orificio de salida del intestino, culo; ~ **polyp** pólipo anal; ~ **pruritus** prurito anal; ~ **reflex** reflejo anal; ~ **sex** coito anal; ~ **sphincter** esfínter anal

analagous idéntico, completamente igual, coincidente, análogo

analeptic analéptico, medicamento de efecto estimulante en la psique

analgesic calmante, analgésico, droga analgésica; ~ **ointment** pomada analgésica; ~ **state** estado analgésico

analogous análogo, de acción parecida; ~ **organs** órganos análogos

analyser analizador

analysis análisis, descomposición

analyte analizado, analito

analytical analítico; ~ **chemistry** química analítica; ~ **function** función analítica; ~ **instrument** instrumento analítico; ~ **method** método analítico; ~ **procedure** procedimiento analítico; ~ **process** proceso analítico; ~ **system** sistema analítico; ~ **test** análisis

anamnesis anamnesis, historia previa de las enfermedades de un paciente

anaphylactic anafiláctico; ~ **shock** anafilácticoshock anafiláctico, choque anafiláctico

anaphylactoid reaction reacción anafilactóide

anaphylatoxin anafilactotoxina, anafilotoxina

anastomosis anastomosis, comunicación natural o artificial entre dos vasos o nervios; ~ **clamp** clamp intestinal de anastomosis

anastral mitosis mitosis de médula ósea

anatomic anatómico, del cuerpo; ~ **pathology** anatomía patológica

anatomical anatómico, del cuerpo; ~ **pathologist** anatomopatólogo; ~ **pathology** anatomía patológica

anatomist's snuff-box tabaquera anatómica

anatomo-pathologist anatomopatólogo

anatomy anatomía

anatoxin anatoxina, toxoide

and y

androgen andrógeno, hormona que produce caracteres masculinos

androgenic andrógeno, que produce caracteres masculinos; ~ **hormone** andrógeno, hormona que produce caracteres masculinos

androgynous andrógino

androgyny androginismo, seudo-hermafrodismo masculino

andropause andropausia

androstenedione androstenodiona

anemia anemia, escasez de sangre o deficiencia en la sangre de glóbulos rojos

anemic anémico, falta de sangre, ferriprivo

anergia anergia, carencia de actividad, falta de reacción

anesthesia anestesia, disminución parcial o total de la sensibilidad dolorosa

anesthesiologist anestesista

anesthetic anestético, droga que produce anestesia

anesthetize, to anestesiar, insensibilizar

aneuploidization aneusoploidia

aneuploidy aneuploidía

aneurin tiamina, vitamina B1, aneurina

aneurysm aneurisma, dilatación de una arteria o del corazón

aneurysmal bladder vejiga aneurismal, vejiga aneurismática

Angelica archangelica Angelica archangelica;
~ **root** Angelica archangelica

angiitis angiitis, inflamación de un vaso
sanguíneo o linfático

angina angina, cinanquia; ~ **decubitus** angina
de decúbito; ~ **herpetica** angina herpética,
herpes gutural; ~ **in the chest** angina de
pecho, angina del pecho, angina péctoris;
~ **pectoris** angina de pecho, angina del pecho,
angina péctoris

anginal anginoso, relativo a la angina; ~ **pain**
dolor anginoso

angiocardiogram angiocardiograma

angioedema edema angioneurótico,
angioedema

angiography angiografía

angiokeratoma angioqueratoma

angioma angioma

angiomyoma of the skin angioma de la piel

angioneurotic angioneurótico; ~ **edema** edema
angioneurótico, angioedema, forma de edema
violento y breve

angiopathy angiopatía, enfermedad de los vasos
sanguíneos

angioplasty angioplastia

angiosarcoma argiosarcoma; ~ **of the liver**
angiosarcoma hepatitico

angiospastic angioespástico; ~ **diathesis**
diátesis angioespástico

angiotensin angiotensina; ~ **converting**
enzyme enzima de conversión de la
angiotensina, enzima convertidora de
angiotensina

angitis angiitis, inflamación de un vaso
sanguíneo o linfático

angle ángulo

angry enfadado

angular angular; ~ **cheilitis** estomatitis angular,
queilitis; ~ **cheilosis** estomatitis angular,
queilitis; ~ **stomatitis** estomatitis angular,
queilitis

anhydrosis anhidrosis, falta de transpiración

anhydrous anhidro, que no tiene agua;
~ **calcium iodate** yodato (m) de calcio,
anhidratato; ~ **dextrose** dextrosa anhidra

animal animal, bestia; ~ **hair** pelo de animales;
~ **protein factor** cobalamina, vitamina B12,
cianocobalamina

anionic aniónico, con carga negativa

aniseiconia aniseiconía, anisoiconia

anisocoria anisocoria, desigualdad del diámetro
de las pupilas

anisole anisol, metoxibenzeno

anistreplase anistreplasa

ankle tobillo; ~ **bone** astrágalo, taba, tobillo;
~ **joint** maléolo, tobillo

ankylosing anquilosante; ~ **spondylitis**
espondilitis anquilosante, la enfermedad de
Bechterew; ~ **spondylitis deformans**
espondilitis deformante

ankylosis anquilosis, inmovilidad de
movimiento en una coyuntura

ankylostomiasis anquilostomiasis

annealing hibridación de ácidos nucleicos

anniversary date fecha del aniversario

annoyance fastidio, molestia, enfado

annular cartilage cartílago cricoides, cartílago
cricoideo

anodontia anodoncia

anogenital anogenital, perteneciente a la región
del ano y los genitales

anomalous anormal, anómalo

anomaly anomalía, desviación de la norma,
irregularidad

anopheline mosquito mosquito anofeles,
mosquito portador del paludismo

anorectal anorectal, referente al ano y al último
trozo del intestino grueso

anorectic agent fármaco anorexígeno,
inhibidor de apetito, depresor de apetito

anorexia anorexia, inapenencia, falta de apetito
o ansia de adelgazar, pérdida de apetito

anorexiant fármaco anorexígeno, inhibidor de
apetito, depresor de apetito

anorexic anoréxico, anoréctico, anorexígeno,
anorexigénico

anosmia anosmia, pérdida o disminución del
sentido del olfato

anovulatory anovular, que no va acompañado
por el desprendimiento de un óvulo

anoxia anoxia, insuficiencia de oxígeno en los
tejidos

antacid antiácido, sustancia que fija los ácidos
gástricos

antagonist antagonista (m/f), músculo que
produce movimiento contrario al de otro

músculo, sustancia que anula la acción de otra, sustancia que anula la acción de otra

antagonistic hostil, antagónico

antecedent antecedente (m), circunstancia anterior en la historia del enfermo

anterior anterior

anterograde anterógrado, dirigido hacia adelante

anthelmintic antihelmíntico, sustancia que destruye los gusanos intestinales

anthrax ántrax (m), inflamación purulenta de la piel, furúnculo

anthropometry antropometría

anthroposophy antroposofía

antiacid antiácido,

antiadrenergic antiadrenérgico

antiallergic antialérgico

antianginal droga antianginosa

anti-antibody antianticuerpo

antiarrhythmic antiarrítmico, medicamento para el tratamiento de la irregularidad del pulso cardíaco

antiasthmatic antiasmático, medicamento para el tratamiento del asma

antibacterial antibacteriano, que destruye las bacterias; ~ **peptide** péptido antibacteriano

antibiogram antibiograma, estudio de la sensibilidad de un microbio frente a diversos antibióticos

antibiotherapy antibioterapia, tratamiento con antibióticos

antibiotic antibiótico; ~ **-associated colitis** colitis asociada a antibióticos, colitis seudomembranosa; ~ **resistance** resistencia a antibióticos; ~ **therapy** terapia antibiótica, tratamiento antibiótico

antibody anticuerpo; ~ **anti-core** anticuerpo contra el núcleo

anticholinergic anticolinérgico, sustancia que bloquea los nervios parasimpáticos

anticholinesterase activity actividad anticolinesterásica

anticoagulant anticoagulante, sustancia que impide la coagulación

anticoding strand cadena intranscrita

anticodon anticodón

anticomplementary anticomplementario

anticonvulsant anticonvulsivo, sustancia que

evita o reduce convulsiones

anti-D immunoglobulin inmunoglobulina anti-D

antidepressant antidepresivo, droga antidepresiva, sustancia que alivia la depresión

antidiabetic antidiabético, sustancia que reduce la concentración de azúcar en la sangre

antidiuretic antidiurético, sustancia que disminuye la cantidad de orina

antidopaminergic antidopaminérgico

antidote antídoto, contraveneno

anti-edema agent fármaco antiedema

antiemetic antiemético, medicamento contra los vómitos

antiepileptic antiepiléptico, medicamento contra la epilepsia, anticomicial

antiestrogen drug antiestrogénico, que impide o contrarresta el efecto de las hormonas estrogénicas

antiestrogenic antiestrogénico, que impide o contrarresta el efecto de las hormonas estrogénicas

antifebrile antitérmico, antifebril

antifibrinolysin antiplasmina, inhibidor de alfa 2-plasmina, antifibrinolisina

antifibrinolytic antifibrinolítico

antiflatulents carminativos

antifoaming agent antiespumante

antifungal antifúngico, que destruye los hongos; ~ **therapy** terapia anti-hongo

antigen antígeno, sustancia considerada como extraña por el organismo; ~ **-presenting cell** célula presentadora de antígeno; ~ **-specific memory cell** célula de memoria del antígeno

antigenic antigénico; ~ **approach** enfoque poliantigénico; ~ **determinant** determinante antigénico, epítope; ~ **drift** deriva antigénica; ~ **peptide** péptido antigénico; ~ **receptor** receptor antigénico; ~ **reversion** reversión antigénica; ~ **shift** cambio antigénico; ~ **site** sitio antigénico; ~ **specificity** especificidad antigénica

antigenicity inmunogenicidad

antiglobulin antiglobulina, suero antiglobulinas humanas, suero Coombs

antihemophilia factor A factor VIII de la coagulación, factor anti-hemofílico; ~ **factor**

deficiency déficit del factor antihemofílico; **~ globulin** factor VIII de la coagulación, factor anti-hemofílico

antihistamine antihistamínico, sustancia que combate la acción de la histamina

anti-HIV serology serología anti-VIH

anti-human globulin immune serum suero antiglobulinas humanas, suero Coombs; **~ globulin serum** suero antiglobulinas humanas, suero Coombs

antihyperlipidemic agent fármaco hipolipidemiante

antihypertensive antihipertensivo, sustancia que disminuye la presión sanguínea

antiinfective antiinfeccioso, que combate la infección

anti–inflammatory antiinflamatorio, que impide o detiene la inflamación; **~ ointment** pomada antiinflamatoria

antiinfluenza vaccine vacuna antigripal

antilymphocyte globulin globulina antilinfocitaria; **~ serum** suero antilinfocitario

antimessenger RNA RNA antisentido

antimetabolite antimetabolito

antimicrobial antimicrobiano, que impide el desarrollo de los microbios

antimicrosomal antimicrosómico; **~ antibody** anticuerpo antimicrosómico

antimitochondrial antimitocondrial; **~ antibody** anticuerpo antimitocondrial

antimitotic antimitótico, sustancia que impide la división y crecimiento de células

antimony antimonio; **~ pneumoconiosis** neumoconiosis por antimonio; **~ -potassium tartrate** tartrato de antimonio y potasio

antimycobacterial antimicobacteriano

antimycotic antimicótico, sustancia que destruye los hongos; **~ skin gel** gel dérmico antimicótico

antineoplastic antineoplásico, que impide el crecimiento de tumores; **~ therapy** terapia antineoplásica

antinephritic medicine medicamento nefrítico

antinuclear antinuclear; **~ antibody** anticuerpo antinuclear

antioestrogenic antiestrogénico, que impide o contrarresta el efecto de las hormonas estrogénicas

antioxidant antioxidante, sustancia que previene el deterioro de un producto por oxidación; **~ food additive** aditivo alimentario antioxidante

antiparasitic antiparasitario

anti-pernicious factor cobalamina, vitamina B12, cianocobalamina

antiphlogistic antiflogístico, sustancia que combate la inflamación

antiplasmin antiplasmina, inhibidor de alfa 2-plasmina, antifibrinolisina

antiplatelets inhibidores de agregacion plaquetaria

antiproliferative antiproliferativo, que actúa en contra del crecimiento y la división de células

antipruritic antipruriginoso, que impide el escozor o picor

antipsychotic neuroléptico, calmante del sistema nervioso, antipsicótico

antipyretic antipirético, sustancia que reduce la fiebre; **~ analgesic** analgésico antipirético

antiretroviral antirretroviral; **~ agent** antirretroviral, agente anti-retrovírico, fármaco anti-retroviral; **~ therapy** tratamiento antirretroviral, terapia antirretroviral

antisense oligonucleotide oligonucleótido antisentido, fármaco anti-senso; **~ RNA** RNA antisentido; **~ strand** cadena antisentido

antiseptic antiséptico, desinfectante; **~ gargle** colutorio antiséptico

anti-serotonin drug fármaco antiserotoninérgico

antiserum antisuero, suero que contiene anticuerpos frente a una enfermedad concreta; **~ avidity** avidez de un antisuero

anti-skid antiderrape, antipatinante, antideslizante, antirresbaladizo; **~ -spasm** espasmolítico, medicamento que sirve para resolver los espasmos; **~ -streptococcic serum** suero antiestreptocócico; **~ -TB drug** tuberculostático, medicamento que inhibe el crecimiento del bacilo de la tuberculosis

antispasmodic antispasmódico, medicamento que combate contracturas, calambres y convulsiones

antistreptolysin antiestreptolisina

antitermination antiterminación

antithermic antitérmico, antifebril

antithrombin antitrombina

antithrombotic antitrombótico, que impide la formación de tapones de sangre y los disuelve

antitissue antibodies anticuerpos antistitulares

antitoxin antitoxina, anticuerpo que actúa como contraveneno

antitrypsin antitripsina

antitumor antitumorígeno, que contrarresta la formación de tumores

antitussive antitusivo, bequico

antiviral antiviral, antivírico

anti-wrinkle antiarrugas

antrum antro; ~ **pyloricum** antro pilórico

anuresis anuria, ausencia de eliminación de orina

anuria ausencia de eliminación de orina

anus ano, sieso, orificio de salida del intestino

anxiety ansiedad, angustia, desesperación, disforia; ~ **neurosis** neurosis de ansiedad; ~ **psychosis** psicosis ansiosa; ~ **reaction** neurosis de ansiedad

anxiolitic ansiolítico, tranquilizante, medicamento contra la ansiedad

anxiolytic ansiolítico, tranquilizante, medicamento contra la ansiedad; ~ **benzodiazepine** loracepam, tranquilizante

anxious ansioso; ~ **, to be** tener ansias, tener angustias

any algún, cualquier

anybody alguien

aorta aorta, la arteria aorta

aortic aórtico; ~ **aneurysm** aneurisma aórtico; ~ **arch syndrome** anomalía del arco aórtico, síndrome del cayado aórtico; ~ **bioprosthesis** bioprótesis aórtica, endoprótesis; ~ **coarctation** coartación de la aorta; ~ **dissection** aneurisma disecante; ~ **impression** impresión aórtica; ~ **insufficiency** enfermedad de Corrigan; ~ **septal defect** ventana pulmonar; ~ **sinus** sinus aórtico; ~ **stenosis** estenosis aórtico; ~ **valve prolapse** prolapso de la válvula aortica; ~ **window** ventana aórtica

aortography aortografía

aortopulmonary window ventana pulmonar

apathetic lánguido, indiferente, apático, perezoso, despistado

apathy apatía, falta de sentimiento o emoción, indiferencia

ape fissure cisura simiesca, cisura perpendicular externa

Apgar index índice de Apgar, test de Apgar; ~ **score** índice de Apgar, test de Apgar

aphasia afasia, imposibilidad o dificultad para hablar

aphonia afonía, perdida de la voz

aphonic afónica; ~ **bronchophony** broncofonía afónica

aphthous aftoso; ~ **fever** fiebre aftosa; ~ **ulcer** llaga ulcerosa en la boca, afta

apical apical; ~ **granuloma** granuloma apical

apicoectomy apicectomía, apectomía

apiectomy apicectomía, apectomía

aplasia aplasia, desarrollo incompleto o defectuoso de un órgano o tejido; ~ **of the urinary bladder** aplasia vesical

aplastic anemia anemia aplástica, pancitopenia

apnea apnea, suspensión de la respiración, parada respiratoria

apocrine glands glándulas apocrinas

apolipoprotein apolipoproteína

apomorphine apomorfina

apoplexy apoplejía, ictus, accidente cerebrovascular agudo

apoptosis apoptosis

apostematous glandular cheilitis queilitis glandular apostematosa

apparatus artilugion, aparato, dispositivo, aparejo

appendicitis apendicitis (f), mal del apendis

appendix apéndice, afijo

appetite apetito; ~ **suppressant** farmaco anorexigeno, inhibidor de apetito, depresor de apetito; ~ **-stimulating** estimulante del apetito

apple manzana; ~ **juice** jugo de manzana; ~ **sauce** compota de manzanas, puré de manzana

application aplicación, administración de un medicamento o empleo de una medida física

apprehension aprensión, preocupación

approximate aproximado

approximately aproximadamente

apraxia apraxia; ~ **of urinary bladder** apraxia vesical

apricot albaricoque, chabacano
April abril
aprotinin aprotinina
aquarium granuloma granuloma de los aquarios
aqueous acuoso, que contiene agua; **~ humor** humor acuoso; **~ solution** disolución acuosa
arabinose arabinosa
arachnidism aracnidismo
arachnoid aracnoide; **~ granulations** granulaciones aracnoideas
arachnoiditis aracnoiditis
arachnoid cyst quiste aracnoideo
arbitrary arbitrario; **~ standard** patrón arbitrario
arbovirus arbovirus
arc welder's pneumoconiosis siderosis
ARDS síndrome de insuficiencia respiratoria del adulto
areic aréico
arginase arginasa
arginine arginina
arhinencephaly holoprosencefalia
arm brazo
armpit arca, axila, sobaco
aromatic aromático, de buen olor
arrest detención, secuestro; **~ of bleeding** hemostasia
arrhythmia arritmia, falta de ritmo regular, pulso irregular
arrhythmogenic arritmogénico, que produce pulso irregular
arsenic arsénico; **~ dermatosis** dermatitis arsenical; **~ melanosis** melanodermia del arsénico
art of healing arte médico
arterial arterial, relativo a las arterias; **~ bleeding** hemorragia arterial; **~ blood** sangre arterial; **~ blood gases** gases de la sangre arterial; **~ carbon dioxide tension** presión parcial del dióxido de carbono en la sangre arterial; **~ embolectomy** embolectomía arterial; **~ homograft** transplante arterial homoplástico; **~ hyperemia** hiperemia activa, hiperemia arterial; **~ oxygen saturation** saturación oxihemoglobinada, saturación del sangre arterial con oxígeno; **~ prosthesis** prótesis arterial, prótesis vascular; **~ pulse** pulso arterial; **~ puncture** punción arterial; **~ vasoconstriction** vasoconstricción arterial
arteriography arteriografía, radiografía de algunas arterias
arteriolar arteriolar, relativo a las ramificaciones de las arterias
arteriole arteriola
arteriosclerosis arteriosclerosis
arteriosclerotic arteriosclerótico; **~ confusion** confusión arteriosclerótica
arteriovenous arteriovenoso, relativo a una arteria y una vena
arteritis arteritis
arthralgia artralgia, dolor de las articulaciones
arthritis artritis, inflamación de una o más articulaciones
arthrocentesis artrocentesis
arthrodesis artrodesis
arthroempyesis empiema articular, empiema en las coyunturas
arthrogryposis artrogriposis
arthrokleisis artrodesis
arthropathy artropatía, enfermedad de las articulaciones
arthroplasty artroplastia
arthropod artrópodo
arthroscopy artroscopía
arthrosis artrosis, anomalía en una articulación por desgaste
articular articular, relativo a una articulación; **~ resection** resección articular
articulation articulación, la nitidez fonética
artificial artificial, no naural, sintético, facticio; **~ ductus arteriosus Botalli** conducto arterioso artificial; **~ fats** grasas artificiales; **~ heart** corazón artificial; **~ heart valve** prótesis valvular cardiaca; **~ incubator** incubadora para prematuros; **~ insemination by donor** inseminación artificial a partir de un donante; **~ larynx** laringe artificial; **~ leech** sanguijuela artificial; **~ leg** pierna artificial, prótesis de la extremidad inferior; **~ limb** prótesis, miembro artificia; **~ neuron** neurona artificial; **~ respiration** respiración asistida, respiración artificial; **~ respirator** respirador, aparato de respiración artificial; **~ skin** piel

artificial; ~ **tears** soluciones oftálmicas, lágrimas artificiales; ~ **tooth** diente artificial

artificially ventilated respiración artificial, bajo ventilación pulmonar

arylsulfatase arilsulfatasa

asbestos amianto, asbesto; ~ **carcinoma** carcinoma secundario a asbestosis; ~ **dermatitis** dermatitis por agujas de amianto; ~ **dust** polvo de amianto; ~ **-induced cancer** cáncer inducido por el amianto

asbestosis asbestosis

Ascaris ascárid, el lobriz intestinal, el ascaride, el gusano redondo

ascending ascendente; ~ **colon** colon ascendente

Aschoff bodies nódulos reumáticos; ~ **~ Rokitansky sinus** seno de Aschoff-Rokitansky; ~ **-Tawara node** nudo de Aschoff-Tawara

ascites ascitis, acumulación de cierto líquido en el vientre

ascitic fluid líquido ascítico

ascorbate ascorbato, ácido ascórbico

ascorbic acid ácido ascórbico, ascorbato

asepsis asepsia, ausencia de gérmenes infecciosos, prevención de infección

aseptic aséptico, libre de gérmenes, estéril; ~ **bursitis** bursitis aséptica; ~ **filling** envasado aséptico; ~ **meningitis** meningitis aséptica, meningitis viral; ~ **operation** operación aséptica; ~ **osteonecrosis** osteonecrosis aséptica

asleep, to be estar dormido, dormir

asparaginase asparraginasa

asparagine asparragina

aspartame aspartamo

aspartate aspartato

Asperger Syndrome enfermedad de Asperger

aspergillosis aspergilosis

asphyxia asfixia, ahogarse

asphyxiate, to sofocar, ahogar, sofocar

aspiration succión, aspiración; ~ **biopsy** biopsia con aguja, punción biopsia; ~ **pneumonia** neumonía por aspiración

aspiratory myringotomy miringotomía de aspiración

aspirin aspirina, ácido acetilsalicílico

assay prueba, ensayo, análisis, examen, exploración

assertiveness asertividad; ~ **training** entrenamiento en asertividad, terapia de afirmación

assessment valorización

assign, to asignar, destinar

assigned value valor asignado

assimilate, to metabolizar, asimilar, digerir

assimilation test prueba de asimilación

assist, to asistir, ayudar, apoyar

assistant ayudante; ~ **medical technician** ayudante técnico médico

associated concomitante, acompañante

association asosiación, acoplamiento, coordinación, unión; ~ **neuron** interneurona

asthenia astenia, cansancio físico intenso, debilidad corporal general, falta de fuerza

asthenopia astenopia, cansancio de los ojos

asthma asma, broncoespasmo, espasmo de los bronquios; ~ **etiology** étiología de asthme; ~ **medication** antiasmático, medicamento para el tratamiento del asma

asthmatic asmático; ~ **bronchitis** bronquitis asmática, bronquitis obstructiva crónica

astigmatism astigmatismo

astringent astringente, que produce sequedad en la piel

astrocyte astrocito

astrocytes astroglia, microglia, astrocitos

astrocytoma astrocitoma

astroglia astroglia, microglia, astrocitos

asymmetric asimétrico

asymptomatic asintomático, que no presenta síntomas; ~ **carrier** portador asintomático

asystole asistolía, paro cardíaco

at en, a; ~ **home** en casa; ~ **midnight** a medianoche; ~ **night** por la noche; ~ **noon** a mediodía; ~ **rest** en reposo; ~ **the back** detrás; ~ **the front** delante

ataxia ataxia, falta de coordinación de los movimientos voluntarios; ~ **-telangiectasia** telangiectasia, dilatación permanente de grupos de capilares y vénulas superficiales

ataxic gait marcha atáxica

atelectasis atelectasia, colapso pulmonar

atelectatic atelectásico; ~ **congenital bronchiectasia** broncoectasia atelectásica congénita; ~ **crepitation** crepitación atelectásica

atheroma ateroma, ateromasia

atheromatosis ateromatosis, aterosclerosis, depósito de placas de grasa en las arterias

athetosis atetosis, movimiento involuntario e incoordinado en los miembros y la cara

athlete atleta; ~ **foot** pie de atleta; ~ **hunch back** cifosis de los deportistas

athrepsia marasmo, retraso del desarrollo, transtorno del crecimiento, síndrome de carencia afectiva, síndrome de declive, fracaso en medrar

ativan loracepam, tranquilizante

atlantoaxial atlantoaxial; ~ **joint** articulación atlantoaxial

atmospheric pressure presión atmosférica

atomic atómico; ~ **absorption** espectrometría de absorción atómica; ~ **mass** masa atómica; ~ **mass constant** constante de masa atómica; ~ **mass unit** unidad de masa atómica; ~ **number** número atómico; ~ **weight** peso atómico

atomizer atomizador, nebulizador

atonic atónico

atony atonía, ausencia o deficiencia de la tensión de un tejido o un órgano

atopic atópico; ~ **dermatitis** dermatitis atópica

atopy atopia

atoxic atóxico, no venenoso, no nocivo

ATPase ATPasa, adenosino-trifosfatasa

atrazine atrazina

atresia atresia, ausencia de una apertura, conducto o canal normal del organismo, como el ano, intestino o vagina; ~ **of the small intestine** atresia del intestino delgado

atrial atrial, relativo a una cámara superior del corazón; ~ **fibrillation** fibrilación ventricular; ~ **flutter** fibrilación ventricular

atrioventricular atrioventricular, relativo a una cámara superior y un ventrículo del corazón; ~ **bundle** fascículo de His; ~ **dissociation** disociación auriculoventricular; ~ **node** nudo de Aschoff-Tawara

at-risk patient paciente en riesgo

atrium atrio, cámara superior del corazón una de las

atrophic atrófico; ~ **cirrhosis** cirrosis atrófica; ~ **gastritis** gastritis atrófica; ~ **muscular**

disorders trastornos musculares atroficos, miotonía atrófical la enfermedad de Steiner; ~ **rhinitis** rinitis atrófica

atrophy atrofia, disminución del tamaño; ~ **of the cerebral cortex** atrofia de la corteza cerebral; ~ **of the optic nerve** atrofia del nervio óptico, atrofia óptica

atropine atropina, un parasimpaticolítico

attack ataque, arrebato, exabrupto; ~ **of cough** quinta de la tos

attend, to asistir, atender

attending physician médico adscrito, médico tratante, médico que atiende, médico curante

attention deficit disorder trastorno de déficit de atención

attentive observador, atento, cuidadoso

attenuance Atenuancia

attenuate, to atenuar, reducir

attenuated Atenuado; ~ **vaccine** vacuna atenuada, vacuna con virus atenuados

attenuation atenuación; ~ **coefficient** coeficiente de atenuación

attraction afinidad, analogía, semejanza

atypical atípico, irregular, anormal

audible respiration Resuello

auditory auditivo, relativo al oído y a la audición; ~ **apparatus** prótesis auditiva; ~ **brainstem evoked potentials** potenciales evocados auditivos del tronco cerebral; ~ **canal** conducto auditivo, conducto acústico; ~ **cortex** corteza auditiva; ~ **disorder** hipoacusia, trastorno de la audición, sordera parcial; ~ **fatigue** fatiga auditiva; ~ **nerve** nervio coclear, nervio auditivo; ~ **perception** percepción auditiva; ~ **vertigo** síndrome de Menière

August agosto

aunt tía

aura aura, sensación que precede un ataque como el epiléptico

aural aural, percibido por el oído; ~ **vertigo** síndrome de Menière

auricular auricular, relativo a la oreja, relativo a una de las dos cámaras superiores del corazón

aurotherapy crisoterapia

auscultation auscultación, acción de escuchar con estetoscopio

authorization autorización

autism autismo
autistic autisto; **~ behavior** comportamiento autista; **~ children** niños autistas; **~ introversion** introversión autista; **~ thinking** pensamiento autista
autoagglomeration autoaglomeración
autoagglutinin autoaglutinina
autoantibody autoanticuerpo
autoantigen autoantígeno
autoclave autoclave
autoimmune autoinmune, relacionado con fenómenos inmunológicos frente a elementos del propio cuerpo; **~ disease** enfermedad de autoinmunidad, enfermedad autoinmunitaria; **~ gastritis** gastritis atrófica; **~ hemolytic anemia** anemia hemolítica autoinmune; **~ reaction** respuesta de autoinmunidad, reacción de índole autoinmunitaria; **~ response** respuesta de autoinmunidad, reacción de índole autoinmunitaria; **~ thyroiditis** tiroiditis autoinmune
autolobectomy autolobectomía
autologous autólogo; **~ transfusion** autotransfusión; **~ transplantation** trasplante autólogo, autotrasplante
automated automatizado; **~ cytology** citología automatizada; **~ DNA sequencer** máquina de secuenciación automática del ADN; **~ operating room** quirófano, sala de operaciones
automation automatización
automatism automatismo
automutilation automutilación, autolesión
autonomic autónomo, independiente; **~ nervous system** sistema nervioso autónoma
autonomous autónomo; **~ replicating sequence** secuencia de replicación autónoma
autoplasty autoplastia
autopsy autopsia, necropsia; **~ room** sala de autopsias
autoradiograph autorradiografía
autoradiography autorradiografía
autosomal autosómico
autosome autosoma, cromosoma autosómico
autotopoagnosia autotopoagnosia
autotroph autótrofo
autumn otoño
auxiliary muscle músculo auxiliar

avant-garde vanguardia
avascular avascular
average medial, mediana; **~ erythrocyte volume** volumen eritrocítico medio
aviator's ear barotraumatismo del oído
Avogadro's constant constante de Avogadro; **~ number** número de Avogadro
avulsion desgarro
a whole entero, un
axial axial; **~ compression** compresión axial; **~ loading** carga axial
axillary lymph node ganglio linfático de la axila
axon reflex reflejo axónico
axonal axónico; **~ degeneration** degeneración axónica; **~ reorganization** remodelación axónica
azathioprine azatioprina
azidothymidine AZT, cidovudina, azidotimidina, Retrovir
azithromycin azitromicina
azlocillin azlocilina
azoospermia azoospermia, falta de espermatozoos en el semen
azotemia azotemia, exceso de cuerpos nitrogenados en la sangre
AZT AZT, cidovudina, azidotimidina, Retrovir
Azulfidine salazopirina

B

babesiosis piroplasmosis, babesiasis, babesiosis
Babinski's sign signo de Babinski, respuesta de Babinski
baby bebé; **~ bottle** mamadera, biberón; **~ milk** leche para lactantes, fórmula adaptada; **~ powder** polvos para bebés; **~ teeth** dientes de leche, primera dentición
bacillus bacilo, bacteria en forma de bastoncillo
back espalda; **~ brace** braguero, corset lumbrosacro, faja, corsé, espaldera, respaldo; **~ massage** masaje de la espalda, masaje del dorso; **~ mutation** mutación restauradora; **~ of the hand** dorso de la mano, nudillo; **~ pain** dorsalgia, notalgia; **~ pressure** presión de retorno, presión de retrógrada, contrapresión; **~ support** braguero, corset

lumbrosacro, faja médica, corsé, respaldo
backache dorsalgia, dolor en la espalda, lumbalgia
backrub masaje de la espalda, masaje del dorso
backward hacia atrás; ~ **spasm** opistótonos
backwards retrógrado, que va hacia atrás, que degenera, deteriora
bacon tocino
bacteremia bacteriemia, presencia de bacterias en la sangre
bacteria (pl) bacterias
bacterial bacteriano; ~ **cast** cilindro bacteriano; ~ **dissemination** propagación bacteriana; ~ **dissociation** disociación bacteriana; ~ **embolism** embolia bacilar; ~ **emulsion** emulsión bacteriana; ~ **examination** examen bacteriologico; ~ **fimbriae** fimbrias bacteriales; ~ **pneumonia** neumonopatía bacteriana, neumonía bacteriana; ~ **pollution** contaminación bacteriana; ~ **suspension** suspensión bacteriana; ~ **translocation** translocación bacteriana
bactericidal bactericida; ~ **activity test** prueba de la actividad bactericida
bactericide bactericida (m), sustancia que destruye las bacterias
bacteriemia bacteriemia, presencia de bacterias en la sangre
bacteriological bacteriológico, relativo al estudio de las bacterias
bacteriology bacteriología; ~ **laboratory** laboratorio de bacteriología
bacteriophage bacteriófago, fago
bacterioproteins bacterioproteínas
bacteriostatic bacteriostático, sustancia que reduce la reproducción de bacterias
bacteriotoxemia bacteriemia, presencia de bacterias en la sangre
bacterium bacteria
bacteriuria bacteriuria
bacteroid semejante a una bacteria
bad mal, malo, -a; ~ **breath** halitosis, mal aliento, ozostomía; ~ **habit** vicio, habito malo
bagassosis bagazosis
balance equilibrio
balanitis balanitis, inflamación del miembro viril
bald calvo

baldness alopecia, calvicie, jiricua, caída general o parcial de cabellos o pelos
ball-and-socket joint articulación cotiloidea; ~ **of the foot** punto del pie; ~ **thrombus** trombus esferico
ballistocardiography balistocardiografía
Ballobes balloon balon gastrico
balloon balón; ~ **angioplasty** angioplastia con balón, la angioplastia de globo; ~ **atrial septostomy** septostomía de balón; ~ **catheter** catéter balón
balm alivio, aligeramento, remedio, desahogo
balneotherapy balneoterapia
bamboo spine columna vertebral en forma de bambú
banana plátano, banano
band banda; ~ **shift** desplazamiento de banda
bandage venda, vendaje, envoltura
banding pattern diagrama de bandas
barbecue azado
barber's itch tiña de la barba, sicosis de la barba
barbiturate barbiturato
barbituric acid ácido barbitúrico
barefoot descalzo, sin zapatos
barium bario; ~ **enema** enema de bario, exploración intestinal con bario; ~ **sulfate** sulfato de bario
barley itch eccema de los graneros, prurito de los cereales
Barnes speculum espéculo de Barnes
baroreceptor barorreceptor
baroreflex barorreflejo
barotitis barotraumatismo del oído
barotrauma barotraumatismo
Barr body cuerpo de Barr
Barré-Liéou syndrome osteofitosis vertebral, síndrome de Barré-Liéou
Barrett's esophagus esófago de Barrett
barrier barrera, obstrucción
Bartholin glands glándula de Bartholin
bartholinitis bartolinitis
basal basal, situado cerca de una base, normal; ~ **cell** célula basal; ~ **cell carcinoma** carcinoma basocelular, basaloma; ~ **ganglia** ganglios basales; ~ **metabolic rate** metabolismo de ayuno, tasa de metabolismo basal; ~ **metabolism** metabolismo de ayuno, tasa de metabolismo basal

basaloid carcinoma carcinoma basaloide

basaloma carcinoma basocelular, basaloma

base portador, excipiente, base, fundamento, parte inferior, vehículo; ~ **quantity** magnitud de base

Basedow's disease enfermedad de Basedow, bocio basedowificado

baseline línea de base, situación basal

basilar basilar; ~ **artery** arteria basilar; ~ **artery migraine** migraña basilar, jaqueca de la arteria basilar; ~ **membrane** membrana basilar; ~ **meningitis** meningitis basal; ~ **migraine** migraña basilar, jaqueca de la arteria basilar

basis base, fundamento, parte inferior

basophil basofilocito, basófilo; ~ **adenoma** adenoma basófilo; ~ **degranulation test** prueba de degranulación; ~ **leucocyte** basofilocito, basófilo

basophilic cell basofilocito, basófilo

basophilocyte basofilocito, basófilo

batch culture cultivo discontinuo; ~ **operation** operación por grupos

bath mitt paño para lavarse, manopla

bathroom aseo, servicio, baño, privada

bathtub tina, bañera

Batten's disease distrofia miotónica de Steinert, enfermedad de Steinert, miotonía atrófica, distrofia miotónica

Batten–Steinert syndrome distrofia miotónica de Steinert, enfermedad de Steinert, miotonía atrófica, distrofia miotónica

battered wife mujer maltratada, víctima de la violencia doméstica

Battle incision laparotomía de Battle, incisión quirúrgica de la pared abdominal

Bayes' theorem teorema de Bayes

B-cell linfocito B, célula B; ~ **lymphocyte** linfocito B

BCG vaccination vacuna BCG

be, to ser; ~ **cross-eyed, to** ser bizco, turnio; ~ **down** estar depresivo; ~ **present, to** asistir, estar presente; ~ **short of breath, to** resuello; ~ **unwell, to** estar destemplado, estar bascoso, estar mareado, estar friolero, tener escalofríos, tener malestar

beans frijoles, porotos

beard barba, barbilla; ~ **hair** barba y los bigotes

because porque

become, to quedar; ~ **hot, to** quedar caliente; ~ **numb, to** entumecer, entorpecer, envarar

bed cama; ~ **rest** reposo en cama, guardando cama; ~ **side test** determinación junto a la cabecera del paciente

bednet mosquitero, red protectora contra los insectos

bedpan bacinilla, basín, chata, pato

bedridden postrado en cama

bedsore escara, úlcera por decúbito

bedtime hora de acostarse

bedwetting enuresis, emisión involuntaria de la orina

bee abeja; ~ **sting** picadura de abeja

beef carne de vaca (f)

beer cerveza

before antes (de); ~ **an operation** preoperatorio; ~ **birth** prenatal

beginner neófito, principiante

behavioral sciences ciencias del comportamiento, ciencias del conducto

behaviorism behaviorismo, conductismo

belch eructo, regüeldo; ~ **, to** eructar, regoldar

belching eructo

Bell's palsy parálisis facial, parálisis de Bell, prosopoplejía

bell-shaped epiphysis epífisis acampanada

belly barriga, panza, vientre; ~ **ache** dolor de vientre

Bence Jones protein proteína de Bence Jones

bend backwards, to doblarse por atrás; ~ **inward, to** doblarse, flexionarse; ~ **over, to** inclinarse, agacharse, doblarse

bends enfermedad por descompresión, mal de descompresión

benefit policy póliza estimada

benign benigno, de poca gravedad, de curso favorable, carente de agresividad; ~ **lymphogranulomatosis** sarcoidosis, sarcoide de Boeck; ~ **lymphoreticulosis** enfermedad por arañazo de gato; ~ **polyp** pólipo benigno; ~ **prostatic hyperplasia** hiperplasia prostática benigna; ~ **prostatic hypertrophy** hipertrofia prostática benigna; ~ **tumor** tumor benigno

bent fracture fractura por flexión forzada

benzaldehyde benzaldehído

benzodiazepine benzodiazepina

benzoyl peroxide peróxido de benzoilo

benzoylcholinesterase colinesterasa

benzyl alcohol bencílico

berry aneurysm aneurisma sacular

beryllium disease beriliosis

beside al lado

Besnier–Boeck disease enfermedad de Schaumann

beta beta; ~ **-antagonist** betabloqueador, betabloqueante; ~ **-endorphin** betaendorfina; ~ **-hemolysis** hemolisis beta; ~ **-hemolytic streptococci** estreptococos betahemolíticos, estreptococos piógenos; ~ **-lactam antibiotic** betalactámico, antibiótico betalactámico; ~ **-lactamase** beta-lactamasa; ~ **-oxidation** betaoxidación

betablocker betabloqueador, betabloqueante

betamethasone betametasona

betamimetic betamimético

better mejor

Betz ligament pliegue faringoepiglótico, ligamento de Betz

bias error sistemático

bicarbonate bicarbonato, hidrogenocarbonato

biceps músculo bíceps, bíceps

bicipital bicipital; ~ **tendonitis** tendinitis bicipital

bicornuate bicórneo

bid dos veces al día

Biett disease enfermedad de Biett, lupus eritematoso discoide

bifurcation bifurcación

big gordo; ~ **toe** dedo gordo del pie, hallux

bigeminy bigeminismo

biguanide biguanida

bi-ischial diameter diámetro biisquial

bilateral bilateral, que tiene dos lados, relativo a dos lados; ~ **temporal lobectomy** lobectomía temporal bilateral

bile bilis; ~ **acid** ácido biliar; ~ **duct** vía biliar, canal biliar, conducto colédoco; ~ **pigment** pigmento biliar

bilharziasis bilharziosis

biliary biliar, relativo a la vesícula biliar y a la hiel; ~ **calculus** cálculo biliar, colelitiasis; ~ **cirrhosis** cirrosis biliar; ~ **colic** cólico hepático; ~ **concretion** cálculo biliar, colelitiasis; ~ **duct** vía biliar, canal biliar,

conducto colédoco; ~ **dyspepsia** dispepsia bílica; ~ **obstruction** obstrucción biliar

bilirubin bilirrubina; ~ **encephalopathy** encefalopatía bilirrubínica, kernicterus, la encefalopatía de bilirrubina; ~ **glucuronid** glucurrónido de bilirrubina; ~ **index** índice ictérico

bill factura, cobro, cuenta

billowing mitral leaflet syndrome prolapso mitral

bind, to astringir

binder vendaje abdominal, faja

binding capacity capacidad enlazante; ~ **site** centro de unión

binocular binocular; ~ **loupe** lupa binocular, lentes binoculares; ~ **magnifying glass** lupa binocular, lentes binoculares; ~ **microscope** microscopio binocular

bioassay bioesayo, ensayo biológico, bioanálisis

bioavailability biodisponibilidad, medida de actividad de un medicamento ingerido

bioavailable biodisponible; ~ **metabolite** metabolito biodisponible

biocenosis biocenosis, comunidad biótica

biochemical bioquímico, relativo a la química de los procesos vitales y organismos vivos; ~ **catalyst** catalizador bioquímico; ~ **engineering** ingeniería bioquímica; ~ **feedback** retroalimentación bioquímica; ~ **genetics** genetica bioquímica; ~ **oxygen demand** demanda bioquímica de oxígeno, necesidad bioquímica de oxígeno; ~ **pharmacology** farmacología bioquímica; ~ **profile** perfil bioquímico; ~ **quantity** magnitud bioquímica

biochemistry bioquímica, química biológica

biodegradable biodegradable

biodegradation biodegradación

bioelectronics bioelectrónica

bioenergy bioenergía

bio-engineer ingeniero biomédico

bioengineering bioingeniería

bioequivalence bioequivalencia

bioequivalent bioequivalente, sustancia farmacológica con potencia y efecto similares a otra

bioethics bioética

biofeedback biofeedback, bioretroalimentación

biofilm biopelicula
bioflavenoid bioflavenoide
biogenic biogénico; ~ **amine** aminas biogénicas, aminas biógenas; ~ **amine receptor** receptor de amina biogénica; ~ **polyamines** poliaminas biogénicas, poliaminas biógenas
biological biológico; ~ **chemistry** bioquímica; ~ **clock** reloj biológico; ~ **dosimetry** dosimetría biológica; ~ **effects** efectos biológicos; ~ **fluid** líquido biológico; ~ **half-life** semivida biológica; ~ **hematology** hematología clínica; ~ **ligands** ligandos biológicos; ~ **limit value** valor biológico límite; ~ **oxidation** oxidación biológica; ~ **quantity** magnitud biológica; ~ **stability** estabilidad biológica; ~ **testing** bioensayo, ensayo biológico, bioanálisis; ~ **therapy** terapia biológica; ~ **warfare** guerra biológica
bioluminescence bioluminiscencia
biomaterial biomaterial
biomechanics biomecánica
biomedical biomédico; ~ **imaging** imaginería biomédica
biomedicine biomedicina
biometrics biometría
biometry biometría
biomicroscope biomicroscopio
biomicroscopy biomicroscopia
bionanotechnolgy nanomedicina
bionic implant implante biónico
bionics biónica, electrónica biológica
bio-oxidation oxidación biológica
bioprosthetic heart valve válvula cardiaca de origen animal
biopsy biopsia; ~ **sample** muestra de biopsia
biorhythm biorritmo, el ciclo periódico de fenómenos fisiológicos del cuerpo
biosafety bioseguridad
biosensor biosensor
biosphere biósfera, biosfera
biosynthesis biosíntesis; ~ **of amino acids** biosíntesis de aminoácidos
biotechnology biotecnología, biotécnica
biotelemetry telemetría médica
biotic biótico; ~ **factor** factor biótico
biotin biotina, vitamina H
biotoxicology biotoxicología
biotransformation biotransformación, trasformación química de un compuesto en el organismo
biotype biotipo
biotyping biotipificación
biotypology biotipología
biphasic difásico, que ocurre en dos fases
biphosphonate bifosfonato
bipolar bipolar; ~ **manic-depressive illness** enfermedad maniacodepresiva bipolar
bird pájaro
Birkett synovial protrusion hernia sinovial de Birkett
birth nacimiento, parto; ~ **attendant** comadrona, matrona, partera; ~ **canal** conducto pélvico, canal del parto; ~ **control** contracepción, anticoncepción, prevención del embarazo; ~ **control pill** píldora anticonceptiva; ~ **defect** patología perinatal, defecto congénito, defecto de nacimiento; ~ **injury** lesión obstétrica, traumatismo del nacimiento; ~ **trauma** lesión obstétrica, traumatismo del nacimiento; ~ **weight** peso al nacer
birthmark marca de nacimiento
biscuit, cookie galleta
bite, to morder, picar; ~ **block** abreboca, abrebocas; ~ **one's nails, to** morderse las uñas, comerse las uñas; ~ **wound** mordedura, herida causada por mordedura
biteguard surco dental primitivo, tablilla, gotiera, bruxismo, plana relajación, ferula oclusal
bitter amargo
black negro; ~ **and blue** lívido; ~ **caries** caries nigra; ~ **disease** hepatitis necrotizante, peste negra de los ovinos; ~ **eye** ojo morado, moretón, ojo a la funerala; ~ **lung disease** enfermedad pulmonar minera, antracosis; ~ **measles** sarampión negro; ~ **mold** moho negro; ~ **out, to** desmayarse, perder el conocimiento; ~ **widow spider** araña viuda negra
blackhead grano, espinilla, granito, barro
blackout visión negra, desmayar
bladder ampolla, vesícula, vejiga, bullón, roncha; ~ **calculus** cálculos vesicales; ~ **examination** cistoscopia, observación del interior de la vejiga mediante un aparato

adecuado (el cistoscopio); ~ **stones** cálculos vesicales

Blalock incision incisión de Blalock; ~ **suture ligature** sutura ligadura de Blalock; ~**-Taussig operation** intervención de Blalock-Taussig, operación de Blalock-Taussig

blanching blanqueamiento

bland diet régimen de comidas no picantes, la dieta blanda gastrica

blank en blanco, sin grabar, vago; ~ **value** valor del blanco

blanket cobija

blast cell hemocitoblasto, hematogonia, hemoblasto

blastocyst blastocito, blástula

blastocyte blastocito, blástula

blastomere blastomero

blastomycosis blastomicosis

blastula blastocito, blástula, blastocisto

bleach cloro, blanqueador, lejía

bleb ampolla, vesícula, vejiga, bullón, roncha

bleed, to sangrar; ~ **profusely, to** morir desangrado; ~ **to death, to** morir desangrado

bleeder hemofílico

bleeding desangramiento, hemorragia, sangrado, sangría; ~ **time** tiempo de sangría

blennorrhagia blenorragia, gonorrea

blepharelosis blefarelosis

blepharitis blefaritis, inflamación del borde libre de los párpados

blepharo–adenitis blefaroadenitis

blepharochalasis blefarocalasia, ptosis atrófica

blepharoconjunctivitis blefaroconjuntivitis

blepharomelasma blefaromelasma

blepharoplasty blefaroplastia

blind ciego; ~ **intubation** intubación ciega; ~ **spot** escotoma, pérdida de la facultad visual en zonas bien circunscritas del campo visual

blinding filariasis oncocercosis, una forma filariasis en America Central y del Sur y en África

blindness amaurosis, ceguera

blink one's eye, to destellar, parpadear, pestañear

blister ampolla, vesícula, vejiga, bullón, roncha; ~ **from burns** flictena, ampolla por quemadura; ~ **pack** blister, envase con comprimidos recubiertos de plástico

blistered bullar, con bullas o ampollas

bloating flatulencia, meteorismo, timpanitis

block bloqueo, obstrucción, atoro, atoramiento, atascamiento

blockage bloqueo, obstrucción, atoro, atoramiento, atascamiento; ~ **of sympathetic trunk** bloqueo del tronco simpático

blocked esophagus obstrucción esofágica

blood sangre; ~ **acidosis** acidosis, aumento de la acidez en líquidos y tejidos del cuerpo; ~ **agar** agar sangre; ~ **analysis** cuadro hemático; ~ **blister** vesicula de sangre; ~ **brain barrier** barrera hematoencefálica; ~ **capillary** vaso capilar sanguíneo; ~ **cell count** recuento sanguíneo, hematimetría, hemograma, fórmula sanguínea; ~ **cell production** hemopoyesis; ~ **clot** coágulo de sangre, trombo, cuajaron de sangre; ~ **congestion** congestión, hiperemia pasiva; ~ **count** hemograma; ~ **count quotient** valor globular; ~ **crossmatching** pruebas cruzadas sanguíneas; ~ **culture** cultivo sanguíneo, hemocultivo; ~ **diagnosis** diagnóstico hematológico; ~ **disease** hemopatía, enfermedad de la sangre; ~ **donor** donante de sangre, dador de sangre, donador de sangre; ~ **expander** expansor plasmático, sustancia que se inyecta para aumentar el volumen sanguíneo; ~ **film** extensión sanguíneo; ~ **flow** corriente sanguínea, flujo sanguíneo, torrente sanguíneo; ~ **gas analysis** gasometría sanguínea, determinación de los gases sanguíneos; ~ **glucose level** nivel de glucosa en sangre; ~ **glucose measuring** vigilancia de la glucosa sanguínea; ~ **glucose monitoring** vigilancia de la glucosa sanguínea; ~ **growth factor** factor hematopoyético; ~ **in the urine** hematuria, orina sanguinolenta; ~ **lancet** lanceta; ~ **letting** sacar sangre, sacar muestra de sangre; ~ **morphology** morfología sanguínea; ~ **picture** recuento sanguíneo, hematimetría, hemograma, fórmula sanguínea; ~ **plasma** plasma sanguíneo, plasma hemático; ~ **plasma donor** donante de plasma; ~ **platelet** plaqueta; ~ **platelet aggregation** aglutinación de las plaquetas; ~ **poisoning** toxemia, intoxicación de la sangre; ~ **preparation** preparación sanguínea; ~ **pressure** presión sanguínea, presión arterial; ~ **pressure meter** esfigmomanómetro; ~ **protein** plasmaproteína, proteína del plasma; ~ **purification** depuración de la sangre; ~ **relationship** parentesco, consanguinidad; ~ **relative** pariente, familiar; ~ **replacement** refrescamiento de sangre; ~ **sample** prueba de sangre; ~ **sedimentation** sedimentatción de la sangre; ~ **serum** suero sanguíneo; ~ **spots** púrpura; ~ **substitute** sustituto de la sangre, sustitutivo de la sangre, substituto sanguíneo; ~ **sugar** glucosa; ~ **sugar level** nivel de glucemia, nivel de glicemia; ~ **sugar regulation** control de la glucemia; ~ **test** analisis del sangre (m); ~ **toxemia** toxemia de la sangre; ~ **transfusion** transfusión de sangre; ~ **type** tipo de sangre, grupo sanguíneo; ~ **urea nitrogen** nitrógeno y urea sanguínea; ~ **vessels** vasos sanguíneos; ~ **viscosity** viscosidad de la sangre; ~ **volume** volumen sanguíneo

blood-brain barrier barrera hematoencefálica
bloodcreatinine creatinina plasmática
blood-deprived brain cell célula cerebral isquémica, célula cerebral privada de irrigación sanguínea
blood-forming tissue tejido hematopoyético
blood-group AB grupo sanguíneo AB
bloodletting extracción de sangre, sangría
bloodpoisoning intoxicación de la sangre, sepsis
bloodstream corriente sanguínea, flujo sanguíneo, torrente sanguíneo
blood-sucking hematófago, hematofágico
bloody sangriento, ensangrentado, cubierto de sangre; ~ **cataract** catarata sanguínea; ~ **stool** defecación sanguinolenta, sangre en el excremento, la hematoquezia; ~ **urine** orina sanguinolenta
blow sacudida, golpe; ~ **one's nose, to** sonarse las narices
blue azul; ~ **urine** orinas azules
blue-dot cataract catarata azul
bluish skin cianosis, coloración azulada de la piel y de las mucosas
blunt end extremo romo
blurred borroso, poco nítido; ~ **vision** visión borrosa, vista empañada
blushing eritema emotivo, rubor, ruborícese,

enrojecimiento
BMI índice de Quetelet, índice de masa corporal
B.O. sobaquina, olor corporal, olor fétido asociado con la transpiración rancia
Boder-Sedgwick syndrome telangiectasia, dilatación permanente de grupos de capilares y vénulas superficiales
body cuerpo; ~ **fluid** líquido biológico; ~ **hair** vello, los pelos; ~ **language** lenguaje corporal, mímica, expresión por medio de gestos, de ideas o pensamientos; ~ **mass index** índice de Quetelet, índice de masa corporal; ~ **odor** sobaquina, olor corporal, olor fétido asociado con la transpiración rancia; ~ **part** región, parte del cuerpo; ~ **scheme** esquema corporal; ~ **temperature** temperatura corporal; ~ **weight** masa corporal
Boeck's sarcoid sarcoidosis, enfermedad de Schaumann, sarcoide de Boeck
boil furúnculo, chichón, bola
boiling water agua hirviente, agua hirviendo
boil-like pustuloso
bolus bolus
bolus infusion inyección rápida
bone hueso, los huesos; ~ **chip bed** cama del injerto óseo; ~ **chips** astillas de hueso, lascas; ~ **densitometer** densitómetro de huesos; ~ **densitometry** densitometría de huesos; ~ **density** masa ósea; ~ **density test** densitometría de huesos; ~ **deossification** desosificación; ~ **dissolving** osteólisis, destrucción o muerte del hueso; ~ **formation** osificación; ~ **fragments** astillas de hueso, lascas; ~ **graft** injerto óseo; ~ **hook** gancho de huesos; ~ **lysis** lisis ósea; ~ **marrow** médula ósea; ~ **marrow biopsy** biopsia de médula ósea; ~ **marrow metaphase** metafase de la médula ósea; ~ **marrow mitosis** mitosis anastral; ~ **marrow transplant** transplante de médula ósea; ~ **mass** masa ósea; ~ **metastasis** metástasis ósea; ~ **pins** clavos ortopédicos; ~ **plate** placa de osteosíntesis; ~ **regeneration** regeneración ósea; ~ **scan** cintigrama óseo; ~ **tissue** tejido óseo; ~ **wires** hilos orthopedicos
bony huesudo, huesoso
booster repetidor, elevador; ~ **shot** inyección secundaria, revacunación, inyección de

refuerzo

borborygmus borborigmo, gorgoteo en el vientre

border límbico, relativo a un borde o margen

borderline case caso limítrofe, caso borderline; ~ **psychosis** trastorno de la personalidad esquizotípica

born deaf sordo de nacimiento

Bornholm disease enfermedad de Bornholm

Borrelia burgdorferi Borrelia burgdorferi; ~ **infection** borreliosis, infección por borrelia

borreliosis borreliosis, infección por borrelia

bosom senos, pechos, chichis

both los dos, ambos

bothriocephalosis botriocefalosis

bothriocephalus anemia anemia botriocefálica

bottle botella

bottle-feed, to dar la mamadera al néné

botulinum botulismo; ~ **toxin** toxina botulínica

Bouillaud's disease cardiopatía reumática

Bourgery ligament ligamento posterior oblicuo de la rodilla, ligamento de Bourgery

Bourneville disease enfermedad de Bourneville, esclerosis cerebral tuberosa, epiloia; ~ **syndrome** enfermedad de Bourneville, esclerosis cerebral tuberosa

bovine bovino; ~ **spongiform encephalopathy** encefalopatía espongiforme bovina, enfermedad de las vacas locas

bowel intestino; ~ **ischemia** isquemia, deficiencia del riego sanguíneo de una zona; ~ **movement** deposición, defecación, las heces; ~ **resection** resección del intestino delgado

boxer's encephalopathy encefalopatía de los boxeadores

boy niño

Bozeman tampon forceps fórceps para manejar tampones

Bozzolo disease mieloma múltiple, plasmocitoma, mielomatosis, enfermedad de Kahler, enfermedad de Huppert el plasmocitoma, enfermedad de Bozzolo

bra sostén, corpiño

braces (dental) frenos, ganchos dentales, bandas; ~ **(limbs)** abrazaderas

brachial braquial; ~ **artery** arteria braquial

bradikinin bradicinina

bradycardia bradicardia, lentitud anormal del ritmo cardíaco

bradykinesia bradiquinesia, lentitud anormal de los movimientos

bradypnea bradipnea, respiración lenta

brain encéfalo, cerebro; ~ **abscess** absceso cerebral; ~ **aneurysm** aneurisma cerebral, aneurisma intracraneal; ~ **concussion** conmoción cerebral, concusión del cerebro; ~ **damage** lesión cerebral difusa, trastorno del cerebro; ~ **dead** clínicamente muerto; ~ **death** muerte cerebral; ~ **disease** enfermedad cerebral, encefalopatía; ~ **dysfunction** trastorno del cerebro; ~ **injury** traumatismo cerebral; ~ **magnetic resonance spectroscopy** electroscopia por resonancia magnética cerebral, ERM cerebral; ~ **mapping** mapeo cerebral, cartografía cerebral; ~ **MRS** electroscopia por resonancia magnética cerebral, ERM cerebral; ~ **pacemaker** estimulador del cerebro; ~ **scan** escanografía cerebral; ~ **scanning** electroencefalografía; ~ **stem crisis** crisis epiléptica del tronco cerebral; ~ **stem seizure** crisis del tronco cerebral; ~ **stimulator** estimulador del cerebro; ~ **tumor** tumor del cerebro, el tumor cerebral; ~ **waves** ondas cerebrais

brainstem tronco encefálico, tronco cerebral; ~ **evoked responses** potenciales evocados auditivos

branch rama, ramo, sección; ~ **migration** prolongación del apareamiento

branching dendrítico, ramificado, relativo a las dendritas (fibras nerviosas)

brand quemadura

brassiere sostén, corpiño

Brazilian pemphigus pénfigo brasileño

bread pan

break v romper(se), fracturar(se), quebrar(se)

break n fractura, rotura, quebradura; ~ **and reunion model** modelo de rotura y reunión; ~ **bone fever** calentura roja; ~ **down** degradación; ~ **open, to** reventarse, romper, explotar; ~ **out** erupción, sarpullido

breakdown subdivisión, desglose, descomposición

breakfast desayuno

breaking nicotine addiction métodos para

quebrar la adicción a la nicotina y tabaco

breakthrough bleeding metrorragia, pérdida sanguínea uterina que no sea menstrual, hemorragia intermenstrual

breast pecho, seno, mama; ~ **bone** esternón, hueso del pecho; ~ **cancer** cáncer de mama, cáncer mamario, cáncer del pecho, cáncer del seno; ~ **cancer screening** cribado mamográfico, mamografía, mamograma; ~ **feed a baby, to** lactar, amamantar, criar con pecho; ~ **feeding** lactancia materna, amamantamiento, lactación; ~ **milk** leche materna; ~ **pain** mastodinia, dolor de la mama; ~ **surgery** mamoplastia

breast–conserving surgery cirugía conservadora de la mama

breast–fed infant lactante, bebé, lactente

breastfed, to dar el pecho

breastfeeding mother madre lactante, madre lactente

breast–related mamario, relativo a la mama

breath resuello

breathe, to respirar; ~ **in, to** inhalar, aspirar, respirar; ~ **out, to** espirar, exhalar

breathing ventilación, aireación por la respiración; ~ **apparatus** máscara de protección respiratoria, mascarilla respiratoria, careta respiratoria; ~ **exercise** ejercicio respiratorio; ~ **in** inspiración; ~ **out** expiración; ~ **test** examen respiratorio

breathlessness respiración entrecortada, falta de hálito, estar sin aire, desalentado

breech trasero, posaderas, nalgas; ~ **birth** presentación de nalgas, presentación pélvica; ~ **delivery** presentación de nalgas, presentación pélvica; ~ **presentation** presentación de pie, presentación podálica, presentación pélvica

Brenner ureter cystoscope cistoscopio ureteral de Brenner

bridging fibrosis fibrosis con bridging

brief transitorio, pasajero

brightfield microscopy microscopía de campo claro

broad amplio; ~ **spectrum** amplio espectro, que es activo contra múltiples grupos de gérmenes

Broca's aphasia afasia motora, afasia motora del habla, afasia de Broca

broken–off tooth raigón dental

bromatoxism intoxicación alimentaria, intoxicación alimenticia

bromelain bromelaína de tronco

bromhidrosis bromhidrosis

bromide acne acné brómico

bromine bromo; ~ **cachexia** bromismo, brominismo; ~ **pemphigus** pénfigo brómico; ~ **pregnancy test** prueba del bromo para embarazo

brominism bromismo, brominismo

bromocresol purple púrpura de bromocresol

bromocriptine bromocriptina

bronchial bronquial, relativo a los bronquios; ~ **asthma** broncoespasmo, asma; ~ **brushing** raspado bronquial; ~ **catheter** catéter de balón; ~ **chondroma** condromia bronquial; ~ **congestion** congestión bronquial; ~ **endometriosis** endometriosis bronquial; ~ **fibroma** fibroma bronquial; ~ **fremitus** vibraciones bronquiales, frémito en los bronquios; ~ **hyperreactivity** hiperreactividad bronquial; ~ **lavage** lavado bronquial; ~ **pneumonia** bronconeumonía, inflamación pulmonar; ~ **tree** árbol bronquial, vías respiratorias

bronchiectasis bronquiectasia, dilatación de los bronquios

bronchiolar bronquiolar; ~ **emphysema** enfisema bronquiolar

bronchiolitis bronquiolitis; ~ **obliterans** bronquiolitis obliterante

bronchitis bronquitis, catarro de pecho

bronchoblastomycosis broncoblastomicosis

bronchoconstriction broncoconstricción, contracción de los bronquios, opresión en el pecho

bronchodilatation broncodilatación, dilatación de los bronquios, broncolisis

broncho–dilating preparation preparacion broncodilatadora

bronchodilator broncodilatador

bronchogenic broncógeno

bronchography broncografía

broncholysis broncodilatación, dilatación de los bronquios, broncolisis

bronchopneumonia bronconeumonía, inflamación pulmonar

bronchopulmonary broncopulmonar, relativo a los bronquios y a los pulmones; ~ **dysplasia** displasia broncopulmonar

bronchoscope broncoscopio, tubo incurvado que sirve para explorar visualmente los bronquios

bronchospasm broncoespasmo, espasmo de los bronquios

bronchus bronquio

broth caldo

brother hermano; ~ **-in-law** cuñado

Brucella dermatitis dermatitis melitocócica; ~ **hepatitis** hepatitis brucelosis; ~ **sepsis** septicemia melitocócica

brucellosis brucelosis

bruise moretón, magulladura, contusión, lesión interna por golpe, compresión o choque, cardenal

bruising moretón, magulladura, contusión, lesión interna por golpe, compresión o choque, cardenal

brush one's teeth, to cepillarse los dientes

bruxism bruxomanía

buboes secas, bubas, bubón

bubonic plague peste bubónica, resultando de la infección de pasteurella pestis

buccal bucal, relativo a la boca o a la mejilla; ~ **cannula** cánula bucal; ~ **cavity** cavidad bucal; ~ **glands** glándulas bucales

buccopharyngeal bucofaríngeo, relativo a la boca y a la garganta; ~ **membrane** membrana bucofaríngea

Buck fascia fascia de Buck

buckle at the knees aflojarse, falsear, colapsarse

Buckley paste pasta de Buckley

Bucky diaphragm diafragma de Bucky, antidifusor de rejilla móvil

Buday sepsis septicemia de Buday

buffalo hump joroba de búfalo, grasa dorsocervical

buffer tampón, buffer, amortiguador; ~ **capacity** capacidad tamponadora; ~ **solution** substrato tampón; ~ **substrate** substrato tampón

buffered solution solución de carga, solución tamponada

buffy coat capa leucocitaria, célula mononuclear de cultivo

bulb of vestibule bulbo del vestíbulo

bulbar bulbar, relativo al bulbo

bulbous bulbar, relativo al bulbo

bulge protuberancia, bulto, comba, abultamiento

bulge, to abultar, hinchar, abombar

bulimia bulimia

bulla ampolla, vesícula, vejiga, bullón, roncha

bullet bala; ~ **wound** herida de bala, herida por arma de fuego

bullous bullar, con bullas o ampollas; ~ **eczema** penfigoide bulloso, eczema penfigoide; ~ **pemphigoid** penfigoide bulloso, eczema penfigoide

bully matón, valentón; ~ , **to** intimidar, tiranizar

bump one's head, to darse en la cabeza; ~ , **to** chocar, sacudir

bundle haz de fibras, cordón, tracto

bunion juanete, bunio

BUN concentración de urea en plasma/suero

Burkitt's lymphoma linfoma de Burkitt, tumor de Burkitt, pseudolinfoma, hiperplasia linfoide reactiva

burn quemadura; ~ **ointment** pomada para quemadura; ~ **victim** gravemente quemado; ~ **wounds** quemaduras

burning (sensation) ardor; ~ **pain** escozor, escocimiento, dolor ardiente

burnout agotamiento psíquico, síndrome de desgaste personal

burns quemadura

burp, to reventarse, romper, explotar

burp the baby, to hacer eructar al bébé

bursa-derived lymphocyte linfocito B, célula B; ~ **equivalent lymphocyte** linfocito B, célula B; ~ **of infraspinatus muscle** bolsa del músculo infraespinoso

bursal lymphoid cell linfocito B, célula B

bursatti infección por spirurida

bursitis bursitis, inflamación de una bolsa articular

burst, to reventarse, romper, explotar

Burton's line ribete de Burton, línea de Burton

but pero, sino

butanoic acid ácido butanoico, ácido butírico

butter mantequilla

buttocks nalgas

butylalcohol alcohol butílico
butyric acid ácido butanoico, ácido butírico
buzzing zumbidos, zumbido de oídos, ruido de aleteo
by de, a desde, mediante, en, aa; ~ **mouth** peroral, por boca
bypass bipás, abocamiento
byssinosis bisinosis

C

cabbage repollo
cacaesthesia disestesia
cachet sello
cachexia caquexia, adelgazamiento extremo, debilitación general, marasmo
cadaver cadáver
cadaveric rigidity rigor mortis
cadherins caderinas, moleculas de adhesión hepática
cadmiosis intoxicación broncopulmonar por cadmio, pneumonía química producida por cadmio
cadmium cadmio; ~ **pneumonitis** intoxicación broncopulmonar por cadmio, pneumonía química producida por cadmio
caduceus caduceo
caesarean operación cesárea, cesárea
Caesarean section operación cesárea, cesárea
café au lait spots manchas de café con leche
caffein cafeína
cake biscocho, pastel, torta
calabar swelling nódulos de calabar, tumor de Calabar, edema ambulante
calcanean spur espolón calcáneo
calcaneodynia calcaneodinia, dolor en el talón
calcaneum calcáneo
calcar avis calcariavis, espolón de Morand, hipocampo menor
calcemia concentración de calcio en plasma, calcemia, tasa de calcio en la sangre
calcidiol calcidiol
calcifediol calcifediol
calciferol calciferol
calcification calcificación, calcinosis; ~ **of the cardiac valve** calcificación valvular del corazón
calcinosis calcinosis, calcificación
calcitonin calcitonina
calcitriol calcitriol
calcium calcio; ~ **antagonist** calcioantagonista; ~ **ATPase** bomba de calcio; ~ **chloride** cloruro cálcico; ~ **deposits** depósitos de calcio, focos de calcificación; ~ **gluconate** gluconato cálcico; ~ **hydrogen carbonate** calciohidrogenocarbonato; ~ **in the urine** calciuria, presencia de calcio en la orina; ~ **ion** ion calcio; ~ **lactate** lactato de calcio, E327, lactato cálcico; ~ **metabolism** metabolismo del calcio; ~ **phosphate** fosfato cálcico; ~ **phosphate calculus** cálculo de fosfato de calcio; ~ **phosphate crystals** cristales de fosfato de calcio; ~ **pump** bomba de calcio
calciuria concentración de calcio en orina, calciuria
calculus cálculo, piedra; ~ **vesicalis** cálculo vesical
calendula officinalis calendula officinalis
calf pantorrilla, chamorro
calibrate calibrar
calibrated flask matraz aforado; ~ **loop** asa calibrada; ~ **pipet** pipeta aforada
calibration calibración; ~ **curve** curva de calibración; ~ **function** función de calibración; ~ **material** material de calibración; ~ **standard** patrón de calibración
calibrator calibrador
call bell timbre
callosity callosidad, tejido calloso
callous calloso, endurecido
callouses callosidad, tejido calloso
calm down, to calmarse
Calmette–Guerin's bacillus Mycobacterium bovis (avirulento)
calomel calomel, calomelanos (purgante), cloruro mercurioso; ~ **allergy** alergia inducida por calomelanos; ~ **disease** alergia inducida por calomelanos
caloric caloría; ~ **stimulation** prueba calórica (de Barany); ~ **test** prueba calórica
calpain calpaina
calusterone calusterona, un andrógeno antineoplástico

calvaria calvaria, bóveda del cráneo, calota craneal

calvarial plastic surgery cirugía de la bóveda craneal

cAMP AMP cíclico, adenosina monofosfato cíclico

Camper ligament aponeurosis perineal profunda

camphor oil aceite alcanforado

camphorated oil aceite alcanforado

campylobacter campilobacter; **~ pylori** Helicobacter pylori

can (to be able to) poder

canal of epididymis conducto epididimario

cancellous esponjoso

cancer carcinoma, tumor nocivo, cáncer; **~ –causing** carcinogénico, que provoca o produce cáncer; **~ induced** cáncer inducido; **~ specialist** oncólogo; **~ staging** estadiaje del cáncer

cancerous canceroso; **~ infiltration** infiltración cancerosa; **~ tissue** tejido canceroso

candela candela

candida candida; **~ mycosis** moniliasis, candidiásis

candidiasis candidiasis, algodoncillo, afta, infección por un hongo del género candida

cane bastón, bordón

canker sore afta, llaga ulcerosa en la boca, úlcera en la boca

cannabis cannabis, haschis

cannula cánula, tubo que se introduce en el organismo

cantus galli laringismo estriduloso

cap remate

capacitance capacitancia

capacity capacidad

capillaropathy angiopatía capilar, capiloropatía

capillary capilar; **~ bleeding** hemorragia capilar; **~ blood pressure** presión capilar; **~ dilation** ectasia capilar; **~ embolism** embolia capilar; **~ fistula** fístula capilar; **~ hemangioma** hemangioma capilar, nevo flameo, capiloropatía; **~ leak syndrome** síndrome de salida capilar; **~ permeability** permeabilidad capilar; **~ porosity** porosidad capilar; **~ pulse** pulso capilar; **~ puncture** punción de la vejiga, punción vesical; **~ serum**

electrophoresis electroforesis de la sangre capilar; **~ thrombosis** trombosis capilar

capitulum capítulo, cabeza; **~ of humerus** cabeza del húmero, capítulo humeral

capneic incubation incubación capneica

capnophilic capnófilico

caprolactam caprolactama

capsaicin capsaicina

capsid cápsida

capsular capsular; **~ cataract** catarata capsulolenticular; **~ glaucoma** glaucoma capsular; **~ hemiplegia** parálisis capsular, síndrome de la cápsula interna; **~ paralysis** parálisis capsular, síndrome de la cápsula interna; **~ pattern** padrono capsular

capsule cápsula

capsulectomy capsulectomía

capsulo-ganglionic hemorrhage hemorragia intracapsular

Captopril captopril

caput brevae cabeza corta (del bíceps crural); **~ musculi** cabeza del músculo

carbamazepine carbamazepina

carbamoyl carbamoil

carbazole carbazole

carbenicillin carbenicilina

carbohydrate carbohidrato, glucósido, glúcido; **~ assimilation test** prueba de la asimilación de glúcidos

carbohydrated antigen antígeno carbohidratado

carbohydrates carbohidratos

carbon carbono; **~ dioxide** dióxido de carbono; **~ monoxide** monóxido de carbono; **~ monoxide haemoglobin** hemoglobina-monóxido de carbono; **~ monoxide poisoning** oxicarbonemia; **~ tetrachloride** tetracloruro de carbono

carbonate dehydratase carbonato-deshidratasa

carboxyhemoglobin carboxihemoglobina

carboxyhemoglobinemia carboxihemoglobinemia

carboxylesterase carboxilesterasa

carboxypeptidase carboxipeptidasa

carcinoembryonic antigen antígeno carcinoembrionario, ACE

carcinogen agente carcinógeno

carcinogenic cancerígeno, carcinogénico, que

provoca o produce cáncer, oncogénico;
~ **virus** virus cancerígeno

carcinoid carcinoide; ~ **tumor** tumor carcinoide

carcinoma carcinoma (m), tumor nocivo, cáncer

cardiac cardíaco, relativo al corazón; ~ **anxiety** palpitación cardíaca, vahídos, angustia cardíaca; ~ **arrest** asistolia, parada cardíaca, paro cardíaco; ~ **arrhythmia** arritmia cardiaca, alteraciones del ritmo cardíaco; ~ **atrophy** atrofia cardíaca; ~ **automatism** automatismo cardíaco; ~ **catheterization** cateterismo cardíaco; ~ **compression** compresión cardíaca; ~ **cycle** ciclo cardíaco; ~ **death** muerte cardíaca; ~ **defect** lesión cardíaca; ~ **deficiency** deficiencia cardíaca; ~ **disorder** afección cardíaca; ~ **enzymes** enzimas cardíacas; ~ **glycoside** glucósido cardiotónico; ~ **infarction** infarto de miocardio; ~ **innervation** inervación cardíaca; ~ **insufficiency** insuficiencia cardíaca; ~ **massage** masaje cardíaco; ~ **minute ouput** gasto cardíaco, volumen minuto del corazón, rendimiento cardíaco; ~ **neurosis** astenia neurocirculatoria; ~ **output** gasto cardíaco, volumen minuto del corazón, rendimiento cardíaco; ~ **output index** índice del rendimiento cardíaco; ~ **pacemaker** marcapasos cardíaco, aparato cardiocinético; ~ **palpitation** palpitación cardíaca, vahídos, angustia cardíaca; ~ **region** zona cardíaca; ~ **rescussitation** reanimación cardíaca; ~ **shadow** silueta cardíaca; ~ **shock** shock cardiogénico; ~ **stimulant** estimulante cardíaco; ~ **syncope** síncope cardíaco; ~ **tamponade** taponamiento cardíaco; ~ **ultrasound** ultrasonido cardíaco; ~ **valvuloplasty** valvuloplastia cardíaca; ~ **work** trabajo del corazón; ~ **zone** zona cardíaca

cardial cardial; ~ **glands** glándulas cardiales; ~ **insufficience** insuficiencia del cardias; ~ **sphincter** esfínter del cardias

cardialgia cardialgia

cardiectomy resección del cardias

cardiogenic cardiogénico, que es consecuencia de una deficiencia del corazón; ~ **shock** shock cardiogénico

cardiologica cardiológico

cardiology cardiología

cardiomegaly cardiomegalia, aumento del tamaño del corazón

cardiomyopathy cardiomiopatía, trastorno crónico que afecta al músculo cardíaco

cardiopathy cardiopatía, dolencia o afección cardíaca

cardiopulmonary cardiopulmonar, relativo al corazón y pulmones; ~ **resuscitation** resucitación cardiopulmonar, reanimación cardiopulmonar

cardiorespiratory cardiorrespiratorio, relativo al corazón y a la respiración

cardiorrhexis rotura cardíaca

cardioselective cardioselectivo, que actúa selectivamente sobre el corazón

cardiospasm cardiospasmo, acalasia del esófago

cardiotomy cardiotomía

cardiotonic cardiotónico, que tiene efecto tónico en el corazón

cardiotoxic cardiotóxico, tóxico para el corazón

cardiotoxicity cardiotoxicidad

cardiovascular cardiovascular, relativo al corazón y a los vasos; ~ **collapse** colapso cardiovascular, fallo cardiovascular; ~ **deconditioning** descondicionamiento cardiovascular; ~ **failure** colapso cardiovascular, fallo cardiovascular; ~ **imaging** imaginería cardiovascular

cardioversion cardioversión, restablecimiento del ritmo sinusal del corazón

care atención, cuidado; ~ **givers** cuidadores, enfermeros, médicos, etc. que cuidan al paciente; ~ **of premature infants** cuidados del prematuro

career profesión, carrera f profesional; ~ **counseling** orientación profesional, consejería profesional

caregivers cuidadores, enfermeros, médicos, etc. que cuidan al paciente

caries prophylaxis profilaxis dental

carina puncture punción de la carina, punción del espolón traqueal; ~ **tracheae** carina de la tráquea, espolón traqueal

cariology cariología

carminatives carminativos

carotenoid carotenoide

carotid carótida; ~ **artery** arteria carótida,

arteria del cráneo, artéria carótida primitiva; ~ **body** glomus carotídeo, cuerpo carotídeo; ~ **pulse** pulso carótido; ~ **sinus death** muerte por reflejo del seno carotídeo; ~ **sinus nerve** nervio del seno carotídeo; ~ **sinus pressure test** prueba de la compresión del seno carotídeo, maniobra de valsalva; ~ **sinus reflex** reflejo del seno carotídeo, reflejo senocarotídeo; ~ **syncope** síncope sinocarotídeo

carpal carpo; ~ **bones** huesos del carpo; ~ **joint** articulación carpiana; ~ **tunnel** canal carpiano, túnel carpiano; ~ **tunnel syndrome** síndrome del tunel carpiano

Carpue Operation rinoplastia de Carpue

carpus carpo, parte de la mano constituida por dos filas de cuatro huesos, articulación de la muñeca; ~ **curvus** deformidad de Madelung

carrier portador, excipiente, vehículo de transmisión de la infección; ~ **cell** fagocito; ~ **of infection** vector de enfermedad; ~ **protein** proteína transportadora; ~-**culture** cultivo portador

carrot zanahoria

carry, to llevar; ~-**over** contaminación; ~-**over inhaler** pipeta de inhalación

cartilage cartílago

cartilaginous cartilaginoso; ~ **joint** articulación cartilaginosa, anfiartrosis, juntura cartilaginosa

cartridge vial, ampolla, pequeña ampolla o frasco de vidrio, envase de vidrio o plástico

carving knife cuchillo de trinchar

caryotype cariotipo

case caso, maleta; ~ **history** fichas clínicas, fichas médicas; ~ **management** manejo de casos, administración de casos; ~ **of relapse** recaída, reincidencia

casein caseína

cash al contado, en efectivo

cassette casete; ~ **mechanism** mecanismo de casete

cast yeso, enyesadura, cilindro (urinario)

castor oil aceite de ricino

castration castración, extirpación de los órganos sexuales

casualty siniestrado, accidentado, persona accidentada

casuistics casuística, registro y estudio de los casos de una determinada enfermedad

cat gato; ~ **bite phlegmon** flemón por mordedura de gato; ~ **scratch disease** enfermedad del arañazo de gato; ~ **scratch fever** enfermedad del arañazo de gato

catabolic catabólico; ~ **degradation** degradación catabólica; ~ **hormones** hormonas catabólicas; ~ **pathway** vía catabólica; ~ **repression** represión catabólica, regulación del catabolismo

catabolism catabolismo, degradación de las sustancias alimentarias en el organismo

catabolite activator protein proteína activadora del catabolismo; ~ **repression** represión catabólica, regulación del catabolismo

catalase catalasa; ~ **test** prueba de la catalasa

catalepsy catalepsia

cataleptic rigidity rigidez cataléptica; ~ **rigor mortis** rigor mortis cataléptico

catalyse, to catalizar, acelerar una reacción química

catalyst catalizador

catalytic catalítico; ~ **activity** actividad catalítica; ~ **activity concentration** concentración de actividad catalítica; ~ **activity flow rate** caudal de actividad catalítica; ~ **activity fraction** fracción de actividad catalítica; ~ **activity rate** caudal de actividad catalítica; ~ **centre** centro catalítico; ~ **concentration** concentración catalítica; ~ **content** contenido catalítico; ~ **elements** elementos catalyticos; ~ **flow rate** caudal catalítico; ~ **fraction** fracción catalítica; ~ **peroxidase** peroxidasa catalítica; ~ **rate** caudal catalítico

catamnesis catamnesis

cataphoresis cataforesis

cataplexy cataplexia, cataplejía, el embotamiento súbito de la sensibilidad en una parte del cuerpo

cataract catarata, cristalino, enturbiamiento de la lente transparente del ojo

catarrh catarro, resfriado, coriza

catarrhal croup asma de Millar

catastrophic catastrófico

catatonia catatonía, un trastorno caracterizado

por

catatonic catatónico

catch a cold, to resfriado, catarro; **~ a cold, to** resfriarse

catecholamine catecolamina

catharsis catarsis

cathartic catártico

cathepsin catepsina

catheter cathéter, tubo, sonda; **~ ablation** ablacion por cateter, ablación por radiofrecuencia, ablación eléctrica transvenosa

catheterization cateterismo, introducción de una sonda en una cavidad hueca

cathexis catexis

cathisophobia acatisia, tasicinesia

cation catión - un ion cargado positivamente

caucasian caucasiano, blanco

caudal caudal, relativo o en dirección hacia la cola

caumesthesia caumestesia

causal causal, causativo

causation causalidad, etiología

causative causativo, causal

caustic cáustico, quemante, corrosivo; **~ soda** hidroxido de sodio, la soda cáustica; **~ soda** lejía de sosa, sosa líquida, hidróxido sódico líquido, NaOH

cauterization cauterización

cautery cauterio

cavernous cavernoso; **~ angioma** angioma cavernoso; **~ cancer** cáncer cavernoso; **~ hemangioma** hemangioma cavernoso; **~ sinus** seno cavernoso; **~ sinus thrombosis** trombosis del seno cavernoso

CA virus virus de la parainfluenza

Cavitron ultrasonic surgical aspirator aspirador ultrasónico

cavity cavidad, espacio hueco; **~ dental** caries; **~ of the mouth** cavidad bucal propiamente dicha

CBC hemograma

cCMP CMP cíclico

CD4 antigen molécula CD4, antigeno CD4; **~ molecule** molécula CD4, antigeno CD4; **~ receptor** receptor CD4, molécula CD4, receptor T4

CD8 antigen antigeno CD8

cDNA clone clon de cDNA; **~ library** genoteca

de cDNA

CEA antígeno carcinoembrionario

cecocolostomy cecolostomía

cecostomy cecostomía

cecropin cecropina

cefaclor cefaclor

cefadroxil cefadroxilo

cefalexin cefalexina

cefaloridine cefaloridina

cefamandol cefamandol

cefazolin cefazolina

cefixime cefixima

cefmenoxime cefmenoxima

cefmetazole cefmetazol

cefonicid cefonicido

cefoperazone cefoperazona

cefotaxime cefotaxima

cefotetan cefotetano

cefoxitin cefoxitina

cefradine cefradina

cefsulodin cefsulodina

ceftazidime ceftazidima

ceftizoxime ceftizoxima

ceftriaxone ceftriaxona

cefuroxime cefuroxima

celiac celíaco; **~ disease** enfermedad celíaca; **~ syndrome** enfermedad celíaca

cell célula; **~ biology** biología celular, citobiología; **~ border** borde de la célula; **~ count** concentración de células, medida de la concentración de células, recuento de células; **~ culture** cultivo celular; **~ cycle kinetics** cinética del ciclo celular; **~ disruption** rotura celular; **~ division** mitosis, division de una célula; **~ drinking** pinocitosis; **~ fractionation** fraccionamiento celular; **~ line** línea celular; **~ membrane** membrana celular, membrana de una célula; **~ morphology** morfología celular; **~ reproductive death** muerte de la célula; **~ surface** membrana celular, membrana de una célula; **~ survival rate** índice de supervivencia celular; **~ technology** tecnología celular

cellular celular; **~ nucleotide** nucleótido celular; **~ oncogen** protooncogen, protooncogén; **~ plasminogen activator** activador del u-plasminógeno; **~ protein**

kinase proteína quinasa celular
cellulase celulasa
cellulite celulitis
cellulitis celulitis (f), inflamación del tejido bajo la piel
Celsius temperature temperatura Celsius
centimeter centímetro
centimorgan centimorgan
central central; ~ **choroiditis** coroiditis central; ~ **choroidoretinitis** coriorretinitis macular; ~ **motor neuron** neurona superior, neurona cortical; ~ **nervous system** sistema nervioso central; ~ **vacuum cleaner system** aspirador central de basuras, aspirador limpiador
centrifugal centrífugo; ~ **force** fuerza centrífuga; ~ **radius** radio centrífugo
centrifugation centrifugación
centrifuge centrifugadora, centrífuga
centrifuged hemolisate centrifuga el hemolizado
centrilobular hepatocyte enlargement hipertrofia de los hepatocitos
centriole centriolo, orgánulo citoplásmico que suele formar parte del centrosoma
centromere centrómero, cinetocoro; ~ – **telomere translocation** translocación centrómero-telómero
centrosome centrosoma
cephalalgia cefalalgia, dolor de cabeza, migraña
cephalea cefalalgia, dolor de cabeza; ~ **nodularis** cefalea induratíva, cefalea nodular
cephalexin cefalexina
cephalic vein vena cefálica
cephaloglycin cefaloglicina
cephaloridine cefaloridina
cephalosporin cefalosporina
cephalosporinase b-lactamasa
cephalothin cefalotina
cephradine cefradina
ceramidase ceramidasa
cerclage of the patella sutura patelar
cerebellar cerebeloso; ~ **astrocytoma** astrocitoma cerebelar; ~ **catalepsy** catalepsia cerebelosa; ~ **cortex** corteza cerebelosa; ~ **gait** marcha cerebelosa; ~ **syndrome** síndrome cerebeloso; ~ **tremor** temblor cerebeloso
cerebellum cerebelo

cerebral cerebral, relativo al cerebro; ~ **abscess** absceso cerebral; ~ **aneurysm** aneurisma cerebral, aneurisma intracraneal; ~ **atrophy** atrofia cerebral; ~ **congestion** congestión cerebral; ~ **dominance** dominancia cerebral, escritura en espejo; ~ **engorgement** congestión cerebral; ~ **hemisphere** hemisferio cerebral; ~ **hemorrhage** hemorragia cerebral; ~ **hernia** herniación cerebral, hernia cerebral; ~ **herniation** herniación cerebral, hernia cerebral; ~ **hypophysis** hipófisis cerebral, cuerpo pituitario; ~ **infarction** infarto cerebral; ~ **infectious embolism** embolia cerebral, embolio cerebral; ~ **lobectomy** lobectomía cerebral; ~ **lymphoma with tumorous lesion** linfoma cerebral con lesión tumoroso; ~ **MRI** IRM cerebral, RM cerebral; ~ **palsy** parálisis cerebral; ~ **revascularization** revascularización cerebral; ~ **rupture** ruptura cerebral; ~ **thrombosis** trombosis cerebral; ~ **toxoplasmosis** toxoplasmosis cerebral; ~ **ventriculography** ventriculografía cerebral
cerebroside–sulfatase cerebrósido-sulfatasa
cerebrospinal cerebrospinal, relativo al cerebro y a la médula espinal; ~ **fluid** líquido cefalorraquídeo, líquido cerebroespinal
cerebrovascular cerebrovascular, que afecta a los vasos cerebrales; ~ **accident** apoplejía, ictus, accidente cerebrovascular agudo; ~ **disease** enfermedad cerebro-vascular
cerebrum cerebro, encéfalo; ~ encéfalo, cerebro
certifiable certificable
certificate value valor certificado
ceruloplasmin ceruloplasmina, ferroxidasa
cerumen cerumen
cervical cervical; ~ **cancer** cáncer del cuello del útero; ~ **cap** capuchón cervical, capuchón en bóveda, casquete cervical, diafragma pesario; ~ **collar** collarín cervical, minerva; ~ **denervation** bloqueo del tronco simpático cervical, desnervación del tronco simpático cervical; ~ **dystocia** distocia cervical; ~ **mucus** moco cervical; ~ **osteoarthritis** osteoartrosis cervical; ~ **rib** costilla cervical; ~ **smear** muestra de exudado cervical, secreción cervical, frotis cérvico-vaginal; ~ –**vaginal swab** toma cervicovaginal, citología vaginal,

frotis vaginal; **~ vertebra** vértebra cervicala

cervicectomy traquelectomía

cervicitis cervicitis, inflamación del cuello del útero

cervicobrachial cervicobrachial; **~ neuralgia** neuralgia cervicobrachial

cervicodorsal algia algia cervicodorsal; **~ algia** algia cervicodorsal

cervix cervix; **~ uteri** cuello uterino, cervix uterino, cuello de matriz

cesarian section sección cesárea

cestode tenia, solitaria, cestodo

CF test prueba de fijación del complemento

CFU partícula formadora de colonia, unidad formadora de colonia

CG coriogonadotropina

chafing intertrigo, acción inflamatoria de los pliegues cutáneos, rozadura

chain cadena; **~ reaction** reacción en cadena; **~ terminator** finalizador de cadena

chair presidente, coordinador

chairman presidente, coordinador

chairperson presidente, coordinador

chalazion chalazion, calacio

chalazodermia dermatolisis, chalazodermia

chalcosis of lens (ophthalmology) catarata en flor de tornasol

challenge testing prueba de provocación

change cambio, cambiar; **~ in bowel movement** cambios en la evacuación; **~ in cognitive function** alteración de la función cognitiva; **~ in color** cambio de color

channel canal

chaperone chaperona; **~ protein** carabina molecular, proteína celadora

chaperonine chaperonina

chapped lips labios agrietados, labios partidos

character trait rasgo, característica

characteristic rasgo, característica, característico

Charcot–Leyden crystals cristales asmáticos de Charcot-Leyden

charge carga; **~ number** número de carga; **~ nurse** enfermera supervisora, jefa de turno

charged tRNA tRNA cargado

charlatan matasanos, farsante, charlatán

charlatanism charlatanería, curanderismo

charlatanry curanderiá, charlatanismo, charlatanería

charley horse agujeta, calambre

chattering of teeth castañetear de dientes

chatty hablador, locuaz, parlanchín

Chauveau bacillus Clostridium chauvoei

Chayes attachment puente fijo desarmable de Chayes, puente de Chayes

check cheque; **~ list** lista de comprobaciones; **~ pessary** pesario; **~ , to** examinar; **~up** chequeo médico, reconocimiento médico

cheek mejilla, cachete; **~ bone** pómulo, hueso malar

cheeks nalgas

cheese queso

cheiloplasty plastía del labio

cheiloschisis labio cucho, labio leporino, labio fisurado

cheiropompholyx dishidrosis, quiroponfólix, eccema dishidrótico, ponfólix

CHE colinesterasa

chelating agent quelante como la penicilamina

chelation quelación

cheloid queloide, cicatriz elevada

cheloma queloide, cicatriz elevada

chemical químico; **~ analysis** análisis químico; **~ burns** quemaduras químicas; **~ castration** castración química; **~ cystitis** cistitis química; **~ immunosuppressive** fármaco inmunosupresor; **~ ionization** ionización química; **~ pathology** bioquímica clínica, química clínica; **~ pneumonia** neumonitis química, neumonía química; **~ pneumonitis** neumonitis química, neumonía química; **~ potential** potencial químico

chemiluminiscence quimioluminiscencia

chemist boticario, farmacia

chemistry química

chemoattractant quimiotáctico

chemokine quimiocina

chemoluminescence quimiluminiscencia, quimioluminiscencia

chemometrics quimiometría

chemonucleolysis chemonucleolisis

chemoprevention quimioprofilaxia, quimioprofilaxis

chemoreceptor quimiorreceptor

chemosis quemosis; **~ of conjunctiva** quemosis, edema de la membrana mucuosa que recubre el globo ocular

chemotaxis quimiotaxis, quimiotactismo

chemotherapeutic quimioterápico, medicamentos que atacan a los microbios parasitarios o a las células de un cáncer

chemotherapy quimioterapia, tratamiento de un cáncer por sustancias químicas

chest pecho, tórax; ~ **compression** compresión del pecho; ~ **deflection** deformación del tórax, deformación de la caja torácica; ~ **pain** dolor en el tórax, dolor torácico; ~ **x-rays** radiografía de tórax; ~ **-wall ECG** electrocardiograma de la pared torácica

chew, to masticar; ~ **coca leaves** masticar hojas de coca

chewable masticable; ~ **tablets** pastillas masticables

chewing masticación

chi ji, qi, energía vital

chi square test prueba de la ji al cuadrado, prueba de la c2

chicken pollo

chickenpox (varicella) varicela, viruela loca; ~ **vaccine** vacuna contra la varicela; ~ **virus** virus varicella-zóster, herpesvirus 3 humano

chigger nigua, pique, chico

chilblains fenómeno de Raynaud

child niño, -a; ~ **bearing** procreación, reproducción; ~ **bearing period** periodo fértil de la mujer, temporada de cría; ~ **born to HIV-positive mother** hijo de madre seropositiva; ~ **death rate** tasa de mortalidad infantil; ~ **development** pedología, desarrollo de los niños; ~ **murder** infanticidio; ~ **psychiatrist** especialista en psiquiatría infantil y juvenil; ~ **psychologist** psicología cognitiva

childbirth nacimiento, parto

childhood disintegrative disorder trastorno generalizado del desarrollo de la infancia; ~ **neurosis** neurosis infantil

children's hospital hospital infantil

chillblains sabañón, congelación, pernio

chills escalofríos, fríos

chimera quimera

chimeric gene gen quimérico

chin mentón

chiropodist ortopedista

chiropractic quiropráctica; ~ **adjustment** ajuste quiropráctico

chiropractor quiropráctico

chitinase quitinasa

chlamydia clamidia, enfermedad venérea; ~ **trachomatis** clamidia trachomatis

chlamydospore clamidospora

chloasma cloasma, manchas irregulares que aparecen generalmente en la cara; ~ **hepaticum** cloasma hepático

chloracne acné clórica

chloral hydrate hidrato de cloral

chlorambucil clorambucil

chloramphenicol cloranfenicol

chlordiazepoxide clorodiazepóxido

chlorhexidine clorhexidina

chloride cloruro

chlorinated hydrocarbons organoclorados

chlorine cloruro

chlorofluorocarbon hidrocarburos de fluoruro, clorofluorocarbono

chloroform cloroformo, triclorometano; ~ **poisoning** intoxicación por cloroformo

chlorophyll body cloroplasto, plasto clorofílico

chloroplast cloroplasto, plasto clorofílico

chloroquine cloroquina, un antimalárico

chlorosis clorosis, amarilleo, amarillez, estar clorótico

chlorotrianisene clorotrianiseno, estrógeno

chlorpheniramine clorfenamina

chlorpromazine clorpromazina

chlorpyrifos clorpirifós, clorpirifos

chlorthalidone clortalidona, un diurético

chlorzoxazone clorzoxazona, un relajante de las musculatura esquelética

choanae coanas

choanal polyp polipo coanal

choke on, to atragantarse; ~ **, to** sufocar, ahogar, sofocar

cholagogue colagogo

cholangiography colangiografía, radiografía de contraste de los conductos biliares

cholangitis colangitis, inflamación de las vías biliares

cholechromeresis hipersecreción de los pigmentos biliares

cholecystectomy colecistectomía, extirpación de la vesícula biliar

cholecystitis colecistitis, inflamación de la vesícula biliar; **~ glandularis proliferans** colecistitis glandular proliferativa

cholecystography colecistografía, estudio radiológico de la vesícula biliar

cholecystokinin pancreozimina

choledochoduodenal coledocoduodenal; **~ fistula** fístula coledocoduodenal

cholelithiasis colelitiasis, cálculos biliares

cholemic chloasma cloasma colemico

cholera cólera; **~ infantum** cólera infantil; **~ toxin** toxina del cólera

choleraphage bacteriófago anticolérico

choleretic colerético, una sustancia que favorece la producción de hiel

cholestasis colestasis (f), retención de hiel en los conductos

cholestatic colestático; **~ hepatosis** hepatosis colestática; **~ icterus** ictericia colestática

cholesteremia concentración de colesterol en plasma, colesteremia

cholesterin colesterol

cholesterol colesterol, colesterina; **~ acyltransferase** esterol-O-aciltransferasa; **~ esterase** esterol-esterasa; **~ -lowering agent** fármaco rebajador del nivel de colesterol; **~ oxidase** colesterol-oxidasa

cholesterolemia colesteremia, colesterolemia, concentración de colesterol en plasma/suero

cholic acid ácido cólico

choline esterase colinesterasa; **~ activity** actividad de colinesterasa; **~ kinase** colina-cinasa; **~ oxidase** colina-oxidasa

cholinergic colinérgico

chondral cartilaginoso; **~ callus** callo cartilaginoso

chondriosome mitocondria, mitocondria, plastosoma

chondritis condritis

chondroblast condroblasto

chondrocalcinosis condrocalcinosis

chondrocyte condrocito

chondrodysplasia condrodisplasia

chondrofibroma condrofibroma

chondroitin condroitina, condroitin; **~ sulfate** sulfato de condroitina

chondrolipoma condrolipoma

chondromalacia condromalacia; **~ patella** condromálacia de la rótula

chondromatosis condromatosis

chondromyxofibroma condromyixfibroma de los huesos

chondrosarcoma condrosarcoma

chondrosis condrosis

chondrosteoma osteocondroma, exostosis osteocartilaginosa

chorea corea, exceso de movimientos voluntarios; **~ fibrillaris** corea fibrilar; **~ gravidarum** corea gravidarum

chorio–adenoma destruens mola maligna, coriodemona, mola hidatiforme invasiva

choriocapillaris capa coreocapilária

choriogonadotropin coriogonadotropina

choriomammotropin coriomamotropina

chorionic coriónico; **~ gonadotrophin** gonadotropina coriónica, coriogonadotropina; **~ somatomammotropin** coriomamotropina, lactogeno placentario; **~ villi** vellosidades coriónicas; **~ villi cell** células de las vellosidades coriónicas

chorionitis corionitis

chorioretinitis corioretinitis

choroid sclerosis esclerosis coroidiana

choroidoretinitis corioretinitis

chromaffin cromafin, cromafínico; **~ cell** célula cromafin; **~ paraganglions** paraganglios cromafines; **~ system** sistema cromafinico

chromatid cromátide

chromatin cromatina; **~ body** cuerpo de Barr

chromatogram cromatograma

chromatograph cromatógrafo

chromatography cromatografía

chrome ulceration pigeonnau

chromomere cromómero

chromophile cromafin

chromophore cromóforo

chromosomal cromosómico; **~ aberration** aberración cromosómica; **~ abnormality** aberración cromosómica, anomalía cromosómica; **~ bridge** puente cromosómico; **~ illness** enfermedad cromosómica; **~ inheritance** herencia cromosómica; **~ region** región de los cromosomas, región cromosómica; **~ sex** sexo cromosómico

chromosome cromosoma; **~ analysis** análisis

cromosómico; ~ **banding** bandeo cromosómico; ~ **count** recuento de cromosomas, número cromosómico; ~ **damage** defecto cromosómico, defecto del cromosoma; ~ **defect** defecto cromosómico, defecto de los cromosomas; ~ **disorder** trastorno de los cromosomas; ~ **erosion** erosión cromosómica; ~ **exchange** intercambio de cromosomas; ~ **jumping** desplazamiento rápido sobre el cromosoma; ~ **map** mapa cromosómico, mapa genético; ~ **set** dotación cromosómica

chromosomopathy enfermedad cromosómica

chronaxy cronaxia

chronic persistente, perseverante, crónico; ~ **active hepatitis** hepatitis crónica activa; ~ **bleeding** hemorragias crónicas; ~ **bronchitis** bronquitis crónica, catarro de pecho; ~ **case** caso crónico; ~ **fatigue syndrome** síndrome de fatiga crónica, encefalomielitis miálgica; ~ **granulomatous disease** enfermedad granulomatosa crónica; ~ **hepatitis** hepatitis crónica; ~ **kidney failure** insuficiencia renal permanente, fallo crónico del riñón, fallo permanente del riñón; ~ **lymphocytic leukemia** leucemia linfoide crónica; ~ **myelogenous leukemia** leucemia mieloblástica crónica, leucemia mielocítica, leucemia mielógena; ~ **neutrophilic leukemia** leucemia neutrofílica crónica; ~ **obstructive bronchitis** bronquitis asmática, bronquitis obstructiva crónica; ~ **obstructive lung disease** enfermedad pulmonar obstructiva crónica, enfermedad pulmonar permanente, bronconeumopatía crónica obstructiva; ~ **obstructive pulmonary disease** EPOC, enfermedad pulmonar obstructiva crónica; ~ **otitis** otitis crónica; ~ **pain** dolor persistente, dolor crónico; ~ **pharyngitis** faringitis crónica; ~ **polychondritis** policondritis recidivante; ~ **renal disease** enfermedad renal crónica; ~ **renal failure** insuficiencia renal aguda; ~ **respiratory disease** enfermedad crónica respiratoria; ~ **toxic encephalopathy** encefalopatía tóxica crónica

chronotropic cronotropo, que concierne a la regularidad y frecuencia de un ritmo cardíaco

chrysotherapy crisoterapia

chubby sobrepeso, pasado de peso, gordo, grueso, gordinflón, petacón, excesode peso

chylomicron quilomicrón

chyluria quiluria

chyme quimo

chymotrypsin quimotripsina

cianocobalamin cobalamina, vitamina B12, cianocobalamina

cicatrization cicatrización

ciclosporin ciclosporina

CIE inmunoelectroforesis bidimensional, contrainmunoelectroforesis

cigarette cigarrillo

ciliary muscle músculo ciliar

ciprofloxacin ciprofloxacino

circadian circadiano; ~ **rhythms** ritmo circadiano

circulating circulante; ~ **antibody** anticuerpo circulante; ~ **immune complex** inmunocomplejo circulante; ~ **monocyt** monocito circulante; ~ **virus** virus circulante

circulation circulación; ~ **of blood** circulación de sangre; ~ **problems** trastorno circulatorio

circulatory circulatorio; ~ **disorder** trastorno circulatorio

circumcision circuncisión

circumference circumferencia

circumscribed circunscrito; ~ **scleroderma** esclerodermia circunscrita

cirrhosis induración granular, cirrosis; ~ **of the kidney** cirrosis renal; ~ **of the liver** cirrosis hepática

cisplatin cisplatino, cis-diaminodicloroplatino

cisterna cisterna

cistron cistrón

citrate citrato

citrated whole human blood, CWHB sangre humana citrada

citric acid ácido cítrico

citronnella toronjil

citrulline citrulina

city ciudad

civil status estado civil

CK creatina-cinasa

claim for compensation acciones por daños y perjuicios; ~ **for damages** acciones por daños y perjuicios; ~ **for Medicare payment** reclamación de pago de Medicare

clap gonorrea, chorro, infección de la mucosa urinaria y genital

clapping golpear, percusión

clarithromycin claritromicina

clasmatocytic sarcoma sarcoma de macrofagos

classic clásico, típico, característico; **~ migraine** jaqueca clásica

classical clásico; **~ pathway** vía clásica

classification clasificación

classifying clasificación

claudication claudicación, cojera

claustrum claustro; **~ virginale** himen

clavacin patulina

clavicle clavícula, hueso del cuello

claviformin patulina

clavulanic acid ácido clavulánico

clavus callo, garras, uñas

clean aséptico, libre de gérmenes, estéril; **~ , to** raspar, fregar, afretar

cleanliness asepsia, ausencia de gérmenes infecciosos, prevención de infección

clearance depuración, aclaramiento; **~ of inuline** depuración de inulina

clearing factor lipase lipoproteina-lipasa; **~ upper respiratory passages** desobstrucción de las vías respiratorias superiores

cleavage escisión

cleft lip labio cucho, labio leporino, labio fisurado; **~ of vertebral arches** fisura vertebral; **~ palate** paladar hendido, boquinete, labio cucho

clench one's fist, to apretar el puño

Clérambault-Kandinsky complex síndrome de Clérambault-Kandinsky

click (valve) chasquido

clicking crujido, trueno, chasquido; **~ of a joint** trueno de una articulación; **~ hip** cadera de resorte

climacteric climatérico; **~ hypertension** hipertensión climatérica

climacterium climaterio, menopausia

climbing stairs subiendo una escalera

clindamycin clindamicina

clinic hospital, clínica

clinical clínico; **~ analysis** análisis clínico; **~ assay** ensayo clínico; **~ biochemistry** bioquímica clínica; **~ biology** biología clínica,

biología médica; **~ chemistry** química clínica; **~ examination** reconocimiento clínico; **~ experiment** ensayo clínico; **~ immunology** inmunología clínica; **~ judgement** juicio clínico; **~ laboratory** laboratorio clínico; **~ laboratory sciences** ciencias de laboratorio clínico; **~ microbiology** microbiología clínica; **~ model** modelo clínico; **~ oncology** oncología clínica; **~ outbreak** foco clínico; **~ outcome** resultados clínicos; **~ pathologist** patólogo; **~ pathology** ciencias de patología clínica; **~ pelvimetry** pelvimetría clínica, medición del tamaño del canal del parto; **~ performance characteristic** caraterística semiológica; **~ pharmacological study** estudio clínico-farmacológico; **~ pharmacology** farmacología clínica; **~ picture** cuadro clínico, síndrome clínico; **~ psychologist** psicología médica, psicología clínica; **~ records** fichas clínicas, expedientes, récords médicos; **~ symptomatology** cuadro clínico, síndrome clínico; **~ syndrome** cuadro clínico, síndrome clínico; **~ toxicology** toxicología clínica; **~ trial** ensayo clínico

clinician clínico, médico interno

clinomania clinomanía

clitoral clitorídeo, clitoral

clitoris clítoris, pepa; **~-related** clitorídeo, clitoral

cloaca cloaca, parte posterior de los intestinos del embrión

clog, to estreñir

clomiphene clomifeno; **~ test** prueba de estimulación con Clomifeno

clone clono

clonic clónico, relativo a la convulsión; **~ reflex** reflejo clónico

clonidine clonidina

cloning clonación; **~ efficiency** eficacia de clonado

clonorchiasis clonorchis sinensis, clonorquíasis

clonorchis sinensis clonorchis sinensis, clonorquíasis

clopidogrel clopidogrel

closed cerrado; **~ chest cardiac massage** masaje cardíaco externo; **~ circle DNA** DNA

circular cerrado; ~ **circuit** circuito cerrado;
~ **fracture** fractura cerrada, fractura simple;
~ **reading frame** marco de lectura cerrado

closing oclusión, cierre

clostridiopeptidase colagenasa microbiana

Clostridium botulinum Clostridium botulinum;
~ **histolyticum collagenase** colagenasa
microbiana

clot coágulo; ~ **–dissolving drug** fármaco
disolvente del coágulo; ~ **–retraction time**
tiempo de retracción del coágulo

clothing ropa, ropas

clotting coagulación (f), formación de tapones
de sangre; ~ **factor** factor de coagulación;
~ **factor IX** factor IX de la coagulación;
~ **time** tiempo de coagulación

cloudy urine orina turbia

cloxacillin cloxacilina

cluster agrupación, concentración, haz, racimo,
grupo, masa, nudo; ~ **headache** cefalalgia
histamínica, migraña en racimos de Horton,
cefalalgia nocturna paroxística

C-mitosis mitosis alterada por la colchicina

CMV citomegalovirus; ~ **retinitis**
(cytomegalovirus retinitis) retinitis por
citomegalovirus

CNS sistema nervioso central; ~ **depressant**
neurodepresor

coagglutination coaglutinación; ~ **test** prueba
de la coaglutinación

coagulase coagulasa; ~ **test** prueba de la
coagulasa

coagulate, to coagular

coagulated mass masa coagulada, cruor
sanguinis, crúor, la sangre desfibrinada

coagulation coagulación; ~ **factor** factor de la
coagulación; ~ **factor I** fibrinógeno; ~ **factor**
II protrombina, factor II de la coagulación
sanguínea

coagulopathy coagulopatía

coagulum coágulo de sangre, coágulo
sanguíneo

coal tar coáltar, alquitrán de hulla; ~ **workers'**
pneumoconiosis enfermedad pulmonar
minera, antracosis

coaptation coaptación, coadaptación; ~ **plate**
placa de coadaptación

coarctation coartación

coated tablet pastilla revestida

coating on tablets queratinizado, recubierto
por una sustancia resistente a la secreción
gástrica

cobalamin cobalamina, vitamina B12,
cianocobalamina

cocaine cocaína; ~ **esterase** carboxilesterasa;
~ **plant** coca

coccidioidin coccidioidina

coccidioidomycosis coccidioidosis,
coccidiodomicosis

coccidiosis coccidiosis

coccus coco

coccygeal bone cóccix, hueso coccígeo

coccygectomy coccigectomía

coccyx colita, rabadilla, hueso coccígeo, cóccix

cochlea cóclea

cochlear coclear, perteneciente al caracol óseo
del oído interno; ~ **implant** implante coclear;
~ **nerve** nervio coclear, nervio auditivo

codeine codeína

coding strand cadena transcrita, hebra
codificadora

codon codón, conjunto de tres nucleótidos que
codifica un aminoácido; ~ **bias** preferencia
codónica

coefficient coeficiente; ~ **of variation**
coeficiente de variación

coelia disease enfermedad celíaca

coenzyme coenzima

cofactor cofactor

coffee café; ~ **with milk** café con leche

cognate sequence secuencia cognada; ~ **tRNA**
tRNA cognado

cognition cognición

cognitive cognitivo, relativo al conocimiento (la
percepción, pensamiento, etc.);
~ **development** desarrollo psíquico;
~ **disorders** trastornos cognitivos, disfunción
cognitiva; ~ **dissonance** disonancia cognitiva;
~ **dysfunction** trastornos cognitivos,
disfunción cognitiva; ~ **function** función
cognitiva, función cognoscitiva; ~ **handicap**
deficiencia cognitiva; ~ **impairment**
discapacidad cognitiva, disfunción cognitiva;
~ **neuroscience** neurociencia cognitiva;
~ **psychologist** psicología infantil; ~ **skills**
destrezas cognitivas; ~ **therapy** terapia

cognitiva

coherent thought coherencia del pensamiento

cohesive cohesivo; **~ end** extremo cohesivo

cohort cohorte

coil DIU

coin moneda; **~ -like** numular, en forma de moneda

coitus coito, cópula carnal; **~ interruptus** coito interrumpido, cópulo carnal

colchicine colchicina; **~ mitosis** mitosis alterada por la colchicina

cold catarro, resfriado, coriza, frío; **~ cream** cold cream, cólcren; **~ room** cámara frigorífica; **~ sore** herpes simple; **~ sweat** sudor frío; **~ water shock** hidrocución; **~ , to be** tener frío; **~ , to catch a** acatarrarse, resfriarse, tomar frío

colectomym pancolectomía, colectomía

coledochoduodenal coledochoduodenal; **~ anastomoses** anastomosis coledochoduodenal

colic cólico, calambre en el vientre; **~ of the stomach** gastralgia, dolor de estómago

colicin typing tipificación con colicina, colicinotipia

coliform bacteria bacteria coliformes, colibacteria, colibacilo

colistin colistina

colitis colitis, inflamación del intestino grueso

collagen colágeno; **~ disease** enfermedad del colágeno, conectivitis, colagenosis, conectivopatía

collagenase colagenasa microbiana

collapse colapso, caída rápida de la tensión sanguínea

collapsible wheelchair silla de ruedas plegable

collarbone clavícula, hueso del cuello

collective colectivo; **~ medical practice** medicina de grupo

Colles fracture fractura de Colles

colliers' anthracosis enfermedad pulmonar minera, antracosis

collodion collodion

colloid goiter bocio coloideo, adenoma gelatinoso; **~ osmotic pressure** presión coloidosmótica; **~ tumor** mixoma, mucosidad tumoral, mixoblastoma, **~ tumor** mixoma, tumor coloide, tumor gelatinoso, tumor

mucoso, mixoblastoma

colloidal coloidal; **~ mercury** mercurio colloidal; **~ osmotic pressure** presión osmótica coloidal

collum arcus vertebrarum pedículo vertebral

collyrium loción para los ojos, colirio

coloboma of the iris coloboma del iris

Colomiatti's bacillus Corynebacterium xerosis

colon colon, intestino grueso; **~ disease** colopatía, enfermedad o trastorno del intestino grueso; **~ enlargement** megacolon, colon anormalmente grande o dilatado

colonic colónio, del colon; **~ diverticulosis** divertículos del colon; **~ fistula** fístula cólica, fístula colónica; **~ flora** flora intestinal; **~ irrigation** irrigación colónica; **~ lavage** irrigación colónica

colonopathy colopatía, enfermedad o trastorno del intestino grueso

colonoscopy colonoscopía

colony colonia

color color; **~ -blind** daltónico; **~ blindness** discromatopsia, daltonismo; **~ , to** manchar, macular

colorectal colorrectal, referente al intestino grueso y su parte final; **~ cancer** neoplasia del colon y recto; **~ dragging resection** resección colorrectal transanal; **~ surgery** cirugía colorectal

colored tumescence tumor pigmentario

coloring coloración, tinción

colostomy colostomía, un ano artificial en la pared abdominal; **~ bag** bolsa de colostomía

colostrorrhea calostrorrea

colostrum calostro

colpitis vaginitis, colpitis, una infección vaginal; **~ mycotica** vaginitis micótica, colpitis micótica

colpomycosis micosis vaginal

colpomyiasis miasis vaginal

colposcopy colposcopia

column columna; **~ chromatography** cromatografía en columna

columnar epithelium célula cilíndrica del epitelio

coma coma

comatose comatoso

combination combinación; ~ **chemotherapy** poliquimioterapia

combined sinérgico

come, to venir; ~ **back, to** regresar; ~ **to consciousness, to** volver en sí conocimiento

comedomastitis comedomastitis

comedone comedón, espinilla

comfort alivio, aligeramento, remedio, desahogo

commensal comensal; ~ **microorganism** microorganismo comensal

commit suicide, to matarse, suicidarse

common general; ~ **cold** resfrío, catarro, constipación, resfriado común; ~ **integument** integumento común; ~ **wart** mezquino, verruga común

commotion conmoción, sacudida violenta

communicable contagioso, transmisible; ~ **disease** enfermedad transmisible, enfermedad contagiosa

community comunidad; ~ **health care** centro comunitario de salud, los servicios de salud comunitario; ~ **health center** centro comunitario de salud, los servicios de salud comunitario

comorbidity comorbilidad

company doctor médico de la empresa

comparative comparativo; ~ **study** estudio comparativo

comparatively relativamente

compatible compatible

compensate, to compensar, resarcir

compensated compensado; ~ **acidosis** acidosis compensada; ~ **cardiac insufficiency** insuficiencia cardíaca compensada; ~ **heart failure** insuficiencia cardíaca compensada; ~ **ionization chamber** camara de ionización compensada

compensation compensación, indemnización

competitive competitivo; ~ **immunoassay** inmunoanálisis competitivo; ~ **inhibition** inhibición competitiva

complaint queja

complement complemento; ~ **component** componente del complemento; ~ **factor B** factor B de complemento; ~ **factor P** properdina; ~ **fixation** fijación del complemento; ~ **fixation reaction** reacción de fijación del complemento

complementary complementario; ~ **deoxyribonucleic acid** ácido desoxirribonucleico complementario; ~ **DNA** DNA complementario; ~ **ribonucleic acid** ácido ribonucleico complementario

complete entero; ~ **blood count** hemograma, recuento sanguíneo; ~ **podalic extraction** gran extracción podálica

complex complejo, grupo, conjunto; ~ **locus** locus complejo; ~ **of symptoms** cuadro clínico, síndrome clínico

complexion cutis, tez

compliance cumplimiento, observancia

compliant wrist muñeca compliante

complicated complicado; ~ **pneumoconiosis** neumoconiosis complicada

complication complicación

component componente; ~ **noise rating** medida de ruidos compuestos; ~ **transposon** transposón compuesto

compound compuesto; ~ **fracture** fractura abierta, fractura compuesta, compuesto

comprehension comprensión

compromise solución de compromiso, equilibrio entre dos cosas, compensación recíproca, solución transaccional

compromised host paciente comprometido

compulsory treatment tratamiento obligatorio

computer computadora; ~ **screen** pantalla de la computadora; ~ **tomography** tomografía computada, diagnóstico por imágenes

computerized informatizado, computadorizado; ~ **records** archivos del fichero médico

concatemer concatémero

concatenate, to concatenar

concealed oculto, escondido, tapado

concentration concentración; ~ **gradient** gradiente de concentración; ~ **in tissues** concentración tisular

conception concepción

concern aprensión, preocupación

conchoscope concoscopio, espéculo nasal, rinoscopio

conclusion conclusión; ~ **by analogy** conclusión por analogía

concomitant concomitante, acompañante;
~ **hydrocephalus** hidrocefalia concomitante;
~ **meningitis** meningitis concomitante;
~ **radiation** radiación concomitante;
~ **therapy** terapia concomitante

concrete concreto

concussion conmoción, sacudida violenta

condenser condensador

condition condición, estado general, capacidad
física de un individuo

condom condón, hule, preservativo

conductance conductancia

conduction conducción, transmisión; ~ **of nerve
impulses** transmisión del impulso nervioso

conductivity conductividad

conductometry conductimetría

conduit of waste in enclosed piping
conducción a los desagües

condyloma condiloma; ~ **acuminatum**
condiloma acuminado, verrugas genitales;
~ **latum** condiloma plano

conference congreso, reunión, simposio

confidentiality privacidad, espacio personal,
derecho civil a la libertad contra intrusión en
los asuntos

confined to bed postrado en cama

confinement puerperio; ~ **to bed** reposo en
cama, guardando cama

confirmatory test prueba confirmatoria

confluence of the sinuses confluencia sinusal,
confluente posterior, confluente torcular

confused confuso

confusion confusión, pensamiento incoherente

congelation urticaria urticaria a frigore

congenital congénito, innato, connatural;
~ **adrenal hyperplasia** hiperplasia adrenal
congénita, HAC, síndrome adrenogenital;
~ **alalia** mutismo, la incapacidad de hablar o
negativa para hacerlo; ~ **aneurysm** aneurisma
congénito; ~ **cardiopathy** cardiopatía
congénita; ~ **colectasia** megacolon congénito,
congenital colectasia; ~ **defect** defecto
congénito; ~ **disability** discapacidad cognitiva,
disfunción cognitiva; ~ **glaucoma** glaucoma
infantil; ~ **heart defect** cardiopatía

congénitiva, defecto congénito del corazón;
~ **hydronephrosis** hidronefrosis congénita;
~ **megaureter** megauréter, megalouréter;
~ **myotonia** ataxia muscular de Thomsen,
miotonia congénita; ~ **obliterating
bronchiolitis** bronquiolitis obliterante
congénita; ~ **polycystic disease** poliquistosis
renal

congestion congestión

congestive congestivo; ~ **atelectasis** síndrome
de insuficiencia respiratoria del adulto;
~ **heart failure** insuficiencia cardíaca
congestiva; ~ **prostatitis** prostatitis congestiva

conical flask matraz de Erlenmeyer

conidiophore conidióforo

conjoined twins gemelos unidos

conjugal conyugal

conjugated conjugado; ~ **vaccine** vacuna
conjugada

conjugation conjugación, ligamiento

conjunctiva conjuntiva

conjunctival conjuntival; ~ **asthenopia**
astenopía conjuntival; ~ **fornix** fórnix
conjuntival

conjunctivitis conjuntivitis

connective conjuntivo; ~ **cells** células
conjuntivas, fibroblastos; ~ **disease**
enfermedad del colágeno, conectivitis,
colagenosis, conectivopatía; ~ **fibers** fibras del
tejido conjuntivo; ~ **tissue** tejido conjuntivo

Conn's syndrome hiperaldosteronismo,
producción excesiva de aldosterona por la
glándula suprarrenal

consciousness conciencia, conocimiento

consensus sequence secuencia de consenso;
~ **value** valor consensual

conservative conservador, sin intervención
quirúrgica; ~ **recombination** recombinación
conservativa; ~ **surgery** cirugía conservadora

conserve, to conservar

constant constante

constantly constantemente, permanente

constipate, to constipar

constipated, to be tener estreñimiento

constipation constipación, estreñimiento,
entablazón

constituents constituyentes

constitutional constitucional; **~ diagnosis** dianostico constitucional; **~ symptom** síntoma constitucional

constitutive enzyme enzima constitutivo; **~ gene** gen constitutivo; **~ mutation** mutación constitutiva

constrict, to astringir

constriction constricción, estrangulamiento; **~ of air passages** broncoconstricción, contracción de los bronquios, opresión en el pecho

constructive criticism feedback, retroalimentación, retroacción; **~ pericarditis of pulmonary artery** síndrome de Gouley

consulting physician médico consultante, médico de consulta

consumption consumo; **~ coagulopathy** coagulopatía de consumo, coagulacion intravascular diseminada

contact contacto; **~ allergen** alergeno de contacto; **~ hypersensitivity** hipersensibilidad de contacto; **~ lens** lente de contacto

contagious contagioso, transmisible, pegajoso; **~ carbuncle** carbunco, pústula maligna, carbunco contagioso; **~ disease** enfermedad transmisible, enfermedad contagiosa

container envase

contaminated clothing ropas manchadas o salpicadas

contamination contaminación

content contenido

contingency contingencia

continue, to continuar

continuing source epidemic epidemia de foco persistente, brote de foco persistente

continuous continuo; **~ erection** priapismo, erección anormal y persistente; **~ flow** flujo continuo; **~ method** método continuo; **~ operation** operación continua

contraception contracepción, anticoncepción, prevención del embarazo

contraceptive contraceptivo, anticonceptivo

contractile contráctil; **~ vacuole** vacuola contráctil

contractility contractilidad (f), capacidad de contraerse

contraction contracción; **~ stress test** prueba de provocación con oxitocina

contracture contractura, contracción persistente e involuntaria de uno o más músculos

contraindication contraindicación

contrast medium medio de contraste, medio para visualización radiográfica; **~ sensitivity** sensibilidad de contraste

contrivance artilugion, aparato, dispositivo, aparejo

control control; **~ group** grupo de referencia, grupo testigo; **~ material** material de control

controlled controlado; **~ hypotension** hipotensión controlada; **~ hypothermia** hipotermia inducida, hipotermia provocada

contusion moretón, magulladura, contusión, lesión interna por golpe, compresión o choque, cardenal; **~ of the eyeball** contusión ocular; **~ of the heart** contusión cardíaca, el traumatismo cardíaco cerrado

contusive contundente

convalescence convalecencia

convalescent convaleciente; **~ home** casa de convalecencia; **~ serum** suero de convaleciente

conventional convencional, conforme con la norma

conversion conversión, histeria, transformación de las emociones en manifestaciones corporales; **~ reaction** reacción de conversión

convert, to convertir(se)

convulsion convulsión, espasmo

convulsions convulsiones, acceso, arrebato

convulsive cough tos espasmódica; **~ yawn** casmodia

cookie galleta

Coombs reaction reacción de Coombs, test de Coombs, prueba de Coombs; **~ serum** suero antiglobulinas humanas, suero Coombs; **~ test** test de Coombs, prueba de Coombs, reacción de Coombs

coordination coordinación

COPD EPOC, enfermedad pulmonar obstructiva crónica

cope with, to hacer frente a, enfrentar, superar

copper cobre; **~ oxide** óxido cuprico; **~ sulfate** sufato de cobre

coprological examination examen coprológico

coproporphyrin coproporfirina

count

copulate, to tener relaciones sexuales, hacer uso de, juntarse con, practicar el coito, copular, usar

copy DNA DNA complementario

cor pulmonale corazón pulmonar

coracoid process apófisis coracoides, coracoideo

cordotomy cordotomía

core núcleo

corelation correlación, relación recíproca o mútua

corium flap colgajo de corión

corn callo; ~ **syrup** jarabe de glucosa

cornea córnea; ~ **globata** córnea globosa; ~ **guttata** distrofia de las células endoteliales de la córnea, córnea guttata; ~ **transplant** queratoplastia, trasplantación de la córnea

corneal corneal; ~ **abrasion** abrasión corneal, ulceración del epitelio corneal producida por fricción; ~ **astigmatism** astigmatismo corneal; ~ **dystrophy** distrofia de la córnea; ~ **microscope** microscopio quirúrgico, microscopio operatorio, microscopio para el estudio de la córnea; ~ **neovascularization** neovascularización de la córnea; ~ **puncture** paracentesis de la córnea; ~ **tonometry** tonometría; ~ **ulcer** úlcera de la córnea

coronary coronario, relativo a arterias y venas del corazón; ~ **angioplasty** angioplastia coronaria; ~ **artery bypass graft** cortocircuito cardiopulmonar; ~ **artery disease** coronariopatía; ~ **artery insufficiency** insuficiencia coronaria; ~ **axial cuts** cortes axiales coronarios; ~ **bypass surgery** cirugía de derivación coronaria, by-pass coronario, puente coronario; ~ **heart disease** cardiopatía coronaria

coroner investigador de muertes violentas o accidentes

corpora candicantia cuerpo mamilar, plexo mamilar

corpus callosum cuerpo calloso; ~ **luteum** cuerpo lúteo

correction correctivo

correspond, to corresponder

corrosion corrosión

corrosive cáustico, corrosivo; ~ **esophagitis** esofagitis corrosiva; ~ **gastritis** gastritis corrosiva, gastritis química

cortex corteza; ~ **of suprarenal gland** corteza suprarrenal, corteza adrenal

cortical cortical, relativo a la corteza; ~ **adenoma** adenoma cortical; ~ **alexia** alexia motora; ~ **attack** acceso cortical; ~ **audiometry** audiometría por potenciales evocados, audiometría electroencefalográfica; ~ **delineation** delineación cortical; ~ **epilepsy** epilepsia cortical; ~ **motor aphasia** afasia de Broca

corticoid corticoid; ~ **therapy** corticoterapia

corticoliberin corticoliberina

corticosteroid corticoide

corticotrophin corticotrofina

corticotropin coticotropina, hormona ACTH, hormona adrenocorticotropa; ~ **releasing hormone** hormona liberadora de corticotropina, factor liberador de corticotropina

cortisol cortisol

cortisone cortisona

Corvisart syndrome síndrome de Corvisart, tetralogía de Fallot

corynebacterium corynebacterium; ~ **xerosis** corynebacterium xerosis

cos end extremo cos

cosmetic cosmético; ~ **dentistry** estetica dental; ~ **prosthesis** prótesis cosmetica; ~ **surgery** cirugía estética, cirugía plastica

cosmid cósmido

cost-effectiveness analysis análisis coste-efectividad

cosyntropin cosintropina

cot value cot

cotton algodón; ~ **ball holder** pinzas para manejar el algodon; ~ **wad** guata, tampon de algodon

couch potato haragán

cough tos; ~ **suppressant** antitusivo, bequico; ~ **syrup** jarabe para la tos; ~ **, to** toser

coughing up blood expulsión de sangre de los pulmones

coulomb coulomb

coulometry culombimetría

coumadin cumadina

counseling asesoramiento, consejo

counselor consejero, asesor

count cuenta, recuento

counteract, to contrarrestar, cancelar, neutralizar

counterclockwise en el sentido contrario a las agujas del reloj

counterimmunoelectrophoresis contrainmunoelectroforesis

counterstain contracoloración

countertranscript contratranscrito

counting chamber cámara de recuento, hemocitómetro, hematímetro

country país

couple pareja

course grip sujeción de una pelota

cousin primo, -a

cover slip cubreobjetos

coverage for illness cobertura de los riesgos de enfermedad

cowbane cicuta acuatica, cicuta virosa

cowpox viruela

cow's milk leche de vaca

COX ciclooxigenasa, prostaglandina-endoperóxido-sintasa

coxa cuadril

coxalgia coxalgia

coxarthrosis coxartrosis

coxsackie myocarditis mocarditis por virus Coxsackie; ~ **virus** virus Coxsackie

CPAP (continuous positive airway pressure) presión positiva continua de las vías respiratorias

C peptide péptido C

CPK creatina-cinasa

CPR reanimación cardiopulmonar

CPS carbamoil-fosfato-sintasa

crab louse piojo ladilla

crack fisura, grieta, brecha, rañura; ~ , **to** tronar, crepitar

cramp calambre; ~ **in the calf** calambre en la pantorilla

cranial craneano, relativo al cráneo; ~ **index** índice cefálico, tamaño del cráneo; ~ **parietal bones** huesos parietales; ~ **vault** calvaria, bóveda del cráneo, calota craneal

craniocerebral craneoencefálico; ~ **trauma** traumatismo craneoencefálico

craniofacial craneofacial

craniometaphyseal dysplasia displasia metafisiaria

cranium cráneo, calavera

cranky irritable, quisquilloso, susceptible, colérico, irascible, arrebatadizo, gruñon

crater cráter

craving vicio, habito malo; ~ **for something** antojos de ....

crawl, to gatear, arrastrarse

crawling gatear, reptante

C-reactive protein proteína-C-reactiva

cream crema

creamed cereals papillas

creatinase creatinasa

creatine creatina; ~ **kinase** creatina-cinasa

creatinemia creatinemia, presencia de creatina en la sangre

creatininase creatininasa

creatinine creatinina; ~ **clearance** depuración de creatininio; ~ **deaminase** creatinina-desaminasa

creatininemia concentración de creatininio en plasma/suero

creatininium creatininio

credibility verosimilitud

credit card tarjeta de crédito

creeping eruption larva migrans; ~ **myiasis** miiasis rampante

crepitation crepitación; ~ **of the skin** crepitación cutánea

crepitus redux crepitación de retorno

CRF corticoliberina

crib death Síndrome de Muerte Infantil Súbita (SIMS)

crichothyrocotomy cricotirocotomía

cricoid cartilage cartílago cricoides, cartilago cricoideo

crime delito, crimen; ~ **lab** laboratorio de criminialística

crisis crisis; ~ **intervention** intervención en la crisis

crisscross inheritance herencia alternativa

criterion criterio, regla

critical critico; ~ **illness** enfermedad critica

criticality criticality

Crohn's disease enfermedad de Crohn, ileitis regional, enteritis regional

cromonema cromonema

crooked torcido, chueco

cross cruz; ~ **infection** infección cruzada,

contagio mutuo, cruz; ~ **link** unión cruzada; ~ **match** prueba de histocompatibilidad cruzada; ~ **matching** pruebas cruzadas; ~ **reaction** reacción cruzada; ~ **resistance** resistencia cruzada

crossallergy alergia cruzada, alergia a sustancias emparentadas

crossed immunoelectrophoresis inmunoelectroforesis cruzada; ~ **vestibular dysreflexia** pararreflexia vestibular cruzada

cross-hybridization hibridación por cruzamiento

crossover entrecruzamiento, recombinación cruzada; ~ **administration of placebo** administración cruzada de un placebo; ~ **electrophoresis** electroforesis cruzada; ~ **fixation** fijación entrecruzada

cross-reactive antibodies anticuerpos que presentan reacciones cruzadas

crotalase venombina A

crotch aldilla, entrepiernas, ingle

croup garrotillo, crup laríngeo, crup diftérico, laringotraqueíta, infección vírica aguda del conducto respiratorio

croupous cruposo; ~ **cough** tos crupal

crown corona

CRP proteína C reactiva

cruciate ligament ligamento cruciforme

crude petroleum jelly petrolatum, vaselina en bruto

cruel inhumano, cruel

cruent cataract catarata sanguínea

cruor masa coagulada, cruor sanguinis, crúor, la sangre desfibrinada

crural crural; ~ **anastomosis** anastomosis crural; ~ **hernia** hernia femoral; ~ **nerve** nervio femoral, nervio crural; ~ **neuralgia** neuralgia crural; ~ **ring** anillo crural

crus of cerebrum pedúnculo cerebral; ~ **of clitoris** raíces de los cuerpos cavernosos del clítoris

crust postilla, costra

crusta phlogistica capa leucocitaria, célula mononuclear de cultivo

crutch muleta, sobaqueras

Cruveilhier fascia aponeurosis pélvica; ~ **valve** válvula de Bianchi, pliegue de Hasner

cry, to llorar

crybaby llorón, gimoteador, llorona

cryoanesthesia anestesia por frío

cryo-anesthesia anestesia por frío, crioanestesia

cryogen criógeno, líquido de refrigeración

cryogenic agent agente criogénico; ~ **gas** gas criogénico

cryogenics ciencia criógenica, criogenia

cryoglobulin crioglobulina

cryoprecipitable protein proteína crioprecipitable

cryosurgery criocirugía

cryptococcosis criptococosis

cryptogamic disease micosis, enfermedad causada por hongos, enfermedad de mohos

cryptorchism criptorquidea, testículo no descendido

cryptosporidiosis criptosporidiosis

crystal violet stain tinción con cloruro de metilrosanilina

crystallization cristalización, formación de cristales

crystallize, to cristalizar

crystalluria cristaluria, presencia de cristales en la orina

CS coriomamotropina

C-section operación cesárea, cesárea

CSF protein content concentración de proteína en líquido cefalorraquídeo; ~ **sugar** concentración de glucosa en líquido cefalorraquídeo

CT scan of the brain TC cerebral; ~ **scanning** tomografía computada; ~ **scanning (computed tomography)** TC (tomografía computada)

cubic centimeter centímetro cúbico

cubital cubital; ~ **syndrome** síndrome cubital

cucumber pepino

cuff manguito de presión

culdocentesis culdocentesis

culdoscopy culdoscopia

culture cultivo; ~ **medium** medio de cultivo

cumbersome engorroso, molesto

cumulative cumulativo, acumulativo

cuneate piramidal, cuneiforme

cuneiform cartilage cartílago cuneiforme, cartílago de Wrisberg

cupboard armario

cupric oxide óxido cuprico

curable diseases enfermedades curables

curarize, to curarizar, colocar al organismo bajo la acción del curare, una sustancia que afloja los músculos

curative curativo, sanativo

curb, to reprimir, represar

cure restablecimiento, curación, recuperación, restitución; ~ **, to** curar

curettage abrasión, erosión dentaria, desgaste; ~ curetaje, raspado

current actual

curvature curvatura

curve curva

Cushing syndrome Cushing syndrome; ~ **syndrome II** síndrome del ángulo pontocerebeloso; ~ **syndrome of the newborn** síndrome de Cushing del recién nacido; ~ **trocar** trocar de Cushing

cushion almohada

custody of children custodia de los hijos, guardia y custodia de los niños

cut incisión, cortada, cortadura, corte

cutaneous cutáneo, relativo a la piel; ~ **amebiasis** amebiasis cutánea; ~ **ankylostomiasis** anquilostomiasis cutánea; ~ **larva migrans** larva migrans; ~ **leishmaniasis** leishmaniasis cutánea; ~ **papilla** papila dérmica; ~ **penetration** penetración cutánea; ~ **reflex** reflejo cutáneo; ~ **T-cell lymphoma** linfoma de célula T cutaneo

cutis anserina cutis anserina; ~ **laxa** cutis laxa, dermatolisis, chalazodermia; ~ **marmorata** cutis marmorato, livedo reticularis, mancha amoratada de la piel; ~ **rhomboidalis nuchae** cutis rhomboidalis nuchae

cut-off point valor discriminante

cutting incisivo, penetrante; ~ **edge** vanguardia; ~ **enzyme** enzima cortadora; ~ **face** cara de corte; ~ **sequence** secuencia de corte

cyanide cianuro

cyanosis cianosis, coloración azulada de la piel y de las mucosas

cyanotic cianotica; ~ **congenital heart disease** cardiopatía congénita cianotica

cyanthoate ciantoato

cyanuria orinas azules

cybernetics cibernética

cybrid cíbrido

cyclamate ciclamato

cyclazocine ciclazocina

cycle ciclo

cyclic cíclico, regular, repetido; ~ **adenosine monophosphate** AMP cíclico, adenosina monofosfato cíclico

cyclizine hydrochloride clorhidrato de ciclina, piperazina

cyclooxygenase prostaglandina–endoperóxido-sintasa

cyclopentolate ciclopentano

cycloheptadine ciproheptadina

cyclophosphamide ciclofosfamida

cycloplegia cicloplejía, parálisis del músculo ciliar (acomodación del ojo)

cycloplegic ciclopléjico

cyclopropane ciclopropano - un gas anestético potente, inflamable y explosivo

cyclosporiasis ciclosporiasis

cyclosporin A ciclosporina A

cyclothymic ciclotímico; ~ **personality** personalidad ciclotímica

cylindroma carcinoma adenoide quístico, cilindroma

cylindruria cilindruria

cyphosis cifosis

cyst quiste, tumor de contenido líquido, cisto; ~ **count** recuento de quistes

cystectomy cistectomia, extirpación de la vejiga

cysteine cisteína; ~ **-containing peptide** péptido que contiene la cisteína

cystic quístico; ~ **fibrosis** fibrosis quística mucoviscidosis; ~ **glioma** glioma quístico; ~ **goiter** bocio quístico; ~ **kidney** enfermedad renal poliquística; ~ **myxoma** mixoma quístico

cysticercosis cisticercosis, teniasis por Taenia solium, infección por Taenia solium

cystine cistina

cystinosis cistinosis

cystitis cistitis, una inflamación de la vejiga urinaria

cystoid cistoide; ~ **macular edema** edema quística macular

cystolithiasis cistolithiasis

cystometry cistometría

cystoscope cistoscopio

cystoscopy cistoscopia, observación del interior de la vejiga mediante un aparato adecuado (el cistoscopio)
cystotomy cistotomía perineal
cytarabine citarabina
cytidine citidina
cytobiology biología celular, citobiología
cytochemistry citoquímica
cytochrome citocromo; ~ **oxidase** citocromo-oxidasa
cytode procariota
cytogenetics citogenética
cytoglobulinic dissociation disociación citoglobulínica
cytokine citoquina, citocina
cytokinesis citocinesis
cytology citología
cytomegalovirus citomegalovirus; ~ **encephalitis** encefalitis por citomegalovirus; ~ **infection** infección por citomegalovirus
cytometry citometría
cytopathic citopático; ~ **effect** efecto citopático
cytopathology citopatología
cytoplasm citoplasma, parte de la célula no ocupada por el núcleo
cytoplasmic citoplasmático; ~ **abnormality** anomalía del citoplasma; ~ **inheritance** herencia citoplasmática, herencia plasmática
cytoprotective agent protector citogénico; ~ **resection** cirugía citorreductora; ~ **therapy** cirugía citorreductora, terapia citorreductora
cytosine citosina; ~ **arabinoside** citarabina, arabinósido de citosina
cytostatic citostático, sustancia que detiene la multiplicación de las células
cytotoxic citotóxico, lesivo para la célula; ~ **effect** acción cito-tóxica; ~ **T cell** linfocito T citotóxico, célula T asesina; ~ **T lymphocyte** linfocito T citotóxico, célula T asesina
cytotropic immunoreaction inmunorrespuesta citotáctica
Czerny myomectomy miomectomía Czerny

D

DaCosta's disease astenia neurocirculatoria; ~ **syndrome** astenia neurocirculatoria
dandruff caspa
Dandy's operation operación de Dandy
dangerous arriesgado, aventurado, peligroso
dapsone dapsona
dark oscuro; ~ **field microscopy** microscopia del campo oscuro
date fecha; ~ **of birth** fecha de nacimiento; ~ **of expiration** fecha de caducidad; ~ **of injury** fecha de la lesión, fecha del accidente
daughter hija (f)
daunorubicin daunorrubicina, la daunomicina
Davaine's bacillus Bacillus anthracis
day día; ~ **after tomorrow** pasado mañana; ~ **before yesterday** anteayer; ~ **blindness** hemeralopía, ceguera diurna; ~ **care center** guardería infantil, jardín de infantes
daydream, to soñar despierto
daytime diurno
DBS (deep brain stimulation) estimulación del cerebro profundo
D&C (dilation & curettage) dilatación y curetaje uterina
DD (differential diagnosis) diagnóstico diferencial
DDS (drug delivery system) sistema de administración de medicamentos
DDT DDT, dicloro-difenil-tricloroetano, el diclorofenil tricloroetano
dead muerto, difunto; ~ **body** cadáver
deadly fatal
deaf sordo
deafness sordera, deterioro de la capacidad auditiva; ~ **due to acoustic trauma** sordera por trauma acústico; ~ **due to occupational noise** sordera profesional
deal with, to hacer frente a, enfrentar, superar
death muerte; ~ **by drowning** muerte por sumersión; ~ **by hanging** ahorcadura, ejecución en la horca; ~ **by lightning** muerte por electrocución; ~ **by suffocation** muerte por asfixia, ahogamiento; ~ **from aspiration** muerte por asfixia de deglución; ~ **rate** tasa de mortalidad

deathbed lecho de muerte

debatable dudoso, discutible, cuestionable

debilitating debilitante; ~ **chronic pain** extenuante dolor crónico; ~ **disease** enfermedad debilitante, trastorno incapacitante; ~ **disorder** enfermedad debilitante, trastorno incapacitante; ~ **migraine** cefalea incapacitadora

debilitation debilidad, extenuación; ~ **of the will** abulia, debilitación de la voluntad

débridement desbridamiento, extirpación de tejido infectado, lesionado o necrosado

debrisoquine debrisoquina

debulking (of a tumor) cirugía citorreductora, terapia citorreductora

decadic absorbance absorbancia decimal; ~ **attenuance** atenuancia decimal

decaffeinated coffee café descafeinado

decarboxylase deficiency disease enfermedad por déficit de decarboxilasa

decarboxylation descarboxilación

decay caries, deterioro localizado del diente; ~ **constant** constante de desintegración

deceased muerto, difunto, fallecido

deceit curandería, charlatanismo, charlatanería

december diciembre

decerebration descerebración

decidua graviditatis decidua gravídica; ~ **menstrual** decidua menstrual

deciduous teeth dientes de leche, primera dentición

deciliter decilitro

declarative memory memoria declarativa, memoria explícita

decolorizer decolorante

decompensation descompensación, fallo

decomposition subdivisión, desglose, descomposición; ~ **of fatty acids** degradación de ácidos grasosos

decompression descompresión; ~ **sickness** enfermedad por descompresión, mal de descompresión

decompressive operation operación de descompresión

decongestant descongestivo

decontaminate, to descontaminar

decontamination descontaminación

decorum decoro, respeto

decrease disminución; ~ **in blood pressure** disminución de la presión sanguínea; ~ **in the pulse rate** disminución de las pulsaciones

decrepit decrépito, desvaído, endeble, vetusto

decubitus decúbito; ~ **angina** angina de decúbito; ~ **ulcer** escara, úlcera por decúbito

deep hondo; ~ **cut** herida por arma blanca, cuchillazo, cortadura profunda; ~ **knee bend** flexión de piernas; ~ **sleep** sueño profundo

deer fly fever tularemia

defecate, to hacer del cuerpo, defecar

defecation deposición, defecación, las heces

defect falta, fallo

defective hearing hipoacusia, trastorno de la audición, sordera parcial; ~ **phage** fago defectuoso; ~ **virus** virus defectuoso

defense defensa; ~ **mechanism** mecanismo de defensa

defibrillation desfibrilación

defibrillator desfibrilador

deficiency deficiencia, defecto, falta

deficient judgement alteración del juicio, debilidad mental

deficit déficit, falta

definite definitivo; ~ **recovery** curación definitiva

definitive host huésped definitivo; ~ **measurement procedure** procedimiento de medida definitivo; ~ **method** método definitivo; ~ **value** valor definitivo

deformity deformidad, dismorfia

degenerating neurons degeneración de las neuronas, decadencia neural

degeneration degeneración

degenerative degenerativo; ~ **eczema** dermatosis degenerativa; ~ **osteoarthritis** osteoarthritis degenerativa

degloving of the skin escoriación dérmica, despegamiento cutáneo

deglutition deglución; ~ **tuberculosis** tuberculosis con puerta de entrada digestiva, tuberculosis por deglución

Degos–Delort–Tricot syndrome papulosis atrófica maligna

degradation degradación; ~ **product** producto catabólico, producto de degradación

degree grado; ~ **Celsius** grado Celsius; ~ **of dissociation** grado de disociación

dehiscence dehiscencia
dehumanizing deshumanización
dehydration deshidratación, carencia de agua en el cuerpo
dehydrocortisone prednisona, dehidrocortisona
dehydroepiandrosterone deshidroepiandrosterona
dejection evacuación intestinal, defecación, deyeción
delay atraso, retraso, demora; ~ **, to** atrasar, impedir, retrasar
delayed retardado, retrasado; ~ **hypersensitivity** hipersensibilidad retardada, hipersensibilidad tardía; ~ **puberty** pubertad tardía, pubertad retrasada; ~ **shock** shock retardado
delaying retardo, retraso
deleterious deletéreo, perjudicial; ~ **mutation** mutación deletérea
deletion deleción
delicate delicado; ~ **child** niño enfermizo, niño delicado
delirious, to be delirar
delirium delirio onírico, demencia vesánica, onirismo
deliver a baby, to aliviarse, alumbrar, dar a luz, acostar
delivery nacimiento, parto
delta hepatitis hepatitis viral delta; ~ **theory** teoría delta
deltacortisone prednisona, dehidrocortisona
delusional delirante; ~ **idea** idea delirante
delusions of grandeur megalomanía, delirio de grandeza
dementia demencia, debilidad mental; ~ **precoz** parafrenia
demoralized desmoralizado
demulcent (adjective) demulcente, emoliente, calmante, que ablanda y relaja las zonas inflamadas o que ablanda la piel
demyelination desmielinación
denaturing desnaturalizante
denaturation desnaturalización
denature, to desnaturalizar
dendriceptor receptor dendrítico
dendritic dendrítico, ramificado; ~ **carcinoma of the mamma** cáncer dendrítico de mama; ~ **keratitis** queratosis folicular estafilocócica,

queratitis dendrítica; ~ **spine** espina dendrítica
denervation desnervación; ~ **of the sympathetic trunk** bloqueo del tronco simpático, desnervación del tronco simpático
dengue fever dengue, fiebre de los tres días, colorado, calentura roja, pantomima; ~ **virus** virus de la fiebre Dengue, virus del dengue
dens serotinus muela del juicio
dense denso; ~ **connective tissue** tejido conjuntivo denso
density densidad
dental dental; ~ **aesthetics** estetica dental; ~ **calculus** cálculo dental, sarro dental; ~ **caries** caries; ~ **clinic** clínica de odontólogo, consulta del dentista; ~ **floss** hilo dental, hilo de higiene dental; ~ **granuloma** granuloma apical; ~ **hyperesthesia** hiperestesia dentaria; ~ **impression** impresión de la dentadura; ~ ~ **implant framewor** armadura de implantación dental; ~ **infundibulum** cornete dentario; ~ **papilla** papila papila, papila dental; ~ **pathology** patología dentaria; ~ **plaque** placa dental, sarro dental; ~ **plaque index** índice de placa dental; ~ **prosthesis** surco dental primitivo, tablilla, gotiera, bruxismo, plana relajación, ferula oclusal; ~ **pulp** pulpa dentaria; ~ **root cyst** conducto periodontal
dentalgia dentalgia
dentine cauterization cauterización dentinaria; ~ **hypersensitivity** hipersensibilidad de dentina, sensibilidad de la dentina
dentist dentista
dentistry odontología
dentition dentición, brote de un diente
dentritic dentrítico; ~ **cell** celulas dentríticas; ~ **inhibition** inhibición dendrítica
denture dentadura postiza, dientes postizos
Denué ligament ligamento radiocubital
Denver classification clasificación de Denver
deodorant desodorante
deoxyadenosine desoxiadenosina
deoxycorticosterone desoxicorticosterona
deoxycytidine desoxicitidina
deoxygenated blood sangre desoxigenada
deoxygenation desoxigenación
deoxyguanosine desoxiguanosina
deoxyribonuclease desoxirribonucleasa

deoxyribonucleic acid ácido desoxirribonucleico

deoxyribonucleotide desoxirribonucleótido

dependence-producing drug droga adictiva, droga toxicomanígena, droga causante de dependencia

dependent dependiente

depersonalization alienación, despersonalización, sensación de extrañeza personal

depigmentation despigmentación

depilating tweezers pinzas para depilar

depilatory depilatorio

depletion depleción

depolarization despolarización

depressant depresor

depressed deprimido

depression depresión, derrumbamiento o disminución; **~ of a cataract** depresión de una catarata

depressive state estado depresivo

deprivation privación (f), falta o carencia

depth profundidad; **~ perception** percepción de la profundidad

De Quervain's tenosynovitis tenosinovitis de De Quervain

derepression desrepresión

derivative derivado

derived derivado; **~ quantity** magnitud derivada; **~ unit** unidad derivada

derma piel, cutis, cuero

dermabrasion dermabrasión

dermal dérmico; **~ absorption study** estudio de absorción dérmica; **~ actinomycosis** actinomicosis cutánea; **~ corrosion** corrosión dérmica, cauterización dérmica; **~ flora** flora dérmica; **~ papilla** matriz del pelo; **~ sarcoma** sarcoma dérmico

dermatitis dermatitis, inflamación de la piel; **~ actinica** radiodermitis, dermatitis radiográfica; **~ hiemalis** dermatitis hiemalis, pruritis invernal

dermatochalasis cutis laxa, dermatolisis, chalazodermia

dermatofibroma dermatofibroma

dermatological dermatológico

dermatologist dermatólogo

dermatology dermatología

dermatolysis cutis laxa, dermatolisis, chalazodermia

dermatomycosis dermatomicosis, enfermedad de la piel cuasada por hongos

dermatopathology dermatopatologia

dermatopathy dermatopatía

dermatophyte dermatofito

dermatophytosis dermatofitosis

dermatosclerosis dermatosclerosis, esclerodermia

dermatosis dermatosis, enfermedad de la piel

dermis dermis

dermite pustuleuse miliaire staphylococcique dermatitis pustulosa miliar estafilocócica

dermographia dermografía, dibujo en la piel, reacción local de la piel a una irritación mecánica o efecto de presión

dermoid cyst quiste dermoide

Dermo-Jet injector inyector a presión, inyector dermo-jet

descending descendente; **~ colon** colon descendente; **~ degeneration** degeneración centrifuga

desensitization desensibilización, disminución de la sensibilidad, insensibilización; **~ therapy** desensibilización, terapia que tiende a reducir una alergia

desiccant desecante, secante

designer drugs drogas sintéticas

designing patient-specific prescriptions prescripciones particularizadas

desinfectant antiséptico, desinfectante

desmectasia desmectasia, tirón, tendon desgarrado

desmocranium desmocráneo

desmoid desmoide, ligamentoso

desogestrel desogestrel

desquamation descamación, exfoliación, formación exagerada de escamas en la piel

desquamative intermenstrual gingivitis gingivitis descamativa catamenial

dessicate, to secarse, enjugar, resecar, descar, enjugar, limpearse

dessication desecación

destabilizing protein proteína desestabilizadora

destructive destructivo; **~ placental mole** mola maligna, coriodemona, mola hidatiforme invasiva

detachment desprendimiento, separación

detect, to detectar, discernir, distinguir, localizar, descubrir

detectability detectabilidad

detection detección, investigación, descubrimiento; ~ **limit** límite de detección

detector detector

detergent detergente

determination determinación

detorsion detorsión, antitorsión; ~ **arch-support (for the foot)** cambrillon detorción del pie, mecanismo de soporte del arco

detoxication destoxificación

detoxify, to desintoxicar

detoxifying desintoxicador

detrimental dañino, nocivo, dañoso, pernicioso, desfavorable; ~ **, to be** deletéreo, perjudicial

developmental disorder trastorno del desarrollo, discapacidad del desarrollo; ~ **handicap** trastorno del desarrollo, discapacidad del desarrollo; ~ **psychology** psicología evolutiva

deviant desviado; ~ **child** niño inadaptado

deviation anomalía, desviación de la norma, irregularidad

device artilugion, aparato, dispositivo, aparejo

devil's grip enfermedad de Bornholm

dexametasone dexametasona

dexfenfluramine dexfenfluramina

dextran dextrano

dextri-maltose maltodextrina

dextrin dextrina

dextrocardia dextrocardia

dextromanual diestro

dextrose glucosa, dextrosa, azúcar de uva; ~ **monohydrate** dextrosa monohidratada

DFP isofluorfato

DHEA (dehydroisoandrosterone) DHEA (dehidroisoandrosterona)

DHF (dengue hemorrhagic fever) fiebre hemorrágica causada por el virus dengue

diabetes diabetes; ~ **drug** antidiabético; ~ **insipidus** diabetes insipida; ~ **mellitus** diabetes mellitus

diabetic diabético; ~ **acidosis** acidosis

diabética; ~ **diet** dieta para diabéticos; ~ **foods** alimentos para diabéticos; ~ **glycosuria** glucosuria diabética; ~ **ketoacidosis** cetoacidosis diabética, exceso de ácidos y cuerpos cetónicos en la sangre; ~ **neuropathy** neuropatía diabética; ~ **retinopathy** retinopatía diabética

diacetylmorphine heroína, diacetilmorfina

diacylglycerol diacilglicerol

diagnosis diagnóstico

diagnostic diagnóstico; ~ **aid** herramienta de dianóstico; ~ **imaging** diagnóstico por imágenes, imaginería diagnóstica; ~ **procedure** procedimiento de dianóstico; ~ **radiology** diagnóstico radiológico; ~ **sensitivity** sensibilidad diagnóstica; ~ **specificity** especificidad diagnóstica; ~ **tool** herramienta de dianóstico; ~ **workup** diagnóstico profundo

diakinesis diacinesis

dialysis dialysis, hemodiálisis

diameter diámetro

diamine oxidase amina-oxidasa (cuprífera)

diapedesis diapédesis

diapedetic bleeding hemorragia por diapédesis

diaper rash dermatitis del pañal

diapers pañales

diaphoresis diaforesis, sudoración

diaphragm diafragma; ~ **pessary** capuchón cervical, capuchón en bóveda, casquete cervical, diafragma pesario

diaphragmatic diafragmático; ~ **breathing** respiración diafragmática; ~ **hernia** hernia diafragmática; ~ **sinuses** senos costodiafragmáticos

diaphragmatocele hernia diafragmática

diaphyseal aclasis aclasia diafisaria

diaphysis diáfisis

diarrhea diarrea, soltarse del estómago; ~ **with yellow-ochre feces** diarrea de heces ocres

diastematomyelia diastematomelia

diastole diástole

diastolic diastólico; ~ **murmur** murmullo distólico; ~ **pressure** diastólico, relativo a la diástole, estadio de relajación del corazón; ~ **volume** volumen diastólico

diathermy diatermia

diathesis diátesis (f)

diazinon diazinón
dichotomy dicotomía, bifurcación
dicloxacillin dicloxacilina
dicumarol dicumarol
dideoxycitidine zalzitabina, didesoxicitidina
didymus didimo
die, to morir
diencephalic diencefálico; ~ **coma** coma diencefálico
diencephalon diencéfalo
dienestrol dienestrol
diet dieta; ~ **pill** píldora de dieta; ~ , **to be on** estar de dieta, estar a régimen
dietary nutricional; ~ **deficiency** trastorno de la nutrición, trastorno nutricional, problema nutricional
diethylcarbamazine dietilcarbamazina
dietician nutricionista, asesor dietético
difference diferencia; ~ **scale** escala de diferencias
differential diferencial; ~ **blood count** recuento diferencial leucocitario, fórmula leucocitaria; ~ **white blood cell count** fórmula leucocitaria
differentiation diferenciación, modificación; ~ **medium** medio de diferenciación
difficulty dificultad
diffraction grating red de difracción
diffuse difuso; ~ **abscess** flemón; ~ **cerebrosclerosis** esclerosis cerebral difusa; ~ **choroiditis** coroiditis difusa, coroiditis diseminada; ~ **interstitial pulmonary fibrosis** fibrosis intersticial pulmonar difusa; ~ **lymphoma** linfoma difuso, linfosarcoma
diffusion difusión; ~ **coefficient** coeficiente de difusión
diflorasone diacetate diacetato de diflorasona
digest, to metabolizar, asimilar, digerir
digestible digerible, digestible
digestion digestión, asimilación
digestive digestivo; ~ **enzyme** fermento digestivo; ~ **tract** tracto alimentario, vía digestivo, tracto intestinal, aparato digestivo
digitalis digitálico; ~ **units** unidades de digital
digitalization digitalización
digitoxin digitoxina
diglyceride lipase lipoproteína-lipasa
digoxin digoxina

dihydroergotoxin dihidroergotoxina
dihydrofolate reductase dihidrofolato-reductasa
diisopropyl fluorophosphate isofluorfato
dilatation dilatación, ensanchamiento, agrandamiento o expansión de un órgano hueco
dilate, to dilatar
diltiazem diltiazem
diluent diluyente
diluted aguado, diluído
diluter diluidor
dimension dimensión
dimensionless quantity magnitud adimensional
dimercury dichlorid calomel, calomelanos (purgante), cloruro mercurioso
dimethylmorphine tebaína, paramorfina
dimorphic dimórfico; ~ **fungi** hongo dimórfico
dinner cena, comida
dinoprostone dinoprostona
diphenylhydantoin fenitoína
diphtheria difteria; ~ **toxin** toxina diftérica
diphtheritic croup garrotillo, crup laríngeo, crup diftérico, laringotraqueítis, infección vírica aguda del conducto respiratorio
diphtheroide difteroide
diphyllobothriasis difilobotriasis
diplococcus diplococo
diploid diploide
diploma diploma
diplomelituria diplomelituria
diplopagus diplopagos
diplopia diplopia, visión doble
diplotene diplotena
dipstick tira reactiva
dipyridamole dipiridamol
dipyrone dipirona
direct directo; ~ **agglutination test** prueba de la aglutinación directa; ~ **bilirubin** bilirrubina esterificada; ~ **fluorescent-antibody test** prueba directa del anticuerpo fluorescente; ~ **fluorescent-antigen detection** detección directa del antígeno fluorescente; ~ **immunofluorescence test** prueba directa de inmunofluorescencia; ~ **lead** derivación directa; ~ **repeat** repetición directa; ~ **wet mount** preparación en fresco
directed dirigido; ~ **mutagenesis** mutagénesis

dirigida
dirty sucio, puerco
disability incapacidad, inhabilidad, invalidez;
~ **benefit** beneficio de incapacidad, prestación
de invalidez; ~ **insurance** seguro de
incapacidad, el seguro de invalidez
disabled minusválido, disminuidodis,
discapacitado; ~ **person** incapacitado,
minusválido, persona con impedimento,
persona con desventaja
discharge flujo, secreción, excreción;
~ **psychosis** psicosis de liberación, psicosis de
alta; ~ **pus** supuración, formación de pus; ~ **,
to** dar el alta; ~ **vaginal** desecho vaginal
discoid discoide, en forma de un disco; ~ **lupus
erythematosus** lupus eritematoso discoide,
enfermedad de Biett
discomfort molestias, incomodidad, malestar
discopathy hernia discal
discouraged desalentado
discover, to detectar, discernir, distinguir,
localizar, descubrir
discrepancy diferencia, discrepancia, disparidad
discrete discreto; ~ **flow** flujo discreto;
~ **transport** transporte discreto
discrimination threshold umbral discriminante
discromatopsis discromatopsia, daltonismo
disease enfermedad; ~ **–free interval** periodo
de remisión, remisión de los síntomas;
~ **prediction** predicción de la enfermedad;
~ **prevention** profilaxis, prevención;
~ **progression** progresión de enfermedad,
empeoramiento; ~ **vector** vector de
enfermedad
diseased state morbididad, tasa de enfermos en
una población
disengagement desinterés, desencajamiento
disgusting repugnante, repulsivo
disheartened desanimado, desmoralizado,
desalentado
disimpaction of the bowel desencajamiento,
desprendimiento intestinal
disinfect, to desinfectar, esterilizar
disinfectant antiséptico, desinfectante

disinfection desinfección; ~ **of clothing**
desinfección de la vestimenta; ~ **of hands**
desinfección de las manos; ~ **of instruments**
desinfección de los instrumentos;
~ **treatment** tratamiento de desinfección
disinhibition desinhibición
disintegration desintegración; ~ **constant**
constante de desintegración; ~ **of
intelligence** pérdida de inteligencia, carencia
intelectual, desintegración de la inteligencia
disjunction disyunción
disk herniation hernia discal, la exostosis
diskectomy meniscectomía
disk-shaped discoide, en forma de un disco
dislocation dislocación, luxación, esguince,
torcedura; ~ **of the kneecap** luxación de la
rótula, luxación patelar
disopyramide disopiramida
disorder alteración, trastorno; ~ **of cholesterol
metabolism** trastorno del metabolismo de
colesterol
disorientation desorientación
disoriented desorientado
dispenser dispensador
dispersed repeat repetición dispersa
dispersion diseminación, disperción
displaced desplazado
displacement desplazamiento; ~ **analysis**
análisis por desplazamiento; ~ **of the vocal
cords** deslocamiento de las cuerdas vocales
display, to visualizar
disposable diaper bragapañal; ~ **suture stapler**
grapadora desechable para sutura; ~ **syringe
and needle** jeringuilla desechable, aguja
hipodérmica desechable
disposition disposición
dissecting disecante; ~ **aneurysm** aneuisma
disecante
disseminate diseminación, siembra, dispersión
de la infección
disseminated diseminado;
~ **bronchopneumonia** bronconeumonía
diseminada, inflamación pulmonar difusa;
~ **choroiditis** coroiditis difusa, coroiditis
diseminada; ~ **encephalomyelitis**
encefalomielitis diseminada; ~ **erythematosus
lupus** lupus eritematoso diseminado,

enfermedad de Biett; ~ **histoplasmosis**
histoplasmosis diseminada; ~ **intravascular**
coagulation coagulación intravascular
diseminada, CID
dissemination diseminación, dispersión
dissimilation catabolismo, disimilación
dissociated verbal amnesia afasia de Broca
dissociation disociación, desdoblamiento;
~ **constant** constante de disociación
dissolution disolución
dissolvent disolvente, solvente
distal distal, alejado
distend, to distender
distended abotagado, hinchado, hipatado,
turgente
distension distención, estiramiento; ~ **luxation**
luxación por distensión
distichia distiquiásis, distiquia
distichiasis distiquiásis, distiquia
distill, to destilar
distorted deforme
distortion distorsión
distractibility distractibilidad
distraction osteogenesis osteogénesis por
distracción
distraught distraído, irritado, olvidadizo
distress aflicción
distribution distribución; ~ **coefficient**
coeficiente de distribución; ~ **constant**
constante de distribución
disturb, to perturbar, molestar, desconcertar
disuse atrophy trastornos musculares atroficos,
miotonía atrófica la enfermedad de Steiner
diuresis diuresis, gasto urinario
diuretic diurético
diurnal diurno
divergence divergencia; ~ **angle** ángulo de
divergencia
divergent divergente; ~ **promoter** promotor
divergente; ~ **squint** exotropia; ~ **strabismus**
exotropia
diverticula divertículos
diverticular concretion cálculo intradivertícular
diverticulitis diverticulitis
diverticulum divertículo
diverting ileostomy ileostomia de descarga
dividing wall septum, tabique de separación
Division of Workers' Compensation División de

Compensación Laboral
divorced divorciado
dizygotic pregnancy embarazo dicigótico;
~ **twins** gemelos fraternos
dizziness mareos, vértigo, vahído
dizzy mareado, aturdido, ligeramente
indispuesto, delirante; ~ , **to be** estar mareado
DNA ácido desoxirribonucleico;
~ **amplification** amplificación de DNA;
~ **damage** lesión del DNA; ~ **-directed DNA**
polymerase DNA-polimerasa dirigida por
DNA; ~ **-directed RNA polymerase** RNA-
polimerasa dirigida por DNA; ~ **fingerprint**
huella genética, dermatoglifia del ADN,
impronta genética; ~ **ligase (ATP)** DNA-ligasa
(ATP); ~ **melting** fusión del DNA; ~ **mutagenic**
repair reparación mutágena del DNA;
~ **packaging** empaquetamiento del DNA;
~ **photolysis** fotólisis del ADN; ~ **polymerase**
transcriptasa inversa, ADN polimerasa;
~ **polymerase chain reaction** reacción en
cadena de la polimerasa de ADN; ~ **probe**
sonda de ácidos nucleicos; ~ **profiling**
tipificación del ADN; ~ **repair** reparación del
ADN; ~ **repair enzyme** DNA-ligasa;
~ **replication** replicación del ADN;
~ **restriction** restricción del ADN; ~ **sequence**
polymorphism polimorfismo de una secuencia
de DNA; ~ **sequencing** secuenciación del
ADN; ~ **synthesizer** sintetizador de ADN,
sintetizador de oligonucleótides; ~ **test** prueba
de ADN
DNCB (dinitrochlorobenzene)
dinitroclorobenceno
do, to hacer
doctor doctor, médico; ~ **-patient**
confidentiality confidencialidad entre médico
y paciente
doctor's assistant asistente de médico,
ayudante de médico, auxiliar de médico;
~ **fee** honorario, honorarios médicos; ~ **office**
consultorio de medicina, consultorio médico,
practica médica; ~ **orders** lo que manda el
médico; ~ **practice** consultorio médico,
consulta; ~ **waiting room** sala de espera
document documento, formulario; ~ , **to**
documentar, constatar
doddering decrépito, desvaído, endeble, vetusto

Döderlein's bacillus Lactobacillus acidophilus
dog perro; ~ **bite** mordedura de perro
domain zona
domestic doméstico; ~ **aid** ayuda en las tareas domésticas; ~ **violence** violencia doméstica, la violencia familiar
dominance dominancia
dominant dominante; ~ **hemisphere** hemisferio dominante
donor donante; ~ **site** centro donador
dopamine dopamina; ~ **agonist** agonista de la dopamina; ~ **antagonist** antagonista de la dopamina; ~ **receptor** receptor de dopamina, receptor dopaminérgico
dope oneself, to doparse
doping dosificación, dopaje
Doppler scanning estudio Doppler; ~ **shift** efecto Doppler; ~ **ultrasonography** ultrasonido, la ultrasonografía Doppler
dormancy letargo, fase de latencia, somnolencia o indiferencia
dorsal dorsal
dorsalgia dorsalgia, notalgia
dorsiflexion dorsiflexión
dorsum manus dorso de la mano, nudillo
dosage dosificación; ~ **effect** efecto de la dosis; ~ **form** primera forma farmacéutica; ~ **regimen** posología, esquema de administración del medicamento; ~ **schedule** esquema (f) de administración del medicamento; ~ **unit** primera forma farmacéutica
dose dosis; ~ **equivalent** dosis equivalente; ~ ~ **effect curve** curva de dosis y respuesta
dosimetry dosimetría
dot punto; ~ **blot** transferencia en mancha
double doble; ~ **-blind comparative trial** ensayo en doble-ciego; ~ **blind study** prueba doble ciego, estudio doble ciego; ~ **diffusion test** prueba de la doble difusión; ~ **helix** doble hélice; ~ **helix of DNA** doble hélice de ADN; ~ **lipid layer** bicapa lipídica; ~ **strand** cadena doble; ~ **-stranded DNA** DNA bicatenario, ADN de doble cadena; ~ **thoracotomy** toracotomía doble; ~ **vision** diplopía, visión doble
down abajo; ~ **mutation** mutación

lentificadora; ~ **-promoter mutation** mutación lentificadora; ~ **syndrome** síndrome de Down, mongolismo trisomia 21; ~ **time** periodo improductivo
downstream río abajo
doxapram doxapram
doxazosin mesylate doxazosin, mesilato de doxazosin
doxepin doxepina
doxorubicin adriamicina, doxorrubicina
doxycycline doxiciclina
D-penicillamine D-penicilamina, dimetilcisteína
dragging agotado, debilitado, quemado, cansado
drain/ toilet cleaner limpiador de tubería / baños
drainage drenaje
dramamine dramamina
drawback inconveniente
drawing blood sacar sangre, sacar muestra de sangre
dress a wound, to hacer apósito en una herida; ~ , **to** vestirse
dressing vendaje
Dressler's syndrome síndrome de Dressler, síndrome postinfarto de miocardio
drift deriva
drink, to beber
Drinker respirator respirador electrofrénico, pulmón de acero, pulmón artificial, respirador de Drinker
dripfeeding perfusión
drop gota; ~ **foot** pie pendular, pie péndulo
droperidol droperidol
droplet infection infección por gotitas
drought estiaje, sequía
drown, to ahogarse
drowning ahogamiento
drowsiness sonolencia, modorra
drowsy sueño, soñoliento, amodorrado, adormilado; ~ , **to be** amodorrado, tener sueño
drug medicamento, fármaco, droga; ~ **abuse** consumo de drogas, abuso de fármacos; ~ **addict** adicto a drogas, drogadicto; ~ **addiction** adición a las drogas, dependencia de drogas, narcomanía; ~ **clinic** clínica para toxicómanos, centro de desintoxicación, centro

de tratamiento para drogadictos; ~ **habit** habituación a las drogas; ~ **incompatibility** incompatibilidad de medicamentos; ~ **oxidation** oxidación del medicamento; ~ **precursor** producto precursor; ~ **screening** ensayos bioquímicos de rastreo; ~ **store** farmacia, botica; ~ **use** consumo de drogas, abuso de fármacos; ~ **withdrawal** abstinencia

druggist boticario, farmácia

drug-induced inducido por drogas

drugs drogas

drunk borracho; ~ **, to be** estarborracho

drunkenness embriaguez, intoxicación alcohólica, ebriedad

dry seco; ~ **chemistry** química en fase sólida, reactivos en fase sólida; ~ **eyes** xeroftalmía, sequedad del globo ocular; ~ **medium** medio seco; ~ **mouth** xerostomía; ~ **out, to** secarse, enjugar, resecar, desecar; ~ **skin** piel seca

dryness desecación, sequedad, seco

Duchenne-Erb paralysis paralisia de Duchenne Erb; ~ **muscular dystrophy** distrofia muscular de Duchenne

duck feet pie valgo

Ducrey's bacillus Haemophilus ducreyi

duct conducto

ductus cholidocus conducto biliar

dull sordo

dumbness mutismo, incapacidad de hablar o negativa para hacerlo

Dunlop oxygen insufflator insuflador de oxígeno de Dunlop

duodenal duodenal; ~ **contents** contenido duodenal; ~ **papilla, minor** papila de Santorini; ~ **ulcer** úlcera duodenal

duodenalileostomy duodenoilostomía

duodenectomy duodenectomía

duodeno-pancreatectomy duodenopancreatectomía

duodenum duodeno

duplex dúplex

duplication replicación, duplicación

Dupuytren's contracture enfermedad de Dupuytren

dura mater duramadre (f); ~ **of the brain** duramadre encefálica

durapatite durapatita

Duret-Berner lesion of the brain hemorragia cerebral de Duret-Berner

during durante; ~ **the operation** peroperatorio, intraoperatorio

dust polvo; ~ **cell** macrofago alveolar; ~ **collector** eliminador de polvo, aspirador de polvo; ~ **eliminator** eliminador de polvo, aspirador de polvo

DVT, deep vein thrombosis trombosis venosa profunda

dwarf enano, enana

dwarfism enanismo, microsomia

D-xylose D-xilosa

dydrogesterone didrogesterona

dynamic ileus íleo dinámico

dysaemia disemia, dishematosis

dysarthria disartria

dyscrasia discrasia

dysdiemorrhysis disdiemorrisis

dysentery disentería

dysesthesia disestesia

dysfunction disfunción, perturbación del funcionamiento de un órgano; ~ **of the immune response** mala respuesta inmunitaria, el trastorno de la respuesta inmunitaria

dysfunctional disfuncional

dysgenesis malformación, disgenesia

dysgeusia disgeusia, perversión del gusto

dysglobulinemia disglobulinemia

dysgonic disgónico

dyshidrosis dishidrosis, quiroponfólix, eccema dishidrótico, ponfólix

dyshidrotic dishidrótico; ~ **eczema** dishidrosis, quiroponfólix, eccema dishidrótico, ponfólix

dyskinesia discinesia, dificultad de los movimientos; ~ **algera** discinesia dolorosa

dyslexia dislexia

dysmenorrhoea dismenorrea, trastorno de la menstruación

dysmetria dismetría

dyspareunia dispareunia

dysparodontia periodontoclasia, gingivopericementitis, paradontólisis

dyspepsia dispepsia

dysphonia disfonía; ~ **spastica** disfonía espástica, disfonía espasmódica

dysphoria disforia

dysplasia displasia

dysplastic displásico; **~ naevus** nevo displásico; **~ naevus-cell-naevus syndrome** síndrome de nevo displásico

dyspnea disnea

dysreflexia disreflexia, trastorno neuromuscular

dystonia distonía, falta de tensión normal

dystopia distopia

dystrophia distrofia; **~ adiposa corneae** xantomatosis de la córnea, distrofia adiposa de la córnea

dystrophin distrofina

dystrophy distrofia, falta de crecimiento de un organismo o tejido

dysuria disuria, emisión dolorosa de la orina

E

each cada

ear (outer) oreja; **~ drops** gotas óticas, gotas para otoplias

earache dolor de oído, otalgia

eardrum tímpano, cavidad del oído medio; **~ rupture** rotura del tímpano, la perforación del tímpano

earlobe lóbulo de la oreja

early temprano, precoz; **~ acromegaly** acromegalia precoz; **~ detection** detección precoz; **~ diagnosis** dianóstico precoz, detección precoz; **~ menopause** menopausia precoz; **~ rheumatic lesion** lesión reumática temprana

earplug tapón de oídos, tampon obturador

earwax cerumen

easy fácil

eat, to ingerir, comer

eating disorder trastorno alimentar

ebb and flow flujo y reflujo

Eberth's bacillus Salmonella typhi

Ebola fever fiebre de Ebola; **~ virus** virus Ebola

eburnation osteoesclerosis, eburnación

ECA peptidil-dipeptidasa A

ecchymosis cardenal, equimosis

ECG electrocardiograma, ECG

echinacea echinacea

echinococcosis equinococosis, hidatidosis; **~ of the liver** echinococosis hepática; **~ of the lung** hidatidosis pulmonar, equinocococia pulmonar

echo eco; **~ image** fantasma, efecto de eco

echocardiogram ecocardiograma, diagnóstico no invasivo que permite visualizar el funcionamiento cardiaco a través de ultrasonidos.

echocardiography ecocardiografía

echography ecografía

echo-guided fine-needle biopsy punción exploradora guiada por ecografía

echopathy ecopatia

echopraxia ecopatia

eclampsia eclampsia, convulsiones y caída de la tensión en mujeres embarazadas; **~ neonatorum** eclampsia infantil, eclampsia del recién nacido; **~ of a newborn child** eclampsia infantil, eclampsia del recién nacido

ECMO (extracorporeal membrane oxygenation) oxigenación de la membrana extracorpórea

ecological ecológico; **~ amplitude** amplitud ecológica; **~ scope** impacto ecológico; **~ succession** sucesión ecológica, sustitución de una comunidad por otra

ecstasy pills éxtasis

ectasia ectasia

ectoderm ectodermo, más externa de las tres capas celulares primarias del embrión

ectodermal ectodérmico; **~ dysplasia** síndrome de displasia ectodérmica, el síndrome de Siemens, el síndrome de Weech, la displasia ectodérmica congénita

ectolysis ectólisis

ectoparasite ectoparásito

ectopia ectopia; **~ of urinary bladder** ectopia vesical

ectopic ectópico, que se encuentra o se produce fuera del lugar habitual; **~ pregnancy** embarazo tuboabdominal, embarazo ectopico, embarazo extrauterino, embarazo cornual

ectoplasm ectoplasma

eczema eczema, una enfermedad de la piel; **~ vesicles** vesículas de eccema/eczema

edema edema

edematous edematoso, envarado

edge-related límbico, relativo a un borde o margen

editor director (de una edición)

educational educativo; **~ program** programa de instrucción, programa educativo; **~ psychologist** psicopedagogía

EEG (electroencephalogram) electroencefalograma, EEG

effacement of the cervix borramiento cervical

effect efecto, resultado

effective eficaz; **~ concentration** concentración eficaz

effectiveness biodisponibilidad

effector efector

efferent eferente; **~ motor aphasia** afasia de Broca; **~ nerve** nervio eferente; **~ neuron** neurona eferente; **~ path** vias eferentes

efficacious efectivo, eficaz

efficacy efectividad, la eficacia

efficiency eficacia, eficiencia

efficient eficaz

effluent efluente

effort esfuerzo; **~ syndrome** astenia neurocirculatoria; **~ urticaria** urticaria por esfuerzo

effusion efusión (f), derrame (m)

eflectance eflectancia

egg óvulo, huevo pequeño; **~ white** blanquillo

eggshell hilus silicosis con calcificación periférica con aspecto de cáscara de huevo

EIA enzimoinmunoanálisis

eight ocho

eighteen dieciocho

eighth octavo

eighty ochenta

ejaculate, to eyacular

ejaculation eyaculación

ejection excreción, expulsión, eyección, eyaculación; **~ click** soplo de expulsión; **~ fraction** fracción de eyección; **~ murmur** soplo cardíaco sistólico, soplo sistólico

elastic elástico, saltarín, flojo; **~ bandage** venda elástica, apósito contentivo; **~ cartilage** cartílago elástico

elasticity elasticidad

elastin elastina

elbow codo; **~ joint** articulación cubital

elder care ayuda a los ancianos, asistencia a la vejez

elderly ancianos, personas mayores

elective electivo, selectivo

electric eléctrico; **~ capacitance** capacitancia eléctrica; **~ charge** carga eléctrica; **~ conductance** conductancia eléctrica; **~ conductivity** conductividad eléctrica; **~ current** corriente eléctrica; **~ current density** densidad de corriente eléctrica; **~ field strength** fuerza del campo eléctrico; **~ mobility** movilidad eléctrica; **~ resistance** resistencia eléctrica; **~ resistivity** resistividad eléctrica; **~ shock** choque eléctrico, descarga eléctrica; **~ shock therapy** electrochoc para el tratamiento de afecciones mentales o nerviosas; **~ wheelchair** silla de ruedas eléctrica

electrical activity of the brain actividad eléctrica del cerebro

electricity electricidad

electro-anesthesia electroanestesia

electroblotting electrotransferencia por adsorción

electrocardiographic monitoring equipment equipo de control de electrocardiografía

electrocardiography electrocardiografía

electro-cerebral inactivity silencio electroencefálico

electrocoagulation electrocoagulación

electrocution electrocución

electrode electrodo; **~ potencial** potencial de electrodo

electrodermal response reflejo psicogalvanico

electrodialysis electrodiálisis

electroejaculation electroeyaculación

electroencephalography electroencefalografía

electroendosmosis electroendósmosis

electroexcision excisión por bisturí eléctrico

electrogravimetry electrogravimetría

electrokaryotipe electrocariotipo

electrokinetic potential potencial electrocinético, potencial zeta

electrolysis electrólisis

electrolyte electrólito

electromedical electromédico; **~ device** aparato electromédico, equipo electromédico; **~ equipment** aparato electromédico, equipo electromédico

electromotive force fuerza electromotriz

electromyogram electromiograma (EMG)

electromyography electromiografía
electron microscope microscopio electrónico
electrones electrónes
electroneural therapy terapia neurovegetativa
electronvolt electronvolt
electropathology electropatología
electrophoresis electroforesis
electrophoretic electroforético; **~ mobility** movilidad electroforética
electrophthalm prótesis visual, prótesis de Norzewski, electroftalmo
electrophysiological electrofisiológico
electrophysiology electrofisiología
electroporation electroporación
electropulsation electropulsación
electrostatic electrostática; **~ charge** carga electrostática; **~ force** fuerza electrostática
electrotherapeutics electroterapia, terapia por estimulación electrica
electrotome bisturí electrónico
element elemento
elementary elemental; **~ charge** carga elemental
elephantiasis elefantiasis; **~ pyodermatica** elefantiasis piodérmica; **~ syphilitica** elefantiasis sifilítica; **~ tuberosa** elefantiasis tuberosa, elefantiasis verrugosa
elevated elevado
eleven once
eleventh once (date), onceavo, undécimo
eliciting factor factor causante
elimination eliminación; **~ diet** regimen de eliminación; **~ phase** fase de eliminación
ELISA elisa
elixir elixir
elongation elongación
eluate, to eluato
eluent eluyente
elution elución; **~ chromatography** cromatografía de elución; **~ curve** curva de elución
elutriate, to elutriar, decantar
elutriation elutriación, decantación; **~ of antibodies** decantación de anticuerpos
emaciation adelgazamiento, emaciación
embassy embajada
embolism embolia
embolization embolización

embolus émbolo
embryo embrión; **~ biopsy** biopsia del embrión, biopsia embrionaria; **~ flushing** lavado del útero; **~ transfer** transferencia de embriones
embryonal embrionario; **~ connective tissue** tejido conjuntivo embrionario, mesénquima
embryonic embrionario; **~ stem cell** célula madre embrionaria, célula cepa embrionaria; **~ vestige** vestigio embrionario
emergency emergencia; **~ eye wash fountain** fuente para el lavado de emergencia de los ojos; **~ kit for burns** botiquín de emergencia para quemaduras; **~ laboratory** laboratorio de urgencias; **~ life support** reanimación de urgencia; **~ medical assistance service** servicio de asistencia médica de urgencia; **~ operation** cirugía de urgencia, operación de urgencia; **~ physician** médico de urgencia; **~ room** sala de emergencia, sala de primeros auxilios, servicio médico de urgencia; **~ service** sala de emergencia, sala de primeros auxilios, servicio médico de urgencia; **~ surgery** cirugía de urgencia, operación de urgencia
emesis emesis, vómito
emetic emético, sustancia que provoca el vómito
emission emisión; **~ spectroscopy** espectroscopía de emisión
emittance emitancia
emmenagogues emenagogos
emmetropia emetropía, visión normal
emollient emoliente, que ablanda la piel; **~ poultice** cataplasma emoliente
emotion sentimiento, emoción
emotional afectivo, emocional; **~ blush** eritema emotivo, rubor, ruborícese; **~ bonding** relación afectiva, vinculación afectiva; **~ climate** clima afectivo, ambiente emocional; **~ devastation** angustia; **~ life** vida afectiva; **~ shock** choque psíquico, shock afectivo; **~ stress** ansiedad psíquica, estrés psicológico
empathy empatía
emphysema enfisema
emphysematous enfisematoso; **~ cholecystitis** colecistitis enfisematosa
empiric empírico, que se basa en la experiencia
employee empleado

empowerment capacitación, empoderamiento

emprosthotonos emprostótonos

emptying evacuación, vaciado de un órgano hueco o un absceso

empyema empiema, colección de pus en una cavidad natural

emulsification emulsificación; ~ **test** prueba de emulsificación

emulsify, to emulsionar, disolver una sustancia en otra

emulsion emulsión

ENA antígeno nuclear extraíble

enalapril enalapril

enanthem enantema, manchas rojas en las mucosas

encapsidation encapsidación

encephalic encefálico; ~ **angioma** angioma cerebral

encephalitis encefalitis (f), inflamación del cerebro

encephalopathy enfermedad cerebral, encefalopatía

encephalotrigeminal angiomatosis angiomatosis encefalotrigeminal, angiomatosis encefalotrigeminal

enchondroma encondroma

enchondromatosis encondromatosis

encode codificar

encopresis encopresis, incontinencia de los feces, de origen psicológica

encysted hernia hernia inguinal enquistada; ~ **peritonitis** absceso intraperitoneal; ~ **tumor** lupia

endarterectomy limpieza de la luz de las arterias

endemic endémico, que se presenta como propio de una población; ~ **disease** enfermedad endémica; ~ **goiter** bocio endémico; ~ **hematuria** esquistosomiasis urinaria; ~ **typhus** tifus exantemático endémico

end-labeling marcaje terminal

endocardiac endocardico, intracardiaco

endocardial endocardico; ~ **cushion** relieve endocardico; ~ **fibro-elastosis** fibroelastosis endocardico

endocarditis endocarditis

endocardium endocardio

endocervical endocervical; ~ **mucus** moco endocervical

endocrine endocrino, que secreta hormonas; ~ **adenomatosis** adenomatosis endocrina; ~ **cachexia** caquexia endocrina; ~ **disrupter** perturbador endocrino; ~ **exophthalmos** exoftalmia de origen endocrino; ~ **gland** glándula endocrina; ~ **system** sistema endocrino

endocrinologist endocrinológico - médico que atiende pacientes con problemas de las glándulas endocrinas

endocrinology endocrinología

endodontics endodoncia

endodontist endodontista

endoenzyme endoenzima

endogenote endogenote

endogenous endógeno, que se desarrolla u origina dentro del organismo

endolysin endolisina

endometrial endometrial; ~ **biopsy** biopsia de endometrio, biopsia endometrial; ~ **breakthrough bleeding** metrorragia perterapéutica; ~ **hyperplasia** hiperplasia del endometrio

endometriosis endometriosis

endometritis endometritis

endometrium mucosidad del útero

endomyocardial endomiocárdica; ~ **biopsy** biopsia endomiocárdica; ~ **fibrosis** fibrosis endomiocárdica

endonuclease endonucleasa

endoparasite endoparásito

endopeptidase endopeptidasa, la proteinasa

endoplasma plasma granuloso

endoplasmic reticulum retículo endoplásmico; ~ **rough surfaced** ergastoplasma, retículo endoplasmático granular

endorphin endorfina

endoscope endoscopio

endoscopic endoscópico; ~ **retrograde cholangiopancreatography** colangiopancreatografía retrógrada endoscópica; ~ **surgery** cirugía endoscópica

endoscopy endoscopia, inspección de una cavidad del cuerpo por medio del endoscopio

endosteal anesthesia anestesia endostal

endostosis endostosis

endothelial endotelial; ~ **cell** célula endotelial; ~ **corneal dystrophy** distrofia de las células endoteliales de la córnea, córnea guttata

endothelium endotelio, capa interna que reviste las cavidades cardíacas y los vasos sanguíneos y linfáticos

endotoxic endotóxico, relativo a las endotoxinas

endotracheal endotraqueal, intratraqueal; ~ **intubation** intubación endotraqueal, intubación intraqueal; ~ **tube** catéter de intubación

endovascular endovascular; ~ **ultrasonography** ecografía endovascular

endoxin endoxina

end-stage kidney disease enfermedad renal en etapa final

endurance aguante, resistencia, fuerza vital, vitalidad; ~ **training** aguante, resistencia, endurecimiento, induración

enema enema, lavativa

energetic energético, relativo a la energía

English inglés

engraftment implantación exitosa del injerto, pega del trasplante, prendimiento del trasplante

enhanced reforzado

enhancer intensificador; ~ **element** secuencia de control, elemento de facilitación genética

enlarged lymph nodes agrandamiento de los nódulos linfáticos, aumento de los ganglios linfáticos

enlargement aumento; ~ **of the heart** aumento del tamaño del corazón

enlarging distensión, estiramiento

enophthalmos enoftalmia

enoxacin enoxacina

enrichment culture caldo de enriquecimiento; ~ **medium** medio de enriquecimiento

E.N.T ORL, otorrinolaringología

enteral entérico; ~ **diarrhea** diarrea entérica; ~ **hormones** hormonas intestinales; ~ **nutrition** nutrición enteral

enteric entérico; ~ **coated** queratinizado, recubierto por una sustancia resistente a la secreción gástrica; ~ **-coated tablet** pastilla con cubierto entérico; ~ **hormone** hormona gastrointestinal

enteritis enteritis (f), inflamación del intestino delgado

enterocolitis enterocolitis

enterohepatic enterohepático, que se refiere al intestino y al hígado

enteroinvasive enteroinvasor

enterokinase enteropeptidasa

enteropathic enteropático; ~ **acrodermatitis** acrodermatitis enteropática; ~ **AIDS** enteropatía en el SIDA

enteropathogenic enteropatógeno

enteropathy enteropatía

enteropeptidase enteropeptidasa

enterotoxigenic enterotoxigénico

enterotoxin enterotoxina

enterovirus enterovirus

enthalpy entalpía

entitic entítico, entésico

entity entidad, ente

entropion entropión; ~ **correction** corrección de entropión

entropy entropía

entry entrada; ~ **exclusion** bloqueo de entrada; ~ **site** centro aceptor

enucleation enucleación, extirpación

enuresis enuresis, emisión involuntaria de la orina

environment entorno, ambiente

environmental ambiental; ~ **degradation** deterioro del medio ambiente

enzymatic enzimático; ~ **activity** actividad enzimática; ~ **adaptation** adaptación enzimática; ~ **coagulation** coagulación enzimática; ~ **concentrate** concentrado enzimático; ~ **reaction** reaccion enzimática

enzyme enzima; ~ **activity** actividad enzimática; ~ **degradation** degradación enzimatica; ~ **electrode** electrodo enzimático; ~ **hydrolysis** hidrólisis enzimática; ~ **immunoassay** enzimoinmunoanálisis; ~ **-linked immunosorbent assay** elisa

enzymic synthesis síntesis de las enzimas

eosine eosina

eosinophil eosinofilocito, eosinófilo; ~ **adenoma** adenoma eosinófilo; ~ **granulocyte** granulocito eosinófilo; ~ **pleurisy** pleuresía eosinófila

eosinophilia eosinofilia

eosinophilic adenoma adenoma eosinófilo;
~ **granuloma** granuloma eosinófilo;
~ **infiltrate** infiltrado eosinófilo

eosinophilocyte eosinofilocito, eosinófilo

epdidymitis epididimitis

ephedrine efedrina

ephemeral fever fiebre efímera

epicanthus epicanto

epicondylalgia epicondilalgia

epicondyle epicóndilo

epicondylitis epicondilitis

epicranium cuero cabelludo, casco de la cabeza

epicutaneous epicutáneo; ~ **test** test
epicutáneo, prueba epicutánea

epidemic epidémico; ~ **diaphragmatic
pleurodynia** enfermedad de Bornholm;
~ **disease** epidemia

epidemiological epidemiólogo, relativo al
estudio de la distribución de enfermedades

epidemiology epidemiología; ~ **of the
outbreak** características epizoóticas del brote

epidermal epidérmico, relativo a la piel; ~ **graft**
injerto de la piel, borde dérmico

epidermolysis bullosa epidermólisis ampollosa

epididymis epididimo

epidural epidural, extradural; ~ **anesthesia**
raquianestesia epidural, anestesia epidural;
~ **injection** inyección epidural

epigastralgia epigastralgia, dolor alrededor del
estómago

epigastric epigástrico; ~ **fossa** fosa epigástrica;
~ **hernia** hernia epigástrica

epigenetic epigenético; ~ **carcinogen** agente
carcinógeno epigenético; ~ **environment**
actividad epigenética, el mecanismo
epigenético

epiglottis epiglotis

epilepsy epilepsia

epiloia enfermedad de Bourneville, esclerosis
cerebral tuberosa, epiloia

epinephrine epinefrina, adrenalina

epiphyseal epifisario

epiphysis glándula pineal, epífisis

episiotomy episiotomía, corte vaginal,
perineotomía

episode episodio; ~ **of transient shift** acceso de
traslocación transitoria

epistaxis epistaxis, sangrar por la nariz

epithelial epitelial; ~ **attachment** inserción
epitelial; ~ **neoplasm** neoplasia epitelial;
~ **tissue** tejido epitelial

epithelioid epitelioide

epithelioma epitelioma

epithelium epitelio, la piel y las mucosas

epitope determinante antigénico, epítope

EPO eritropoyetina

Epsom salt sal de Epsom, sal de Selditz

Eppstein–Barr disease mononucleosis
infecciosa, angina monocítica; ~ **virus** virus de
Epstein-Barr

Epstein nephrosis nefrosis de Epstein,
síndrome nefrótico; ~ **nephrosis therapy**
tratamiento para la nefrosis de Epstein;
~ **syndrome** nefrosis de Epstein, síndrome
nefrótico

epulis épulis, un tumor benigno de la encía

equatorial plate placa ecuatorial

equilibrium equilibrio, ~ **constant** constante de
equilibrio

equivalent equivalente, de igual valor; ~ **dose**
bioequivalente, sustancia farmacológica con
potencia y efecto similares a otra

ERA (evoked response audiometry) ERA,
audiometría electroencefalográfica,
audiometría por potenciales evocados

eradicate, to erradicar

eradication erradicación, eliminación; ~ **of the
outbreak** erradicación del brote

Erasmus' syndrome síndrome de Erasmus

**ERCP (endoscopic retrograde
cholangiopancreatography)**
colangiopancreatografía retrógrada
endoscópica

ergastoplasma ergastoplasma, retículo
endoplasmatico granular

ergocalciferol ercalciol

ergoloid mesylate mesilatos ergoloides

ergometric ergométrico; ~ **bicycle** bicicleta
ergométrica

ergonomics ergonometría

ergot alkaloids alcaloides del ergot

ergotherapy ergoterapia, terapia ocupacional

ergotism ergotismo, intoxicación producida por
el cornezuelo del centeno

ergotoxin ergotoxina

eritrasma eritrasma

Erlenmeyer flask matraz de Erlenmeyer
Ermengen's bacillus Clostridium botulinum
erosion erosión
error error
eructate, to eructar, regoldar
eructation eructo, regüeldo
eruption erupción, sarpullido
erysipelas erisipela
erysipeloid erisipeloide
erythema eritema, enrojecimiento;
~ **chronicum migrans** eritema cronico
migrans; ~ **infectiosum** eritema infeccioso,
quinta enfermedad; ~ **multiforme** eritema
multiforme; ~ **nodoso** eritema nudoso
erythematous eritematoso; ~ **blepharitis**
blefaritis eritematosa
erythrasma eritrasma
erythrocyanosis eritrocianosis
erythrocyte eritrocito, glóbulo rojo; ~ **cast**
cilindro sanguíneo; ~ **count** recuento de
eritrocitos, volumen eritrocítico; ~ **membrane**
membrana eritrocítica; ~ **monocyte**
megacariocito; ~ **sedimentation rate**
eritrosedimentación; ~ **stroma** estroma
eritrocítica
erythrodermia eritrodermia; ~ **ichthyosiforme**
congenitum eritrodermia ictiosiforme
erythrogenic toxin veneno de la escarlatina
erythroid enrojecido, rojizo; ~ **progenitor cells**
células progenitoras eritroides
erythromelalgia eritromelalgia, enfermedad de
Mitchell
erythromycin eritromicina
erythropoiesis eritropoyesis
erythropoietin eritropoyetina
erythrosedimentation eritrosedimentación
escaped beat extrasístole, latido prematuro del
corazón
escherichia coli escherichia coli, E.coli
esculin agar agar-esculina
Esmarch bandage torniquete (de Esmarch)
esophageal esofágico; ~ **achalasia**
cardioespasmo, acalasia del esófago; ~ **cancer**
cáncer del esófago, neoplasma del esófago;
~ **diverticulum** divertículo esofágico;
~ **intubation** intubación gástrica, intubación
gastrointestinal; ~ **manometry** manometría
esofágica; ~ **neoplasm** cáncer del esófago,

neoplasma del esófago; ~ **reflux** reflujo al
esófago, regurgitación del estómago al
esófago; ~ **regurgitation** reflujo al esófago,
regurgitación del estómago al esófago;
~ **stenosis** estenosis esofágica, constricción del
esófago; ~ **stricture** estenosis esofágica,
constricción del esófago; ~ **varices** varices
esofágicas
esophagitis esofagitis, inflamación del esófago
esophagogastrectomy esofagogastrostrectomía
esophagostomy esofagostomía
esophagus esófago, tragante, gaznate,
tragadero
especially especialmente, particularmente, sobre
todo
espundia espundia, leishmaniosis
cutaneomucosa americana
ESR eritrosedimentación
ESRD enfermedad renal en etapa fina
essential esencial; ~ **amino acid** aminoácido
esencial; ~ **hemorrhagic thrombocythemia**
trombocitemia hemorrágica esencial; ~ **trace**
element oligoelemento
esthesioneuroblastoma neuroblastoma
olfatorio, estesioneuroblastoma
estradiol estradiol
estrogen estrógeno; ~ **suppressant**
antiestrogénico, que impide o contrarresta el
efecto de las hormonas estrogénicas;
~ **gestagen mixture** asociación estrógeno-
progestativa
ESWL (extracorporeal shock-wave
lithotripsy) litotripsia extracorporal con onda de
choque
etanidazole etanidazol
ethacridine lactate lactato de etacridina
ethanol etanol
ethanolamine etanolamina
ether éter; ~ **narcosis** narcosis por éter,
eterización
ethical ético; ~ **drugs** medicamento que se
puede conseguir únicamente con receta;
~ **evaluation** valoración ética
ethnicity raza, etnicidad
ethosuximide etosuximida
ethylacetic acid ácido butanoico, ácido butírico
etiology etiología, cause de una enfermedad
etoposide etoposida

eugenic eugenésico; ~ **sterilization** esterilización eugénica

eugenics eugenesia

euglycemia euglucemia - un nivel normal de glucosa en la sangre

eugonic eugónico

eukaryotic eucariota

eukkaryote célula eucariota

euphoria agitación, euforia, inquietud y actividad aumentada

euphrasy eufrasia

Eustachian tube tubo de Eustaquio, tubo auditivo

euthanasia eutanasia

euthyroid eutiroide; ~ **hypometabolism** hipometabolismo eutiroide

evacuation defecación, evacuación, expulsión de los excrementos; ~ **cystoscope** cistoscopio aspirador; ~ **of the stomach** evacuación del estómago, vaciar el estómago

evaluation valorización, evaluación

evaporation evaporación

evaporator evaporador, nebulizador

evening noche

eventration eventración

eversion eversión, vuelta de adentro hacia afuera

every cada

evidence evidencia; ~ **-based medicine** medicina basada puramente en las evidencias

evident manifiesto, ostensible, evidente

evisceration evisceración; ~ **of orbit** evisceración de la órbita

evoke, to evocar

evoked evocado; ~ **potential** potencial evocado; ~ **response audiometry** audiometría por potenciales evocados, audiometría electroencefalográfica

evolution evolución

Ewing's sarcoma sarcoma de Ewing

exacerbation agravamiento, empeoramiento, exacerbación

exaggerate, to exagerar

examination examen, exploración, inspección; ~ **table** mesa de reconocimiento, mesa para reconocimiento clínico

examine, to pesquisar, buscar, escudriñar, examinar, indagar, investigar

examining doctor inspector médico, médico asesor

exanthema salpullido, erupción de la piella, rash, exantema, roncha

exarthrosis exartrosis

excess exceso

excessive excesivo, desmesurado; ~ **gastric acid secretion** acidez gástrica; ~ **salivation** ptialismo, sialorrea; ~ **sweating** hiperhidrosis, sudación exagerada

excimer laser láser de excímero

excipient excipiente

excise, to extirpar

excision escisión, extirpación, resección; ~ **of a cancerous tumor** excisión de un tumor maligno, extirpación de un tumor canceroso; ~ **of an aneurysm** excisión de aneurisma

excitation estimulación, sobreexcitación, sensibilidad exagerada, excitación; ~ **energy** energía de excitación

excitatory postsynaptic potential potencial postsináptico de excitación

exclusion exclusión; ~ **chromatography** cromatografía de exclusión

exclusive exclusivo, que excluye, único, solo, absoluto, total

excoriation excoriación

excrement heces, excrementos, deposiciones

excrescence excrecencia

excretion secreción, flujo, excreción; ~ **pyelography** pielografía, urografía

excretory excretor; ~ **duct** conducto excretor; ~ **urography** urografía intravenosa

exercise ejercicio físico, movimiento; ~ **-induced asthma** asma inducida por exercicio

exeresis exéresis

exertion esfuerzo

exertional asthma asma inducida por exercicio; ~ **dyspnea** disnea por esfuerzo; ~ **headache** cefalea postejercicio

exfoliation areata linguae lengua geográfica

exfoliation exfoliación, desprendimiento en escamas o capas; ~ **syndrome** glaucoma capsular, síndrome de exfoliación

exfoliative exfoliativo; ~ **cheilitis** estomatitis angular, queilitis; ~ **cytodiagnosis** citodiagnóstico exfoliativo; ~ **cytology** citodiagnóstico exfoliativo, citología exfoliativa

exhale, to espirar, exhalar

exhaust fan bomba de vacío, aspirador, eyector

exhausted sin fuerzas, agotado, debilitado

exhauster bomba de vacío, aspirador, eyector

exhaustion lasitud, debilidad, cansancio, agotamiento, laxitud

exit of gunshot wound orificio de salida de un proyectil

exocoelom exoceloma, celoma extraembrionario

exocrine exocrino, que secreta hacia afuera

exocytosis exocitosis

exoenzyme exoenzima

exogenote exogenote

exogenous exógeno, por causas externas; ~ **aneurysm** aneurisma exógeno; ~ **retrovirus** retrovirus exógeno

exon exón

exonuclease exonucleasa

exophoria exoforia, heteroforia

exophthalmos exoftalmía, propulsión del globo del ojo

exophytic exofítico; ~ **tumor** carcinoma exofítico, tumor exofítico

exostosis exostosis; ~ **multiplex cartilaginea** exostosis múltiple hereditaria, exostosis múltiple cartilaginosa

exotoxin exotoxina

exotropia exotropía

expander extensor

expanding expansivo; ~ **cancer** carcinoma invasivo, cáncer invasivo

expansion dilatación, ensanchamiento, agrandamiento o expansión de un órgano hueco; ~ **of consciousness** perdida de la consciencia

expansive expansivo; ~ **querulous paranoia** queromanía expansiva

expectant expectante; ~ **mother** mujer embarazada

expectorant expectorante

expectoration esputo

experimental experimental; ~ **pathology** patología experimental; ~ **standard desviation** desviación típica experimental; ~ **variable** variable experimental

expert experto; ~ **opinion** dictamen experto

expiration espiración

expiratory espiratorio; ~ **depth** profundidad espiratoria, volumen espiratorio; ~ **dyspnea** disnea espiratoria; ~ **reserve volume** volumen de reserva espiratoria, volumen de reserva espiratoria

explanation interpretación

explicit declarativo, explícito; ~ **memory** memoria declarativa, memoria explícita

expression expresión; ~ **of the recessive phenotype** expresión del fenotipo recesivo

expressive expresivo; ~ **aphasia** afasia motora, afasia motora del habla, afasia de Broca; ~ **gesture** gesto expresivo

expulsion expulsión; ~ **of the placenta** expulsión de la placenta

exsiccosis deshidratación, carencia de agua en el cuerpo

extended prolongado; ~ **care** cuidado prolongado, cuidados a largo plazo, tratamiento adicional; ~ **DNA** DNA expandido

extension extensión (f), despliegue; ~ **treatment** tratamiento por extensión

external externo, situado fuera de, de fuera, extraño; ~ **cardiac compression** masaje cardíaco externo; ~ **envelope glycoprotein** glicoproteína de la envoltura externa, la proteína de envoltorio del VIH; ~ **heart massage** masaje cardíaco de Oertel; ~ **hospital doctor** médico autorizado, médico externo de hospital; ~ **quality assessment** evaluación externa de la calidad; ~ **quality control** control externo de la calidad

exteroceptive exteroceptivo; ~ **reflex** reflejo exteroceptivo

extinction extinción, absorbancia

extirpate, to extirpar

extirpation desprendimiento, extirpación, ablación

extracapsular extracapsular

extracellular extracelular, situado fuera de las células; ~ **fluid** fluido extracelular, líquido extracelular; ~ **hyperhydration** hiperhidratación extracelular; ~ **liquid** fluido extracelular, líquido extracelular; ~ **matrix** matriz extracelular

extracerebral extracerebral

extracorporeal extracorporal, situado fuera del

cuerpo, desviado fuera del cuerpo;
~ **photochemotherapy** fotoferesis;
~ **photopheresis** fotoferesis

extract extracto, preparación concentrada de una droga; ~, **to** extraer

extractable residuo extraíble; ~ **nuclear antigen** antígeno nuclear extraíble

extraction extracción, extirpación quirúrgica

extradural epidural, extradural

extra-embryonic extraembrionario

extra-hepatic cholestasis colestasis extrahepatica, obstrucción del conducto biliar extrahepatico

extra-marital birth nacimiento fuera del matrimonio

extrapyramidal extrapiramidal

extrarenal extrarrenal, situado fuera del riñón

extrasystole extrasístole, latido prematuro del corazón

extra-uterine extrauterino; ~ **chloasma** cloasma extra-uterino

extravasation extravasación, derrame de sangre

extravascular extravascular, situado fuera de un vaso

extreme extremo, que está alejado; ~ **fever** hiperpirexia, fiebre extremadamente elevada; ~ **leanness** adelgazamiento, emaciación; ~ **sleepiness** clinomanía

extremity extremidades

extrinsic extrínseco; ~ **allergic alveolitis** neumopatía por hipersensibilidad, alveolitis alérgica, alveolitis alérgica extrínseca; ~ **asthma** asma bronquial extrínseca; ~ **coagulation pathway** coagulación extrínseca; ~ **coagulation system** sistema extrínseco de coagulación, coagulación extrínseca

extrusion erupción

extumescence tumefacción, hinchamiento

exudate exudado, líquido que aparece en una superficie inflamada

exudation exudación

exudative exudativo; ~ **enteropathy** enteropatía exudativa; ~ **pleurisy** pleuresía exudativa

eye ojo; ~ **chart** cuadro de agudeza visual, tabla oftálmica; ~ **compress** c0900ataplasma

ocular; ~ **drops** loción para los ojos, colirio; ~ **inflammation** iridociclitis, inflamación del iris y del cuerpo ciliar; ~ **injury** lesión ocular; ~ **irritation** iritis, inflamación del iris; ~ **ointment** pomada oftálmica, gel ocular; ~ **patch** parche de ojo; ~ **socket** cuenca, órbita del ojo

eyeball globo del ojo

eyebrow ceja

eyedropper pipeta, cuenta-gotas

eyelashes pestañas

eyelid párpado

eyestrain astenopía, cansancio de los ojos, cansancio de los órganos visuales

eyewash colirio

F

face cara, rostro; ~ **down** estar boca abajo, estar postrado, acostado boca abajo, prono; ~ **lift** ritidoplastia, ritidectomia

facet faceta ósea

facial facial, relativo a la cara; ~ **artery** arteria facial; ~ **erythrosis** acné rosácea, rosácea, eritrosis facial; ~ **expression** mímica; ~ **hyperhidrosis** hiperhidrosis facial; ~ **massage** masaje facial; ~ **muscles** músculos faciales; ~ **neuralgia** neuralgia facial; ~ **paralysis** parálisis facial, parálisis de Bell, prosopoplejía

facilitation facilitación

factitious artificial, no naural, sintético, facticio

factor factor, causa; ~ **VIII** factor VIII de coagulación, factor antihemofílico A; ~ **VIII deficiency** hemofilia A

factory fábrica; ~ **worker** trabajador en una fábrica

facultative facultativo; ~ **anaerobe** anaerobio facultativo; ~ **parasite** parásito facultativo; ~ **symptom** síntoma facultativo

fæces las heces, excrementos, deposiciones

fagicladosporic acid ácido fagicladospórico

failure fallo, fracaso, insuficiencia; ~ **of treatment** fracaso terapéutico, insuficiencia del tratamiento

faint desmayo; ~, **to** desmayarse, perder el

conocimiento

fainting soponcio, patatús, desmayar; ~ **spell** desmayo

fair complected tez blanca; ~ **-skinned** tez blanca

faith healer curandero, sanador; ~ **healing** curación por creencia, curación por la fé

fall caída, disminución, otoño

fall asleep, to adormecerse

fallopian tube trompa de falopio

Fallot's tetralogy síndrome de Corvisart, tetralogía de Fallot

false ~ **aneurysm** aneurisma falso; ~ **membrane** seudomembrana; ~ **memory** ilusión mnésica, falsa memoria; ~ **negative** negativo falso; ~ **neuroma** neuroma falso; ~ **positive** positivo falso; ~ **posture** postura mala; ~ **pregnancy** seudociesis, seudoembarazo; ~ **rib** falsa costilla; ~ **tumor** tumor fantasma, pseudotumor, tumor falso

familial familiar

familiar conocido

family familia; ~ **case history** historia de caso familiar; ~ **doctor** médico generalista, especialista en medicina familiar y comunitaria; ~ **history of cancer** antecedente familiar de cáncer; ~ **planning** planificación familiar, planificación de la familia, asistencia sanitaria genésica; ~ **relationship** parentesco, consanguinidad

Fanconi's anemia anemia de Fanconi, síndrome de Fanconi

fangotherapy barro termal, barro terapéutico, sedimentos curativos, fangoterapia

farad farad

Faraday constant constante de Faraday

farmer ranchero; ~ **lung** pulmón del granjero

farsighted, far-sighted présbite

far-sightedness presbiopía, presbicia

fart viento, pedo; ~ **, to** pedar, arrojar flatos

farting flatulencia, presencia abundante de gaz en el estómago o el intestino

fascia aponeurosis, fascia; ~ **bulbi** cápsula de Tenon

fasciculation fasciculación

fase, to perturbar, molestar, desconcertar

fast rápido; ~ **, to** ayunar

fastidious mimado, maniático; ~ **anaerobe** anaerobio exigente

fasting en ayunas; ~ **cure** cura de hambre; ~ **metabolism** metabolismo de ayuno, tasa de metabolismo basal

fat gordo, lípido, sobrepeso; ~ **cell** célula cebada; ~ **embolism** embolia grasa; ~ **necrosis** necrosis grasa, esteatonecrosis; ~ **replacers** substitutos de grasa, grasas artificiales

fatal pernicioso, peligroso, aniquilante, grave, maligno, fatal; ~ **injury** lesión mortal, accidente mortal

father padre; ~ **-in-law** suegro

fatigue lasitud, debilidad, cansancio, agotamiento, laxitud

fat-soluble liposoluble

fatty grasoso, graso, grasiento; ~ **acid** ácido graso; ~ **degeneration** esteatosis, acumulación excesiva de glóbulos grasos en los tejidos; ~ **foods** comidas grasas; ~ **heart** gordura sobre el corazón; ~ **lymphoid tissue** tejido conjuntivo; ~ **tissue** tejido adiposo, tejido grasoso

FBC hemograma completo

fear miedo, temor; ~ **of abandonment** miedo al abandono; ~ **of castration** ansiedad inducida por la castración

febrile febril, relativo a la fiebre, con fiebre

February febrero

fecal fecal; ~ **culture** coprocultivo; ~ **matter** heces, excrementos, deposiciones; ~ **occult blood test** búsqueda de sangre oculta en las deposiciones

feces las heces, excrementos, deposiciones

fee factura, cobro, cuenta

feeblemindedness retraso mental, la retardación mental, la oligofrenia, la debilidad mental, la imbecilidad, la demencia, el trastorno mental

feedback feedback, retroalimentación, retroacción

feeding alimentación; ~ **by a stomach tube** alimentación por sonda

feel, to sentir(se), palpar, tener ganas (de); ~ **bloated, to** estar envarado; ~ **nauseous, to** estar nauseabundo; ~ **out of sorts, to** estar destemplado, estar bascoso, estar mareado, estar friolero, tener escalofríos, tener malestar

feeling sensación, sentimiento, palpación;
~ **nauseated** náusea, asco, basca, ganas de vomitar; ~ **of inadequacy** autodesvalorización, falta de amor proprio; ~ **of worthlessness** autodesvalorización, un sentimiento de insuficiencia, falta de amor proprio; ~ **sick** náusea, asco, basca, ganas de vomitar

feign illness, to fingirse enfermo, hacerse el enfermo

felon panadizo

female femenina; ~ **circumcision** circuncisión de la mujer; ~ **infibulation** infibulación de la mujer

feminine feminina; ~ **hygiene product** producto para la higiene femenina; ~ **hyperestrogenism** hiperestrinismo femenino

femoral femoral; ~ **artery** arteria femoral; ~ **calcar** calcar femoral; ~ **hernia** hernia femoral; ~ **nerve** nervio femoral, nervio crural; ~ **ring** anillo crural

femorocele hernia femoral

femur fémur; ~ **load cell simulator** simulador dinamométrico del fémur

fenfluramine fenfluramina

fenugreek fenogreco, heno griego, alholva

fermentation fermentación; ~ **test** prueba de la fermentación

ferredoxin ferredoxina

ferriprive ferriprivo

ferritin ferritina

ferrocene–lidocaine complex complejo ferroceno-lidocaína

ferrochelatase ferroquelatasa

ferrocyanide hexacianoferrato (II)

ferroxidase ferroxidasa, ceruloplasmina

fertile fértil

fertilisation fecundación

fertility fertilidad; ~ **rate** tasa de fertilidad

fertilize, to fecundar

fertilized ovum zigoto, óvulo fecundado

Feseri's bacillus Clostridium chauvoei

fetal fetal; ~ **alcohol syndrome** síndrome del alcoholismo fetal; ~ **chondrodystrophy** acondroplasia, condrodistrofia fetal de Kaufmann, acondrodisplasia; ~ **damage** daño

fetal; ~ **death** muerte fetal; ~ **distress** sufrimiento fetal; ~ **erythroblastosis** eritroblastosis fetal; ~ **hemoglobin** hemoglobina fetal; ~ **hydrops** hidropesía fetal, eritroblastosis fetal; ~ **icterus** ictericia fetal; ~ **injury** lesión fetal, daño fetal; ~ **jaundice** ictericia fetal; ~ **malnutrition** insuficiencia placentaria; ~ **organ maturity** madurez de los organos fetales; ~ **rachitis** raquitismo fetal; ~ **retention** retención del feto muerto; ~ **rickets** raquitismo fetal

fetalism fetalismo

fetoplacental fetoplacentario

fetotoxic fetotóxico, venenoso para el feto

fetus feto

fever fiebre, calentura, pirexia; ~ **blister** ampolla febril; ~ **inducing** pirógeno, que produce fiebre

feverish febril, afiebrado, enfebecido, acalenturado

few pocos

FIA inmunofluorescencia

fiber fibra; ~ **optic laryngoscope** laringoscopio fiberoptico

fibrillar fibrilar; ~ **chorea** corea fibrilar

fibrillation fibrilación

fibrin fibrina; ~ **cross-linking** entrecruzamiento de fibrina; ~ **degradation products** productos de degradación de la fibrina

fibrinase plasmina

fibrinogen adj fibrinógeno, f trombina; ~ **split products** productos de la degradación del fibrinógeno

fibrinolysin plasmina

fibrinolysis fibrinolisis

fibrinolytic fibrinolítico; ~ **diathesis** diatesis fibrinolítica

fibrinoplastin fibrinoplastina

fibrinous fibrinoso; ~ **exudate** exudado fibrinoso

fibroadenoma fibroadenoma, adenoma fibroso, adenofibroma

fibroblast fibroblasto; ~ **interferon** interferón del fibroblasto, interferón beta

fibrocystic fibroquístico; ~ **mastitis** mastopatía fibroquística

fibrolipoma lipofibroma

fibroma fibroma, una formación compuesta de

tejido fibroso o conjuntivo y vasos
fibromatosis fibromatosis
fibromyalgia fibromiálgica, encefalomielitis miálgica, síndrome de fatiga crónica
fibronectin fibronectina
fibrosing fibroso; ~ **osteochondroma** osteocondroma fibroso, osteocondrofibroma
fibrosis fibrosis; ~ **of the myocardium** fibrosis del miocardio
fibrositis reumatismo muscular, fibrositis
fibrous fibroso; ~ **ankylosis** anquilosis fibrosa; ~ **capsule of liver** capsula fibrosa del higado, capsula fibrosa perivascularis; ~ **struma** estruma fibroso
fibula peroné
fibular notch incisura fibularis tibiae
ficain ficaina
Fick's bacillus Proteus vulgaris
fifteen quince
fifth quinto; ~ **disease** eritema infeccioso, quinta enfermedad
fifty cincuenta
fig wart verrugas genitales, condiloma acuminado
fight riña
filamentous filiforme
filarial elephantiasis elefantiasis filariensis, elefantiasis de les árabes
filiform filiforme; ~ **papillae** papilas filiformes
fill-in reaction reacción de relleno
filling (in teeth) empaste
film-coated (pill, tablet) revestido con una tapa de película
filter filtro; ~ **flas** matraz de filtración; ~ **hybridization** hibridación sobre filtro
filtration filtración
fimbriae fimbria, ribetes falopianos/uterinos
fimbrial adhesion adherencia de la fimbria; ~ **pregnancy** embarazo tuboabdominal, embarazo ectopico, embarazo extrauterino, embarazo cornual
fimbriate franjeado; ~ **hymen** himen franjeado, himen denticular
final terminal; ~ **stage** fase terminal
finasteride finasterida
find, to encontrar, hallar
findings hallazgos, resultados, observaciones
fine bien, bueno; ~ **motor skills** fina destreza

motora, fina motricidad
finger dedo; ~ **contracture** contractura de los dedos; ~ **splint** férula digital, a tala do dedo, tablilla digital
fingernail uña
fingerprint huella digital
fingerprinting obtención de la huella genética
fingertip yema del dedo
fire fuego
firm to the touch firme al tacto
first primero, en primer lugar, principal, principio, originario, primario; ~ **aid** primeros auxilios, curas médicas de urgencia; ~ **aid kit** botiquín de urgencia, maletín de urgencia, caja de urgencia; ~ **aid oxygen generator** generador de oxígeno de emergencia; ~ **menses** menarca, menarquía, fecha de la primera menstruación; ~ **name** nombre; ~ **pass** de primer paso; ~ **period** menarca, menarquía, fecha de la primera menstruación; ~ **vaccination** primovacunación, vacunación que se efectúa por primera vez
fish pescado
fishmeal worker's lung pulmón de harina de pescado
fission fisión
fissura fisura, hendedura, cisura, surco, grieta
fist puño; ~ , **to make a** cerrar la mano, apretar el puño
fistula fistula; ~ **of small intestine** fistula del intestino delgado; ~ **of the cavernous sinus** fistula del seno cavernoso de la carotida
fistulous gluteal blastomycosis blastomicosis fistulosa glútea
fit adj arrebato, f convulsión; ~ , **to have a** pataleta, acceso, ataque, crisis
fitness aptitud, buena salud; ~ **center** gimnasio; ~ **training** entrenamiento
fitting a (urine) bag cateterismo, introducción de una sonda en una cavidad hueca
five cinco; ~ **hundred** quinientos
fixation fijación; ~ **plate** grapa de fijación, placa
fixed fijo; ~ **bridgework** puente dental, dentadura parcial fija; ~ **coronary artery occlusive disease** oclusión permanente de la arteria coronaria; ~ **partial dental bridge** puente dental, dentadura parcial fija

flabby fláccido, flojo

flaccid fláccido, laxo, flojo, blando, débil; ~ **part of tympanic membrane** membrana fláccida, membrana de Shrapnell

flagellar flagelar; ~ **stain** tinción flagelar

flame llama; ~ **atomic absorption spectrometry** espectrometría de absorción atómica de llama; ~ **atomic emission spectrometry** espectrometría de emisión atómica de llama; ~ **photometry** espectrometría de emisión atómica de llama

flank ijar, ijada; ~ **pain** dolor del costado, mal de ijar, dolor de bazo, punzada en el costado

flank, to flanquear

flanking sequence secuencia flanqueadora

flash-back recurrencia; ~ **phenomenon** fenómeno de recurrencia

flat plano

flatulence flatulencia, presencia abundante de aire en el estómago o el intestino

flatulent aventado, flatulento; ~ **colic** cólico flatulento, cólico gaseoso

flatus viento, pedo

flavin flavina; ~ **-adenine dinucleotide** dinucleótido de flavina y adenina; ~ **mononucleotide** mononucleótido de flavina

flavone flavona

flavonoids flavonoides

flavor sabor

flaw falta, fallo

flea pulga; ~ **bite** picadura de pulga, de piojo

flesh carne; ~ **-eating disease** fasciitis necrotizante, necrólisis epidérmica tóxica; ~ **wound** desgarro

fleshy growth carnosidad

Fletcher factor precalicreína

flex, to doblarse, flexionarse

flexible flexible; ~ **fiberscope** fibroscopio flexible, endoscopio de fibra óptica, laparoscopio; ~ **wrist** muñeca compliante

flexion flexión

Flexner's bacillus Shigella flexneri

flight surgeon cirujano ortopedista

floccose flocoso

floor of the pelvis perineo

floppy-valve syndrome prolapso mitral

flossing the teeth limpiarse los dientes con hilo dental, usar hilo dental

flow flujo; ~ **cytometry** citometría de flujo; ~ **injection** inyección en flujo

flu gripa, gripe, flu, influenza; ~ **vaccine** vacuna antigripal

fluconazole fluconazol

flucytosine flucitosina

fluid liquor, líquido, solución; ~ **removal** paracentesis, drenaje; ~ **retention** retención hídrica

flunitrazepam flunitracepam

fluor albus flúor albus, flujo blanco, pérdidas blancas, excreción vaginal

fluorescein fluoresceína

fluorescence immunoassay fluoroinmunoanálisis, inmunofluorescencia; ~ **polarization immunoassay** fluoroinmunoanálisis de polarización

fluorescent fluorescente; ~ **-antibody test** prueba del anticuerpo fluorescente; ~ **stain** tinción fluorescente

fluorine flúor

fluorodeoxyglucose fluorodeoxiglucosa

fluoroimmunoanalysis fluoroinmunoanálisis

fluorometry fluorimetría

fluoroscope fluoroscopio, aparato de radioscopia, roentgenoscopio

fluoroscopic screen pantalla radioscópica

fluoroscopy fluoroscopía

fluorouracil fluorouracilo

fluoxetine fluoxetina

fluphenazine flufenazina

flush rubor, enrojecimiento; ~ **, to** tirar al retrete, enjuagar

flutter aleteo del corazón, flúter

fluvastatin fluvastatina

fluvoxamine fluvoxamina

flux flujo

fly screen mosquitero, red protectora contra los insectos

foam espuma; ~ **inhibitor** antiespumante

focal focal; ~ **sepsis** sepsis focal; ~ **spots** focos

foci focos

focus foco; ~ **elimination** eliminación del foco

Fogarty balloon catheter catéter balón de Fogarty, sonda de Fogarty

folacin ácido fólic, B9, folacin, folate

folate folato

fold arruga, doblez, pliegue; ~ **of skin or tissue** pliegue, reborde de tejido, plica

folic acid ácido folic, B9, folacin, folate

follicle folículo; ~ **lymphocyte** linfocito folicular; ~ **ripening** maduración del folículo; ~ **-stimulating hormone** hormona foliculoestimulante, folitropina; ~ **-stimulating-hormone-releasing factor** foliberina

follicular folicular; ~ **blepharitis** blefaritis folicular; ~ **dentritic cells** celulas dentricas foliculares; ~ **ileitis** ileítis folicular; ~ **keratosis** queratosis folicular; ~ **tonsillitis** angina folicular, la angina lacunar

folliculitis foliculitis, inflamación de uno o más folículos pilosos; ~ **superficialis staphylogenes** foliculitis superficial estafilocócica

follitropin hormona foliculoestimulante, folitropina

follow-up recordatorio, continuación, seguimiento, catamnesis; ~ **treatment** cuidados posteriores, fase posterior al tratamiento, servicios de terapia de convalescencia

fomite fómite

fontanelle fontanela, espacio no osificado del cráneo en el recién nacido

food alimento; ~ **and Drug Administration (FDA)** Administración de medicamentos y alimentos, Organismo para el control de alimentos y medicamentos, la Dirección de alimentos y drogas/fármacos; ~ **-borne illness** enfermedad transmitida por alimentos; ~ **chain** cadena alimentaria; ~ **hygiene** higiene de los alimentos, higiene alimenticia; ~ **poisoning** intoxicación alimentaria, intoxicación alimenticia; ~ **sanitation** higiene de los alimentos, higiene alimenticia; ~ **-related** alimentario

foot pie, (animal term: pata, zarpa); ~ **and mouth disease** fiebre aftosa; ~ **infection** tiña podal, infección superficial crónica con hongos de la piel del pie; ~ **rot** panadizo interdigital; ~ **splint** férula del pie

footling presentation presentación de pie, presentación podálica

footprint impronta (del pie)

footprinting obtención de la impronta

footwear calzado

for para, por

foramen caecum of tooth orificio ciego de la dentadura; ~ **magnum** foramen magnum

force fuerza; ~ **of morbidity** fuerza de morbilidad

forced forzado; ~ **abduction** abducción forzada; ~ **expiratory volume** volumen expiratorio forzado (en un segundo)

forceps hierros, pinzas

forearm antebrazo

forehead frente, testera, testuz

foreign extraño; ~ **antigen** antígeno extraño, antígeno ajeno; ~ **body macrophage** macrófago para cuerpos extraños; ~ **matter** partículas

forensic forense; ~ **chemistry** química médico-legal; ~ **medicine** medicina legal y forense, medicina legal; ~ **serology** serología forense

forerunner antecedente, precursor, circunstancia anterior en la historia del enfermo, que precede

foreskin prepucio, pliegue que cubre el pene o el clítoris

form documento, formulario

formal neuron neurona artificial

formaldehyde formaldehído, formol

formate formiato

formative tissue tejido indiferente

formication parestesia, sensación de hormigueo, pinchazos

forming metheamoglobin producción de metahemoglobina

formol formol, formaldehído

fornix fórnix; ~ **cerebri** trígono cerebral

forward hacia a delante; ~ **mutation** mutación directa

foster family familia adoptiva; ~ **home** casa de crianza, hogar de adopción, casa de acogida; ~ **parents** padres adoptivos, familia de acogida

foul adj pestilente, fénido, malísimo, f falta; ~ **breath** halitosis, mal aliento, ozostomía; ~ **-smelling sweat** bromhidrosis

four cuatro

fourteen catorce

fourth cuarto

fourty cuarenta

FPIA fluoroinmunoanálisis de polarización

fractile fractil

fraction fracción, parte de un todo, cociente entre dos cantidades

fractionation fraccionamiento; ~ **of human blood plasma** fraccionamiento de plasma

fracture fractura; ~ **healing** regeneración ósea

fragile frágil; ~ **X syndrome** síndrome del X frágil

fragment fragmento; ~ **ion** ión fragmento

frail deformado, endeble, canijo, delicado; ~ **consumptive** héctico, hético

frame-shift mutation mutación del marco de lectura

Francisella tularensis pasteurella tularensis

fraud matasanos, farsante, charlatán

fraudulence curanderiá, charlatanismo, charlatanería

fraudulent fraudulento; ~ **claim** reclamación fraudulenta, reclamo fraudulento

freak deformado, monstruo

freckled pecoso, cubierto de pecas

free libre; ~ **-electron laser** láser de electrones libres; ~ **energy** energía libre; ~ **exudate** exudado libre; ~ **fatty acids** ácidos grasos no esterificados; ~ **floating anxiety** neurosis de ansiedad; ~ **moisture** humedad libre, vapor libre de agua; ~ **of odor** exento de olor; ~ **radical** radical libre, radicales libres; ~ **radical inhibitor** inhibidor de radicales libres

freeing up movilización

freeze-drie producto liofilizado, producto preparado mediante congelación y deshidratación; ~ **-drying** liofilización, criodesecación

freeze, to tener frío; ~ **to death, to** helarse

freezing to death muerte por hipotermia

frequency frecuencia

frequently con frecuencia

fresh semen esperma fresco, semen fresco

friction frotamiento, fricción; ~ **factor** factor de fricción

frictional coefficient coeficiente de fricción

Friday viernes

fried frito

Friedewald's formula fórmula de Friedewald

Friedlander's bacillus Klebsiella pneumoniae

friend amigo, -a

fright susto, espanto

frigidity frigidez, insensibilidad sexual

fringed franjeado

fringes ribete, franjas

from de, a desde, mediante, en, a

frontal frontal, de frente; ~ **lobe** lóbulo frontal

frontoparietal frontoparietal; ~ **operculum** opérculo frontoparietal, opérculo rolándico

frost escarcha, helada; ~ **erythema** eritema por frío

frostbite congelación

froth in mouth babaza

frozen congelado; ~ **semen** esperma ultracongelado; ~ **shoulder** hombro congelado, capsulitis adhesiva

fructaldolase B fructosa-bisfosfato-aldolasa

fructokinase fructocinasa

fructosamine fructosamina

fructose fructosa; ~ **-bisphosphatase** fructosa-bisfosfatasa; ~ **1-phosphate aldolase** fructosa-bisfosfato-aldolasa; ~ **tolerance test** prueba de tolerancia a la fructosa

fruit fruta

frusemide furosemida

FSH folitropina; ~ **-RF** foliberina

FTA anticuerpo fluorescente antitreponémico

Fuchs coloboma coloboma de Fuchs; ~ **dimple** surco de Fuchs; ~ **epithelio-corneal dystrophy** distrofia epitelocorneal de Fuchs; ~ **furrow** surco de Fuchs; ~ **stomata** lagunas de Fuchs; ~ **syndrome** síndrome oculomucocutáneo de Fuchs

fuchsin fucsina, un colorante rojo

full lleno, completo; ~ **blood count** hemograma completo; ~ **-time nursing care** servicio (cuidado) de enfermería de tiempo completo

fullness llenado; ~ **of the bladder** llenado vesical

fumigate fumigar

function función

functional funcional; ~ **adaptation** adaptación funcional; ~ **capacity evaluation** evaluación de capacidad laboral; ~ **orthodontic appliance** aparato ortodóncico funcional; ~ **psychosis** psicosis funcional; ~ **rehabilitation** reeducación funcional, rehabilitación funcional; ~ **test** prueba funcional

fundamental fundamental, fundamental
fundoplication fundoplicación
fungal hongo (m), tumor en forma de hongo;
~ **disease** micosis, enfermedad causada por
hongos, enfermedad de mohos; ~ **infection**
infección de hongos
fungemia fungemia
fungible fungible
fungicide fungicida
fungistatic fungistático, que inhibe el
crecimiento de los hongos
fungus hongo, fungus
funnel embudo
funny gracioso; ~ **bone** olécranon, hueso del
codo
furosemide furosemida
furrow surco, fisura
furuncle furúnculo, chichón, bola, forúnculo,
divieso
furunculosis furunculosis (f), aparición de
furúnculos
fusiform gyrus convolución fusiforme
fusion fusión
fusional fusional; ~ **movement** vergencia
fusional; ~ **vergence** vergencia fusional
fussy mimado, maniático

G

gadget artilugion, aparato, dispositivo, aparejo
gait modo de andar, andadura
galactokinase galactocinasa
galactopoiesis lactogénesis, galactogénesis
galactorrhea galactorrea
galactose galactosa; ~ **oxidase** galactosa-
oxidasa
galactosemia galactosemia, galactocinasa, la
deficiencia de enfermedad por deficiencia de
udpglucosa 4-epimerasa
galactosidase galactosidasa
galenical galénico, preparado a partir de drogas
vegetales en vez de sustancias químicas
gall hiel, caradura; ~ **bladder** vesícula biliar;
~ **bladder disease** bilis, mal de hiel, la
colecistitis; ~ **duct** conducto biliar
galley proof galerada

gallstone cálculo biliar, colelitiasis; ~ **ileus** íleo
biliar
galtonian inheritance herencia poligenica
galvanocautery galvanocauterio
gamete gameto, célula generadora;
~ **intrafallopian transfer** transferencia
intratubaria de gametos, transferencia de
gametos en las trompas; ~ **recognition**
reconocimiento de gametos
gamma globulin gamaglobulina; ~ **globulin
prophylaxis** profilaxia por gamaglobulina;
~ **globulin transfer** transferencia
transplacentaria de gammaglobulina; ~ **GT** g-
glutamiltransferasa; ~ **-indicator diagnosis**
diagnóstico por gammagrafía; ~ **interferon**
interferón gamma, interferón inmune;
~ **radiation** rayos gamma; ~ **rays** rayos gamma
gammagraphy gammagrafía
ganciclovir ganciclovir
ganglion ganglio, engrosamiento localizado en
un nervio o vaso linfático
ganglioneuroblastoma ganglioneuroblastoma
ganglioneuroma ganglioneuroma, ganglioma
ganglionic ganglionar; ~ **blocking agent**
agente bloqueante ganglionar; ~ **neuroma**
ganglioneuroma, ganglioma
gangrene necrólisis, gangrena, necrosis
gangrenous gangrenoso; ~ **cholecystitis**
colecistitis gangrenosa
gapped DNA DNA incompleto
garden jardín
gargle, to hacer gárgaras
gargling gargarismo
Gartner's bacillus Salmonella enteriditis
gas flatulencia, meteorismo;
~ **chromatography** cromatografía de gases;
~ **gangrene** gangrena gaseosa; ~ **-liquid
chromatography** cromatografía gas-líquido;
~ **-permeable lenses** lentes gas-permeables;
~ **sterilizer** esterilizador por gas
gash cuchillada, cortadura profunda, inciso
gasoline gasolina
gasp, to jadear, acezar, resollar, quedar sin
aliento
gasping for breath jadeo, respiración
superficial y rápida, hacer esfuerzos para
respirar
gastralgia gastralgia, dolor de estómago

gastric gástrico; ~ **acid** ácido gástrico; ~ **balloon** balón gástrico; ~ **bubble** balón gástrico; ~ **cancer** cáncer gástrico, cáncer de estómago; ~ **contents** contenido gástrico; ~ **glands** glándulas gástricas; ~ **ileus** íleo gástrico; ~ **inhibitory peptide** polipeptido inhibidor gástrico; ~ **intubation** intubación gástrica, intubación gastrointestinal; ~ **juice** jugo gástrico; ~ **lavage** lavado del estómago, lavado gástrico, purga; ~ **lymph node** ganglio linfático gástrico; ~ **lymphatic nodule** nódulo linfático gástrico; ~ **mucosa** mucosa gástrica, revestimiento del estómago; ~ **surface of the liver** superficie gástrica del hígado; ~ **ulcer** úlcera gástrica; ~ **wall** pared del estomago

gastricine gastricsina

gastrin gastrina

gastritis gastritis, inflamación del estómago

gastrocnemius muscle músculo esqueletico, los músculos gemelos de la pierna

gastroduodenal gastroduodenal, relativo al estómago y al intestino delgado simultáneamente

gastroenteritis gastroenteritis, inflamación del estómago y del intestino delgado

gastroenterocolitis gastroenterocolitis

gastroenterostomy gastroenterostomía

gastroesophageal gastroesofágico, relativo al estómago y al esófago

gastrogavage alimentación por sonda

gastrointestinal gastrointestinal, relativo al estómago y a los intestinos; ~ **absorption** absorción gastrointestinal; ~ **bleeding** hemorragia gastrointestinal; ~ **hormone** hormona gastrointestinal; ~ **scan** gammagrafía gástrica; ~ **scintigraphy** gammagrafía gástrica; ~ **tolerance** tolerancia gastrointestinal; ~ **tract** tracto intestinal, tubo digestivo, aparato digestivo

gastrooesophageal gastroesofágico, relativo al estómago y al esófago

gastroscope gastroscopio

gastroscopy gastroscopia

gastrostomy gastrostomía

gastrula blastoporo; ~ gástrula, arquenteron, blastoporo, intestino primitivo

gastrulation gastrulación

gated imaging imagen de compuerta

gauze gasa; ~ **dressing** apósito de gasa; ~ **strip for bandages** venda de gasa para apósito

gavage feeding alimentación por sonda

G-CSF (Granulocyte–Colony Stimulation Factor) G-CSF, factor estimulador de colonias de granulocitos

Geiger–Müller counter contador Geiger

gelatinous mucoso, gelatinoso; ~ **tumor** mixoma, tumor coloide, tumor gelatinoso, tumor mucoso, mixoblastoma

gender sexo, género; ~ **selection** predeterminación del sexo

gene gen; ~ **bank** genoteca; ~ **cloning** clonación de genes; ~ **coding for degradation of xenobiotics** gen que codifica la degradación de xenobióticos; ~ **coupling** apareamiento génico; ~ **deletion** deleción génica; ~ **disruption** interrupción génica; ~ **dosage** dosis génica; ~ **library** genoteca; ~ **manipulation** manipulación génica; ~ **tagging** marcado génico; ~ **targeting** reconocimiento génico; ~ **tracking** seguimiento génico; ~ **translocation** translocación de un gen

genealogy árbol genealógico, estudio genealógico, genealogía

general general; ~ **anesthesia** anestesia general; ~ **medical practice** consultorio de medicina general; ~ **physical examination** reconocimiento médico, exploración, examen, seguimiento médico; ~ **practitioner** médico de familia, médico generalista

generalized generalizado; ~ **anxiety** ansiedad generalizada; ~ **tonic–clonic seizure** gran mal, epilepsia generalizada

generic genérico; ~ **medication** medicamento genérico; ~ **medicine** medicamento genérico

genetic genético, relativo a los genes o a la herencia; ~ **adaptation** adaptación genética; ~ **background** contexto genético; ~ **carrier** vector genético; ~ **change** cambio genómico; ~ **cleaving** segmentación; ~ **code** código genético, clave genética; ~ **counseling** consejo genetico; ~ **disjunction** disyunción genética; ~ **engineering** ingeniería genética, manipulación genética; ~ **footprint** huella genética, dermatoglifia del ADN, impronta genética; ~ **imprint** huella genética,

dermatoglifia del ADN, impronta genética;
~ **information** información genética;
~ **inversion** inversión genética; ~ **load** carga
genética; ~ **manipulation** ingeniería genética,
manipulación genética; ~ **map** mapa
cromosómico, mapa genético; ~ **mapping**
cartografía genética; ~ **marker** marcador
genético; ~ **oncology** oncología genetica;
~ **polymorphism** polimorfismo genético;
~ **predisposition** predisposición genética;
~ **protein engineering** ingeniería de
proteínas; ~ **screening** detección genética,
tamizaje genética; ~ **therapy** terápia genética,
genoterapia; ~ **toxicology** toxicología
genética; ~ **transcription** transcripción
genética; ~ **transfer** transferencia genética;
~ **units** unidades genéticas; ~ **variability**
variabilidad genética

genetically geneticamente, por ingeniería
genética; ~ **engineered hemoglobin**
hemoglobina modificada por ingeniería
genética; ~ **modified organism** organismo
modificado genéticamente

geneticist genetista

genetics genética

genital genital, relativo a los órganos sexuales;
~ **canal** conducto genital; ~ **diseases** afección
genitales; ~ **herpes** herpes genital; ~ **pruritis**
prurito genital; ~ **region** entresijo; ~ **wart**
condiloma acuminado, verrugas genitales

genitalia vergüenzas, genitales

genitals genitales, partes (nobles, ocultas,
privadas), vergüenzas, genitales

genitourinary genitourinario

genome genoma; ~ **mutation** mutación de
genomio, mutación génica

genomic genómico; ~ **change** cambio
genómico; ~ **imprinting** huella genómica;
~ **library** genoteca genómica, biblioteca
genómica; ~ **mismatch scanning** rastreo
genómico de malapareamiento; ~ **resource**
recurso de origen genómico

genomics genómica

genotype genotipo

gentamicin gentamicina

genupectoral genupectoral

geographic geográfico; ~ **tongue** lengua
geográfica

GERD (gastroesophageal reflux disease)
enfermedad por reflujo gastroesofágico (GERD)

geriatric geriátrico, relativo a la medicina que
trata de las enfermedades de la vejez; ~ **nurse**
enfermera geriatrica

geriatrician geriatra, un médico especializado
en geriatría

geriatrics geriatría

germ microorganismo, microbio; ~ **carrier**
portador de gérmenes; ~ **gene therapy** terápia
germinal; ~ **plasm** germoplasma; ~ **vector**
portador de gérmenes, portador de la
infección; ~ **warfare** guerra biológica

German alemán; ~ **measles** rubéola, sarampión
alemán, sarampión de los tres días

germanium germanio

germicidal germicido, germicida

germinal germinal; ~ **center** centro germinal;
~ **epithelium** epitelio germinal, epitelio
germinativo; ~ **tissue** tejido embrionario

germs gérmenes, micróbios

gerontological gerontológico

gerontology gerontología, estudio de la vejez

Gerstmann-Sträussler-Scheinker syndrome
síndrome de Gerstmann-Sträussler-Scheinker

gestation gestación, embarazo; ~ **nephrosis**
nefrosis gravidica; ~ **tetany** tetania gravidica

gestational gravidico; ~ **myocardiopathy**
miocardiopatía gravidica; ~ **protein** proteína
gravidica

gesticulate, to manotear, gesticular

gestodene gestodén

get, to recibir, obtener, contraer (illness), tener,
conseguir; ~ **a haircut, to** hacerse cortar el
pelo; ~ **an erection, to** tener una erección,
tener la tiesa; ~ **goosebumps, to** enchinarse
(la piel); ~ **hot, to** calentarse, quedar caliente;
~ **sick again, to** sofrir una recaída, sofrir una
reincidencia; ~ **up, to** levantarse; ~ **well, to**
recuperarse, restablecerse, sanarse

getting well restablecimiento, curación,
recuperación, restitución

GFR caudal de filtración glomerular

g-glutamyltransferase g-glutamiltransferasa

GGT gamma glutamyl transpeptidase GGT,
gamma glutamil transferasa

GGTP (gamma glutamyl transpeptidase)
gamma-GT (gamma glutamil transpeptidasa),

g-glutamiltransferasa

GH somatotropina, hormona del crecimiento

Ghon–Sachs bacillus Clostridium septicum

ghost image fantasma, efecto de eco

GH–RF somatoliberina

giant gigante, enorme; **~ cell arteritis** arteritis de células gigantes, arteritis temporal, vasculitis sistémica; **~ cell fibroma** fibroma de células gigantes; **~ cell granuloma** granuloma de células gigantes; **~ cell of bone marrow** megacariocito; **~ cell sarcoma** sarcoma gigantocelular; **~ cell tumor** tumor de células gigantes; **~ hypertrophic gastritis** gastritis hipertrófica gigante

Giardia lamblia infection giardiasis, lambliasis

giardiasis giardiasis, lambliasis

Gibbs free energy energía libre de Gibbs

Gibson glioma glioma de Gibson

giddy, to be estar mareado

Giemsa stain tinción de Giemsa

GIFT transferencia intratubaria de gametos, transferencia de gametos en las trompa

Gilchrist disease blastomicosis norteamericana

Gilles de la Tourette syndrome síndrome de Gilles de la Tourette

gingivitis gingivitis, inflamación de las encías

gingivopericementitis periodontoclasia, gingivopericementitis, paradontólisis

Ginkgo biloba ginkgo biloba

ginseng ginseng, panax

Giordano–Giovanetti diet dieta de Giordano-Giovanetti

girl niña

give, to dar; **~ a medical certificate, to** dar la baj; **~ birth, to** aliviarse, alumbrar, dar a luz, acostar

giving birth parto

glabella glabella

glabellar glabellar; **~ lines** líneas glabellares

glandular glandular; **~ cheilitis** queilitis glandular; **~ fever** mononucleosis infecciosa, angina monocítica; **~ kallikrein** calicreína hística; **~ phlegmon** flemón glandular

glans penis glándulas del pene

Glanzmann's thrombasthenia trombastenia de Glanzmann, un trastorno congenito de sangramiento

glass vaso

glasses espejuelos, gafas, lentes

glassy vítreo, cristalino

glaucoma glaucoma; **~ tolerance test** prueba de carga para el diagnóstico de glaucoma

glaucosuria orinas azules

glenohumeral glenohumeral

glenosporosis blastomicosis por glenospora, glenosporosis

gliadin gliadina, una sustancia proteica que se obtiene del gluten del trigoy del centeno

glial glial; **~ cells** células gliales del cerebro; **~ reticulum** retículo glial

gliclazide gliclazida, un farmaco hipoglicemico sulfonilurea que estimula la secreción de insulina

glimepiride glimepirida

glioblastoma multiforme glioblastoma multiforme

glioma glioma, tumor cerebral que está compuesto de células gliales malignas; **~ of the optic nerve** glioma del nervio óptico

glipizide glipizida, un antidiabético oral

Glisson's capsule capsula fibrosa del higado, capsula fibrosa perivascularis

global mundial, global; **~ aphasia** afasia completa; **~ cardiac insufficiency** insuficiencia cardiaca global

globin globina

globular globular

globulin globulina

glomerular glomerular, relativo a la parte filtrante del riñón; **~ filtrate** filtrado glomerular; **~ filtration** filtración glomerular; **~ filtration rate** velocidad de filtración glomerular, caudal de filtración glomerular; **~ lesion** lesión glomerular

glomeruli glomérulos

glomerulonephritis glomerulonefritis, enfermedad renal con inflamación de los glomérulos, filtros del riñón

glomerulus glomérulo

glomus typmpanicum paraganglios no cromafines, paraganglios parasimpáticos

glossitis glositis, glossitis, inflamación de la lengua

glossodynia glosodinia, dolor en la lengua

glossolalia glosolalia, la emisión de palabras en un leguaje desconocido que suele producirse en estado de éxtasis

glossopharyngeal glosofaríngeo; ~ **nerve** nervio glosofaríngeo

glottis glotis; ~ **stroke** cierre glótico, glotis traumática; ~ **-closing muscles** músculos constrictores de la glotis

gloves guantes

glucagon glucagón; ~ **liver function test** prueba de la fusión hepática con glucagón

glucan glucano

glucemia concentración de glucosa en plasma/suero

glucocerebrosidase glucosilceramidasa

glucocorticoid glucocorticoide

glucogenic glucógeno; ~ **cardiomegaly** cardiomegalia glucógena

glucokinase glucocinasa, hexocinasa

gluconate kinase gluconocinasa

gluconokinase gluconocinasa

glucosamine glucosamina

glucose glucosa, dextrosa, azúcar de uva; ~ **1-dehydrogenase** glucosa-1-deshidrogenasa; ~ **-galactose malabsorption** malabsorción de glucosa y galactosa; ~ **isomerase** glucosa isomerasa; ~ **metabolic rate** tasa metabólica de glucosa; ~ **oxidase** glucosa-oxidasa; ~ **-6-phosphatase** glucosa-6-fosfatasa; ~ **-6-phosphate dehydrogenase deficiency** déficit de glucosa-6-fosfato deshidrogenasa; ~ **resorption** resorción de glucosa; ~ **syrup** jarabe de glucosa; ~ **tolerance** tolerancia a la glucosa; ~ **tolerance test** prueba de tolerancia a la glucosa

glucosidase glucosidasa

glucosuria concentración de glucosa en orina, excreción de glucosa en orina

glucuronic glucurónico; ~ **acid** ácido glucurónico

glucuronidase glucuronidasa

glucuronosyltransferase glucuronosiltransferasa

glutamate glutamato

glutamic acid ácido glutámico

glutaminase glutaminasa

glutamine glutamina

glutathione glutatión; ~ **reductase (NADPH)** glutatión-reductasa (NADPH); ~ **reductase deficiency anemia** anemia por carencia de glutatión-reductasa; ~ **synthase** glutatión-sintasa; ~ **synthetase** glutatión-sintasa

gluten gluten (m); ~ **disintegration** desintegración del gluten; ~ **induced enteropathy** enfermedad celíaca; ~ **tolerance test** prueba de tolerancia al gluten

glutethimide glutetimida, un fármaco sedante

glutinous mucoso, gelatinoso

glycated hemoglobin glicohemoglobina

glycemia glucemia

glycerol glicerol; ~ **kinase** glicerol-cinasa

glyceryl trinitrate nitroglicerina

glycine glicina; ~ **tolerance test** prueba de tolerancia a la glicina

glycogen glucógeno; ~ **-storage disease** glucogenosis; ~ **synthase** glucógeno-sintasa

glycogenosis glucogenosis

glycohemoglobin glicohemoglobina

glycopeptide glicopéptido

glycophorin glicoforina

glycoprotein glucoproteína

glycopyrrolate glucopirrolato

glycosaminoglycan glicosaminoglicano, mucopolisacárida

glycoside glucósido; ~ **hydrolase** glicósido hidrolasa

glycosuria glucosuria, presencia de la glucosa en la orina

glycosylated hemoglobin glicohemoglobina

glycosylation glicosilación

GM-CSF (granulocyte-macrophage-colony stimulation factor) GM-CSF

GMP (guanosine 5'-monophosphate) guanosina 5'-monofosfato

gnathology gnatología

gnathospasm trismo, imposibilidad de apertura total de la boca, trismus

go, to ir

goal gol, meta; ~ **of treatment** meta del tratamiento

going pallid blanqueamiento

goiter estruma, bocio, engrosamiento del tiroides

gold oro; ~ **miner's disease** silicosis de los obreros de las minas de oro

Goldberg-Maxwell-Morris syndrome seudohermafroditismo

golfer's elbow epicondilitis por humedad, codo

de tenista
gomphosis gonfosis, gonfiasis
gonad gónada
gonadal gonadal, relativo a las glándulas
  sexuales; ~ **dysgenesis** disgenesia gonadal;
  ~ **dysgenesis XO** síndrome de Turner
gonadorelin gonadorelina, hormona de
  liberación de la gonadotrofina
gonadotrope gonadotropo, que estimula las
  glándulas sexuales
gonadotrophin gonadotropina; ~ **releasing**
  hormone (GRH) hormona de liberación de la
  gonadotrofina
gonadotropic gonadotropo
gonadotropin gonadotropina; ~ **-releasing**
  factor gonadoliberina
gonads testículos, gonadas masculinas
gonarthrosis artrosis de la rodilla
gonioscopy gonioscopia, examen del ángulo de
  la cámara anterior del ojo
gonococcus Neisseria gonorrhoeae
gonorrhea blenorragia, gonorrea, chorro
gonosomal gonosómico; ~ **heredity** herencia
  gonosómica
good bien (adv), bueno (adj); ~ **taste** decoro,
  respeto
Goodpasture's syndrom estenosis de la válvula
  pulmonar, síndrome de Goodpasture
goose flesh cutis anserina
gout gota, tofo
Gowers contraction signo de Gowers;
  ~ **disease** enfermedad de Gowers, síndrome de
  Gowers; ~ **hemoglobinometer**
  hemoglobinómetro de Gowers; ~ **syndrome**
  enfermedad de Gowers, síndrome de Gowers
gown camisón
Graafian follicle folículo de Graaf, folículo
  ovárico
grade grado
Gradenigo's syndrome síndrome de Gradenigo
gradual gradual, poco a poco
Graf pneumothorax neumotórax de Graf
graft injerto; ~ **rejection** rechazo de un injerto
grafting trasplante
grain itch eccema de los graneros, prurito de los
  cereales
gram gramo; ~ **negative** gramnegativo;
  ~ **positive** grampositivo; ~ **stain** tinción de

Gram, coloración de Gram
grand mal gran mal, epilepsia generalizada
grandfather abuelo
grandmother abuela
granular granular; ~ **induration** induración
  granular, cirrosis; ~ **layer of epidermis** capa
  queratohialina, capa granulosa de la
  epidermis; ~ **plasma** plasma granuloso;
  ~ **vaginitis** colpitis granular de las vacas
granulated granulado, preparación
  farmacéutica en forma de gránulos
granulation granulación; ~ **tissue** grano
  exuberante, tejido de granulación
granules granulado
granulocyte granulocito
granulocytopenia granulocitopenia
granuloma granuloma; ~ **annulare** granuloma
  anular
granulomatous granulatomoso; ~ **interstitial**
  pulmonary disease enfermedad intersticial
  pulmonar granulatomosa; ~ **liver damage**
  lesión hepática granulomatosa
grape uva; ~ **sugar** glucosa, dextrosa, azúcar de
  uva
grasping reflex reflejo de prensión palmar
gratuitous gratuito; ~ **inducer** inductor
  gratuito
gravidity gravidez, embarazo, gestación
gravimetry gravimetría
g-ray rayo g
gray gray; ~ **degeneration** degeneración gris;
  ~ **matter in the brain** materia gris del cerebro
grayish blue livido
graze abrasión, erosión dentaria, desgaste,
  raspado
greasy grasoso, graso, grasiento, aceitoso,
  resbaladizo, lúbrico, resbaloso; ~ **blepharitis**
  blefaritis oleosa
great grande
greater trochanter trocánter mayor
green verde
grey gris
grief duelo, luto
grieving duelo, luto
grind, to molar, machar, majar, molturar,
  micronizar, reducir a polvo fino
grinding one's teeth bruxomanía
grip apretón; ~ **strength** fuerza de sujeción

gripe cólico, espasmo abdominal, retortijón
griseofulvin griseofulvina
groan, to gemir, lamentarse
Groenblad-Strandberg syndrome síndrome de Grönblad-Strandberg
grogginess obnubilación
groin aldilla, entrepiernas, ingle
grooming hábitos de limpieza
groove fisura, hendidura, cisura, surco
gross flagrante, ordinario, basto; ~ **mutation** mutación voluminosa
group grupo; ~ **counseling** asesoramiento para grupos; ~ **hospitalization insurance** seguro colectivo de asistencia médica; ~ **practice** medicina de grupo; ~ **psychotherapy** psicoterapia de grupo, terapia de grupo; ~ **therapy** psicoterapia de grupo, terapia de grupo
growth crecimiento, aumento; ~ **factor** factor de crecimiento, promotor del crecimiento; ~ **hormone** somatotropina, hormona del crecimiento; ~ **hormone-releasing factor** somatoliberina; ~ **promotor** factor de crecimiento, promotor del crecimiento; ~ **stimulant** estimulante de crecimiento
GTP, guanosine triphosphate guanosina-trifosfato
guanine guanina
guanosine guanosina
guanylate kinase guanilato-cinasa
gullet esófago, tragante, tragadero, gaznate; ~ **inflammation** esofagitis
gum encía; ~ **inflammation** gingivitis, inflamación superficial de la encía
gummatous abscess úlcera sifilítica
gunshot balazo, tiro, disparo; ~ **wound** herida de bala, herida por arma de fuego
gurgle, to borbotear
gurgling sound ruido de bazuqueo, ruido de molino
gurney camilla con ruedas, portacama rodante, parihuelas
gustation sentido del gusto
gut abdomen, vientre
gutta percha gutapercha
guttate gotas; ~ **infiltration** infiltración en gotas
Guyon's canal syndrome síndrome del canal de Guyon

gynecoid ginecoide; ~ **biotype** biotipo ginecoide; ~ **pelvis** pelvis ginecoide
gynecological ginecológico; ~ **instrument** instrumento para ginecología
gynecologist ginecológico
gynecology ginecología
gynecomastia ginecomastia
gynelogical ginecológico

H

habitual habitual, acostumbrado; ~ **abortion** aborto habitual, trés o más abortos espontáneos consecutivos
habituate acostumbrar, habituar
habituated to corticosteroids dependente de corticosteroides
habituation habituación
habitus habitus; ~ **phthisicus** habitus tísico
hæm hemo; ~ **synthetase** ferroquelatasa
Hageman factor factor XIIa de la coagulación; ~ **factor deficiency** enfermedad de Hageman
hair pelo; ~ **brush** cepillo para el pelo; ~ **bulge** tumescencia pilosa; ~ **cell** célula sensorial de Corti; ~ **-erector muscle** músculo piloerector, músculo erector del pelo; ~ **follicle** folículo piloso; ~ **matrix** folículo piloso, matriz del pelo; ~ **papilla** papila pilosa; ~ **penetration test** prueba de la penetración capilar; ~ **root** folículo piloso, pelo radical
hairball (in stomach) bola de pelo (en el estomago)
hairiness hirsutismo, vellosidad exagerada en la mujer
hairpin horquilla
hairy peludo, cabelludo, piloso
half medio, -a; ~ **-life** semivida; ~ **-life of red corpuscles** vida media de los eritrocitos; ~ **-upright position** posición semiincorporado
halfway house unidad de día, residencia de transición
halisteresis osteohalistéresis, reblandecimiento de los huesos por resorción o aporte insuficiente de sales
halitosis halitosis, mal aliento, ozostomía

hallucination alucinación

hallucinatory alucinógeno; ~ **action** acción alucinógena; ~ **confusion** confusión alucinatoria

hallux hallux; ~ **valgus** hallux valgus

halo effect efecto halo

halogenated halogenado; ~ **hydrocarbon** hidrocarburo halogenado

halon halón

haloperidol haloperidol

halothane halotano

hamamelis hamamelis

hamate bone hueso ganchoso, hueso unciforme

Hamman disease síndrome de Hamman, el enfisema mediastínico de Hamman; ~ **mediastinal emphysema** síndrome de Hamman, el enfisema mediastínico de Hamman

Hammer symptom síntoma de Hammer

hammertoe dedo en martillo

Hammond wire-arch splint férula de arco de Hammond

Hamolsky tri-iodothyronine test prueba de la tri-iodotironina de Hamolsky

hamstring muscles músculos isquiosurales; ~ **tendon** tendón del hueso poplíteo, tendón de la corva, tendón isquirosural

hand mano; ~ **ophtalmoscope** oftalmoscopia manual; ~ **prosthesis** prótesis de la mano

handicap impedimento, incapacidad

handicapped minusválido, disminuidodis, discapacitado; ~ **person** persona con impedimento, persona con desventaja, incapacitado, minusválido

hanging pendiente; ~ **drop** gota pendiente

hangnail padrastro, respigón

hangover resaca, cruda

Hanot cirrhosis cirrosis de Hanot, enfermedad de Hanot; ~ **disease** cirrosis de Hanot, enfermedad de Hanot

Hansen's bacillus Mycobacterium leprae; ~ **disease** lepra

Hantaan virus virus Hantaan, hantavirus

hantavirus virus Hantaan, hantavirus

haphephobia haptofobia, hafefobia

haploid haploide

haplotype haplotipo

hapten hapteno

haptoglobin haptoglobina

haptonomy haptonomía

haptophobia haptofobia, hafefobia

hard duro; ~ **chancre** chancro de Hunter, cancro duro; ~ **glioma** glioma sólido; ~ **palate** paladar duro, bóveda; ~ **ulcer of primary syphilis** induración de Hunter, induración sifilítica

hardened calloso, endurecido; ~ **testicle** testículo endurecido

hardening aguante, resistencia, endurecimiento, induración; ~ **of fats** hidrogenación de grasas; ~ **of the arteries** endurecimiento de las arterias

hare liebre; ~ **lip** labio cucho, labio leporino, labio fisurado

harm, to lastimar, dañar, abusar

harmful adverso, contrario, desfavorable, pernicioso, peligroso, aniquilante, grave, maligno, de evolución fatal; ~ **to your health** dañino, nocivo, dañoso, pernicioso, desfavorable

harmless inocuo, que no causa daño

Harris syndrom hiperinsulinismo espontáneo

Hashimoto thyroiditis tiroiditis de Hashimoto

hashish hachís, hashish, cannabis

Hasner's fold válvula de Bianchi, pliegue de Hasner

have, to haber, tener; ~ **a relapse, to** sofrir una recaída, sofrir una reincidencia; ~ **gas, to** estar envarado; ~ **sex, to** tener relaciones sexuales, hacer uso de, juntarse con, practicar el coito, copular, usar

Haversian canals conductos de Havers; ~ **glands** glándulas de Havers; ~ **system** conductos de Havers

hay heno; ~ **fever** fiebre del heno

hazardous peligroso; ~ **waste** residuo peligroso

HBsAg hepatitis B surface antigen HBsAg, antígeno de superficie de la hepatitis-B

HDL -colesterol colesterol de HDL; ~ **high-density lipoprotein** lipoproteína de alta densidad, HDL

he él

head cabeza; ~ **cold** romadizo; ~ **injury** lesión a la cabeza; ~ **nurse** enfermera supervisora, jefa de turno; ~ **of femur** cabeza del fémur; ~ **of humerus** cabeza del húmero, capítulo humeral; ~ **of muscle** cabeza del músculo

headache cefalalgia, dolor de cabeza; ~ **tablets** pastillas para dolor de cabeza; ~ **, to have a** tener dolor de cabeza

headcap aparato craniocervical de ortodoncia, castillete ortodontico

headgear aparato craniocervical de ortodoncia, castillete ortodontico

heal, to medicinar, curar, medicamentar, medicar, sanar

healing curación, cura, *adj* curativo, sanativo; ~ **mudpack** barro termal, barro terapéutico, sedimentos curativos, fangoterapia; ~ **wound** encarnado, hinchamiento

health salud, sanidad, salubridad; ~ **care** atención médica, prestaciones sanitarias, asistencia sanitaria; ~ **care fraud** fraude en la atención médica, abuso en las prestaciones médicas; ~ **care provider** profesional sanitario; ~ **care services** atención médica, prestaciones sanitarias, asistencia sanitaria; ~ **club** gimnasio; ~ **Department** servicio sanitario; ~ **facilities** instituciones de salud; ~ **food** alimentos saludables; ~ **insurance** seguro de enfermedad; ~ **professional** profesional sanitario, personal sanitario; ~ **worker** profesional sanitario, personal sanitario

healthful curativo, sanativo, salubre, saludable, sano; ~ **living environment** habitación salubre

healthy sano, robusto, de salud fuerte

hearing audición, oído; ~ **aid** audífono, prótesis auditiva, aparato para sordos; ~ **apparatus** aparato para sordos; ~ **disorder** hipoacusia, trastorno de la audición, sordera parcial; ~ **impaired** duro de oído, con un defecto acústico; ~ **-impaired person** sordo, sorda; ~ **impairment** sordera, deterioro de la capacidad auditiva; ~ **relief** relieve acústico

heart corazón; ~ **action** trabajo del corazón; ~ **attack** infarto de miocardio, el ataque cardíaco; ~ **beat** latido, pálpitación; ~ **complaint** precordialgias; ~ **disease** enfermedad del corazón, cardiopatía; ~ **failure** fallo cardíaco; ~ **-lung transplant** transplante cardíaco-pulmonar; ~ **massage** masaje cardíaco externo; ~ **monitor** electrocardiografía; ~ **murmur** soplo del

corazón, soplo cardíaco; ~ **muscle tension** precarga; ~ **palpitation** palpitación cardíaca, vahidos, angustia cardíaca; ~ **throb** palpitación cardíaca, vahidos, angustia cardíaca; ~ **transplant** transplante cardíaco; ~ **trouble** precordialgias; ~ **valve** válvula cardíaca; ~ **valve disease** enfermedad de la valvula cardíaca; ~ **valve prolapse** prolapso de las valvulas cardíacas; ~ **valve replacement** prótesis valvular cardiaca

heartache angustia

heartbeat pulsación, latido rítmico, latido del corazón

heartburn acedías, pirosis, agrior, cardialgia, dolor precordial

heat calor; ~ **capacity** capacidad térmica; ~ **cramps** contractura por calor; ~ **-induced erythema** eritema calórico; ~ **regulation** termorregulación, regulación del calor o de la temperatura; ~ **shock** choque térmico; ~ **sterilization** esterilización por calor; ~ **stress** incomodidad térmica, malestar por causa del frio/del calor; ~ **stroke** golpe de calor, siriasis

heating pad almohada eléctrica, cojín eléctrico

heavy pesado; ~ **metals** metales pesados

heel talón; ~ **bone** calcáneo; ~ **of the foot** talón; ~ **spur** espolón calcáneo; ~ **to toe** marcha de funambulo

Heidenhain gastric mucosa cell célula gástrica de Heidenhain

height altitud, tallo

Heimlich maneuver maniobra de Heimlich

helicobacter pylori Helicobacter pylori

heliosis insolación, asoleada, solanera

heliotropin piperonal

helium hélio

helix helice; ~ **of protein chains** helice de cadenas polimericas de proteína

Heller operation operación de Heller, esofagocardiomiotomía extramucosa; ~ **procedure** operación de Heller, esofagocardiomiotomía extramucosa

hello hola

HELLP syndrome síndrome de HELLP, (H) hemolisis, que es pérdida de glóbulos rojos, (EL) elevado número de enzimas en el hígado, (LP) bajo número de plaquetas

helminth helminto
help, to asistir, ayudar, apoyar
helper auxiliar; ~ **cell** célula T4, linfocito T4,
linfocito coadyuvante, linfocito colaborador;
~ **lymphocyte** célula T4, linfocito T4, linfocito
coadyuvante, linfocito colaborador
helpless feel, to sentirse desamparado
Helsinki Accord acuerdos de Helsinki,
declaración de Helsinki; ~ **Declaration**
acuerdos de Helsinki, declaración de Helsinki
hem hemo; ~ **synthase** ferroquelatasa
hemacytometer chamber cámara
hemocitométrica
hemadynamometer esfigmomanómetro
hemagglutination hemaglutinación;
~ **inhibition** inhibición de la hemaglutinación;
~ **inhibition test** prueba de la inhibición de la
hemaglutinación
hemagglutinin hemaglutinina
hemangioma hemangioma, tumor benigno
constituido por una masa de vasos sanguíneos
hemangiosarcoma hemangiosarcoma
hematemesis hematemesis, vómitos de sangre
hematochezia defecación sanguinolenta, sangre
en el excremento, hematozequia
hematocolpos hematocolpos
hematocrit hematócrito
hematogene hematógeno; ~ **acidose** acidosis
hematógena
hematogone hemocitoblasto, hematogonia,
hemoblasto
hematological hematológico, relativo a la
hematología
hematologist hematólogo
hematology hematología; ~ hematología
hematoma hematoma, acumulación de sangre
extravasada
hematophagous hematófago, hematofágico
hematoplastic hematoplástico
hematopoiesis hematopoyesis
hematopoietic hematopoyético; ~ **stem cell**
célula madre hematopoyética; ~ **system**
sistema hematopoyético; ~ **tissue** tejido
hematopoyético
hematoxilyn and eosin stain tinción con
hematoxilina y eosina
hematuria hematuria, orina sanguinolenta
hemeprotein hemoproteína

hemeralopia hemeralopía, ceguera diurna
hemihypalgesia hipoalgesia unilateral
hemimelia hemimelia
hemiparesis hemiparesia
hemipelvectomy hemipelvectomía
hemiplegia hemiplejía, parálisis total o parcial
de un lado del cuerpo
hemiplegic hemiplégico; ~ **gait** marcha
hemiplégica; ~ **migraine** jaqueca clásica,
migraña hemiplégica, migraña con hemiplejía
hemisomia hemisomía
hemochromatosis hemocromatosis, diabetes
bronceada
hemocytoblast hemocitoblasto, hematogonia,
hemoblasto
hemodialysis hemodiálisis (f)
hemoglobin hemoglobina; ~ **A1**
glicohemoglobina; ~ **electrophoresis**
electroforesis de la hemoglobina; ~ **tolerance
test** prueba de tolerancia a la hemoglobina
hemoglobinopathy hemoglobinopatía
hemoglobinuria hemoglobinuria
hemogram recuento sanguíneo, hematimetría,
hemograma, fórmula sanguínea
hemolysis hemólisis; ~ **shock** choque hemolítico
hemolytic hemolítico; ~ **anemia** anemia
hemolítica; ~ **diseases** enfermedades
hemolíticas; ~ **streptococces** estreptococos
hemolíticos; ~ **uremic syndrome** síndrome
hemolítico-uremico
hemolyzed hemolizado; ~ **blood** sangre
hemolizada
hemopathy hemopatía, enfermedad de la
sangre
hemoperfusion hemoperfusión
hemophilia hemofilia, hemopatía hereditaria
hemophiliac hemofílico
hemophilic hemofílico; ~ **arthritis** artritis
hemofílica
hemopoietic hemopoyético, que forma sangre
hemoptoe hemoptisis severa
hemoptysis hemoptisis (f), expulsión de sangre
de los pulmones
hemorrhage hemorragia
hemorrhagic hemorrágico; ~ **pleurisy** pleuresía
hemorrágica
hemorrhoidal hemorroidal; ~ **proctitis** proctitis
hemorroidal; ~ **prolapse** prolapso hemorroidal

hemorrhoidectomy hemorroidectomía
hemorrhoids / piles hemorroides, almorranas
hemosiderin hemosiderina
hemostasis hemostasia
hemostatic hemostático; ~ **preparation** hemostático
hemotherapy hemoterapia
hemovigilance system sistema de hemovigilancia
hemoximeter hemoxímetro
Henderson-Hasselbach equation ecuación de Henderson-Hasselbach
henna alheña
henry henry
heparin heparina
heparinized heparinizado; ~ **blood** sangre heparinizada; ~ **syringe** jeringuilla heparinizada
hepatic hepático; ~ **amebiasis** amebiasis hepática; ~ **amebic abscess** amibiasis hepática; ~ **cirrhosis** cirrosis del hígado; ~ **clearance** depuración hepática; ~ **colic** cólica hepática; ~ **lobe** lóbulo hepático; ~ **lymph node** ganglio linfático retrohepático
hepatitis A / B / C hepatitis, inflamación del hígado; ~ **antibodies** anticuerpos antihepatitis; ~ **B core antigen** antígeno nuclear de la hepatitis B; ~ **delta virus** virus de la hepatitis D; ~ **virus** virus de la hepatitis A
hepatobiliary hepatobiliar, relativo al hígado y a los conductos biliares; ~ **capsule** capsula fibrosa del higado, capsula fibrosa perivascularis
hepatocellular hepatocelular, relativo a las células del hígado; ~ **cancer** cáncer hepatocelular, el cáncer del hígado, el carcinoma hepatocelular; ~ **carcinoma** carcinoma hepatocelular; ~ **insufficiency** insuficiencia hepatocelular; ~ **toxic hepatitis** hepatitis tóxica hepatocelular
hepatocholangiogastrostomy hepatocholangiogastrostomía
hepatocyte hepatocito; ~ **culture** cultivo de hepatocitos; ~ **genome** genoma del hepatocito
hepatojugular hepatoyugular; ~ **reflux** reflujo hepatoyugular
hepatolenticular hepatolenticular; ~ **degeneration** enfermedad de Wilson, degeneración hepatolenticular
hepatolith cálculo intrahepático
hepatologist hepatólogo
hepatoma cáncer de hígado, hepatoma
hepatomegaly hepatomegalia, aumento del tamaño del hígado
hepatopancreas hepatopáncreas
hepatorenal hepatorrenal; ~ **syndrome** síndrome hepatorrenal
hepatotoxic hepatotóxico, nocivo para las células del hígado
her le, poss, su (s), sus (pl)
herbal de hierbas, herbario; ~ **medicine** producto fitofarmacéutico, fitofármaco, fitoterapia, terapia herbaria, hierbas medicinales; ~ **treatment** fitoterapia, terapia herbaria, hierbas medicinales
here aquí
hereditary hereditario; ~ **disease** enfermedad hereditaria; ~ **keratosis** queratosis hereditaria; ~ **myotonia** ataxia muscular de Thomsen, miotonia congénita
heredity herencia
hermaphroditic hermafrodita
hermaphroditism hermafroditismo
hermetic hermético, impenetrable
hernia hernia; ~ **bandage** braguero para hernia, faja para hernia, vendaje para la hernia; ~ **truss** braguero inguinal
hernial herniario; ~ **aneurysm** aneurisma herniario; ~ **impaction** estrangulación de la hernia; ~ **truss** braguero para hernia, faja para hernia, vendaje para la hernia
herniated herniado; ~ **disc** disco herniado, disco protruído
heroin heroina, diacetilmorfina; ~ **addict** heroinómano; ~ **addiction** heroinomanía, adicción a la heroína, dependencia de heroína; ~ **seizure** confiscación de estupefacientes, incautación de heroína
herpes herpes; ~ **conjunctivae** conjuntivitis flictenular, herpes conjuntival; ~ **infection** infección herpérica, infección por herpes; ~ **sexualis** herpes genital; ~ **simplex** herpes simple; ~ **simplex infection** infección por herpes simple; ~ **zoster** herpes zóster, zona
herpetic herpético; ~ **arteritis** periarteritis herpética; ~ **stomatitis** estomatitis herpética

Herter disease enfermedad celíaca
hertz hertz
Herzberg operation operación de Herzberg
hetacillin hetacilina
heterochylia heteroquilia
heterocyclic heterocíclico; ~ **compound** compuesto heterocíclico; ~ **organic compound** compuesto orgánico heterocíclico
heteroduplex analysis análisis heterodúplex; ~ **mapping** cartografía heterodúplex
heterogeneous xenogénico, heterógeno; ~ **graft** injerto heterólogo, xenotrasplante, heteroimplante; ~ **immunoassay** inmunoanálisis heterogéneo
heterogenic heterogenético; ~ **agglutinins** aglutininas heterogenéticas
heterogenote heterogenote
heterograft heteroimplante, transplante heterólogo
heterologous anafilaxia heteróloga; ~ **insemination** inseminación artificial a partir de un donante; ~ **transplant** injerto heterólogo, xenotrasplante, heteroimplante
heterophoria heteroforia
heteroplasty heteroimplante
heteroproteins heteroproteínas
heteropycnosis heteropicnosis
heteroscedaticity heterocedasticidad
heterothroph heterótrofo
heterotopia ectopia
heterotropia estrabismo manifesto
heterozygote heterocigoto
heterozygous heterocigoso, heterocigoto, heterocigótico; ~ **advantage** ventaja heterocigótica; ~ **strain** cepa heterocigota
hexaclorophene hexaclorofeno
hexahydrate calcium iodate yodato (m) de calcio, exohidratado
hexogen hexógeno
hexokinase hexocinasa
hexose monophosphate shunt via de los pentasofosfatos
Hg mercurio, azogue
hiccup singulto, hipo
hiccups, to have the tener el hipo
hidden oculto, escondido, tapado
high alto; ~ **altitude** respirador de altitud; ~ **altitude cerebral edema** edema cerebral de

gran altura; ~ **altitude headache** dolor de cabeza de gran altura; ~ **altitude hypoxia** hipoxia de altitud; ~ **altitude myopia** miopía de altura; ~ **altitude pulmonary edema** edema pulmonar de gran altura; ~ **blood pressure** hipertonia, tensión aumentada, aumento de la tensión, presión elevada; ~ **cholesterol** alto en colesterol; ~ **-grade differentiated** alto grado diferenciado; ~ **-protein diet** dieta rica en proteínas; ~ **-risk pregnancy** embarazo de alto riesgo
highly potent de gran potencia, muy potente
hilar hiliar; ~ **cells** células hiliares; ~ **cell hyperplasia** hiperplasia de células hiliares
him a él, le
hip pelvis, cadera; ~ **bone** quadrillo; ~ **bone index** índice del hueso ilíaco; ~ **joint arthroplasty** protesis de cadera, artroplastia de la cadera; ~ **joint prosthesis** protesis de cadera, artroplastia de la cadera; ~ **joint replacement** implante osteoarticular de cadera; ~ **pain** coxalgia; ~ **replacement** artroplastia de la cadera; ~ **splint** férula de cadera, aparato corrector de la cadera
hipogastric hipogástrico
hipogastrium hipogastrio
hippocampal commissure comisura del hipocampo
hippocampus hipocampo, asta de Ammon
Hippocratic oath juramento hipocrático
hippocratism hipocratismo
hippurate test prueba del hipurato
Hirschsprung disease megacolon congénito, congenital colectasia, Hirschsprung diseaseco
hirsutism hirsutismo, vellosidad exagerada en la mujer
hirudin tolerance test prueba de tolerancia a la hirudina
hirudiniasis hirudiniasis
his su, sus
His' bundle fascículo de His; ~ **spindle** huso de His
histamine histamina; ~ **H2 receptor** receptor H2 de histamina; ~ **iontophoresis** histaminoiontophoresis; ~ **latex reaction** reacción de la histamina-látex; ~ **test** prueba de la histamina
histaminic histamínico; ~ **headache** cefalalgia

histamínica, migraña en racimos de Horton, cefalalgia nocturna paroxística

histidine histidina; **~ decarboxylase** histidina descarboxilasa

histiocyte histiocito

histiocytosis histiocitosis; **~ X** histiocitosis de celulas de Langerhans

histochemistry histioquímica

histocompatibility histocompatibilidad; **~ genes** genes de histocompatibilidad; **~ test** prueba de histocompatibilidad

histological histológico, relativo a la histología

histology histología

histone histona

histopathology histopatología

histoplasmosis histoplasmosis

histotrophic histótrofo, histotrópico

histrionic histriónico; **~ hemorrhage** hemorragia histriónica, hemorragia del síndrome de Münchhausen

HIV (Human Immunficiency Virus) VIH, Virus de Inmunodeficiencia Humana; **~ antigen** antígeno VIH; **~ human immunodeficiency virus** virus de la inmunodeficiencia humana, HIV; **~ -infected** seropositivo; **~ infection** infección con VIH; **~ positive** seropositivo con VIH; **~ screening test** prueba de detección VIH; **~ wasting syndrome** enteropatía en el SIDA

hives urticaria, habones

H+/K+-ATPase bomba de protones

HLA antigeno leucocitario humano, ALH; **~ -DP** antigenos HLA; **~ histocompatibility system** sistema HLA de histocompatibilidad; **~ typing** tipificación de HLA,

HMGA proteins proteínas HMGA

HMG-AT-hook proteins proteínas HMGA

HMO (health maintenance organization) Organización de Atención Médica

H₂O₂ (hydrogen peroxide) agua oxigenada

hoarse ronco

hoarseness ronquera, afonia

hobbies actividades de tiempo libre, actividades recreativas, recreción

hobble, to cojear, renquear, zalenquear

hobnail liver hígado nodular

Hodgkin's disease enfermedad de Hodgkin

hog cholera peste porcina

hold, to tener, coger, agarrar, abrazar, mantener; **~ the breath, to** suspender/aguantar la respiración

holistic holístico; **~ healing** curación holistica, **~ medicine** salud holistica

hollow cavidad, espacio hueco

holocrine holocrino; **~ secretion** secreción holocrina

holo-endemic pandemia, pandémico

hologynic inheritance herencia gologínica

holoprosencephaly holoprosencefalia

Holter monitoring monitorización Holter, registro Holter

home casa, domicilio, hogar; **~ health aide** asistente para servicios de la salud en el hogar; **~ health care** asistencia médica a domicilio, atención domiciliaria; **~ health service** asistencia médica a domicilio, atención domiciliaria

homeobox homeosecuencia

homeopathic homeopático; **~ dilution** dilución homeopática; **~ dose** dosis homeopática; **~ pharmacology** materia médica, la farmacología homeopática; **~ preparation** preparado homeopático; **~ remedy** medicamento homeopático; **~ stock** cepa homeopática

homeopathy homeopatía

homeostasis homeostasis

homocysteine homocistina

homoduplex homoduplex

homoeomiasmatic remedy remedio homeomiasmático

homogeneous homogéneo, uniforme; **~ immunoassay** inmunoanálisis homogéneo

homogenesis homogenesia, homogénesis

homogenote homogenote

homogeny homogenia, homogénesis

homoioplastic homoplástico; **~ artery transplant** transplante arterial homoplástico

homologous homólogo, igual, adecuado; **~ anaphylaxis** anafilaxia homóloga; **~ graft** aloinjerto, homoinjerto, donación alogénica, trasplante alogénico; **~ immunoglobulin** inmunoglobulina homóloga

homology homología

homoscedasticity homocedasticidad

homozygote homocigoto

homozygotic homocigoso, homocigótico

honorarium honorario, honorarios médicos

hoof-and-mouth disease fiebre aftosa

hooked bone hueso unciforme

hordeolum perilla (del ojo), orzuelo (del ojo); ~ **sty** orzuelo

horizontal horizontal; ~ **tomography** tomografía en decúbito horizontal

Hormann's bacillus Corynebacterium pseudodiphtericum

hormonal hormonal

hormone hormona; ~ **antagonists** antagonistas de hormonas; ~ **receptor** receptor hormonal; ~ **replacement therapy** terapia de sustitución hormonal; ~ **therapy** hormonoterapia

Horton's headache cefalalgia histamínica, migraña en racimos de Horton, cefalalgia nocturna paroxística

hospice care centro de cuidados paliativos, asistencia emocional del morubundo

hospital hospital, clínica; ~ **acquired infection** infección hospitalaria; ~ **-based medicine** medicina hospitalaria; ~ **bed** cama de hospital; ~ **capacity** capacidad hospitalaria; ~ **care** atención médica en hospital; ~ **computer system** red médica local, sistema de informática hospitalaria; ~ **gown** bata de hospital; ~ **information system** sistema de informática hospitalaria; ~ **scrubs** ropas de hospital; ~ **sheet** tela hospital; ~ **waste** residuos de hospitales

hospitalization hospitalización (f), ingreso en un centro médico, admisión en un hospital

host anfitrión, presentador; ~ **cell** célula anfitriona, célula huésped, célula hospedadora; ~ **computer** ordenador central, computadora central

hostile hostil, antagónico

hot caliente; ~ **flashes** calores, sofocos, bochornos, sensación pasajera de calor que experimentan las mujeres menopáusicas; ~ **pack** bolsa de agua caliente; ~ **spot** punto caliente; ~ **tub** bañera de hidromasaje, baño de remolino

hotel hotel

hour hora

house casa

housekeeping gene gen de mantenimiento

housewife ama de casa

how como; ~ **much** cuánto

HPLC cromatografía en fase líquida de alta eficacia

Huggler endoprosthesis endoprótesis de Huggler

human adenovirus humano; ~ **adenovirus** adenovirus humano; ~ **chorionic gonadotrophin** gonadotropina coriónica humana; ~ **dignity** dignidad humana; ~ **fibrinogen** fibrinógeno humano; ~ **growth hormone** hormona del crecimiento; ~ **immunodeficiency virus** virus de la inmunodeficiencia humana; ~ **leukocyte antigen** antígeno leucocitario humano, ALH; ~ **leukocyte antigen test** prueba de antígeno leucocitario humano; ~ **lymphocyte antigen typing** tipificación de HLA; ~ **menopausal gonadotrophin** gonadotropina menopáusica humana; ~ **normal immunoglobulin** inmunoglobulina humana normal; ~ **papiloma virus** virus papova humano; ~ **plasma** plasma sanguíneo, plasma hemático

humanitarian humanitario; ~ **assistance** ayuda humanitaria

humeral humeral, relativo al húmero

humeroscapular humeroscapular

humerus húmero

humidifier humidificador para uso médico; ~ **lung** fiebre de las humidificadoras

humidophilic humidófilo

humor humor, jocosidad, comicidad, hilarida

humoral humoral, relativo a los líquidos corporales

humpbacked joroba, cheposa, corcovado

hunchback joroba, cheposa, corcovado

hundred cien

hunger hambre; ~ **cure** cura de hambre; ~ **edema** edema de hambre; ~ **lymphocytosis** linfocitosis del hambre

Hunter chancre chancro de Hunter, cancro duro; ~ **induration** induración de Hunter, induración sifilítica

Huntingdon's chorea corea de Huntington, enfermedad de Huntington; ~ **disease** corea de Huntington, enfermedad de Huntington

hurt daño; ~ **, to** doler

husband esposo

husky ronco

Hutchinson choroiditis coroiditis senil; ~ –
Gilford disease progeria, infantilismo senil;
~ **melanotic freckle** peca melanotica de
Hutchinson

hyaline hialino; ~ **connective tissue** tejido
conjuntivo hialino

hyalo–enchondroma condroma hialino

hyaloideo–retinal degeneration degeneración
hialoideorretiniana

hybrid híbrido; ~ **cell** célula híbrida; ~ **ion** ion
híbrido, ión anfótero, amfoion, ion dipolar

hybridization hibridación; ~ **of nucleic acids**
hibridación de ácidos nucleicos

hybridoma hibridoma; ~ **tissue culture** cultivo
tisular de hibridomas

hydatid hidátide; ~ **cyst** quiste hidatádico;
~ **fremitus** frémito hidatádico; ~ **thorax** tórax
hidatádico; ~ **torsion** torsión del pedículo de
un hidátide

hydatidosis hidatidosis

hydatiform hidatiforme; ~ **mole** mola
hidatiforma

hydralazine hidralacina

hydramniose hidramnios

hydrargyrosis hidrargirismo, hidrargirosis

hydrarthrosis hidrartrosis

hydration hidratación

hydroalcoholic hidroalcohólico, preparado con
alcoholes diluidos

hydro–appendix hidroapéndice

hydrocarbon hidrocarburo; ~ **chain** cadena
hidrocarbonada

hydrocephalus hidrocéfalo, aumento de líquido
en el cerebro

hydrochloric clorhídrico; ~ **acid** ácido
clorhídrico

hydrochloride clorhidrato

hydrocortisone hidrocortisona; ~ **butyrate**
butirato de hidrocortisona

hydrocution hidrocución

hydrocyanic cianhídrico; ~ **acid** ácido
cianhídrico, cianuro de hidrógeno

hydrogen hidrógeno; ~ **breath test** prueba del
hidrógeno espirado; ~ **carbonate**
hidrogenocarbonato, carbonato ácido de
sodio; ~ **cyanide** ácido cianhídrico, cianuro de
hidrógeno

hydrogenation hidrogenación; ~ **of fats**
hidrogenación de grasas

hydrogenion ion hidrógeno

hydrolase hidrolasa

hydrolisis hidrólisis

hydroncus tumefacción acuosa

hydronephrosis hidronefrosis

hydroparesis paresia edematosa

hydrophallus edema del pene

hydrophilic hidrofílico

hydrophobia hidrofobia

hydrophobic hidrófobo

hydrops hidropesía; ~ **vesicae felleae**
colecistitis hidrópica

hydroretrocortine prednisolona

hydrosalpinx hidrosalpinx

hydrotherapy balneoterapia, hidroterapia

hydrothermal hidrotermal

hydrothorax pleuritis, pleuresía, hidrotórax,
inflamación de la pleura

hydrotis acumulación serosa en oído medio

hydrotropic hidrotrópico

hydrotropy hidrotropía

hydrotubation lavado tubárico

hydroxocobalamin hidroxicobalamina,
hidroxocobalamina

hydroxyapatite durapatita

hydroxychloroquine hidroxicloroquina

hydroxyl hidroxilo; ~ **value** índice de hidróxido

hydroxylation hidroxilasa

hydroxyproline hidroxiprolina

hygiene higiene

hygienic higiénico

hygroma higroma

hygromatosis rheumatica higromatosis
reumática

hymen himen; ~ **of vagina** himen

hymenal atresia himen imperforado, atresia
vaginal

hyoscyamine hioscíamina

hyperacousia hiperacusia

hyperactivity hiperactividad, hiperquinesia,
hiperactividad, actividad motora exagerada

hyperaemia hiperemia, exceso de sangre en los
vasos de un órgano

hyperaesthesia hiperestesia, sensibilidad
exagerada

hyperaldosteronism hiperaldosteronismo

hyperalgesia hiperalgia, sensibilidad exagerada al dolor

hyperbaric hiperbaro, relativo a una presión elevada; ~ **medicine** medicina hiperbárica; ~ **oxygenation** oxigenación hiperbárica

hypercalcemia hipercalcemia; ~ **syndrome** síndrome de hipercalcemia

hypercapnia hipercapnia

hyperchloremic hiperclorémico; ~ **acidosis** acidosis hiperclorémica

hypercholesterolemia hipercolesterolemia

hyperemesis hiperemesis

hyperemia hiperemia

hyperemic hiperémico; ~ **dermatitis** dermatitis hiperémica

hyperesthesia hiperestesia

hyperextension hiperextensión; ~ **of the neck** hiperextensió del cuello

hyperflexion fracture fractura por flexión forzada; ~ **of the knee** hiperflexión de la rodilla

hyperglycemia hiperglucemia

hyperglycemic factor glucagón

hypergonadotrophic hypogonadism hipogonadismo primario

hyperhidrosis hiperhidrosis, sudación exagerada

hyperinsulinemia hiperinsulinemia

hyperkalemia hipercalemia, exceso de potasio en la sangre

hyperkeratosis hiperqueratosis

hyperkinesia hiperkinesia

hyperlipidemia hiperlipidemia, aumento de la cantidad de lípidos en la sangre

hypermetropia hiperopia, hibermetropía

hypernatremia hipernatrémia

hyperopia hiperopia, hibermetropía

hyperopic hiperópico; ~ **astigmatism** astigmatismo hiperópica

hyperorthocytosis hiperortocitosis

hyperostosis hiperostosis, engrosamiento de un hueso

hyperoxalemia hiperoxalemia

hyperoxia hiperoxia, hiperoxemia

hyperparathyroidism hiperparatiroidismo

hyperpathia hiperpatía

hyperpigmentation hiperpigmentación

hyperpituitarism hiperpituitarismo

hyperplasia hiperplasia, aumento del tamaño de un órgano o de un tejido

hyperplastic hiperplástico; ~ **muscular dystrophy** distrofia muscular hiperplástica

hyperprolactinemia hiperprolactinemia

hyperprolinemia iminoglicinuria, hiperprolinemia

hyperpyrexia hiperpirexia, fiebre extremadamente alta

hyperreflexia hiperreflexia, exageración de los reflejos

hypersecretion hipersecreción

hypersensitivity hipersensibilidad; ~ **angiitis** angitis alérgica, angeítis alérgica, angiitis alérgica; ~ **pneumonitis** neumopatía por hipersensibilidad, alveolitis alérgica, alveolitis alérgica extrínseca; ~ **reaction** reacción de hipersensibilidad

hypersexuality hipersexualismo

hypersideremia hipersideremia, sobrecarga de hierro

hypersomnia hipersomnia

hyperstimulation estimulación exagerada

hypertelorism hipertelorismo

hypertension hipertonía, tensión aumentada, aumento de la tensión, presión elevada

hypertensive hipertónico; ~ **encephalopathy** encefalopatía hipertensa

hyperthermia hipertermia

hyperthyroidism hipertiroidismo

hypertonia hipertonía, tensión aumentada, aumento de la tensión, presión elevada

hypertonic hipertónico -ica; ~ **dehydration** deshidratación hipertonica

hypertrichosis hipertricosis (f), aumento del espesor del vello corporal

hypertrophic hipertrófico; ~ **calf** hipertrofia de la pantorrilla; ~ **capillary angioma** angioma capilar hipertrófico; ~ **degenerative arthritis** artrosis deformante; ~ **myocardiopathy** miocardiopatía hipertrófica

hypertrophy hipertrofia, aumento del tamaño de un órgano o tejido

hyperuricemia hiperuricemia, exceso de ácido úrico en la sangre

hypervaccination inyección secundaria, revacunación, inyección de refuerzo

hyperventilation hiperventilación; ~ **alkalosis** alcalosis respiratória

hypervitaminosis hipervitaminosis, estado causado por ingestión excesiva de vitaminas

hypervolemia hipervolemia, aumento anormal de volumen de sangre circulante

hypha hifa

hypnosis hipnosis

hypnotic hipnotico, píldora de dormir, pastilla que induce sueño

hypoacusis hipoacusia, disminución de la audición

hypoaldosteronism hipoaldosteronismo

hypocapnia hipocapnia

hypochondriac hypocondríaco

hypochondriasis hipocondría, preocupación exagerada por la salud

hypochrome hipocromático

hypochromic hipocrómico; ~ **anemia** anemia hipocrómica

hypodense hipodenso

hypodermic hipodérmico, que está o se pone debajo de la piel; ~ **injection** inyeccion subcutanea; ~ **needle** aguja hipodérmica; ~ **syringe** jeringa hipodérmica, aguja hipodérmica

hypoferric anemia anemia ferropénica, la anemia por carencia de hierro

hypogastric plexo hipogástrico; ~ **plexus** plexo hipogástrico

hypoglottis hipoglotis

hypoglycemia hipoglicemia, descenso del nivel de glucosa en la sangre

hypoglycemic hipoglucemiante; ~ **shock** shock hipoglicémico

hypogonadism hipogonadismo, desarrollo sexual insuficiente

hypogonadotrophic hypogonadism hipogonadismo secundario

hypokalemia hipocaliemia, nivel bajo de potasio en la sangre

hypoliquorrhea disminución del líquido cefalorraquídeo

hypomania hipomanía, forma leve de la manía

hypometabolism hipometabolismo

hypopharynx hipofaringe

hypophyseal hipofisario, relativo a la hipófisis; ~ **castration** extirpación terapéutica de la hipófisis; ~ **coma** coma hipofisario

hypophysectomy hipofisectomia

hypophysis hipófisis

hypoplasia hipoplasia, desarrollo insuficiente de un órgano o tejido

hypoproteinemia hipoproteinemia

hypotension hipotensión arterial, hipotonía, presión sanguínea anormalmente baja

hypotensive hipotensivo

hypothalamic hipotalámico

hypothalamus hipotálamo

hypothermia hipotermia, temperatura corporal baja

hypothermic de hipotermia

hypothesis hipótesis, suposición

hypothrepsia inanición, desnutrición, subalimentación, hipotrepsia

hypothyroidism hipotiroidismo, actividad insuficiente de la glándula tiroides

hypotonia hipotonía, tono muscular disminuido, la tensión disminuida

hypotrophy hipotrofia, disminución del tamaño de un tejido o de un órgano

hypouricemia hipouricemia, deficiencia de ácido úrico en la sangre

hypoventilation hipoventilación, respiración lenta y superficial

hypovitaminosis hipovitaminosis, carencia de una o más vitaminas esenciales

hypovolemia hipovolemia, disminución de la cantidad de sangre circulante

hypovolemic hipovolémico; ~ **shock** shock hipovolémico

hypoxanthine hipoxantina; ~ **guanine phosphoribosyl transferase** hipoxantina guanina fosforibosiltransferasa

hypoxemia hipoxemia, contenido bajo de oxígeno en sangre

hypoxia hipoxia, disminución en el suministro de oxígeno a los tejidos

Hyrtl sphincter esfinter de Hyrtl

hysterectomy histerectomia, extirpación quirúrgica del útero,

hysteria histeria, conversión, transformación de las emociones en manifestaciones corporales

hysterical histérico; ~ **dyspepsia** dispepsia histérica; ~ **reaction** reacción histérica

hysterorrhexis rotura uterina

hysterosalpingography histerosalpingografía

hysterosalpingo-oophorectomy
  histerosalpingooforectomía
hysteroscope histeroscopio
hysteroscopy histeroscopia
hysterotrachelectomy histerotraquelectomía

I

iatrogenic yatrogénico, provocado por la intervención médica (diagnóstica, terapéutica); ~ **disease** enfermedad yatrógena; ~ **neurosis** neurosis yatrógena
IBD enfermedad inflamatoria del intestino
ibuprofen ibuprofeno
ice hielo; ~ **pack** bolsa de hielo; ~ **pack anesthesia** anestesia local con hielo
ichthyosiform ictiosiforme
ichthyosis ictiosis, trastorno de la piel que la hace seca y escamosa; ~ **bullosa** ictiosis bulosa; ~ **congenita** ictiosis congénita
icterohemoglobinuria icterohemoglobinuria
icterophthisis caquexia ictérica
icterus ictericia, coloración amarillenta de la piel; ~ **index** índice ictérico
ICU unidad de cuidado intensivo
ideation ideación, concepción
identical idéntico, completamente igual, coincidente, analogo; ~ **twins** gemelos identicos, gemelos monocigotos
identification identificación, psiq, asimilación inconsciente con otra persona; ~ **process** proceso de identificación; ~ **system** sistema de identificación
ideokinetic ideomotor
ideomotor apraxia apraxia ideomotora
ideosynchysis confusión, ideosínquisis
idiomotor ideomotor
idiopathic idiopático, de causa desconocida, primario, espontáneo; ~ **hypoproteinemia** hipoproteinemia idiopática; ~ **thrombocytopenic purpura** púrpura trombocitopénica idiopática
idiosyncrasy idiosincrasia, alergia o sensibilidad exagerada a un medicamento, peculiar a un individuo
idiotope idiotopo

idioventricular idioventricular; ~ **rhythm** ritmo idioventricular
IDT (intradermal test) prueba intradérmica
if si
IgA deficiency deficiencia de IgA, déficit de IgA
IGF-1 factor de crecimiento parecido a la insulina
ileitis ileitis (f), inflamación del íleon, última parte del intestino delgado
ileocecal ileocecal; ~ **resection** resección ileocecal; ~ **volvulus** vólvulo ileocecal
ileocecostomy ileocecostomía
ileocolic ileocólico; ~ **artery** arteria ileocolica; ~ **sphincter** esfinter ileocólico
ileostomy ileostomía
ileum íleon
ileus íleo, obstrucción intestinal, parálisis intestinal, oclusión intestinal
iliac ilíaco; ~ **bursa** bolsa ilíaca; ~ **fossa** fosa ilíaca; ~ **pedicle** pedículo ilíaco; ~ **vessels** vasos ilíocecales
ilium hueso ilíaco, ilion
ill enfermo; ~ , **to be** estar enfermo
illegible ilegible
illness enfermedad
illuminance iluminancia
image imagen
imaging spectroscopy espectroscopía de imágenes
imbalance desequilibrio
IME evaluación médica independiente
iminoglycinuria iminoglicinuria, hiperprolinemia
imipramine imipramina
immaturity inmadurez, estado de no haber alcanzado su desarrollo pleno
immersion inmersión; ~ **foot** pie de inmersión, pie de trinchera; ~ **lens** objetivo de inmersión; ~ **objective** objetivo de inmersión; ~ **oil** aceite de inmersión; ~ **syncope** hidrocución
immiscible inmiscible
immobilization inmovilización, sujeción, restricción física, inmobilización
immobilize, to paralizar, inmovilizar
immortal inmortal
immune inmune, relativo al sistema inmunitario,

insensible, protegido contra una infeccion; ~ **adherence** inmunoadherencia; ~ **cell** inmunocito, célula de memoria; ~ **complex** inmunocomplejo; ~ **deficiency** inmunodeficiencia, defecto immunitaria; ~ **dysfunction** defecto immunitario, inmunodeficiencia; ~ **interferon** interferón gamma, interferón inmune; ~ **response modulator** modulador de la respuesta inmunitaria; ~ **serum** antisuero, suero que contiene anticuerpos frente a una enfermedad concreta; ~ **suppressor response** respuesta supresora; ~ **system** sistema inmunitario, el complejo bioquímico que protege al organismo frente a los gérmenes pathógenos

immunity inmunidad, protección contra las enfermedades infecciosas

immunization vacunación, inmunización

immunoadsorbent inmunoadsorbente; ~ **column** columna inmunoadsorbente

immuno–allergist alergista, especialista en alergias, alergólogo

immunoassay inmunoensayo, inmunoanálisis

immunoblot inmunotransferencia

immunoblotting inmunotransferencia

immunochemistry inmunoquímica

immunocompetent cell inmunocito, célula de memoria

immunocyte inmunocito, célula de memoria

immunocytochemistry imunohistoquímica, imunocitoquímica

immunodiagnostic diagnóstico inmunológico

immunodiffusion inmunodifusión; ~ **radial** inmunodifusión radial

immunoelectrodiffusio inmunoelectrodifusión

immunoelectrophoresis inmunoelectroforesis

immunoelectrophoretic inmunoelectroforético

immunoenzyme inmunoenzima; ~ **techniques** tecnicas para inmunoenzimas

immunofixation inmunofijación

immunofluorescence inmunofluorescencia

immunogenic inmunógeno, agente que induce una respuesta inmunitaria

immunogenicity inmunogenicidad

immunoglobulin inmunoglobulina; ~ **supergene family** inmunoglobulina de la familia supergén

immunohematology inmunohematología

immunohemolysin inmunohemolisina

immunohistochemistry inmunohistoquímica

immunological inmunológico, relativo al sistema inmunitario; ~ **memory** memoria inmunológica

immunology inmunología

immunomodulation inmunomodulación

immunoperoxidase inmunoperoxidasa; ~ **assay** prueba de la inmunoperoxidasa

immunoprecipitation inmunoprecipitación

immunoradiometry inmunoradiometría

immunoreaction inmunorrespuesta

immunostimulant inmunoestimulante

immunosuppressant inmunosupresor, agente que impide que se produzca la respuesta inmunitaria

immunosuppression inmunosupresión

impact sacudida, golpe

impaired minusválido, disminuido, discapacitado; ~ **elderly person** anciano inválido; ~ **judgement** alteración del juicio, debilidad mental

impairment deficiencia, defecto, falta; ~ **of fertility** disturbio ocasionado a la fertilidad, daño ocasionado a la fertilidad; ~ **rating** declaración de discapacidad, escala de valoración de avería

impedance impedancia; ~ **plethysmograph** reógrafo

imperforate imperforado; ~ **hymen** atresia vaginal, himen imperforado

impetiginous impetiginoso; ~ **cheilitis** queilitis impetiginosa

impetigo impétigo, infección purulenta de la piel con vesículas y costras; ~ **follicularis** impétigo folicular; ~ **varicellosa** impétigo varioloso

implantable implantable; ~ **defibrillator** desfibrilador implantable; ~ **infusion pumps** bombas de infusión implantables, bombas peristálticas

implantation implantación, nidación del óvulo fecundado, inserción de un órgano o tejido en un nuevo sitio, inserción de materiales biológicos vivos inertes o radioactivos en el cuerpo

implausible dudoso, discutible, cuestionable

implication implicación
implicit implícito; ~ **memory** memoria no
declarativa, memoria implícita
impotence impotencia, falta del poder de
copulación en el hombre
imprecision imprecisión; ~ **profile** perfil de
imprecisión
impregnation impregnación, fecundación del
óvulo, imbibición
impression impresión; ~ **paste** pasta de
impresión
improper indecoroso, impropio; ~ **posture**
postura mala
impurity impureza
in sobre, en (place), encendido (e.g. radio),
dentro de; ~ **extremis** in extremis, al momento
de la muerte; ~ **situ** in situ, en su lugar
natural; ~ **situ hybridization** hibridación in
situ; ~ **the afternoon** por la tarde; ~ **the
direction of** en dirección; ~ **the evening** al
atardecer; ~ **the morning** por la mañana;
~ **the night** por la noche; ~ **the normal place**
in situ, en su lugar natural; ~ **vitro** in vitro,
que se produce u ocurre en un tubo de
ensayo; ~ **vitro diagnostic medical device**
dispositivo médico para diagnóstico in vitro;
~ **vitro fertilization** fecundación
extracorporal, fecundación in vitro; ~ **vitro
penetration assay** prueba de penetración
cruzada in vitro; ~ **vivo** vivo, que está situado
u ocurre en el cuerpo vivo
inability incapacidad; ~ **to concentrate**
distractibilidad
inaccuracy inexactitud
inactive inactivo, quieto, en reposo; ~ **period**
período latente, período entre la aplicación o
la recepción de un estímulo y la reacción
consiguiente; ~ **plasmid** plásmido desarmado
inactivity anergia, carencia de actividad, falta
de reacción; ~ **atrophy** atrofia por inactividad
inadequacy insuficiencia, función inadecuada
de un órgano o sistema
inadequate inadecuado, no apropiado,
insuficiente; ~ **stimulus** estímulo inadecuado
inanition inanición, desnutrición,
subalimentación; ~ **acetone from fasting**
acetona de ayuno; ~ **atrophy** atrofia por
inanición; ~ **feces** heces de ayuno

inborn innato; ~ **metabolic brain diseases**
enfermedades cerebrales metabolicas innatas;
~ **metabolic disease** trastorno congénito del
metabolismo
incarcerate, to encarcelar
incarcerated hernia hernia estrangulada
incarceration incarceración, enclavamiento
anormal
incest incesto
incidence incidencia, número de casos nuevos,
llegada de energía radiante en una superficie;
~ **of disease** morbididad, tasa de enfermos en
una población
incidental incidental
incipient incipiente; ~ **abortion** aborto
incipiente; ~ **cataract** catarata incipiente
incised wound herida por arma blanca,
cuchillazo, cortadura profunda
incision incisión, corte, abordaje; ~ **guide** guía
de incisión
incisive incisivo, penetrante
inclusion incorporación, unión de una sustancia
al interior del organismo; ~ **body** cuerpo de
inclusión
inclusive inclusivo
incoherent incoherente, confuso, inconexo;
~ **thinking** pensamiento incoherente
income ingresos, renta; ~ **support** ayuda a la
renta, asistencia social
incompatible incompatible, no adecuado para
administración simultánea, que se repele
mútuamente
incompetent incompetente; ~ **cervix**
incompetencia del cuello uterino, insuficiencia
cervical, cérvix insuficiente
incontinence incontinencia, incapacidad de
control de los excrementos, exceso
incorporation incorporación, unión de una
sustancia al interior del organismo
increase m aumento, v aumentar; ~ **in blood
pressure** aumento de la presión sanguínea;
~ **in pulse rate** aceleración del pulso
increased heart rate aumento del ritmo
cardiaco; ~ **secretion of adrenalin** aumento
de la secreción de adrenalina
increasing cumulativo, acumulativo
incubation incubación, período entre contagio y
manifestación de la enfermedad

incurable incurable

independent independiente

index índice; ~ **finger** dedo índice

Indian rhinoplasty rinoplastia india, rinoplastia de Carpue

indicanuria orinas azules

indicate, to indicar

indication indicación,

indicative indicativo

indicator indicador; ~ **electrode** electrodo indicador

indigenous indígeno; ~ **flora** flora indígena

indigestion indigestión, dispepsia, trastorno de la digestión

indirect indirecto; ~ **agglutination test** prueba indirecta de la aglutinación; ~ **bilirubin** bilirrubina no esterificada; ~ **fluorescent-antibody test** prueba indirecta del anticuerpo fluorescente; ~ **hemagglutination test** prueba indirecta de la hemaglutinación

individual individual, referido al individuo

indolence indolencia, ausencia de dolor, pereza

indolent indolente

indomethacin indometacina, un fármaco antiinflamatorio no esteroideo

induce producir, inducir, provocar

induced provocado, inducido; ~ **abortion** aborto provocado; ~ **cardiac arrest** paro cardiaco inducido; ~ **hypothermia** hipotermia inducida, hipotermia provocada; ~ **labor** trabajo de parto inducido

inducer inductor

induction inducción, provocación de un proceso

induration induración, endurecimiento, callosidad

industrial industrial; ~ **injury** lesión laboral, lesión por accidente de trabajo; ~ **medicine** medicina laboral, medicina del trabajo; ~ **psychologist** psicología industrial

indwelling catheter cateterismo permanente, sonda a permanencia; ~ **ureteral catheterism** cateterismo ureteral permanente

inebriated borracho

inert inerte; ~ **gas** gas inerte; ~ **waste** residuos inertes, desperdicios inertes

inertia inercia, inactividad, incapacidad de moverse espontáneamente

infant niño/a; ~ **formula** leche para lactantes, formula adaptada; ~ **milk** leche para lactantes, formula adaptada; ~ **mortality** mortandad, mortalidad infantil

infanticide infanticidio

infantile infantil; ~ **anemia** anemia infantil; ~ **atrophy** atrofia infantil, marasmo; ~ **glaucoma** glaucoma infantil; ~ **language** lenguaje infantil; ~ **paralysis** poliomielitis

infarct infarto

infected infectado; ~ **wound** infección de la herida

infection infección; ~ **rate** tasa de infección

infectious infeccioso; ~ **acne** acné infecciosa; ~ **anemia** anemia infecciosa; ~ **angioma** angioma serpiginoso; ~ **bronchitis** bronquitis infecciosa; ~ **disease** enfermedad infecciosa, enfermedad contagiosa; ~ **exanthema** exantema infeccioso; ~ **hepatitis** hepatitis virica, hepatitis infecciosa; ~ **jaundice** leptospirosis; ~ **mononucleosis** mononucleosis infecciosa, angina monocítica; ~ **waste** desechos infecciosos, residuos de hospitales

infectivity infecciosidad

inferior inferior

inferiority complejo de inferioridad; ~ **complex** complejo de inferioridad

infertility infertilidad, infecundidad

infiltration infiltración

infirm decrépito, desvaído, endeble, vetusto

infirmary enfermería

inflamed inflamado; ~ **lymph nodes** bubas, bubón, incordio

inflammation inflamación; ~ **around the fingernail** panadizo, uñero; ~ **of the kidney** pielitis, inflamación de pelvis renal; ~ **of the oral mucosa** estomatitis, inflamación de la mucosa oral; ~ **of the ovaries** ooforitis; ~ **of the tongue** glossitis; ~ **of the throat** laringitis, inflamación de la laringe

inflammatory inflamatorio; ~ **bowel disease** enfermedad inflamatoria del intestino; ~ **dysmenorrhea** dismenorrea inflamatoria; ~ **infiltrate** infiltrado inflamatorio

inflatable splint férula hinchable

influence influencia; ~ **quantity** magnitud influyente, influencia

influenza influenza, gripe, flu; ~ **vaccine** vacuna antigripal

information información, conocimientos;
~ **service** servicio de referencias, centro de
orientación
informativity informatividad
infrapatellar infrapatelar; ~ **bursa, deep** bolsa
infrapatelar profunda; ~ **bursa,
subcutaneous** bolsa subcutánea infrapatelar,
bolsa pretibial; ~ **bursitis** bursitis infrapatelar
infrapiriforme hernia hernia isquiática
infrared infrarrojo; ~ **microscopy** microscopia
infrarroja; ~ **spectroscopy** espectroscopia
infraroja
infuse, to infundir
infusion infusión; ~ **solvents** solución de
perfusión, soluciones para perfusión;
~ **therapy** tratamiento por perfusión;
~ **urography** pielografía intravenosa,
pielografía por eliminación
ingest, to ingerir, comer
ingestion ingestión, toma
ingredient ingrediente, componente
ingrown encarcerado, estrangulado; ~ **toenail**
uña del pie encarnado
inguinal inguinal, relativo a la ingle; ~ **hernia**
hernia inguinal; ~ **part of the vas deferens**
parte inguinal del conducto deferente;
~ **truss** braguero inguinal
inguinodynia inguinodinia
inhalation inhalación, aspiración de gases o
vapores; ~ **anesthesia** anestesia por
inhalación; ~ **mist** nebulización por
inhalación; ~ **toxicology** toxicología
inalatória, toxicología respiratória
inhalational allergen alergeno respiratorio,
anafilactógeno respiratorio; ~ **favism** favismo
por inhalación
inhale, to aspirar, inhalar
inhaler inhalador, nebulizador
inherent inherente, implantado por naturaleza,
innato
inherited hereditario; ~ **glycogenosis**
glucogenosis hereditaria
inhibin inhibina
inhibition inhibición, atenuación, supresión o
bloqueo de una función o reacción; ~ **of
collagen synthesis** inhibición de la síntesis de
colágeno
inhibitor inhibidor

inhibitory inhibidoro; ~ **concentration**
concentración inhibidora; ~ **postsynaptic
potential** potencial postsináptico de
inhibición; ~ **quotient** cociente inhibidor
in-home nursing care asistencia a domicilio
inhuman inhumano, cruel
initial inicial, que comienza, al principio;
~ **dose** dosis de cebamiento, dosis inicial
initiation codon codón de iniciación
initiator site centro iniciador
injection inyección
injure, to lastimar, dañar, abusar, herir
injured herido; ~ **person** accidentado, persona
accidentada; ~ **worker** trabajador lastimado
injury lesión, daño, desperfecto, traumatismo,
herida, lastimadura
inner interno, intrínseco, situado dentro de una
parte o perteneciente exclusivamente a ella;
~ **ear** oído interno; ~ **ear deafness** sordera
sensorineural, sordera de percepción, sordera
neurosensorial, hipoacusia neurosensorial
innervation inervación, irrigación nerviosa de
un área u órgano; ~ **frequency** frecuencia de
inervación
inoculate, to inocular, vacunar
inoculation vacuna; ~ **hepatitis** hepatitis por
inoculación, hepatitis serica
inoculum inóculo
inoperable inoperable, no curable mediante
operación
inorganic inorgánico, carente de vida,
inanimado; ~ **serum** suero inorgánico
inotropic inotrópico, que afecta la fuerza de las
contracciones musculares
inpatient paciente hospitalizado; ~ **care**
atención médica en hospital
input entrada, input; ~ **rate** velocidad de
procesamiento
insane psicopático, psicótico
insect insecto; ~ **bite** picadura de insecto;
~ **infestation** infestación por insectos, plaga
de insectos; ~ **screening** mosquitero, red
protectora contra los insectos; ~ **sting**
picadura de insectos
insecticide insecticida
insemination inseminación
insensible insensible, inconsciente;
~ **perspiration** perspiración insensible

insert inserto; **~ to** insertar
inserting inserción, implantación, punto de unión de un músculo a un hueso
insertion inserción, implantación, punto de unión de un músculo a un hueso; **~ mutation** mutación por inserción
insertional insercional; **~ mutagenesis** mutagénesis insercional
inside dentro; **~ of the cell membrane** pared interna de la membrana celular
insole plantilla para el calzado
insomnia insomnio, incapacidad para dormir, vigilia anormal
insomniac insomne, sin dormir
inspect, to inspeccionar
inspiration inspiración
instability inestabilidad, falta de solidez, desequilibrio, falta de voluntad firme
instep empeine, cuello del pie
interstitial cell-stimulating hormone lutropina
instill, to instilar
instillation instilación, administración de un líquido gota a gota
instruction instrucción, indicaciones
instrument instrumento
instrumental instrumental; **~ dependability** seguridad instrumental
instrumentation instrumentación
insufferable insufrible, insoportable; **~ pain** dolor insufrible
insufficiency insuficiencia, función inadecuada de un órgano o sistema
insulin insulina; **~-dependent diabetes** diabetes mellitus dependiente de insulina, diabetes de tipo I; **~ growth factor** factor de crecimiento parecido a la insulina; **~-like growth factor** factor de crecimiento insulinoide; **~ shock** choque insulínico
insult insulto, ataque, acceso
insurance (medical) seguro médico; **~ policy** póliza de seguro
intact intacto
integrate, to integrar(se)
integrated integrado; **~ hospital care** asistencia de hospital integrada; **~ retroviral DNA** ADN retrovírico integrado, provirus
integrative integrativo
integrin integrina

integrity integridad, conservación inalterada
integumentary integumentario, que sirve de cubierta, como la piel
intelligence inteligencia
intense intenso, enorme, vehemente; **~ craving** deseo vehemente
intensity intensidad, grado de fuerza o tensión
intensive intensivo; **~ care** cuidados intensivos, medicina intensiva; **~ care nurse** enfermera de cuidados intensivos; **~ care unit** unidad de cuidado intensivo; **~ chemotherapy** quimioterapia de intensificación; **~ therapy** tratamiento intensivo; **~ treatment** tratamiento intensivo
intensivist médico intensivista
intention intención, propósito; **~ tremor** temblor intencional, temblor que aparece al intentar efectuar un movimiento voluntario coordinado
interaction interacción, relación existente entre dos elementos
intercalating intercalable; **~ agent** agente intercalable
intercellular intracelular; **~ cavity** cavidad secretora, cavidad intracelular
interchangeability intercambiabilidad
intercostal intercostal, situado entre dos costillas
intercourse coito, cópula carnal
interdigital interdigital; **~ panaritium** panadizo interdigital
intererence interferencia, estorbo
interference intromisión, interferencia; **~ filter** filtro interferencial; **~ spectroscopy** espectroscopía de interferencia
interferon interferón
interindividual interindividual, de individuos entre sí; **~ biological variability** variabilidad biológica interindividual
intermediary intermediario, que se efectúa u ocurre en una etapa media
intermediate intermedio; **~ host** hospedero intermedio
intermeningeal intermeníngeo; **~ apoplexy** apoplejía intermeníngea
intermenstrual intermenstrual; **~ bleeding** metrorragia, pérdida sanguínea uterina que no

sea menstrual, hemorragia intermenstrual;
~ **pain** dolor intermenstrual, dolor y
hemorragias intermenstruales
intermittent intermitente, que se interrumpe o
cesa y prosigue o se repite, que ocurre a
intervalos separados; ~ **fever** fiebre
intermitente; ~ **hernia** hernia intermitente;
~ **hydrops** hidropesía intermitente;
~ **hyperbilirubinemia** hiperbilirrubinemia
intermitente
intern interno de hospital
internal interno, intrínseco, situado dentro de
una parte o perteneciente exclusivamente a
ella; ~ **energy** energía interna; ~ **medicine**
medicina interna; ~ **parasite** endoparásito;
~ **quality control** control interno de la calidad
international internacional; ~ **non-proprietary
name** nombre farmacéutico internacional;
~ **standard** patrón internacional, norma
internacional; ~ **unit** unidad internacional
interneuron interneurona
internship curso de prácticas en hospitales,
internado
internuncial neuron interneurona
interpersonal interpersonal, de individuos entre
sí; ~ **relations** relaciones humanas, relaciones
interpersonales; ~ **skills** capacidad por
contacto, aptitud comunicativa
interphase interfase, período del ciclo celular en
el que el núcleo de la célula no está en
división, ni mitótica ni meiótica. Cromosomas
se duplican durante la interfase. ~ **nucleus**
núcleo interfásico, núcleo no divisional
interpleural cavity mediastino
interpretation interpretación
interpreter intérprete
interstitial intersticial, situado en los
interespacios de un tejido; ~ **cells of the
testicle** células intersticiales de Leydig; ~ **cell-
stimulating hormone** hormona luteinizante;
~ **collagenase** colagenasa intersticial;
~ **exudate** exudado intersticial; ~ **induration**
induración intersticial; ~ **lymphocytic
pneumonia** pneumonitis intersticial linfoide,
hiperplasia pulmonar linfoide; ~ **pulmonary
emphysema** enfisema pulmonar alveolar
intertrigo intertrigo, acción inflamatoria de los
pliegues cutáneos, rozadura

interureteric interuretero; ~ **fold** pliegue
interuretera
interval intervalo, porción de espacio o de
tiempo entre dos cosas
intervascular intervascular
intervening intermedio; ~ **sequence** secuencia
interpuesta, intermedio
intervention intervención, operación
intervertebral intervertebral, situado entre dos
vértebras contiguas; ~ **disk** disco
intervertebral, cartílago intervertebral;
~ **foramen** foramen intervertebral, agujero
intervertebral
intestinal intestinal, relativo al intestino;
~ **amebiasis** amebiasis intestinal;
~ **amicrobiosis** amicrobiosis intestinal;
~ **bleeding** hemorragia intestinal; ~ **catheter**
sonda intestinal; ~ **colic** cólico intestinal;
~ **decompression tube** sonda intestinal de
descompresión; ~ **flora** flora intestinal, el
conjunto de bacterias que viven en el intestino
grueso; ~ **gases** gases intestinales; ~ **ischemia**
isquemia, deficiencia del riego sanguíneo de
una zona; ~ **lipodystrophy** enfermedad de
Whipple; ~ **loops** asas intestinales; ~ **mucosa**
mucosa intestinal; ~ **obstruction** oclusión
intestinal, íleo, vólvulo, miserere; ~ **parasite**
parásito intestinal, gusano parasito, lombrice
intestinal; ~ **polyp** pólipo del colon; ~ **probe**
sonda intestinal; ~ **tract** tracto intestinal, tubo
digestivo, aparato digestivo; ~ **transit** tránsito
intestinal, paso a través de los intestinos
intestine intestino
intima-pia íntima-pía, combinación de la
íntima de los vasos sanguíneos y de la
piamadre que rodea a las arterias del cerebro
intimate íntimo; ~ **care** higiene sexual
into a dentro
intolerable insoportable, insufrible,
inaguantable
intolerance intolerancia, incapacidad para
soportar un medicamento; ~ **to light**
fotofobia, aversión a la luz
intoxication intoxicación, envenenamiento
intraarachnoid intraaracnoide
intracapsular intracapsular; ~ **hemorrhage**
hemorragia intracapsular
intracellular intracelular; ~ **fluid** líquido

intracelular; ~ **hyperhydratation**
hiperhidratación intracelular
intracranial intracraneal; ~ **aneurysm**
aneurisma intracraneal; ~ **bleeding**
hemorragia intracraneal; ~ **hemorrhage**
hemorragia intracraneal; ~ **hypertension**
hipertensión intracraneal; ~ **insufflation**
insuflación intracraneal; ~ **pressure** presión
intracraneal
intracutaneous intracutáneo, intradérmico;
~ **injection** inyección intracutánea, inyección
intradérmica; ~ **test** prueba intradérmica
intradermal intradérmico; ~ **closure** cierre
intradérmico; ~ **injection** inyección
intracutánea, inyección intradérmica;
~ **inoculation** inoculación endodérmica,
inyección endodérmica; ~ **test** prueba
intradérmica
intraductal intracanicular, ductal;
~ **noninfiltrating carcinoma** carcinoma
intracanicular no infiltrante, carcinoma ductal
in situ
intradural intradural; ~ **bleeding** hemorragia
intradural
intrahepatic intrahepático
intraindividual intraindividual, dentro del
individuo; ~ **biological variability** variabilidad
biológica intraindividual; ~ **biological
variation** variación biológica intraindividual,
variabilidad biológica intraindividual
intraluminal coronary artery stent stent
coronario
intramolecular intramolecular
intramuscular intramuscular, que está situado u
ocurre dentro de un músculo
intraneural endoneural; ~ **injection** inyección
endoneural
intraocular intraocular, que está situado o se
produce dentro del ojo; ~ **pressure** presión
intraocular; ~ **hypotonia** hipotonía ocular
intraoperative peroperatorio, intraoperatorio;
~ **complications** complicaciones
intraoperatorios
intraperitoneal intraperitoneal
intrathecal intratecal, que ocurre dentro de una
túnica
intrathoracic intratorácico; ~ **goiter** bocio
subesternal; ~ **pressure** presión intratorácica

intratracheal intratraqueal
intrauterine intrauterino; ~ **asphyxia** asfixia
intrauterina; ~ **blood transfusion** transfusión
de sangre intrauterina
intravascular intravascular, situado dentro de
un vaso; ~ **erythrocyte aggregation**
agregación eritrocítica, aglutinación
eritrocítica vascular
intravenous intravenoso, situado dentro de una
vena; ~ **cholangiography** colangiografía
intravenosa; ~ **immunoglobulin**
inmunoglobulina intravenosa; ~ **injection**
inyección intravenosa; ~ **urography** urografía
intravenosa
intraventricular bloqueo intraventricular;
~ **block** bloqueo intraventricular
intrinsic intrínseco, situado dentro de una parte
o perteneciente exclusivamente a ella;
~ **coagulation** coagulación intrínseca;
~ **coagulation pathway** sistema intrínseco de
coagulación, coagulación intrínseca
introduction presentación, introducción; ~ **of
fresh blood** refrescamiento de sangre
intron intrón; ~ **splicing** eliminación de intrones
introversion introversión
intrusion intrusión
intubation intubación, introducción de un tubo
en un órgano hueco; ~ **catheter** catéter de
intubación
intussusception intususpeción
inuline inulina
invalidate, to invalidar, debilitar
invasion invasión
invasive invasivo, que penetra, que invade;
~ **cancer** carcinoma invasivo, cáncer invasivo;
~ **carcinoma** carcinoma invasivo, cáncer
invasivo; ~ **hydatiform mole** mola maligna,
coriodemona, mola hidatiforme invasiva;
~ **procedure** procedimiento cruento;
~ **surgery** cirugía invasiva
inverse anafilaxia invertida
inversion inversión; ~ **loop** lazo de inversión;
~ **of uterus during birth** inversión uterina
parcial
invert, to invertir, poner al revés
inverted testicle torsión testicular
invert sugar azúcar invertido, mezcla de
glucosa y fructosa

investigate, to pesquisar, buscar, escudriñar, examinar, indagar, investigar

invoice factura, cobro, cuenta

involucrum involucro

involution (post-partum) involución, retorno del útero a su tamaño natural después del parto; ~ (upon aging) degradación y pérdida funcional de los órganos con el paso de la edad

involutional de involución, involutivo; ~ depression depresión de involución, depresión involutiva

involve, to implicar, involucrar

iodic rhinorrhoea coriza por yodo

iodide peroxidase ioduro-peroxidasa

iodinase ioduro-peroxidasa

iodination yoduración

iodine yodo; ~ deficiency disease enfermedad por carencia de yodo; ~ disinfection yoduración

ion ion

ion par par iónico

ionic iónico; ~ activity actividad iónica; ~ activity coefficient coeficiente de actividad iónica; ~ bond unión iónica, enlace iónico, inmovilización por adsorción; ~ polymerization polimerización iónica; ~ semiconductor semiconductor iónico; ~ strength fuerza iónica

ionization ionisación, ionización

ionizing radiation radiación ionizante

ionogram ionograma

iontophoresis ionoforesis

ipecac ipecacuana, alcaloide de ipecacuana

IPSP potencial postsináptico de inhibición

iridocyclitis iridociclitis (f), inflamación del iris y del cuerpo ciliar

iron hierro; ~ chelation quelación del hierro; ~ chelator quelante del hierro; ~ deficiency carencia de hierro; ~ deficiency anemia anemia por carencia de hierro, anemia ferropénica; ~ deficiency syndrome síndrome sideropénico; ~ -deficient ferriprivo; ~ lung respirador electrofrénico, pulmón de acero, pulmón artificial, respirador de Drinker; ~ metabolism metabolismo del hierro, metabolismo férrico; ~ metabolism disorder trastorno del metabolismo del hierro

irradiance irradiancia

irradiate, to irradiar

irradiated milk leche irradiada

irrational irracional; ~ behavior comportamiento irracional

irrationality irracionalidad

irregular aberrante, anormal, extraño, irregular, que difiere de lo normal; ~ heartbeat arritmia, falta de ritmo regular, pulso irregular

irregularly esporádicamente

irreversible irreversible, sin retorno; ~ inhibitors inhibidores irreversibles; ~ sterility esterilidad irreversible, insuperable

irrigate, to irrigar; ~ a wound irrigación de una herida

irrigation irrigación, riego o aporte sanguíneo; ~ cystoscope cistoscopio de irrigación; ~ syringe jeringuilla para irrigación

irritable irritable, quisquilloso, susceptible, colérico, irascible, arrebatadizo, gruñón, sensitivo; ~ bowel syndrome síndrome de colon irritable, colon inestable; ~ colon colon irritable, colon inestable

irritation irritación

ischemia isquemia, deficiencia del riego sanguíneo de una zona; ~ of the colon isquemia, deficiencia del riego sanguíneo de una zona

ischemic isquémico; ~ attack ataque isquémico; ~ brain cell célula cerebral isquémica, célula cerebral privada de irrigación sanguínea; ~ demyelination desmielinización isquémica; ~ heart disease (IHD) enfermedad cardiaca isquémica; ~ myocardial disease enfermedad cardiaca isquemica; ~ necrosis necrosis por coagulación; ~ pain dolor isquémico; ~ seizure ataque isquémico; ~ stroke ataque de isquemia en el cerebro

ischial bone isquión

ischiatic isquiático; ~ hernia hernia isquiática, isquiocele; ~ lymph node ganglio isquiático

ischiocapsular isquicapsular

ischium isquion

ischuria spastica iscuria espasmódica

islets of Langerhans islotes de Langerhans

isoagglutinin isoaglutinina

isoamylase isoamilasa

isoanaphylaxis isoanafilaxia

isoantibody aloanticuerpo

isoelectrical isoeléctrico; **~ point** punto isoeléctrico
isoelectrofocusing isoelectroenfoque
isoenzyme isoenzima
isoform isoforma
isoimmunization isoinmunización feto-materna
isoimmunoreaction isoinmunización
isolate, to aislar
isolation aislamiento; **~ place** local en cuarentena
isoleucine isoleucina
isoniazid isoniacida
isonicotinylhydrazine isoniacida
isonipecaine meperidina
isopregnenone didrogesterona
isopropyl alcohol alcohol isopropílico, alcohol alcanforado
isopters isópteras
isopycnose isopicnosis
isoschizomer isoesquizómero
isosmotic isosmótico
isosorbide dinitrate dinitrato de isosorbide
isotherapy isoterapia
isotonic isotónico; **~ buffered saline solution** solución salina isotónica (tamponada); **~ dehydration** deshidratación isotónica; **~ muscle contraction** contracción muscular isotónica; **~ solution** solución isotónica
isotope isótopo
isozyme isoenzima
isthmic ístmico; **~ spondylolisthesis** espondilolistesis, un movimiento de las vértebras de la columna vertebral
isthmus istmo; **~ uteri** istmo del útero
it ello
itch mite sarcoptes scabiei
itching *sub* prurito, picor, picazón, *adj* prurítico, picante, sarnoso, con picazón
itchy prurítico, hormigante, sarnoso, con picazón
iteration iteración
iteron iterón
ithyokyphosis itiocifosis
its esto
IU unidad internacional
IUD (intra-uterine device) alambrito, DIU, dispositivo intrauterino
IV intravenoso, situado dentro de una vena

J

jack sores infección por spirurida
jacuzzi bañera de hidromasaje, baño de remolino
Jamaica neuropathic syndrome síndrome neuropático de Jamaica
Janet syringe jeringuilla para heridas, jeringa de Janet
Janeway lesions lesiones de Janeway, manchas de Janeway, pequeñas máculas eritematosas que se producen en las palmas de las manos o plantas de los pies; **~ spots** lesiones de Janeway, manchas de Janeway, pequeñas máculas eritematosas que se producen en las palmas de las manos o plantas de los pies
Jansen operation operación de Jansen
Jansky-Bielschowsky disease lipofuscinosis ceroide neuronal, idiocia amaurótica familiar
January enero
jar, to chocar, sacudir
jaundice ictericia, coloración amarillenta de la piel
jaw mandíbula; **~ joint** articulación temporomaxilar, articulación temporomandibular; **~ retractor** retractor de mandíbulas
jawbone mandíbulo, quijada, maxilar superior
jejunoileostomy yeyunoileostomía
jejunum yeyuno, porción del intestino delgado comprendida entre el duodeno y el íleon
jelly jalea
jellyfish sting picadura de medusa
jerk, to crisparse
jet injector inyector a presión, inyector dermo-jet; **~ lag** desacomodación horaria, desambientación fisiológica; **~ of water** chorro de água
jewelry joyas
job stress estrés del trabajo
Johne's bacillus Mycobacterium paratuberculosis
joined conjugado
joining agregación, concentración
joint coyuntura; **~ ache** dolores articulares; **~ fluid** líquido sinovial; **~ inflammation** periartritis; **~ replacement implant** sustitución prostética de una articulación,

implante de sustitución osteoartricular

Jolliffe syndrome síndrome de Jolliffe

jolt, to chocar, sacudir

jostle, to chocar, sacudir

joule joule

jugal hueso malar

jugular yugular; **~ vein** vena yugular

juice jugo

July julio

jump, to saltar, lanzarse, tirarse

jumping gene gen saltador

junctional activity gap junctions sin alteración

June junio

Junin virus virus de Junin, virus del mal de los rastrojos

juvenile adolescente, joven, juvenil; **~ -onset diabetes** diabetes mellitus dependiente de insulina, diabetes de tipo I

K

Kahler's disease mieloma múltiple, plasmocitoma, mielomatosis, enfermedad de Kahler, enfermedad de Huppert el plasmocitoma, enfermedad de Bozzolo

kala-azar leismaniosis visceral, kala-azar

kanamycin kanamicina

Kaposi sarcoma sarcoma de Kaposi; **~ syndrome** sarcoma de Kaposi; **~ varicelliform eruption** erupción variceliforme kaposi

karyokinesis cariocinesis

karyolysis cariólisis, cromatólisis, disolución del núcleo celular

karyotype cariotipo

Kawasaki syndrome síndrome mucocutáneo adenopático

keep, to conservar, tener, guardar, reservar, mantener

keloid queloide, cicatriz elevada

kelvin kelvin

keratectomy queratectomia

keratin queratina

keratinocyte queratinocito

keratinous querático

keratitis keratitis, queratitis, inflamación de la córnea del ojo

keratoconjunctivitis queratoconjuntivitis, inflamación de la córnea y la conjuntiva del ojo

keratohyaline layer capa queratohialina, capa granulosa de la epidermis

kerato–iridocyclitis queratoidociclitis

keratolytic queratolítico, un agente que disuelve la capa córnea de la piel

keratoma senilis queratosis senil, queratosis actínicas

keratoplasty queratoplastia, trasplantación de córnea

keratosis queratosis; **~ follicularis** queratosis folicular; **~ follicularis acneiformis** queratosis folicular acneiforme; **~ labialis** queratosis labial; **~ pigmentosa** queratosis pigmentada

ketamine ketamina

ketoacidosis cetoacidosis, exceso de ácidos y cuerpos cetónicos en la sangre

ketoconazole ketoconazol

ketohexokinase cetohexocinasa

ketone body compuesto cetónico, cuerpo cetónicos

ketonuria cetonuria, acetonuria, presencia de cueroops cetónicos en la orina

key llave; **~ enzyme** enzima llave; **~ -hole surgery** cirugía laparoscopica

kickbacks fraude en la atención médica, abuso en las prestaciones médicas

kidney riñón, riñones; **~ dialysis** diálisis (de los riñones); **~ disease** nefropatía, enfermedad del riñón; **~ dish** cubeta para utensiles; **~ inflammation** nefritis, inflamación del riñón; **~ kallikrein** calicreína hística; **~ specialist** nefrólogo; **~ stone** cálculo renal, nefrolito, piedra del riñón; **~ transplant** trasplante de riñón

Kienböck disease enfermedad de Kienböck, mal del semilunar; **~ atrophy** atrofia de Kienboeck

killer matador; **~ DNA DNA** matador; **~ T cell** linfocito T citotóxico, célula T asesina

kilogram kilo

kinase quinasa

kind clase

kindergarden jardín de infancia

kind–of–property tipo de propiedad; **~ –of–quantity** tipo de magnitud

kinesiatrics cinesiterapia, cinesia, cinesis
kinesitherapy cinesiterapia, cinesia, cinesis
kinesthesis cinestesia
kinetic cinético, perteneciente al movimiento o que lo produce; **~ energy** energía cinética
kinetics cinética, estudio de las fuerzas que producen, detienen o modifican los movimientos del cuerpo; **~ of immobilized catalysts** cinética de catalizadores inmovilizados
kinetochore cinetocoro
King medium medio de King
kinin cinina
kininogenin calicreína plasmática
Kinyoun acid-fast stain tinción de ácidorresistencia de Kinyoun
kit equipo de reactivos
Kitasato's bacillus Yersinia pestis
Klauder erysipeloid erisipeloide de Klauder
Klebs-Löffler's bacillus Corynebacterium diphteriae
Klenow enzyme DNA-polimerasa dirigida por DNA
kleptolagnia cleptolagnia, cleptomanía sexual
knead, to amasamiento, amasar; **~ , to** amasamiento, amasar
knee rodilla; **~ -cap** rótula, patela, hueso de la rodilla, choquezuela; **~ jerk reflex** reflejo patelar; **~ pads** rodilleras
kneel, to arodillarse
knife cuchillo; **~ wound** cuchillada, herida por arma blanca, cuchillazo, cortadura profunda
knot ganglio, engrosamiento localizado en un nervio o vaso linfático
knotty nodular
know, to saber, conocer
known sample muestra testigo
knuckle articulación, nudillo; **~ -bending splint** ferula para doblar y inmovilizar los dedos
Koch's bacillus Mycobacterium tuberculosis
Koch-Weeks bacillus Haemophilus influenzae
Koebner phenomenon fenómeno de Koebner
Köhler illumination iluminación de Köhler
Köhler's disease enfermedad de Köhler
koilonychia coiloniquia, uña en cuchara, celoniquia
Koplik's spots manchas de Koplik

Kopp's asthma laringismo, espasmo de la laringe, laringospasmo
Korean hemorrhagic fever fiebre hemorrágica de Corea
Kornberg polymerase DNA-polimerasa dirigida por DNA
Kovacs oxidase test prueba de la oxidasa de Kovacs
Kruse-Sonne's bacillus Shigella sonnei
kufs disease lipofuscinosis ceroide neuronal, idiocia amaurótica familiar
kynureninase cinureninasa
kyphosis cifosis

L

L form forma L
lab tests exámenes médicos, pruebas
label, to etiquetar, poner etiqueta a
labeled atom atomo marcado; **~ water** agua marcada con lantano radioactivo, agua marcada con tritio radiactivo
labelling marcado
labia labios; **~** labios de la vagina
labial labial; **~ dyslalia** dislalia labial; **~ hernia** hernia labial; **~ hyperplasia** hiperplasia labial
labile lábil, inestable, fácilmente modificable o alterable, inconstante; **~ hypertension** hipertensión lábil
labor parto, trabajo; **~ pain** dolor de parto
laboratory laboratorio; **~ assistant** ayudante de laboratorio; **~ medicine** ciencias de laboratorio clínico; **~ test** procedimiento de medida, procedimiento analítico, análisis, prueba analítica
labored breathing respiración laboriosa
labyrinthine hearing loss sordera sensorineural, sordera de percepción, sordera neurosensorial, hipoacusia neurosensorial; **~ vertigo** síndrome de Menière
laceration laceración, desgarro, herida desgarrada
lack deficiencia, defecto, falta; **~ of appetite** inapetencia, anorexia, falta de apetito o ansia de adelgazar, pérdida de apetito; **~ of self-esteem** autodesvalorización, falta de amor

proprio; ~ **of sense of personal worth** anomalía de la personalidad, falta de autoestimación

lackadaisica lánguido, indiferente, apático, perezoso, despistado

lacrimal lagrimal, referido a las glándulas que secretan las lágrimas; ~ **bone** hueso lagrimal; ~ **ducts** conductos lagrimales, canal lacrimal; ~ **fluid** secreción lacrimal; ~ **fold** válvula de Bianchi, pliegue de Hasner; ~ **nerve** nervio lagrimal

lactase b-galactosidasa

lactate lactato; ~ **dehydrogenase** lactato deshidrogenasa; ~ , **to** lactar, amamantar, dar pecho

lactation lactación; ~ **hormone** hormona lactógena, prolactina

lactic láctic; ~ **acid** ácido láctico, ácidos lácticos, lactato; ~ **acid dehydrogenase** D-lactato-deshidrogenasa, L-lactato-deshidrogenasa; ~ **acidosis** acidosis láctica, acumulación de ácido láctico en el cuerpo; ~ **fermentation** fermentación láctica

Lactobacillus acidophilus Lactobacillus acidophilus, Bacillus acidophilus; ~ **plantarum** Lactobacillus plantarum

lactoferrin lactoferrina

lactogenesis lactogénesis, galactogénesis

lactogenic hormone hormona lactógena, prolactina

lactose lactosa

lactotropic hormone prolactina

lactotropin prolactina

lactoylglutathione lyase lactoilglutatión-liasa, metilglioxalasa

lacunar lacunar; ~ **tonsillitis** angina lacunar

lag phase fase de latencia

lagging strand cadena discontinua

LAL test prueba limulus

lamb borrego

lameness claudicación, cojera

laminagraph tomógrafo

laminar laminar; ~ **flow** flujo laminar

laminectomy laminectomía

lampbrush chromosome cromosoma plumoso

lancet for vaccination lanceta para vacunar

land tierra; ~ **mine** mina terrestre

Langerhans cell histiocytosis histiocitosis de células de Langerhans

language lenguaje, lengua, idioma

lanolin lanolina, grasa hecha con lana

lansoprazole lansoprazol

lanugo lanugo

laparoscope fibroscopio flexible, endoscopio de fibra óptica, laparoscopio

laparoscopy laparoscopia, cirugía laparoscopica

laparotomy laparotomía de Battle, incisión quirúrgica de la pared abdominal

lard manteca

large grande; ~ **intestine** intestino mayor, intestino grueso

laryngeal laríngeo; ~ **catalepsy** catalepsia laríngea; ~ **prominence** bocado de Adán, nuez de adán; ~ **spasm** laringismo, espasmo de la laringe, laringospasmo; ~ **speculum** espéculo laríngeo

laryngectomy laringectomía

laryngismus laringismo, espasmo de la laringe, laringospasmo; ~ **stridulus** laringismo estriduloso

laryngitis laringitis, inflamación de la laringe

larynx laringe

laser láser, rayo láser; ~ **angioplasty** angioplastia por láser, angioplastia coronaria con láser; ~ **beam** rayo láser; ~ **scalpel** bisturí láser; ~ **surgery** cirugía con láser

Lassa fever fiebre de Lassa; ~ **virus** virus Lassa

lassitude lasitud, debilidad, cansancio, agotamiento, laxitud

last último, pasado; ~ **name** apellido; ~ **time** última vez; ~ **week** semana pasada

late tardío

latency latencia, fase de latencia; ~ **period** período ventana, etapa de latencia; ~ **stage** período ventana, etapa de latencia

latent latente; ~ **diabetes** diabetes latente; ~ **period** período latente; ~ **time** período latente, período entre la aplicación o la recepción de un estímulo y la reacción consiguiente

later más tarde

lateral lateral, alejado del centro o de la línea media; ~ **angina** faringitis lateral; ~ **deviation** desviación lateral; ~ **root** raíz lateral; ~ **separation** rechazo lateral, separación lateral

latex látex; ~ **agglutination test** prueba de aglutinación con látex; ~ **fixation test** prueba de fijación con látex; ~ **skin-prick test** prick test para látex

laugh, to reírse, reír

laughing gas gas hilarante, óxido nitroso

laughter humor, jocosidad, comicidad, hilaridad

lavatory baño, inodoro, excusado

laxative laxante, purgante, medicamento contra el estreñimiento

layer capa, estrato; ~ **of tissue** estrato de tejido

lazy perezoso, vago; ~ **eye** ambliopía, visión bizcada; ~ **eye syndrome** ambliopía, visión bizcada, visión reducida

LDH lactato deshidrogenasa

LDL lipoproteína de baja densidad; ~ **cholesterol** colesterol de lipoproteínas de baja densidad, colesterol de LDL

L-dopa levodopa, L-dopa

lead plomo; ~ **apron** delantal de plomo, blusón de plomo; ~ **dioxide** lead dioxide, el óxido pulga, el anhídrido plúmbico, PbO2; ~ **-induced laryngeal paralysis** parálisis laríngea saturnina; ~ **-induced parodits** parodits saturnina; ~ **intoxication** gota saturnina, plumbismo, saturnismo crónico; ~ **palsy** parálisis por plomo, parálisis saturnina; ~ **paralysis** parálisis por plomo; ~ **poisoning** gota saturnina, plumbismo, saturnismo crónico; ~ **poisoning anemia** anemia saturnina, discrasia presaturnina

leader líder, jefe/a; ~ **sequence** secuencia guía

leading strand cadena adelantada, hebra conductora, hebra líder

leaky con goteras, que gotea, con fugas; ~ **mutation** mutación parcial

lean back, to doblarse por atrás; ~ **forward, to** inclinarse hacia adelante, agacharse, doblarse; ~ **out of a window, to** inclinarse en una ventana

lecture conferencia, disertación

left izquierda, a la izquierda; ~ **-handed** zurdo, pierna, siniestral, zurda; ~ **to the** a la izquierda; ~ **ventricular assist device, LVAD** aparato estimulador del ventrículo cardíaco; ~ **ventricular extrasystole** extrasístole ventricular izquierda; ~ **ventricular failure** insuficiencia del ventrículo izquierdo,

insuficiencia ventricular izquierda; ~ **ventricular hypertrophy** hipertrofia ventricular izquierda

leg pierna; ~ **prosthesis** pierna artificial, prótesis de la extremidad inferior; ~ **splint** férula para la pierna; ~ **ulcer** úlcera crural

legal legal; ~ **drugs** drogas legales, drogas lícitas; ~ **medicine** medicina legal y forense, medicina legal

legionnaire's disease enfermedad del legionario

leiomyoma leiomioma, mioma

leiomyosarcoma leiomiosarcoma

Leishmania infection leishmaniasis, leishmaniosis

leishmaniasis leishmaniasis, leishmaniosis

leisure ocio, tiempo libre; ~ **activities** actividades de tiempo libre; ~ **time** tiempo libre, descanso

lemon limón; ~ **balm** toronjil

length longitud; ~ **of life** longevidad, larga vida, duración de la vida

lenticular lenticular, con forma de lente; ~ **dermatofibroma** dermatofibroma lenticular

lentigo mola hidatídica, mola hidatidiforme, lentigo

leprosy lepra; ~ **bacterium** bacteria de la lepra

leprotic leproso; ~ **keratitis** queratitis leprosa

leprous de la lepra, leproso; ~ **conjunctivitis** conjuntivitis de la lepra

leptomeningeal cyst quiste aracnoideo

leptospira bacteria Leptospira

leptospirosis leptospirosis

leptotene leptotena

lesbian lesbiana

lesion lesión, herida, daño, desperfecto

less menos

lethal letal, mortal; ~ **concentration** concentración letal; ~ **dose** dosis letal; ~ **dose of radiation** dosis letal de radiación; ~ **gene** gen letal; ~ **threshold dose** dosis umbral letal

lethargic aletargo

lethargy letargo, somnolencia o indiferencia

Letterer-Siwe disease enfermedad Letterer-Siwe

leucine leucina; ~ **aminopeptidase** leucil-aminopeptidasa; ~ **enkephalin** encefalina

leucina; ~ -sensitive hypoglycemia hipoglucemia sensible a la leucina;
~ transaminase leucina-transaminasa

leucocyte leucocito; ~ count recuento leucocitario; ~ diapedesis diapédesis de leucocitos, diapédesis leucocitaria;
~ interferon interferón leucocitario, interferón alfa

leucopenia leucopenia, reducción del número de glóbulos blancos en la sangre

leucyl aminopeptidase leucil-aminopeptidasa;
~ peptidase leucil-aminopeptidasa

leukemia leucemia, leucemia; ~ cell line línea celular leucémica

leukocyte leucocito; ~ adhesion deficiency deficiencia de adhesión leucocitaria de tipo II;
~ elastase elastasa de leucocito

leukocytic leucocítico, perteneciente o relativo a los glóbulos blancos de la sangre

leukocytosis leucocitosis, incremento del número de glóbulos blancos en la sangre

leukoderma leucodermia

leukoerythroblastic anemia anemia leucoeritroblástica

leukogram fórmula leucocitaria

leukokeratosis leucoplasia, leucoplaquia, leucoqueratosis, formación de manchas blancas en las mucosas

leukomonocyte linfocito

leukopenia leucopenia, reducción del número de glóbulos blancos en la sangre

leukoplakia leucoplasia, leucoplaquia, leucoqueratosis, formación de manchas blancas en las mucosas

leukoplasia leucoplasia, leucoplaquia, leucoqueratosis, formación de manchas blancas en las mucosas

leukorrhea leucorrea, exceso de secreción de flujo blanco de la vagina

level concentración, nivel

levodopa levodopa

levonorgestrel levonorgestrel

LH/FSH-RFL gonadoliberina

LHL lutropina

LH-RFL luliberina

liaison enlace, coordinación, relación; ~ group grupo de enlace

libido libido, deseo sexual, naturaleza

library biblioteca

lice piojos, pediculosis, infestación humana por piojos, piojos, cáncanos, sabandija

lichenification liquenificación, engrosamiento de ciertas capas en la piel

lick, to lamer

licofelone licofelone

lidocaine lidocaína

L-iduronidase L-iduronidasa

lie, to echarse, acostarse, tumbarse; ~ down, to acostarse; ~ on the table face up, to acostarse sobre la mesa boca arriba; ~ on your back, to acostarse boca arriba

life vida; ~ expectancy promedio de vida, esperanza de vida; ~ insurance seguro de vida

ligament ligamento

ligamentous desmoide, ligamentoso

ligand ligando

ligase ligasa; ~ chain reaction reacción en cadena por la ligasa

ligation ligación

light ligero, claro; ~ -headed mareado, aturdido, ligeramente indispuesto, delirante;
~ microscope microscopio óptico;
~ microscopy microscopia óptica

lightheadedness mareado, aturdido, ligeramente indispuesto, delirante

lignocaine lidocaína

like mismo, semejante, como

likelihood ratio razón de verosimilitud

limber elástico, saltarín, flojo; ~ up, to precalentarse, aflojarse, entrar en calor

limbic límbico, relativo a un borde o margen;
~ system sistema límbico, agrupación de estructuras dentro del rinencéfalo

limit limitación, límite; ~ of detection límite de detección

limitation limitación, límite

limp, to cojear, renquear, zalenquear

limping cojera, claudicación

Limulus test prueba del Limulus

lincomycin lincomicina

line rágade, fisura, grieta o escara lineal de la piel

linea albicante estrías, veteaduras, vetas

lineality range intervalo analítico

linear linear, relativo a una línea o parecido a ella; ~ accelerator acelerador lineal de partículas

linearity rectilinealidad, linealidad

lineic lineico -ica; ~ **absorbance** absorbancia linéica

lines rágade, fisura de la piel

link, to unir, conectar

linkage conjugacion, ligamiento; ~ **group** grupo de enlace

linked gene gen ligado

linker ligador; ~ **DNA** ADN de unión, ADN de enlace

linking number número total de vueltas

lip labio; ~ **surgery** plastía del labio

lipemia concentración de lípido en plasma, concentración de lípido en suero

lipid lípido, grasas y sustancias similares; ~ **bilayer** bicapa lipídica; ~ **lowering medication** fármaco hipolipidemiante; ~ **membrane** membrana lipídica; ~ **peroxidation** peroxidación lipídica

lipoatrophic lipoatrófico; ~ **diabetes** diabetes mellitus lipoatrofica

lipocyte célula cebada

lipodystrophy lipodistrofia, alteración en el metabolismo de las grasas

lipoid spleno-hepatomegaly enfermedad de Niemann, enfermedad de Niemann-Pick, esfingolipidosis, esfingomielinasa

lipolysis lipolisis

lipoma lipoma

lipomatosis lipomatosis

lipomatous lipomatoso; ~ **nephritis** nefritis lipomatosa

lipophilic lipófilo, soluble en grasa, capaz de disolver las grasas, que tiene predisposición a la obesidad

lipophosphodiesterase fosfolipasa D

lipoprotein lipoproteína, combinación de una grasa y una proteína; ~ **lipase** lipoproteína-lipasa

lipo-soluble liposoluble

liposome liposoma

liposuction liposucción

lipotropic hormone lipotropina

liquid líquido; ~ **chromatography** cromatografía en fase líquida, cromatografía de líquidos; ~ **culture medium** medio de cultivo líquido; ~ **enrichment medium** medio

líquido de enriquecimiento; ~ **-gel chromatography** cromatografía líquido-gel; ~ **-liquid chromatography** cromatografía líquido-líquido; ~ **-liquid extraction** extracción líquido-líquido; ~ **scintillation counter** contador de centelleo líquido

liquifilm película líquida

liquor liquor

lisozime muramidasa sérica

listen, to escuchar

listeria listeria (una bacteria); ~ **monocytogenes infection** listeriosis

listeriosis listeriosis, listeriosis

listless decaído, apático

liter litro

lithium litio; ~ **ion** ion litio; ~ **salts** sales de litio

litocholic acid ácido litocólico

litter camilla, las parihuelas

little pequeño, chico, poco, apenas; ~ **finger** dedo meñique; ~ **toe** dedo pequeño del pie

livedo livedo, punto o mancha de alteración de color sobre la piel

liver hígado; ~ **cell** células hepáticas (cultivadas); ~ **enlargement** hepatomegalia, aumento del tamaño del hígado; ~ **enzymes** enzimas del hígado; ~ **profile** informe del estado del hígado; ~ **scan** gammagrafía hepática; ~ **transplant** transplante hepático

livid lívido

lividity lividez

livor mortis livor mortis, prerigor

load, to cargar

loading dose dosis de cebamiento, dosis inicial; ~ **solution** solución de carga, solución tamponada

lobar lobar

lobate hymen himen lobular

lobe lóbulo

local local, restringido, no general; ~ **anesthesia** anestesia local; ~ **immunity** inmunidad tisular

localization localización, determinación del sitio o lugar de un proceso, restricción a un área limitada

locating localización, determinación del sitio o lugar de un proceso, restricción a un área limitada

lochia loquios, pérdidas vaginales tras el parto

lockjaw trismo, imposibilidad de apertura total de la boca, trismus

locomotor locomotor; ~ **system** aparato locomotor

locoregional locorregional, local y regional

locus locus

Löffler's bacillus Corynebacterium diphtheriae

logit logit

loin lomo

lomefloxacin lomefloxacina

long larga; ~ **-acting drug** fármaco de acción duradera; ~ **life** longevidad, larga vida, duración de la vida; ~ **time ago** hace mucho tiempo; ~ **-term care** atenciones a largo plazo; ~ **-term survivors** sobrevivientes a largo plazo

longevity longevidad, larga vida, duración de la vida

longitudinal longitudinal; ~ **comparision** comparación longitudinal

look, to mirar

loop asa

loose, to perder; ~ **blood** desangramiento, hemorragia, sangrado, sangría; ~ **consciousness, to** perder el conocimiento; ~ **skin** cutis laxa, dermatolisis, chalazodermia; ~ **weight, to** emagrecer, adelgazar

loosening movilización

loperamide loperimida, agente antiperistáltico

loquacious hablador, loquaz, parlanchín

loratidine loratidina

lorazepam loracepam, tranquilizante

loss pérdida; ~ **of appetite** inapetencia, anorexia, falta de apetito o ansia de adelgazar, pérdida de apetito; ~ **of blood** pérdida de sangre, sangrado; ~ **of consciousness** ampliacion de la consciencia; ~ **of hair** caída de cabello; ~ **of intelligence** pérdida de inteligencia, carencia intelectual, desintegración de la inteligencia; ~ **of memory** pérdida de memoria, amnesia; ~ **of strength** astenia, cansancio físico intenso, debilidad corporal general, falta de fuerza; ~ **of voice** afonia, perdida de la voz; ~ **of weight** pérdida de peso

lotion loción

lots bastante, mucho

Lou Gehrig's disease enfermedad de Lou

Gehrig, esclerose lateral amiotrófica

loud fuerte

loudness volumen; ~ **recruitment** hiperacusia

Louis–Bar syndrome ataxia telangiectasia

louse piojo

lovastatin lovastatina

low bajo; ~ **back pain** dolor lumbar bajo, dolor bajo de espalda, dolor de la espalda inferior, presión baja; ~ **backache** dolor lumbar bajo, presión baja; ~ **blood pressure** hipotensión arterial, hipotonía; ~ **-calorie diet** dieta baja en calorías; ~ **-cholesterol diet** dieta pobre en colesterol; ~ **-density lipoprotein** lipoproteína de baja densidad; ~ **-grade fever** febrícula; ~ **plasma volume** bajo volumen plasmático; ~ **point** nadir, punto más bajo; ~ **-tar cigarette** cigarillo con poco contenido de alquitrán; ~ **white blood cell count** neutropenia, disminución del número de leucocitos neutrófilos en la sangre

lower amplitud radiocubital inferior; ~ **back** cintura; ~ **extremities** pierna; ~ **jaw** mandíbulo, quijada, maxilar inferior; ~ **jawbone** mandíbulo, quijada, maxilar inferior; ~ **limbs** pierna; ~ **lobe** lóbulo inferior; ~ **part** base, fundamento, parte inferior

lower, to bajar

lozenge pastilla

luciferase luciferasa

luetic luético, sifilítico

luggage equipaje (m)

Lugol's solution solución de Lugol

lukewarm tibio; ~ **water** agua tibia

luliberin luliberina

lumbago lumbago, dolor en la parte inferior de la columna vertebral

lumbar lumbar, relacionado con la parte inferior de la columna vertebral; ~ **herniated disc** disco lumbar herniado; ~ **portion of the spinal column** porción lumbar de la columna vertebral; ~ **puncture** punción lumbar; ~ **region** cintura; ~ **rigidity** rigidez lumbar; ~ **spine** porción lumbar de la columna vertebral; ~ **splenic puncture** punción medular; ~ **sympathetic** simpático lumbar; ~ **vertebrae** vértebras lumbares

lumen lumen, cavidad o canal dentro de un

órgano en forma de tubo

luminescent luminiscente; ~ **screen** pantalla luminiscente, consta generalmente de sulfuro de zinc mezclado con otros materiales

luminiscence luminiscencia; ~ **immunoassay** luminoinmunoanálisis

luminoimmunoassay luminoinmunoanálisis

luminometer luminómetro

luminous luminoso; ~ **flux** flujo luminoso; ~ **intensity** intesidad luminosa

lump bola/bolita, bulto, chichón, tolondro

lumpectomy tumorectomia, mastectomia segmental

lunatic maníaco, loco, descabellado

lunch almuerzo

lung pulmón; ~ **biopsy** biopsia pulmonar; ~ **cancer** cáncer de pulmón, cáncer broncopulmonar; ~ **capacity** capacidad vital, volumen de gas que puede expulsarse de los pulmones; ~ **collagen** colágeno pulmonar; ~ **disease** enfermedad pulmonar, neumopatía; ~ **mechanics** mecánica pulmonar, mecánica respiratoria; ~ **power** flujo maximal

lupoid lupoide; ~ **panmyelopathy** panmielopatía lupoide

lupus lupino, lupino, de la piel, lupus eritomatoso sistémico; ~ **anticoagulant** anticoagulante lúpico; ~ **pernio** sarcoidosis, enfermedad de Schaumann, sarcoide de Boeck

Luschka's bursa bolsa faríngea

luteal phase fase de secreción

luteinizing hormone hormona luteinizante, lutropina; ~ **–releasing factor** luliberina; ~ **releasing hormone** hormona de liberación de la gonadotrofina

lutropin hormona luteinizante, lutropina

luxation dislocación, luxación, esguince, torcedura; ~ **of the clavicle** luxación de la clavícula; ~ **of the patella** luxación de la rótula, luxación patelar; ~ **of the temporomandibular joint** luxación temporomaxilar

lyase liasa

lycopene licopeno, hidrocarburo no saturado, cristalino y rojo que constituye el pigmento carotenoide de los tomates

lye lejía, lejía de sosa

Lyell's syndrome necrólisis epidérmioca tóxica

lying falso, mentiroso; ~ **face up** acostado boca arriba; ~ **prone** estar boca abajo, estar postrado, acostado boca abajo; ~ **supine** acostado boca arriba, estar supino

Lyme disease enfermedad de Lyme

lymph plasma, linfa, líquido corporal; ~ **corpuscle** linfocito; ~ **glands** linfonódulos, ganglios linfáticos; ~ **node** ganglio linfático; ~ **node disease** linfadenopatía, tumefacción de uno o más ganglios linfáticos; ~ **nodules** linfonódulos

lymphadenectomy adenotomía, linfadenectomía

lymphadenitis linfadenitis

lymphadenopathy linfadenopatía, tumefacción de uno o más ganglios linfáticos

lymphangioleiomyomatosis linfangioleiomiomatosis

lymphangitis linfangitis, inflamación de los vasos linfáticos

lymphatic linfático; ~ **bundle** paquete linfático; ~ **drainage** drenaje linfático; ~ **system** sistem linfático; ~ **vessel inflammation** linfangitis, inflamación de los vasos linfáticos

lymphedema limfoedema

lymphnoduli linfonódulos, ganglios linfáticos

lymphoblast linfoblasto; ~ **interferon** interferón leucocitario, interferón alfa

lymphocyte linfocito; ~ **depletion** depleción grave, colapso ganglionar; ~ **marker** marcador linfocitario

lymphocytic linfocitario, concierne a los linfocitos, células con núcleo redondo; ~ **infiltrate** infiltrado linfocítico; ~ **lymphoma** linfoma linfocítico, linfocitoma, linfoma linfocítico maligno bien diferenciado

lymphocytoma linfoma linfocítico, linfocitoma, linfoma linfocítico maligno bien diferenciado

lymphoedema limfoedema

lymphogenous leukaemia leucemia linfoblástica aguda, leucemia linfocítica, leucemia linfática, leucemia linfógena, leucemia linfoide

lymphogranuloma linfogranuloma; ~ **venereum** linfopatía venérea

lymphoid linfoide; ~ **cancer** linfoma, tumor

maligno originado en el tejido linfoide; ~ **cell** linfocito; ~ **follicle** folículo primario, folículo linfoide; ~ **leucocyte** linfocito; ~ **leukemia** leucemia linfoblástica aguda, leucemia linfocítica, leucemia linfática, leucemia linfógena, leucemia linfoide; ~ **stroma** estroma linfoide

lymphokine linfocina, linfokina, linfoquina; ~ **activated killer** linfocito matador activado por la interleucina

lymphoma linfoma, tumor maligno originado en el tejido linfoide

lymphoreticular linforeticular; ~ **malignancy** neoplasia linforeticular

lymphosarcoma linfosarcoma, linfoma linfocítico, linfocitoma, linfoma linfocítico maligno

lymphotoxin linfotoxina

lyophilisate producto liofilizado, producto preparado mediante congelación y deshidratación

lyophilizate producto liofilizado, producto preparado mediante congelación y deshidratación

lyophilization liofilización, criodesecación

lyophilized liofilizado; ~ **gamma globulin** gammaglobulina liofilizada

lysine lisina

lysis lisis, disolución, desaparición gradual

lysogenic lisogénico

lysogenicity lisogenia

lysogeny lisogenia

lysosome lisosoma

lysozyme lisozima

lytic lítico, que concierne o influye en la destrucción de la célula

M

MacConkey agar agar de MacConkey

maceration maceración, hinchazón o ablandamiento por contacto con líquidos

Machado–Joseph disease enfermedad de Machado-Joseph

machinist maquinista; ~ **disease** enfermedad de los maquinistas, trastorno cervicobraquial laboral

machismo machismo, discriminación sexual adoptada por los hombres

macrobiotic macrobiótico

macrocephaly macrocefalia, megaencefalia

macroconidia macroconidia

macrocythemia macrocitemia, macrocitosis, megalocitosis

macrocytosis macrocitemia, macrocitosis, megalocitosis

macroglobulin macroglobulina

macroglobulinemia macroglobulinemia

macrolide macrólido

macron partícula macroscópica, macrón

macrophage macrófago; ~ **activating factor** factor activador de macrófagos; ~ **chemotactic factor** factor quimiotactico de macrófagos; ~ **migration inhibitory factor** factor inhibidor de la migración de los macrófagos

macrophyte macrofita

macroscopic macroscópico; ~ **properties** propiedades macroscópicas

macula mácula; ~ **lutea** mancha amarilla, mácula lútea

macular macular; ~ **degeneration** degeneración macular

macule mácula, mancha en la retina, mancha

maculopapular maculopapular, consistente en manchas y pápulas

MAF (Macrophage Activating Factor) factor activador de macrófagos

magnesium magnesio; ~ **ion** ion magnesio; ~ **lactate** lactato de magnesio; ~ **sulphate** sulfato magnésico, sulfato de magnesio, sal de magnesio

magnetic magnético; ~ **particle detector** detector de partículas magnéticas; ~ **resonance imaging** proyección de imágenes por resonancia magnética, IRM, MRI, imagen por resonancia magnética; ~ **resonance imaging of the brain** IRM cerebral, RM cerebral; ~ **resonance spectroscopy of the brain** espectroscopia por resonancia magnética cerebral, ERM cerebral

magnifying glass lupa

magnitude cuantía

maidenhair tree ginkgo biloba

main primario, principal, primero, al principio, originario; ~ **ingridient** constituyente principal de un medicamento

maintenance mantenimiento, manutención; ~ **chemotherapy** quimioterapia de mantenimiento, quimioterapia de sostén

major muy importante, fundamental; ~ **histocompatibility antigen** antígeno de histocompatibilidad; ~ **histocompatibility complex (MHC)** complejo principal de histocompatibilidad; ~ **joints** coyunturas principales, articulaciones principales; ~ **medical benefits** beneficios médicos suplementarios; ~ **medical expense insurance** beneficios médicos suplementarios

make, to hacer, confeccionar, preparar, grabar, fabricar; ~ **love, to** tener relaciones sexuales, hacer uso de, practicar el coito, copular, usar

malabsorption malabsorción, trastorno de la absorción intestinal de nutrientes; ~ **syndrome** síndrome de malabsorción

malaise malestar

malar hueso malar

malaria malaria, paludismo

male masculino, varón, andrógeno, que produce caracteres masculinos; ~ **circumcision** circuncisión del hombre; ~ **gonad** testículo, gonada masculina; ~ **impotence** impotencia masculina, falta del poder de copulación en el hombre; ~ **menopause** andropausia

malformation malformación, disgenesia

malfunction disfunción, perturbación del funcionamiento de un órgano

malignancy malignidad, neoplasma maligno

malignant pernicioso, peligroso, maligno; ~ **bubo** bubón maligno; ~ **carbuncle** carbunco, pústula maligna, carbunco contagioso; ~ **epithelioma** cáncer de la piel, cáncer cutáneo, epitelioma; ~ **hypertension** hipertensión maligna; ~ **malaria** fiebre estivootoñal, el paludismo falciparum, paludismo causado por P. falciparum; ~ **melanoma** melanoma maligno, melanocarcinoma, cáncer melánico; ~ **mesothelioma** mesotelioma; ~ **mole** mola maligna, coriodemoma, mola hidatiforme invasiva; ~ **neoplasm** neoplasma maligno; ~ **tumor** neoplasma maligno

malinger, to fingirse enfermo, hacerse el enfermo

malleolar maleolar; ~ **eversion fracture** fractura maleolar por abducción

malnutrition inanición, desnutrición, subalimentación, hipotrepsia, mala nutrición

malpighian cell célula de Malpighi, célula espinosa; ~ **corpuscles** corpúsculos de Malpighi

maltase a-glucosidasa

maltodextrin maltodextrina

mamillary mamilar; ~ **body** cuerpo mamilar; ~ **plexus** plexo mamilar

mamma mamá; ~ **carcinoma** cáncer de mama, cáncer mamario, cáncer del pecho, cáncer del seno

mammaplasty mamoplastia

mammary mamario, relativo a la mama; ~ **gland** glándula mamaria

mammatropic hormone prolactina

mammatropin prolactina

mammogram cribado mamográfico, mamografía, mamograma

mammography screening cribado mamográfico, mamografía, mamograma

mammoplasty mamoplastia

man hombre

manage, to dirigir, administrar, manejar, poder con

managed care asistencia de hospital integrado, los cuidados dirigidos

mandible mandíbulo, quijada, maxilar inferior

mandibular mandibular; ~ **joint** articulación temporomaxilar, articulación temporomandibular

mange mite sarcoptes scabiei; ~ **mites** ácaros de la sarna

mangy tinoso, sarnoso

mania manía

maniac maníaco, loco

manic maníaco, relativo a una manía; ~ ~ **depressive psychosis** enfermedad maniacodepresiva bipolar

manifest manifiesto, ostensible, evidente

manifestation manifestación (f), exteriorización de una enfermedad

manly masculino, varón, andrógeno, que produce caracteres masculinos

M

mannitol manitol; ~ **salt agar** agar con manitol y sal

mannose manosa

manometry medida manométrica, manometría; ~ **of the small intestine** manometría del intestino delgado

Mantoux test prueba de la tuberculina

manual manual; ~ **dexterity** destreza manual; ~ **insufflator** insuflador manual; ~ **resuscitation appliance** aparato de reanimación manual

manubrium manubrio

manufacture producción, fabricación

manufacturer fabricante

many muchos

MAO (monoamine–oxidase) monoanima oxidasa, amina–oxidasa (flavinífera); ~ **inhibitor** inhibidor de la monoaminooxidasa, inhibidor MAO, IMAO

mapping cartografía, aplicación (matemática), función (matemática); ~ **and sequencing the human genome** estudio y secuenciación del genoma humano

maprotiline maprotilina

March marzo

marginal marginal; ~ **gingivitis** gengivite marginal

marigold calendula officinalis

marijuana marihuana

marital conyugal; ~ **rape** violación conyugal, estupro de la esposa; ~ **status** estado civil

marker marcador; ~ **gene** gen marcador

marketing mercadotecnia

marriage matrimonio; ~ **counseling** asesoramiento matrimonial; ~ **counselor** consejero matrimonial

married casado

marrow médula, tuétano; ~ **-related** medular, relativo a la a la médula de cualquier tipo

Martin–Bell syndrome síndrome del X frágil

masculine masculino, varón, andrógeno, que produce caracteres masculinos; ~ **pseudo–hermaphroditism** androginismo, seudo–hermafrodismo masculino; ~ **virile hyperoestrogenism** hiperestrogenismo viril masculino; ~ **woman** virago, hombruna

masculinity virilismo, masculinidad

masculinization virilización, masculinización

mask máscara

mass masa; ~ **concentration** concentración de masa; ~ **fraction** fracción de masa; ~ **number** número de masa; ~ **rate** caudal de masa; ~ **spectrometer** espectrómetro de masas; ~ **spectrometry** espectrometría de masas; ~ **spectroscopy** espectroscopía de masa, espectrometría de masa

massage masaje; ~ **apparatus** aparato para masaje; ~ **therapist** masajista; ~ **, to** sobar, friccionar, hacer masajes

massaging device aparato para masaje

massic másico

massive masivo, grande, amplio, macizo; ~ **progressive pneumoconiosis** neumoconiosis masiva progresiva

mast cell mastocito, célula de Mast

mastectomy mastectomía

mastication masticación

masticatory masticatorio, que afecta a los músculos de la masticación, que debe masticarse

mastitis mastitis, inflamación de la glándula mamaria

mastocyte mastocito, célula de Mast

mastodynia mastodinia, dolor de la mama

mastoid mastoideo; ~ **process** apófisis mastoides

mastoiditis mastoiditis (f), inflamación de la apófisis mastoides, en el oído

masturbate, to masturbarse

masturbation masturbación

materia medica materia médica, la farmacología homeopática

maternal materno; ~ **dystocia** distocia materna; ~ **inheritance** herencia materna

maternity maternidad; ~ **clinic** hospital de maternidad, clínica de maternidad; ~ **girdle** faja de embarazada, faja de embarazo

mating apareamiento

matrix matriz; ~ **metalloproteinase I** colagenasa intersticial

matter materia, sustancia, material

mature maduro; ~ **lymphocyte** linfocito maduro

maudlin lánguido, indiferente, apático, perezoso, despistado

maxillary maxilar, relativo a los huesos de la

cara donde se encuentran fijados los dientes

maximal máximo, efecto o cantidad mayores que pueden lograrse; ~ **allowable error** máximo error tolerable

maximum máximo, acmé de un proceso o una enfermedad; ~ **breathing capacity** ventilación máxima voluntaria; ~ **medical improvement** máxima mejoría médica; ~ **voluntary ventilation** ventilación máxima voluntaria

may poder, deber

May mayo

maybe tal vez

mazindol macindol, agente anorexígeno

mazodynia mastodinia, dolor de la mama

MC antigen antígeno MC

mca anticuerpo monoclonal

McFarland nephelometer nefelómetro de McFarland

MDMA (Ecstasy) MDMA, éxtasis

me me, a mí

meal comida

mean media (aritmética), promedio; ~ **lethal concentration** concentración letal media; ~ **life** vida media; ~ **time** tiempo medio

measles sarampión; ~ **vaccine** vacuna contra sarampión; ~ **virus** virus del sarampión

measurand mesurando

measure, to medir

measurement medida, medición; ~ **procedure** procedimiento de medida; ~ **range** intervalo de medida

measuring medición; ~ **curve** curva de medida; ~ **function** función de medida; ~ **instrument** instrumento de medida; ~ **interval** intervalo de medida; ~ **system** sistema de medida; ~ **tape** cinta para medir

meat carne

meatus of the urethra hoyito del chi

mechanical mecánico; ~ **aspirator** aspirador mecánico

mechanism mecanismo

mechanization mecanización

mechanoreceptor mecanorreceptor

Meckel's cavity cavidad de Meckel; ~ **diverticulum** divertículo de Meckel

meconium meconio, excrementos del recien nacido durante las primeras 24 a 48 horas de vida

medical médico; ~ **acoustics** acústica médica; ~ **anthropology** antropología médica; ~ **assistant** asistente de médico, ayudante de médico, auxiliar de médico; ~ **attention** asistencia médica; ~ **belt** faja médica; ~ **care** asistencia médica, prestaciones sanitarias; ~ **counseling** consejo médico; ~ **device** producto sanitario; ~ **engineering** técnica médica, ingeniería médica; ~ **ethics** ética médica; ~ **evacuation sheet** ficha médica de evacuación; ~ **exam** reconocimiento médico, exploración, examen, seguimiento médico; ~ **examination** reconocimiento médico, exploración, examen, seguimiento médico; ~ **examiner** inspector médico, médico asesor; ~ **fee** honorario, honorarios médicos; ~ **files** fichas clínicas, fichas médicas; ~ **genetics** genética médica; ~ **history** historial médico; ~ **imaging software** sistema informatizado para imágenes médicas; ~ **imaging system** sistema de imágenes médicas, imagen cardíaca; ~ **insurance** seguro de enfermedad, cobertura de los riesgos de enfermedad; ~ **intolerance** intolerancia, incapacidad para soportar un medicamento; ~ **jurisprudence** medicina legal y forense, medicina legal; ~ **laboratory** laboratorio médico; ~ **malpractice** error médico; ~ **microbiologist** microbiólogo médico; ~ **mycology** micología médica; ~ **officer** inspector médico, médico asesor; ~ **pharmaceutical assistance** asistencia medico-farmaceutica; ~ **practice** consultorio de medicina, el consultorio médico, practica médica; ~ **prescription** prescripción, receta médica; ~ **psychology** psicología médica, psicología clínica; ~ **questionnaire** cuestionario médico; ~ **radiology** radiología médica; ~ **records** expedientes, registros, registros médicos, récords médicos, fichero médico; ~ **report** informe médico, relato médico; ~ **research** investigación médica; ~ **residency** residencia médica, especialización en la medicina; ~ **resident** residente; ~ **robot** robot médico; ~ **robotics** robótica quirúrgica, robótica médica; ~ **science** ciencia médica; ~ **social worker** asistente médico social; ~ **specialist** médico especialista; ~ **supplies** dotación médica, botiquín; ~ **terms** términos médicos; ~ **tests** exámenes médicos, pruebas; ~ **treatment** tratamiento médico

median mediano; ~ **effective concentration** concentración eficaz mediana; ~ **effective dose** dosis mediana efectiva

mediastinal del mediastino, mediastino; ~ **cancer** neoplasma del mediastino, tumor del mediastino; ~ **cavity** mediastino; ~ **hernia** hernia mediastínica; ~ **lymph node** ganglio mediastínico; ~ **neoplasm** neoplasma del mediastino, tumor del mediastino; ~ **shift** movimiento del mediastino

mediastinum mediastino

mediate, to mediar, abogar, arbitrar, intervenir

mediator mediador, sustancia química que transmite algo

Medicaid seguro de enfermedad del gobierno, programa de asistencia médica del gobierno de los EE.UU. para los pobres

medicament fármaco, medicamento, medicina

medicamentous medicinal; ~ **mixtures** mezclas medicinales

Medicare seguro de salud del gobierno

medicate, to medicinar, curar, medicamentar, medicar

medicated medicinal, medicado; ~ **elixir** elixir

medication medicación, prescripción o aplicación de medicamentos, medicamento

medicinal medicinal, medicado; ~ **beer** cerveza medicinal; ~ **extract** extracto medicinal; ~ **flask** frasco medicinal; ~ **herbs** hierbas medicinales, plantas medicinales; ~ **leech** sanguijuela medicinal, hirudo; ~ **mud** barro termal, barro terapéutico, sedimentos curativos, fangoterapia; ~ **plants** hierbas medicinales, plantas medicinales

medicine medicina, medicación, prescripción, medicamento; ~ **cart** carrito de medicamentos; ~ **dropper** cuéntagotas medicinal; ~ **man** merolico, curandero; ~ **wagon** carrito de medicamentos

medico-social research investigación médico-social

medifraud fraude en la atención médica, abuso en las prestaciones médicas

Mediterranean anemia anemia mediterránea, talasemia

Medrol metilprednisolona

medulla oblongata bulbo raquídeo, medulla oblongata

medullary medular, relativo a la médula de cualquier tipo; ~ **canal** conducto medular espinal, conducto espinal; ~ **stroma** estroma medular; ~ **syndrome** síndrome medular

medulloblastoma meduloblastoma

mefenamic acid ácido mefenámico

megacaryocyte megacariocito

megacolon megacolon, colon anormalmente grande o dilatado

megakaryoblast megacarioblasto

megakaryocyte megacariocito

megalencephaly macrocefalia, megaencefalia

megaloblastic megaloblástico

megalocornea córnea globosa

megalocytosis macrocitemia, macrocitosis, megalocitosis

megalomania megalomanía, delirio de grandeza

megaloureter megauréter, megalouréter

meiosis meiosis

meiotic meiótico; ~ **disjunction** disyunción meiótica

melaena melena, excremento oscuro conteniendo sangre, vómitos negros

melamine formaldehyde melamina formaldehído

melanin melanina

melanoblast melanoblasto

melanoblastoma melanoma maligno, melanocarcinoma, cáncer melánico

melanocyte melanocito; ~ **–stimulating hormone** hormona estimulante de melanocitos, melanotropina

melanocytic melanocítica

melanoderma melanodermia

melanoma melanoma, cáncer melánico

melanophages melanófagos

melanosis melanosis (f), coloración oscura superficial de la piel o las mucosas

melanotropin release–inhibiting factor melanostatina; ~ **–releasing factor** melanoliberina

melanuria melanuria

melasma blefaromelasma

melatonin melatonina

melibiase a-galactosidasa

melphalan melfalan

melphalanum melfalan

member miembro, pene, cosa

membrane membrana; ~ **protein** proteína de la membrana celular, proteína membranal

membranous membranoso;
~ **glomerulonephritis** glomerulonefritis membranosa

memory memoria; ~ **cell** célula de memoria;
~ **disorder** trastorno de la memoria;
~ **disturbance** trastorno de la memoria; ~ **loss** pérdida de memoria, amnesia; ~ **training** adiestramiento de la memoria

menarche menarca, menarquía, fecha de la primera menstruación

Menetrier disease gastritis hipertrófica gigante

Ménière's disease síndrome de Menière;
~ **syndrome** síndrome de Menière

meningeal meningeo; ~ **herniation** meningocele

meninges meninges

meningioma meningioma

meningiome meningioma

meningitis meningitis, inflamación de las meninges

meningocele meningocele

meningococcal meningitis meningitis cerebroespinal epidémica

meniscus menisco

menopausal menopáusico

menopause climaterio, menopausia;
~ **hypertension** hipertensión climatérica

menorrhagia menorragia, menstruación anormalmente prolongada y aumentada

menotropin menotropina

menstrual menstrual; ~ **bleeding pattern** ciclo menstrual; ~ **calendar** calendario menstrual; ~ **cramps** retortijones, dolores mentruales; ~ **cycle** ciclo menstrual; ~ **flow** menstruación, criterio, regla

menstruation menstruación, criterio, regla

mental mental, psiquico; ~ **anguish** angustia, congoja, ansia, ansiedad psíquica, estrés psicológico; ~ **automatism** síndrome de Clerambault-Kandinsky; ~ **deficiency** retraso mental, retardación mental, oligofrenia, debilidad mental, imbecilidad, demencia, trastorno mental; ~ **deterioration** pérdida de inteligencia, carencia intelectual,

desintegración de la inteligencia; ~ **disorder** retraso mental, retardación mental, oligofrenia, debilidad mental, imbecilidad, demencia, trastorno mental; ~ **distress** angustia, congoja, ansia; ~ **fatigue** fatiga mental, fatiga síquica; ~ **health** salud mental; ~ **health services** servicios de salud mental; ~ **hospital** hospital psiquiátrico; ~ **numbness** obnubilación; ~ **or physical impairment** discapacidad mental o física; ~ **pathology** psicopatología; ~ **retardation** retraso mental, la retardación mental, la oligofrenia, la debilidad mental, la imbecilidad, la demencia, el trastorno mental; ~ **shock** choque psíquico, shock afectivo; ~ **status** estado mental; ~ **status schedule** escala del estado mental; ~ **strain** fatiga mental, estrés

mentally deranged psicótico, deficiente mental; ~ **disabled persons** personas con discapacidad mental, enfermos mentales; ~ **ill person** enfermo mental, pacente mental; ~ **retarded** retardado, atraso mental

menthol mentol

meperidine meperidina, petidina;
~ **hydrochloride** clorhidrato de petidina

mephobarbital metilfenobarbital

mercurial mercurial; ~ **poisoning** hidrargirismo, hidrargirosis

mercurialism hidrargirismo, hidrargirosis

mercuric mercúrico; ~ **chloride** cloruro mercúrico, cloruro de mercurio

mercurous mercurioso; ~ **chloride** calomel, calomelanos (purgante), cloruro mercurioso

mercury mercurio, azogue; ~ **poisoning** hidrargirismo, hidrargirosis

Merkel cell célula de Merkel; ~ **cell carcinoma** carcinoma trabecular, carcinoma de célula de Merkel

merriment humor, jocosidad, comicidad, hilaridad

merycism rumiación

mesenchymal mesenquimal; ~ **cells** células mesenquimales

mesenchyme tejido conjuntivo embrionario, mesénquima

mesenteric mesentérico, relativo al mesenterio; ~ adenitis adenitis mesentérica; ~ lymphadenitis adenitis mesentérica; ~ panniculitis paniculitis mesentérica

messenger mensajero; ~ ribonucleic acid ácido ribonucleico mensajero; ~ RNA RNA mensajero

meta-analysis meta-análisis

metabolic metabólico; ~ acidosis acidosis metabólica; ~ activation system sistema de activación metabólica; ~ alkalosis alcalosis metabólica; ~ diseases enfermedades metabólicas; ~ disturbance trastorno metabólico

metabolism metabolismo, conjunto de reacciones bioquímicas dentro del organismo

metabolite metabolito

metabolization metabolización

metabolize, to metabolizar

metacarpal metacarpiano; ~ bone hueso metacarpiano; ~ hematoma hematoma metacarpiano

metacarpals metacarpos

metacortandracin prednisona, dehidrocortisona

metacortandralone prednisolona

metamyelocyte metamielocito

metanephrine metanefrina

metaphase metafase, estadio de la división nuclear en la mitosis y en la meiosis en que los cromosomas se disponen en el plano ecuatorial del huso; ~ analysis análisis en la metafase; ~ plate placa metafásica

metaphyseal metafisiario; ~ dysplasia displasia metafisiaria

metaphysis metafisis

metaplasia metaplasia, proceso de transformación de células o tejidos en otros distintos

metaproterenol orciprenalina

metastasis metástasis (f), aparición de un cáncer a distancia

metastasize, to metastatizar

metastasizing vesicular mole mola metastásica

metastatic metastásico; ~ gout gota metastásica

metatarsal metatarsiano, del mediopié

meteorism flatulencia, meteorismo, presencia de gas en el vientre o intestino

meter metro

metformin metformina

methadone metadona; ~ hydrochloride clorhidrato de metadona

methamphetamine metanfetamina, pervitin, metilanfetamina

methanol alcohol metílico, metanol, carbinol

metheamoglobin metahemoglobina

methedrine metanfetamina, metilanfetamina

methemoglobinemia metahemoglobinemia, presencia de metahemoglobina en la sangre que da por resultado cianosis

methenamine-silver stain tinción con metenamina y plata

methicillin meticilina; ~ resistance resistencia a la meticilina; ~ resistant resistente a la meticilina

methimazole tiamazol

methione metiona

methionine metionina; ~ adenosyltransferase metionina-adenosiltransferasa; ~ enkephalin encefalina metionina

method método; ~ of measurement método de medición; ~ of treatment método de tratamiento, procedimiento terapéutico

methotrexate metotrexato

methoxyadrenalin metoxiadrenalina

methoxynoradrenalin metoxinoradrenalina

methyl metílico; ~ alcohol alcohol metílico, metanol, carbinol; ~ -cisteine mecisteína; ~ red test prueba del rojo de metilo; ~ salicylate metilsalicilato

methylacetic acid ácido propiónico

methylamphetamine metanfetamina, pervitin, metilanfetamina

methylbutyrase carboxilesterasa

methylcellulose hipromelosa

methyldopa metildopa

methylene metiltioninio; ~ blue cloruro de metiltioninio; ~ blue stain tinción (f) con cloruro de metiltioninio; ~ blue test prueba con azul de metileno

methylergonovine metilergometrina

methylketone metilcetona

methylmorphine codeína, metilmorfina

methylphenidate metilfenidato; ~ hydrochloride hidrocloruro de metilfenilato

methylprednisolone metilprednisolona

meticillin meticilina

metmyoglobin metamioglobina
metoclopramide metoclopramid
metrological metrológico; ~ **sensitivity** sensibilidad metrológica, especificidad metrológica; ~ **variability** variabilidad metrológica
metrology metrología
metronidazole metronidazol
metrorrhagia metrorragia, pérdida sanguínea uterina que no sea menstrual, hemorragia intermenstrual
metrorrhexis rotura uterina
metyrapone metirapona
mezlocillin mezlocilina
MFR melanoliberina
MHC complejo principal de histocompatibilidad; ~ **genes** genes del complejo de histocompatibilidad
micelle micela
Michaelis constant constante de Michaelis
miconazole miconazol
microagglutination microaglutinación; ~ **test** prueba de la microaglutinación
microbe microorganismo, comensal, microbio, gérmen
microbial microbiano; ~ **collagenase** colagenasa microbiana, clostridiopeptida A; ~ **flora** microflora; ~ **genetics** genética microbiana; ~ **strain** cepa microbiana
microbic microbiano
microbiological microbiológico; ~ **discovery** invención microbiológica; ~ **invention** invención microbiológica; ~ **process** procedimiento microbiológico
microbiology microbiología; ~ **laboratory** laboratorio de microbiología
microcalcification microcalcificación
microcautery microcauterio
microcephalia microcefalia
microcephaly microcefalia
microchemistry microquímica
microchip microplaquita
microcirculation microcirculación, flujo de sangre en todo el sistema de vasos minúsculos
microcytic microcítico; ~ **anemia** anemia microcítica
microencapsulation microencapsulación
microfilaments microfilamentos

microfilaria microfilaria, forma prelavaria del helminto filariásico
microflora microflora
microglia astroglia, microglia, astrocitos
microgram microgramo, millonésima parte de un gramo
micrography micrografía, examen con el microscopio
microgravity ingravidez
micrometer micrómetro
micronize, to micronizar, reducir a polvo fino
micronuclei formation test prueba de formación de micronúcleos
microorganism microorganismo, comensal, microbio
microphallus microfallo
micropipette micropipeta
microscope microscopio; ~ **examination** micrografía, examen con el microscopio
microscopic microscópico, de tamaño extremadamente pequeño, perteneciente a la microscopia
microscopy microscopía
microsequencing microsecuenciación
microsomal microsomal, procedente de los microsomas; ~ **aminopeptidase** alanil-aminopeptidasa de membrana
microsomia microsomía
microsporum microsporum
microsurgery microcirugía
microtiter plate placa de microtitulación
microtubule microtúbulo
microvillus microvellosidad
micturition micción, acción de orinar
middle medio; ~ **finger** dedo cordial, dedo corazón
midget enano, enana
midstream urine orina del chorro medio
midwife comadrona, matrona, partera
midwifery profesión de comadrona
Miescher granulatomous cheilitis queilitis granulomatosa de Miescher
migraine migraña, jaqueca, cefalea
mild ligero, subclínico; ~ **epilepsy** ausencia, pérdida momentánea del conocimiento; ~ **pain** dolor ligero, dolor leve
milk leche; ~ **powder** polvos lácteos; ~ **production** lactación, secreción de leche,

período de secreción de leche, amamantamiento; ~ **protein** proteína de la leche, lactoalbúmina; ~ **sugar** lactosa; ~ **teeth** dientes de leche, primera dentición

milker's nodule nódulo del ordeñador

Milkman's syndrome síndrome de Looser Milkman

Millar's asthma asma de Millar

milligram miligramo

millimeter milímetro

million millón

Milroy's disease limfoedema

mime mímica, expresión por medio de gestos, de ideas o pensamientos

mimetic mimético; ~ **substance** substancia mimética

mineral mineral; ~ **oil** aceite mineral, grasa mineral

mineralization mineralización

mineralocorticoid mineralocorticoide

miners' black lung enfermedad pulmonar minera, antracosis

minimal mínimo, más pequeño

minimize, to minimizar

minimum mínimo; ~ **lethal concentration** concentración letal mínima

mini–stroke accidente isquémico transitorio, ataque de isquemia transitoria

minocycline minociclina

minor incidental; ~ **epilepsy** epilepsia minor, eplepsia con ataques poco intensos, petit mal

minors menores de edad

minute minuto; ~ **chromosome** minicromosoma

miosis miosis

miotic miótico; ~ miótico, agente que produce contracción pupilar

mirth humor, jocosidad, comicidad, hilaridad

misalignment desalineación, desajuste, falta de alineación

miscarriage aborto, interrupción del embarazo

miscible miscible

misdivision maldivisión

mismatch malapareamiento; ~ **repair** reparación de un malapareamiento

misoprostol misoprostol

Miss señorita

miss, to perder, dejar pasar

missed–lesion mammogram cribado

mamográfico, mamografía, mamograma

missense mutation mutación sustitutiva

Mitchell disease eritromelalgia, enfermedad de Mitchell

mite ácaro

mitochondrial mitocondrial; ~ **deoxyribonucleic acid** ácido desoxirribonucleico mitocondrial; ~ **DNA** ADN mitocóndrico; ~ **encephalomyopathy** encefalomiopatía mitocondrial; ~ **function** función mitocondrial; ~ **ribonucleic acid** ácido ribonucleico mitocondrial

mitosis mitosis, división de una célula

mitotic mitótico; ~ **index** índice mitótico; ~ **metaphase** metafase mitótica; ~ **spindle** huso acromático, huso mitótico

mitral mitral; ~ **reflux** reflujo mitral; ~ **regurgitation** reflujo mitral; ~ **stenosis** estenosis mitral; ~ **valve** válvula mitral; ~ **valve prolapse** prolapso mitral

mittelschmerz dolor intermenstrual, dolor y hemorragias intermenstruales

mixable miscible

mixed mixto; ~ **astigmatism** astigmatismo mixto; ~ **tumor of salivary glands** tumor mixto de glándulas salivares

MLC test prueba del cultivo linfocítico mixto

MMI (Maximum Medical Improvement) máximo mejoramiento médico, máxima mejoría médica

MMR vacine vacuna contra sarampión-paperas-rubeola

mnemic delusion ilusión mnésica, falsa memoria

MOA (monoamine oxidase) monoamina oxidasa, amina-oxidasa (flavinífera)

moan, to gemir, lamentarse

mobile motor; ~ **cardia** cardias móvil; ~ **phase** fase móvil

mobility movilidad; ~ **of head of femur** movilidad de la cabeza del fémur, signo del pistón

mobilization movilización

Möbius disease diplejía facial congénita, síndrome de Moebius

Möbius syndrome diplejía facial congénita, síndrome de Moebius

mocolytic mucolítico, agente que destruye o

disuelve la mucina
moderate moderado
modifier modificador
modify, to modificar
modulator modulador, sustancia reguladora
Moeller's bacillus Mycobacterium phlei
moist vapor nebulizer inhalador, nebulizador
moisturizer crema hidratante
molal molal
molality molalidad
molar muela (f), molar (adj); ~ **absorption coefficient** coeficiente de absorción molar; ~ **absorptivity** absortividad molar; ~ **concentration** concentración molar; ~ **conductivity** conductividad molar; ~ **glands** glándulas molares; ~ **heat capacity** capacidad térmica molar; ~ **mass** masa molar; ~ **volume** volumen molar
molarity concentración de sustancia
mole mola, pápula, pequeña elevación sólida y circunscrita de la piel; ~ **fraction** fracción de sustancia
molecular molecular, relativo a las moléculas o compuesto por ellas; ~ **absorption spectrometry** espectrometría de absorción molecular; ~ **biology** biología molecular; ~ **chaperone** carabina molecular, proteína celadora; ~ **cloning** clonación molecular; ~ **fluorescence spectrometry** espectrometría de fluorescencia molecular; ~ **genetics** genética molecular; ~ **hybridization** hibridación molecular; ~ **luminiscence spectrometry** espectrometría de luminiscencia molecular; ~ **mass** masa molecular; ~ **mimicry** mimetismo molecular; ~ **nanotechnology** nanotecnología; ~ **oncology** oncología molecular; ~ **pathology** patología molecular; ~ **weight** peso molecular
molluscum contagiosum molusco contagioso; ~ **contagiosum virus** virus del molusco contagioso
moment momento; ~ **of inertia** momento de inercia
momentary closure oclusión, cierre
Monday lunes
money dinero
moniliasis candidiasis urogenital, moniliasis
monitor, to monitorizar, vigilar, controlar

monitoring monitorización, control o supervisión con ayuda de un monitor
monkeypox virus virus monkeypox, virus de la viruela del mono
monoblast monoblasto
monobutyrase carboxilesterasa
monoclonal monoclonal; ~ **antibody** anticuerpo monoclonal; ~ **murine** murino monoclonal, anticuerpo monoclonal A33
monocomponent de un solo componente
monocromator monocromador
monocyte monocito
monocytic monocítico; ~ **angina** mononucleosis infecciosa, angina monocítica
monogamous monógamo
monogamy monogamia
mononeuritis mononeuritis
mononuclear mononuclear; ~ **hepatitis** hepatitis mononuclear; ~ **leukocytosis** mononucleosis infecciosa, angina monocítica
mononucleosis mononucleosis
monotherapy monoterapia, terapia con sólo un medicamento
mono-unsaturated fatty acids monoinsaturados, ácidos grasos monoinsaturados
monounsaturates monoinsaturados, ácidos grasos monoinsaturados
monozygotic monocigótico; ~ **pregnancy** embarazo monocigótico; ~ **twins** gemelos idénticos, gemelos monocigótos
monster monstruo
month mes
mood humor; ~ **-altering** psicotrópico, que afecta al estado mental; ~ **disorder** trastorno afectivo, rastorno de humores
Morax–Axenfeld's bacillus Moraxella lacunata
morbid mórbido, malsano; ~ **anatomy** anatomía patológica; ~ **fear** miedo mórbido; ~ **jealousy** celos mórbidos; ~ **sleepiness** clinomanía
morbidity morbididad, tasa de enfermos en una población; ~ **rate** tasa de morbilidad
more más; ~ **than** más que
Morgan's bacillus Morganella morganii
morgue depósito de cadáveres
morning mañana; ~ **stiffness** rigidez matutina
morphine morfina
morphinomimetic morfinomimético, productos

que tienen un efecto parecido al de la morfina

mortality mortalidad, tasa de muertes en una población; ~ **rate** mortalidad, tasa de muertes en una población

mosquito mosquito; ~ **bite** picadura de mosquito; ~ **netting** mosquitero, red protectora contra los insectos

most la mayor parte (de)

mother madre; ~ **-in-law** suegra; ~ **'s milk** leche materna; ~ **-to-be** mujer embarazada; ~ **-to-child transmission** transmisión perinatal, transmisión vertical, transmisión maternofilial; ~ **tongue** lengua materna

motility motilidad, facultad de moverse espontáneamente; ~ **medium** medio para motilidad

motion movimiento; ~ **-related** cinético, perteneciente al movimiento o que lo produce; ~ **sickness** mareo

motor motor, que mueve; ~ **alexia** alexia motora; ~ **aphasia** afasia motora, afasia motora del habla, afasia de Broca; ~ **asthenopia** astenopía muscular; ~ **cortex** corteza motora; ~ **debility** debilidad motora; ~ **infantilism** debilidad motora

mottling jaspeado, marcas de presión, livedo, punto o mancha de alteración de color sobre la piel

mountain montaña, montón; ~ **fever** fiebre americana, fiebre de picadura de garrapata; ~ **sickness** mal de montaña, mal de altura, soroche, vértigo

moustache bigote, bigotes

mouth boca, trompa; ~ **guard** surco dental primitivo, tablilla, gotiera, bruxismo, plana relajación, ferula oclusal; ~ **speculum** espéculo bucal; ~ **-to-mouth resuscitation** respiración artificial por boca

mouthwash enjuague, enjuague bucal

move to mover; ~ **the bowels, to** defecar, purificar, refinar, clarificar, obrar, evacuar

movement ejercicio físico, movimiento; ~ **-cure** cinesiterapia, cinesia, cinesis; ~ **therapy** cinesiterapia, cinesia, cinesis

moving móvil, en marcha, en movimiento; ~ **apart** extensión, despliegue; ~ **-beam therapy** radioterapia de movimiento

moxalactam latamoxef

Mr. señor

MRI (magnetic resonance imaging) proyección de imágenes por resonancia magnética, IRM, MRI, imagen por resonancia magnética

Mrs. señora

MSH melanotropina

MSU orina del chorro medio

much muchos

mucin mucina

mucinase hialuronato-liasa, hialuronoglucosaminidasa, hialuronoglucuronidasa

mucociliary mucociliar, mucilaginoso; ~ **clearance** depuración mucociliar, flujo mucilaginoso; ~ **transport** depuración mucociliar, flujo mucilaginoso

mucocutaneous mucocutáneo; ~ **leishmaniasis americana** espundia, leishmaniosis cutaneomucosa americana

mucogingival muco-gingival

mucoid mucoide; ~ **degeneration** degeneración mucoide

mucolytic mucolítico, agente que destruye o disuelve la mucina

mucopolysaccharide glicosaminoglicano, mucopolisacarid

mucopurulent mucopurulento, que contiene moco y pus

mucosa membranas mucosas, las mucosas

mucous mucoso; ~ **membranes** membranas mucosas, las mucosas; ~ **tumor** mixoma, tumor coloide, tumor gelatinoso, tumor mucoso, mixoblastoma

mucus mucus, moco

mud packs barro termal, barro terapéutico, sedimentos curativos, fangoterapia

Mueller-Hinton medium medio de Mueller-Hinton

multi-allergy alergia cruzada, alergia a sustancias emparentadas

multicopy plasmid plásmido multicopia

multidose multidosis, dosis múltiple

multifactorial multifactorial; ~ **etiology** etiología multifactorial; ~ **inheritance** herencia poligénica

multinuclear plurinucleado

multinucleated giant cell celula gigante

plurinucleada, célula gigante multinucleada, mieloplaxa

multiparametric analyzer multianalizador

multiparous multípara, que ha parido como mínimo dos hijos

multiple múltiple, de muchas clases, variado; ~ **addiction** toxicomanía múltiple, politoxicomanía; ~ **chemical sensitivity** sensibilidade química multiple; ~ **crossing** cruzamiento múltiple; ~ **drug abuse** toxicomanía múltiple, politoxicomanía; ~ **factor** poligénes; ~ **hereditary exostoses** exostosis múltiple hereditaria, exostosis múltiple cartilaginosa; ~ **myeloma** mieloma múltiple, plasmocitoma, mielomatosis, enfermedad de Kahler, plasmacitoma; ~ **organ failure** insuficiencia de multiples organos; ~ **sclerosis** esclerosis múltiple; ~ **villous adenoma** poliadenoma velloso

multiplex polimerase chain reaction reacción en cadena por la polimerasa múltiplex

multiplexing multiplexado

multiplication proliferación, reproducción, multiplicación

multisite multicéntrico

mumps parotiditis, papaeras, chanza, parótidas, inflamación de la glándula salivar; ~ **vaccine** vacuna contra las paperas; ~ **virus** virus de la parotiditis, virus de las paperas

Munchausen syndrome by proxy síndrome de Münchausen, patomimia, trastornos facticios, Munchausen el síndrome por poder

mupirocin mupirocina

muriatic acid ácido clorhídrico

murine leukemia leucemia murina, leucemia que afecta a las ratas; ~ **typhus** tifus exantemático endémico

muscle músculo; ~ **balance** equilibrio muscular; ~ **building** musculación, ejercicio muscular; ~ **cramp** calambre muscular, espasmo muscular; ~ **denervation** desnervacion muscular; ~ **disease** miopatía, enfermedad muscular; ~ **inflammation** miositis, inflamación de un músculo voluntario; ~ **pain** mialgia, dolor en un músculo o músculos; ~ **phosphorylase** glucógeno-fosforilasa; ~ **relaxant** relajante muscular, miorrelajante; ~ **rupture** rotura

muscular; ~ **spasm** tetania, espasmo muscular; ~ **tension** tono, tensión muscular; ~ **tone** tono, tensión muscular; ~ **training** musculación, ejercicio muscular; ~ **twitch** tirón, tic; ~ **weakness** miastenia, debilidad o fatiga musculares anormales

muscular muscular, bien musculado; ~ **atrophy** atrofia muscular; ~ **dystrophy** distrofias musculares; ~ **rheumatism** reumatismo muscular, fibrositis

musculature musculatura, músculos

musculoskeletal system aparato locomotor

mushrooms hongos

mustache bigote, bigotes

mustard mostaza; ~ **plaster** sinapismo, cataplasmo de mostaza

mutagen mutágeno

mutagenesis mutagénesis

mutagenic mutágeno; ~ **agent** mutágeno; ~ **repair** reparación mutágena

mutagenicity mutagenicidad; ~ **test** prueba de mutagenicidad; ~ **testing** tests de mutagenicidad, estudios de mutagenicidad

mutant mutante

mutation mutación, cambio en el material genético, ~ **of chromosomes** aberración cromosómica; ~ **rate** frecuencia de mutación; ~ **site** centro de mutación

mute mudo

mutilation mutilación; ~ **of female genitalia** ablación ritual del clitoris

mutism mutismo, incapacidad de hablar o negativa para hacerlo

muton mutón

mutual mutuo, común; ~ **help** autoayuda; ~ **infection** infección cruzada, contagio mutuo

muzolimine muzolimina

my mi, ~s (pl)

myalgia mialgia, dolor en un músculo o músculos

myalgic miálgico; ~ **encephalomyelitis** síndrome de fatiga crónica, encefalomielitis miálgica

myasthenia miastenia, debilidad o fatiga musculares anormales; ~ **gravis** miastenia gravis

mycardial miocardico; ~ **ischemia** isquemia miocardica

mycetoma micetoma
mycobacteriosis micobacteriosis
mycobacterium micobacteria; ~ **leprae** bacteria de la lepra; ~ **tuberculosis** Mycobacterium tuberculosis
mycological micológico
mycolysin micolisina
mycoplasma mycoplasma
mycosis micosis, enfermedad causada por hongos, enfermedad de mohos; ~ **fungoides** microtoxicosis, micosis fungoide
mycotic micótico; ~ **aneurysm** aneurisma micótico; ~ **cardiopathy** cardiopatía micótica; ~ **elements** elementos micóticos; ~ **infection** micosis, enfermedad causada por hongos, enfermedad de mohos
mydriasis dilatación pupilar, midriasis
mydriatic midriático, droga que dilata la pupila
myelencephalon bulbo raquídeo, medulla oblongata
myelin mielina; ~ **basic protein** proteína básica de la mielina; ~ **sheath** vaina de mielina
myeloblast mieloblasto
myelocitic mielocítico; ~ **leukemia** leucemia mielocítica, leucemia mielógena, leucemia mieloide, mielocitosis
myelocyte mielocito
myelocytosis leucemia mielocítica, leucemia mielógena, leucemia mieloide, mielocitosis
myelodysplasia mielodisplasia
myelogram mielograma
myeloid mieloide; ~ **cell** célula mieloide, tejido mieloide; ~ **leukemia** leucemia mielocítica, leucemia mielógena, leucemia mieloide, mielocitosis; ~ **tissue** célula mieloide, tejido mieloide
myeloma mieloma, tumor maligno de la médula ósea, mielomatosis
myelomatosis mielomatosis, cáncer de la médula ósea
myelomeningocele mielomeningocele
myelomonocytic mielomonocítico; ~ **leukemia** leucemia mielomonocítica
myelopathy mielopatía
myelosuppression mielosupresión
myelotoxic mielotóxico, que es nocivo para la médula ósea
myiasis miasis

myoadenylate deaminase AMP-desaminasa
myocardial miocardio; ~ **contractility** contractilidad miocardica; ~ **contraction** contracción miocardica; ~ **disease** miocardiopatía; ~ **hypoxia** hipoxia miocardica; ~ **infarction** infarto de miocardio, ataque cardíaco; ~ **insufficiency** insuficiencia cardíaca; ~ **reperfusion** reperfusión miocardica; ~ **revascularization** revascularización miocardica; ~ **sclerosis** miocardiosclerose
myocarditis miocarditis, inflamación del miocardio
myocardium miocardio
myoclonic absence mioclonías del pequeño mal; ~ **seizure** mioclonías del pequeño mal
myoclonus contracciones musculares, mioclonia, contracción involuntaria de los músculos
myoglobin mioglobina
myoma mioma
myomectomy miomectomía
myometrium miometrio, capa muscular de la pared uterina
myoneural neuromuscular; ~ **junction** unión neuromuscular
myopathy miopatía, enfermedad muscular
myopia miopía, vista corta
myopic miope; ~ **astigmatism** astigmatismo miópico; ~ **choroiditis** coroiditis miópica
myosin miosina; ~ **protein** miosina
myositis miositis, inflamación de un músculo voluntario
myotonic miotónico; ~ **dystrophia** distrofia miotónica de Steinert, enfermedad de Steinert, miotonía atrófica, distrofia miotónica
myringitis inflamación infecciosa del tímpano
myxoma mixoma, mucosidad tumoral, mixoblastoma
myxomatous mixomatoso; ~ **angiosarcoma** angiosarcoma mixomatoso

N

N-acetyl penicillamine N-acetilpenicilamina
NADH peroxidase NADH-peroxidasa
nadir nadir, punto más bajo

NADP (methylenetetrahydrofolate dehydrogenase) metilenotetrahidrofolato-deshidrogenasa, NADP

naevo-carcinoma melanoma maligno, melanocarcinoma, cáncer melánico

naevus nevo; **~ pigmentosus** mola hidatidica, mola hidatidiforme, lentigo

nafcillin nafcilina

nail uña; **~ -patella syndrome** sindrome de la uña-patella; **~ pulse** pulso capilar

naked desnudo

nalidixic acid ácido nalidíxico

name nombre, apellido; **~ tag** distintivo de identificación, escudo, insignia de identidad

nanomedicine nanomedicina

nanometer nanómetro, nanon

nanon nanómetro, nanon

nanotube nanotube

nape of the neck nuca

naproxen naproxeno

narcolepsy narcolepsia

narcotic narcótico, agente que produce insensibilidad, estupor o anestesia; **~ analgesics** analgesicos opioides

narrow, to estrecharse, entrecerrarse, reducir(se)

nasal nasal, relativo a la nariz; **~ bones** hueso nasal, huesos nasales; **~ calculus** litiasis nasal; **~ concha** cornete; **~ congestion** congestión nasal; **~ decongestant** descongestivo, sustancia que alivia la congestión nasal; **~ hemorrhage** desangramiento en las narices, almorragia, epistaxis; **~ mucus** moco, moquera, muco nasal; **~ polyp** pólipo nasal; **~ secretion** secreción nasal; **~ sinus** seno nasal; **~ speculum** concoscopio, espéculo nasal, rinoscopio; **~ tone** gangoso, násico, nasalizado

nasogastric nasogástrico; **~ intubation** intubación gástrica, intubación nasogástrica

nasolacrimal nasolacrimal; **~ duct** conducto nasolagrimal

nasopharyngeal naso-faríngeo; **~ catarrh** adenoiditis; **~ cavity** cavidad naso-faríngeo, nasofaringe; **~ fibroma** fibroma nasofaríngeo; **~ neoplasm** neoplasma neofaringeo, carcinoma naso-faríngeo

nasopharyngitis catarro, resfriado, coriza

nasopharynx cavidad naso-faríngeo, nasofaringe

National Institute of Allergy and Infectious Diseases (USA) Instituto Nacional de Alergia y Enfermedades Infecciosas

natremia natremia, concentración de ion sodio en plasma

natriuresis natriuresis, excreción de cantidades anormales de sodio en la orina

natriuria natriuria, concentración de ion sodio en orina, excreción de ion sodio en orina

natural natural, inherente, implantado por naturaleza, innato; **~ killer** célula asesina natural, célula NK, célula citotóxica natural; **~ killer cell** célula asesina natural, célula NK, célula citotóxica natural; **~ medicine** naturopatía

naturopath naturópata, naturista

naturopathic healer curandero homologado

naturopathy naturopatía

nausea náusea, asco, basca, ganas de vomitar

nauseated, to be estar nauseado, vomitar, tener náuseas

navel ombligo

near cerca, junto; **~ care point testing** determinaciones junto a la cabecera del paciente; **~ -sighted** miope; **~ -sightedness** miopía, vista corta

nearest proximal

nebulizer atomizador, nebulizador

neck cuello, gollete, (of animal: pescuezo); **~ brace** collarín cervical, minerva; **~ cramp** espasmo de los músculos cervicales; **~ of femur** cuello del fémur; **~ of the uterus** cervix uterino, cuello de matriz, cuello uterino; **~ spasm** espasmo de los músculos cervicales

necrolysis necrólisis, gangrena, necrosis

necropsy necropsia, autopsia

necrosis necrólisis, gangrena, necrosis

necrotic necrótico; **~ acne** acné necrótica; **~ angina** angina necrótica; **~ bronchitis** bronquitis necrótica; **~ diphtheria** difteria hemorrágica necrotizant; **~ granuloma** acné necrótica; **~ hepatitis** hepatitis necrotizante, peste negra de los ovinos

necrotizing necrosante; **~ arteritis** arteritis necrosante; **~ enterocolitis (of a newborn)** enterocolitis necrotizante, enfermedad adquirida de los recién nacidos; ~ **fasciitis** fasciitis necrotizante, necrólisis epidérmica tóxica; ~ **gingivitis** gingivitis necrótica

need, to necesitar

needle aguja; ~ **biopsy** biopsia con aguja, punción biopsia

needleless injector inyector a presión, inyector dermo-jet

nefrogenic nefrogenico; ~ **diabetes insipidus** diabetes insipida nefrogenica

negative negativo, sin resultado, no positivo, bajo la línea cero; ~ **predictive value** valor predictivo de un resultado negativo

negligible insignificante, despreciable

neighbor vecino

neogenesis neogénesis, regeneración

neomycin neomicina, antibiótico aminoglucósido

neonatal neonatal, relativo al primer mes de vida

neophyte neófito, principiante

neoplasia neoplasia, neoplasma

neoplasm neoplasia, neoplasma

neoplastic neoplásico, relativo a un cáncer; ~ **gingivitis** gengivitis neoplásica; ~ **lesion** lesión neoplásica

nephelometric immunoassay inmunoanálisis nefelométrico

nephelometry nefelometría, turbidimetría

nephew sobrino

nephrectomy nefrectomía, operación consistente en extirpar un riñón

nephritic nefrítico; ~ **abscess** absceso nefrítico; ~ **disease** nefropatía, enfermedad del riñón; ~ **medicine** medicamento nefrítico

nephritis nefritis, inflamación del riñón

nephrocalcinosis nefrocalcinosis

nephrogenic nefrógeno; ~ **blastema** blastema nefrógeno

nephrogenous nefrógeno

nephrolith nefrolito, piedra del riñón, cálculo renal

nephrologist nefrólogo, especialista en nefrología

nephrology nefrología

nephron nefrón

nephropathy nefropatía, enfermedad del riñón

nephrorrhagia nefrorragia, hemorragia renal

nephrotic nefrótico, relativo a una enfermedad del riñón o causado por ella

nephrotomy nefrotomía

nephrotoxic nefrotóxico, que es tóxico para el riñón

nephrotoxicity toxicidad para los riñones, nefrotoxicidad

Nernst equation ecuación de Nernst

nerve nervio; ~ **block** bloqueo nervioso; ~ **cell** neurona; ~ **compression syndrome** sindrome de compresión del nervio; ~ **deafness** sordera sensorineural, sordera de percepción, sordera neurosensorial, hipoacusia neurosensorial; ~ **distribution** inervación, irrigación nerviosa de un área u órgano; ~ **entrapment** atrapamiento neural, mononeuropatía con lesión verviosa y debilidad, sindrome de compresión nerviosa; ~ **gas** gas neurotóxico, gas nervioso; ~ **impulse** impulso nervioso; ~ **inflammation** inflamación de un nervio; ~ **synapse** sinapsis

nervous nervioso; ~ **breakdown** crisis nerviosa; ~ **exhaustion** neurastenia; ~ **system** sistema nervioso; ~ **system disorder** neuropatía, enfermedad nerviosa

nervousness nerviosismo, excitabilidad e irritabilidad excesivas

net adj neto

netilmicin netilmicina

network plexo

Neumann's bacillus Klebsiella pneumoniae

neural neural

neuralgia neuralgia

neuralgic neurálgico; ~ **herpes** herpes neurálgico

neuraminic acids ácidos neuraminicos

neuraminidase neuraminidasa, exo-a-sialidasa

neurasthenia neurastenia

neurectomy neurectomía

neurilemma neurolema, neurilema, células de Schwann

neurilemmoma periférico, neurinoma, neurocitoma

neurinoma periférico, neurinoma, neurocitoma

neuritis neuritis, inflamación de un nervio

neurobiology neurobiología

neuroblast neuroblasto

neuroblastoma neuroblastoma

neurochemical neuroquímico; **~ abnormality** anomalía neuroquímica

neurocirculatory neurocirculatorio; **~ asthenia** astenia neurocirculatoria

neurocysticercosis neurocisticercosis

neurodegenerative neurodegenerativo; **~ disease** enfermedad neurodegenerativa

neurodermatitis neurodermatitis

neuroendocrine neuroendocrino; **~ cancer** cáncer neuroendocrino, carcinoma neuroendocrino; **~ carcinoma** cáncer neuroendocrino, carcinoma neuroendocrino

neurofibromatosis neurofibromatosis, neuroma múltiple, polifibromatosis neurocutánea pigmentaria, enfermedad de Recklinghausen, osteítis fibroquística

neurogenic neurogénico; **~ arcoosteolysis** acro-osteolisis progresiva; **~ dermatrophy** atrofia dérmica neurogénica

neuroglial cells astroglia, microglia, astrocitos

neurohormone neurohormona

neurolemma neurolema, neurilema, células de Schwann

neuroleptanalgesia neuroleptoanalgesia

neuroleptic neuroléptico, antipsicótico, tranquilizante mayor, calmante del sistema nervioso

neurological neurológico; **~ disorder** trastorno neurológico, alteración neurologica, enfermedad nervosia

neuroma neuroma

neuromuscular neuromuscular; **~ blocker** agente bloqueador neuromuscular, agente bloqueante neuromuscular; **~ coordination** coordinación neuromuscular; **~ depolarizing agent** relajante muscular, relajante de acción muscular, miorrelajante, agente despolarizante neuromuscular; **~ disease** enfermedad neuromuscular; **~ junction** unión neuromuscular; **~ prosthesis** prótesis neuromuscular; **~ synapse** sinapsis neuromuscular

neuron neurona

neuronal neuronal; **~ ceroid-lipofuscinosis** lipofuscinosis ceroide neuronal, idiocia amaurótica familiar; **~ cholesterol lipidosis** enfermedad de Niemann, enfermedad de Niemann-Pick, esfingolipidosis,

esfingomielinasa

neuropathic neuropático; **~ arthropathy** artopatía neuropática; **~ bleeding** hemorragia neuropática; **~ osseous atrophy** acro-osteolisis progresiva; **~ pain** dolor neuropático

neuropathology neuropatología

neuropathy neuropatía, enfermedad nerviosa

neurophysiology neurofisiología

neuropil neurópilo

neuropilem neurópilo

neuropsychology neuropsicología

neuroscience neurología, neurociencia

neurosis neurosis

neurosurgeon neurocirujano

neurosurgery neurocirugía

neurosurgical suture needle aguja para sutura en neurocirugía

neurotic neurótico

neurotomy neurotomía; **~ of the peripheral nerv** neurotomía del nérvio periférico

neurotoxic neurotóxico; **~ cytokine** citoquina neurotóxica; **~ gas** gas neurotóxico, gas nervioso

neurotransmitter neurotransmisor

neurotrophic neurotrófico; **~ arthropathy** atropatía neurotrófica; **~ osseous atrophy** acro-osteolisis progresiva

neurotropic neurotropo, neurotrópico, neurofílico; **~ strain** cepa neurotrópica

neurovegetative neurovegetativo; **~ dystonia** distonía neurovegetativa

neutering castración, extirpación de los órganos sexuales

neutralization neutralización; **~ test** prueba de la neutralización

neutropenia neutropenia, disminución del número de leucocitos neutrófilos en la sangre

neutrophil neutrofilo; **~ elastase** elastasa leucocitaria

neutrophilocyte neutrofilocito, neutrófilo

nevirapine nevirapina, Viramune

nevus nevo; **~ arachnoides** araña vascular; **~ depigmentosus** nevus acrómico, nevus despigmentado

new nuevo; **~ user** neófito, principiante

newborn neonatal, relativo al primer mes de vid; **~ baby** recién nacido

Newcastle disease virus virus de la enfermedad de Newcastle

next próximo; ~ **week** próxima semana

niacin ácido nicotínico, niacina, vitamina del complejo B

niacinamid niacinamida, nicotinamida

nick mella; ~ **translation** traslación de mellas

nicking–closing enzyme DNA-topoisomerasa

Nicolaier's bacillus Clostridium tetani

nicotinamide niacinamida, nicotinamida; ~ **mononucleotide** mononucleótido de nicotinamida

nicotine nicotina; ~ **patch** parche de nicotina, parche transdermico; ~ **poisoning** intoxicación por nicotina

nicotinic acid ácido nicotínico, niacina, vitamina del complejo B

nicoumalone acenocumarol

nictitate, to destellar, parpadear, pestañear

nidation nidación, implantación del embrión maduro

niece sobrina

Niemann–Pick disease enfermedad de Niemann, enfermedad de Niemann-Pick, esfingolipidosis, esfingomielinasa

night noche; ~ **blindness** ceguera nocturna, hemeralopía; ~ **guard** surco dental primitivo, tablilla, gotiera, bruxismo, plana relajación, ferula oclusal; ~ **sweats** sudor nocturno

nightly nocturno, nocturnal

nightmare pesadilla

nil nulo

nine nueve

nineteen diecinueve

ninety noventa

ninth noveno

nipple chichi, pezón, tetilla, mamelon, tetilla, mamila

Nissl's bodies corpúsculos cromófilos, cuerpos de Nissl

Nitinol Nitinol

nitrate nitrato; ~ **assimilation medium** medio de asimilación de nitrato; ~ **reductase** nitrato-reductasa, NAD(P)H; ~ **reduction medium** medio de reducción de nitrato

nitrofurantoin nitrofurantoína

nitrogen nitrógeno; ~ **balance** equilibro

nitrogenado, balance de nitrógeno; ~ **equilibrium** equilibro nitrogenado, balance de nitrógeno; ~ **mustard** mostaza nitrogenada

nitroglycerine nitroglicerina; ~ **poisoning** envenenamiento por nitroglicerina, glononismo

nitroimidazole nitroimidazol

nitrosamine nitrosamina

nitrosourea nitrosourea

nitrous oxide gas hilarante, óxido nitroso

NK cell célula asesina natural, célula NK, célula citotóxica natural

NMR (multinuclear nuclear magnetic resonance) espectrómetro multinuclear, resonancia magnética nuclear, RMN

NMR (nuclear magnetic resonance) resonancia magnética nuclear, RMN

no no

Nocard's bacillus Salmonella typhimurium

nociceptor nociceptor

nocturia nicturia

nocturnal nocturno, nocturnal; ~ **amblyopia** ceguera nocturna

nod, to inclinar, asentir

nodding spasm corea de la cabeza

node nódulo, nódulo, perla, nudo

nodose nodular

nodular nodular; ~ **headache** cefalea induratíva, cefalea nodular; ~ **heterotopia** heterotopia nodular

nodule nódulo, perla, nudo

nodus (in the hypodermis) nódulo, perla, nudo

Noguchi leptospira de Noguchi

noise ruido; ~ **-induced hearing loss** sordera por trauma acústico

nominal nominal; ~ **scale** escala nominal

non-allergic contact dermatitis dermatitis no alérgica de contacto; ~ **-coding strand** cadena intranscrita; ~ **-competitive** no competitivo; ~ **-conventional medicine** medicina paralela, medicina alternativa; ~ **-ergot** no cornezuelo; ~ **-esterified** no esterificado; ~ **-gluten enteropathy** enfermedad celíaca; ~ **-Hodgkin's lymphoma** linfoma no Hodgkiniano; ~ **-insulin-dependent diabetes** diabetes que no es dependiente de insulina, diabetes de tipo II; ~ **-invasive method** método no invasivo, procedimiento no invasivo; ~ **-ionizing radiation** radiación no ionizante; ~ **- malignant** benigno; ~ **-narcotic analgesics** analgesicos no opioides; ~ **-organic** inorgánico, carente de vida, inanimado; ~ **- palpable** no palpable, impalpable; ~ **- poisonous** atóxico, no venenoso, no nocivo; ~ **-repetitive DNA** DNA no repetido; ~ **- saturated fatty acids** ácidos grasos insaturados; ~ **-selective** no selectivo; ~ **- specific** inespecífico, no característico; ~ **- steroidal anti-inflammatory drugs** fármacos antiinflamatorios no esteroideos; ~ **-striated muscle** músculo liso, el músculo de contracción involuntaria; ~ **-toxic** atóxico, no venenoso; ~ **-urgent** electivo, selectivo

nonchromafin paraganglia paraganglios no cromafines, paraganglios parasimpáticos
noncompliance incumplimiento (terapéutico)
nonfermenter no fermentador
nonnutrient agar plate placa con agar sin nutrientes
nonsense tonterías; ~ **mutation** mutación sin sentido
nonslip antiderrape, antipatinante, antideslizante, antirresbaladizo
nonspecific inespecífico, no característico
nonsporeforming bacillus bacilo no esporulado
nontropical sprue enfermedad celíaca
Noonan's syndrome síndrome de Noonan
noradrenaline noradrenalina
norepinephrine norepinefrina
norethisterone noretisterona
norfloxacin norfloxacina
norleucine norleucina
normal fisiológico, normal; ~ **saline solution** solución fisiológica; ~ **values** valores de referencia (de la población sana)
normalization normalización
normally normalmente
normotensive normotenso, con la tensión normal
North American blastomycosis blastomicosis norteamericana
northern norte, del norte; ~ **blot** transferencia northern
nortriptyline nortriptilina
nose nariz

nosebleed epistaxis, desangramiento en las narices, sangrar por la nariz, hemorragia nasal
nosocomial nosocomial, relacionado con la hospitalización o con un hospital, hospitalario
nosographic sensitivity sensibilidad nosográfica; ~ **specificity** especificidad nosográfica
nosologic sensitivity sensibilidad nosológica; ~ **specificity** especificidad nosológica
nosology nosología
nostril ventanilla, naric
not no
notalgia dorsalgia, notalgia
notice, to notar
November noviembre
novice neófito, principiante
novobiocin novobiocina
novocain clorhidrato de procaina, novocaína
now ahora
noxious dañino, nocivo, dañoso, pernicioso, desfavorable; ~ **gases** gas tóxico
NSAIDs (non-steroidal anti-inflammatory drugs) fármacos antiinflamatorios no esteroideos, AINE
nuclear nuclear; ~ **deoxyribonucleic acid** ácido desoxirribonucleico nuclear; ~ **magnetic resonance spectroscopy** espectroscopia por resonancia magnética nuclear; ~ **magnetic resonance tomography** resonancia magnética metabólica, RM metabólica; ~ **medicine** medicina nuclear; ~ **ribonucleic acid** ácido ribonucleico nuclear; ~ **sex** sexo cromosómico, sexo nuclear
nuclease nucleasa
nucleic nucleico; ~ **acid** ácido nucleico; ~ **acid denaturation** desnaturalización de un ácido nucleico; ~ **acid hybridization** hibridación de ácidos nucleicos; ~ **acid probe** sonda de ácidos nucleicos; ~ **base** base nucleotídica, base de ácido nucleico; ~ **bases complementarity** complementaridad de las bases nucleicas
nucleohistone nucleohistona
nucleolus nucleolo
nucleophile nucleófilo
nucleoplasm nucleoplasma, carioplasma
nucleoplasma nucleoplasma, carioplasma
nucleoside nucleósido; ~ **analog** análogo

nucleósido, análogo de los nucleósidos; ~ **analogue** análogo nucleósido, análogo de los nucleósidos; ~ **diphosphate** nucleósido difosfato; ~ **–phosphate kinase** nucleósido-fosfato-cinasa

nucleosome nucleosoma

nucleotide nucleótido; ~ **base** base nucleotídica, base de ácido nucleico; ~ **sequencing** secuenciación de nucleótidos, secuencia nucleotídica

nucleus núcleo; ~ **accumbens** nucleus accumbens; ~ **gracilis** núcleo gracilis, el núcleo de Goll

nuclide nucleido

nude desnudo

null cell célula nula; ~ **mutation** mutación completa

nulliparous nulípara; ~ **woman** mujer nulípara

numb, to entumecer, entorpecer, envarar; ~ **up, to** anestesiar, insensibilizar

number número; ~ **concentration** concentración de número; ~ **content** contenido de número; ~ **flow rate** caudal de número; ~ **fraction** fracción de número; ~ **of cases** incidencia

numbness adormecimiento; ~ **of feet** adormecimiento en los pies

numerical numérico; ~ **taxonomy** taxonomía numérica; ~ **value** valor numérico

nummular numular, en forma de moneda

nurse enfermero, enfermera; ~ **case manage** enfermera cargada del caso, enfermera a cargo, enfermera a cargo del caso; ~, **to** lactar, amamantar, dar pecho; ~ **'s aide** asistente de enfermería

nursery guardería, jardín de infancia; ~ **school** guardería infantil, jardín de infantes

nursing enfermería; ~ **a baby** lactancia materna, amamantamiento, lactación; ~ **assistant** asistente de enfermería; ~ **bottle** mamadera, biberón; ~ **home** clínica para convalecientes o ancianos, asilo; ~ **mother** madre lactante

nutation nutación

nutcracker esophagus trastorno de la motilidad esofágica

nutrient nutrimento, alimentación, alimento, nutriente; ~ **agar** agar nutritivo; ~ **artery** arteria nutricia; ~ **broth** caldo nutritivo

nutrition alimento

nutritional nutricional; ~ **anemia** anemia nutricional; ~ **atrophy** atrofia infantil, marasmo; ~ **cachexia** atrofia infantil, marasmo; ~ **claim** declaración de propiedades nutritivas; ~ **disease** enfermedad nutricional; ~ **disorder** trastorno de la nutrición, trastorno nutricional, problema nutricional; ~ **disturbance** trastorno de la nutrición, trastorno nutricional, problema nutricional; ~ **marasmus** marasmo nutricional; ~ **surveillance** vigilancia nutricional

nutritionist nutricionista

nycturia nicturia

nystagmus nistagmo ocular, nistagmo

O

obese obeso

obesity obesidad

ob–gyn doctor obstetra-ginecólogo, médico especializado en obstetricia y genecología

objective objetivo, meta; ~ **medical decision making** toma de decisiones médica objetiva

obligate obligado; ~ **anaerobe** anaerobio obligado; ~ **parasite** parásito estricto

oblique oblicuo

obliterating obliterante; ~ **bronchiolitis** bronquiolitis obliterante

obnubilation adormecimiento, obnubilación, envaramiento, entumecido

observant observador, atento, cuidadoso

observation observación, estudio de un fenómeno, hallazgo, resultado

observe, to apreciar, vigilar, observar

obsession obsesión, idea fija; ~ **(psychology)** fijación

obsessive obsesivo; ~ **–compulsive disorder** trastorno obsesivo-compulsivo; ~ **–compulsive psychoneurosis** trastorno obsesivo-compulsivo

obstetrical obstétrico; ~ **ultrasound** ecografía obstétrica; ~ **vacuum extraction** extracción obstétrica por aspiración

obstetrician and gynecologist obstetra-ginecólogo, médico especializado en obstetricia y genecología

obstetrics obstetricia, profesión de comadrona; **~ and gynecology** obstetricia y ginecología

obstipation constipación, estreñimiento, entablazón

obstreperous intratable, indócil, malmandado

obstruction obstrucción

obstructive obstructivo; **~ bronchitis** bronquitis obstructiva; **~ thrombus** trombo oclusivo

obtundent apaciqua, que calma el dolor

obturator obturador; **~ foramen** agujero obturador; **~ gluteal hernia** hernia obturatriz, hernia obturadora; **~ hernia** hernia obturatriz, hernia obturadora; **~ membrane** membrana obturatriz; **~ muscle** músculo (m) obturador; **~ nerve** nervio obturador

occasional ocasional, de vez en cuando

occipital occipital; **~ bone** hueso del occipital; **~ condyle** cóndilo del occipital; **~ index** índice craneométrico occipital; **~ inductor** inductor occipital; **~ radius** radio occipital; **~ region** región occipital; **~ zone** región occipital

occiput occipucio

occluded ocluido; **~ blood vessel** vaso sanguíneo ocluido

occlusal oclusal; **~ plate** placa de la dentadura postiza; **~ splint** surco dental primitivo, tablilla, gotiera, bruxismo, plana relajación, ferula oclusal

occlusion oclusión, cierre; **~ of the bowel** oclusión intestinal

occlusive oclusivo; **~ arterial disease** arteriopatia oclusiva; **~ bandage** aposito semi-oclusivo; **~ ileus** ileo por obstrucción; **~ thrombus** trombo oclusivo

occult oculto, escondido, tapado; **~ bleeding** hemorragia oculta (en las heces); **~ blood** hemorragia oculta (en las heces); **~ blood in fæces** hemoglobina en heces

occupational profesional, laboral, ocupacional; **~ disability** incapacidad profesional; **~ injury** lesión laboral, lesión por accidente de trabajo; **~ medicine** medicina laboral, medicina del trabajo; **~ safety** seguridad profesional, seguridad en el trabajo; **~ therapist** ergoterapeuta, terapeuta ocupacional,

terapeuta de reeducación; **~ therapy** ergoterapia, terapia ocupacional

ochre ocre; **~ mutation** mutación ocre

OCT (oxytocin challenge test) prueba de provocación con oxitocina

octacosanol octacosanol

October octubre

ocular ocular; **~ biometry** biometria ocular; **~ burn** quemadura ocular; **~ carcinoma** carcinoma ocular; **~ cataplasm** cataplasma ocular; **~ convergence** convergencia ocular; **~ lesion** lesión ocular; **~ micrometer** micrómetro ocular; **~ mycosis** infección fungica del ojo; **~ nystagmus** nistagmo ocular, nistagmo; **~ parallax** paralelaje ocular; **~ prosthesis** ojo artificial; **~ ultrasonography** ecografía ocular; **~ vertigo** vértigo ocular

oculogyric oculógiro

oculomucocutaneous oculomucocutáneo

Oddi's sphincter esfinter hepatopancreatico

odontodynia odontalgia

odontoid odontoide, odontoides; **~ process** apófisis odontoides

odor olor, aroma, fragancia

Oertel heart massage masaje cardíaco de Oertel

of de, a desde, mediante, en, a

offensive ofensivo, insultante, muy desagradable; **~ odor** olor, aroma, fragancia

offspring descendencia, progenie, descendentes, progenitura

ofloxacin ofloxacina

ohm ohm

oil aceite; **~ acne** botones de aceite; **~ ~ immersion lens** objetivo de inmersión en aceite

oily resbaladizo, lúbrico, resbaloso

ointment ungüento; **~ for wounds** ungüento para heridas, pomada para heridas

old viejo; **~ age** senilidad, ancianidad, vejez

oleandomycin oleandomicina

olecranon olécranon, hueso del codo

olfaction olfacción, olfato

olfactory olfato, órgano olfatorio; **~ bulb** bulbo olfatorio; **~ nerve** nervio olfativo; **~ organ** sentido olfativo, órgano olfatorio; **~ system** sistema olfativo

oligodendrocytes oligodendroglia, células

oligodendrogliales
oligodendroglia oligodendroglia, células oligodendrogliales
oligoelement oligoelemento, elemento traza
oligomenorrhea oligomenorrea, menstruación poco frecuente
oligonucleotide oligonucleótido; ~ **fingerprint** huella oligonucleotídica
oligoprobe oligosonda
oliguria oliguria, secreción deficiente de orina
ombudsman ombudsman, defensor del pueblo
omeprazole omeprazol
omphalocele hernia umbilical, exónfalo
omphalo-enteric duct conducto onfalomesentérico
omphalosite onfalocito
omphalotomy omfalotomía
OMR referencias médicas atribuibles
on sobre, en (place), encendido (e.g. radio), dentro de; ~ **the first pass** primer paso; ~ **top** encima de
once una vez
onchocercosis oncocercosis, una forma filariasis en America Central y del Sur y en África
oncofetal antigen antígeno oncofetal
oncogene oncogén
oncogenic oncogénico, cancerígeno, carcinogénico, tumorigénico
oncogenic virus virus oncogenico, oncovirus
oncologist oncólogo
oncology oncología
oncolytic oncolítico
oncotic oncótico
oncovirus virus oncogenico, oncovirus
one uno, -a
onirism delirio onírico, demencia vesánica, onirismo
only sólo, solamente
ontodoid apophysis apófisis odontoides
onychia maligna oniquia maligna
onychlysis onicólisis, destrucción de la uña
onychoclasis onicoclasia, la onicoclasis
onychophagia onicofagia, morderse las uñas
oophorectomy ooforectomía, ovariectomía, castración
oophoritis ovaritis, ooforitis
oozing hemorrhage hemorragia difusa
opale mutation mutación ópalo

opalescent opalescente
opalgia opalgia, neuralgia facial
opal-like opalescente
open abierto; ~ **ductus arteriosus Botalli** conducto arterioso persistente
operate, to operar
operating characteristic curve [en estadística] curva de eficacia; ~ **microscope** microscopio quirúrgico, microscopio operatorio, microscopio para el estudio de la córnea; ~ **room** sala de operaciónes, quirófano
operation operación
operative peroperatorio, intraoperatorio
operator operador
operon operón
ophthalmic oftálmico
ophthalmological oftalmológico
ophthalmologist oculista
ophthalmology oftalmología
ophthalmoplegia oftalmoplejia
ophthalmoplegic ophthalmoplegic; ~ **hemicrania** hemicrania oftalmopléjica; ~ **migraine** diplejía facial congénita, síndrome de Moebius
ophthalmorrhea oftalmorrea
ophthalmoscope oftalmoscopio, esquiascopio
ophthalmotonus presión intraocular
opiate opiata, opioide, opiáce; ~ **antagonist** antagonista de los opiáceos; ~ **receptor** receptor opeaceo
opioid opiata, opioide, opiáceo; ~ **antagonist** antagonista de los opiáceos; ~ **receptor** receptor opeaceo
opisthotonos opistótonos
opium opio; ~ **alkaloids** alcaloides del opio
opportunist species especie oportunista
opportunistic oportunista
opposable medical references referencias médicas atribuibles
opsin opsina
opsonization opsonización
optic óptico; ~ **atrophy** atrofia del nervio óptico, atrofia óptica; ~ **foramen** conducto óptico; ~ **nerve** nervio óptico; ~ **neuritis** neuritis óptica
optical óptico; ~ **density** absorbancia; ~ **-fiber endoscope** fibroscopio flexible, endoscopio de fibra óptica, laparoscopio; ~ **illusion** ilusión

óptica
optician optometrista, óptico
opticociliotomy opticociliotomía
optimal óptimo
optional facultativo
optochin test prueba de la optoquina
optometrist optometrista
or o
oral oral; ~ **candidiasis** candidiasis oral,
muguet; ~ **cholecystogram** colecistografía
oral; ~ **contraceptive** contraceptivo oral;
~ **hygiene** higiene oral; ~ **part of pharynx**
orofaringe; ~ **rehydration therapy** terapia de
rehidratación oral; ~ **thrush** candidiasis oral,
muguet; ~ **vaccine** vacuna oral
orally por vía oral; ~ vía bucal, peroral
orange naranja
orbital orbital; ~ **aneurysm** aneurisma orbital
orchidectomy orquidectomía, orquiectomía
orchiectomy orquidectomía, orquiectomía
orchitis orquitis, inflamación de un testículo
ordinal scale escala ordinal
orexigenic estimulante del apetito
organ órgano; ~ **bank** banco de órganos;
~ **donor** donante de órganos; ~ **dysfunction**
disfunción orgánica, insuficiencia de un
órgano; ~ **transplanation** transplante de un
órgano
organic orgánico; ~ **acid** ácido orgánico;
~ **cerebral involution** involución cerebral
orgánica; ~ **chlorine compound** compuesto
organoclorado; ~ **insufficiency** insuficiencia
orgánica; ~ **solar cell** célula solar orgánica
organism organismo
organogenesis organoplastia, organogénesis
organoleptic organoléptico
orgasm orgasmo
orientation orientación
ornithine ornitina
orofacial orofacial
oropharynx orofaringe
orphan huérfano/a; ~ **disease** enfermedad
"huérfana"; ~ **drug** fármaco marginal,
medicamento huérfano; ~ **illness** enfermedad
"huérfana"
orphon orfón
orthodontic ortodoncico; ~ **appliance**
aparato ortodóncico; ~ **work** ortodoncia,

odontoplastia
orthodontics ortodoncia, odontoplastia
orthodontology ortodoncia, odontoplastia
orthodonture ortodoncia, odontoplastia
orthopedic ortopédico; ~ **footwear** zapatos
ortopédicos; ~ **insert** plantilla ortopédica;
~ **surgeon** médico de aviación
orthopedist ortopedista
orthosis ortesis
orthostatic ortostático
oscheotomy orquidectomía, orquiectomía
osmolality osmolalidad
osmometry osmometría
osmotic osmótico; ~ **coefficient** coeficiente
osmótico; ~ **concentration** concentración
osmótica; ~ **pressure** presión osmótica
osseous huesudo, huesoso; ~ **ankylosis**
anquilosis ósea; ~ **hyperparathyroidism**
hiperparatiroidismo óseo; ~ **tissue** tejido óseo
ossicle osículo, huesecillo
ossification osificación
ossifying osificante
ossifying fibroma osteofibroma
osteitis osteítis, ostitis; ~ **fibrosa cystica**
neurofibromatosis, polifibromatosis
neurocutánea pigmentaria, enfermedad de
Recklinghausen, osteítis fibroquística
osteoarthritis artrosis, osteoartritis; ~ **of the
elbow** artrosis del codo
osteoarthrosis osteoartrosis
osteoblast osteoblasto
osteocalcin osteocalcina
osteocartilaginous osteocartilaginoso;
~ **exostosis** osteocondroma, exostosis
osteocartilaginosa
osteochondrodysplasia osteocondrodisplasia,
osteocondrodisplasia
osteochondrofibroma osteocondroma fibroso,
osteocondrofibroma
osteochondroma osteocondroma, exostosis
osteocartilaginosa
osteoclast osteoclasto
osteoclastic osteoclastic
osteocranium osteocráneo
osteocyte osteocito
osteodensimetry densitometría de huesos
osteodystrophy osteodistrofia, distrofia de los
huesos
osteoesclerosis osteoesclerosis, eburnación

osteogenic osteogénico, osteógeno;
~ **sarcoma**, sarcoma osteógeno, osteosarcoma
osteogenous chondromatosis condromatosis osteogénica
osteohalisteresis osteohalistéresis
osteoid osteoide; ~ **carcinoma** carcinoma osteoide; ~ **osteoma** osteoma osteoide;
~ **tissue** tejido osteoide
osteolysis osteólisis, destrucción o muerte del hueso
osteomalacia osteomalacia
osteometric densitometer densitómetro de huesos
osteomyelitis osteomielitis
osteonecrosis osteonecrosis
osteopathy osteopatía
osteopetrosis osteopetrosis
osteophyte osteófito
osteophytosis osteofitosis
osteoplastic cancer carcinoma osteoide
osteopoikilosis osteopoiquilosis, osteopoiquilia, osteopetrosis
osteoporosis osteoporosis, desmineralización esquelética
osteosarcoma sarcoma osteógeno, osteosarcoma
osteosis cutis osteoma cutáneo
osteosynthesis osteosíntesis
osteotomy osteotomía; ~ **plate** placa ósea
otalgia otalgia, dolor de oído
OTC (over-the-counter drugs, non-prescription medication) medicamento sin presentación de receta médica, de venta libre, medicamento OTC
other otro
otic exudate exudado ótico
otitis otitis, inflamación del oído; ~ **media** otitis media
otophone audífono, prótesis auditiva, aparato para sordos
otoplasty otoplastia
otorhinolaryngology otorrinolaringología, ORL
otorrhea otorrea, otorrhea
otorrhoea otorrea, otorrhea
otosclerosis otosclerosis
otoscope otoscopio
ototoxic ototóxico
our nuestro

out afuera, fuera de; ~ **of breath** sin resuello, sin aliento, jadeante; ~ **of work** sin trabajo
outer exterior; ~ **ears** orejas, los sentidos;
~ **membrane** membrana plasmática, plasmalema
outgrowth excrecencia
outhouse retrete, dependencia
outlier value valor aberrante
outlook prognosis, pronóstico, futuro
outpatient paciente externo, paciente ambulatorio; ~ **care** centro ambulatorio, clínica ambulatoria, tratamiento ambulatorio, atención ambulatoria; ~ **clinic** centro ambulatorio, clínica ambulatoria, tratamiento ambulatorio, atención ambulatoria;
~ **consultation** tratamiento ambulatorio, atendimiento ambulatorio; ~ **treatment** centro ambulatorio, clínica ambulatoria, tratamiento ambulatorio, atención ambulatoria
output rate rendimiento
outside exterior, afuera, fuera de
oval ovalo
ovarian ovárico; ~ **cyst** quiste ovário, quiste ovárico; ~ **endometriosis** endometriosis ovárica, adenoma endometrioide del ovario;
~ **follicle** folículo de Graaf, folículo ovárico;
~ **hormones** hormonas ováricas; ~ **interstitial cells** células tecales
ovariectomy ovariectomía, ooforectomía, ovariotomía normal, castración
ovaries ovarios
ovariprival arthropathy artropatía menopáusica
ovary ovario
over pasado
overall survival rate tasa de supervivencia global
overdose sobredosis, dosis excesiva
overdosing sobredosis, dosis excesiva
overeating hipernutrición, alimentación en exceso
overestimate, to sobreestimar
overexert oneself, to sobrefatigarse
overflow, to rebasar
overhanging end extremo saliente
overlap hybridisation hibridación por superposición

overnight durante la noche

overstate, to exagerar

over-stimulation estimulación exagerada

over-the-counter drugs medicamento sin presentación de receta médica, de venta libre, medicamento OTC

over-the-counter medicine medicamento sin presentación de receta médica, de venta libre, medicamento OTC

overuse syndrome traumatismo provocado por trabajo de movimientos repetitivos

overweight sobrepeso, pasado de peso, gordo, grueso, gordinflón, petacón, excesode peso

ovulation ovulación, desprendimiento natural del óvulo

ovum óvulo, huevo pequeño

oxacillin oxacilina

oxalate oxalato

oxandrolone oxandrolona

oxazepam oxacepán

oxazolidinone oxazolidinona

oxidase oxidasa; ~ **test** prueba de la oxidasa

oxidation oxidación; ~ **-reduction** oxidorreducción, oxidación-reducción

oxidative oxidativo; ~ **decarboxylation** descarboxilación oxidativa; ~ **decomposition** descomposición oxidante; ~ **phosphorylation** fosforilación oxidante, fosforilación oxidativa

oxidoreductase óxidorreductasa

oximeter oxímetro, hemoxímetro

oxolinic acid ácido oxolínico

oxybutynin hydrochloride oxibutinina hidrocloruro

oxycodone oxicodona

oxygen oxígeno; ~ **absorbtion** consumo de oxígeno, capacidad aeróbica; ~ **capacity** consumo de oxígeno, capacidad aeróbica; ~ **deprivation** privación de oxígeno; ~ **free radical** radical libre de oxígeno; ~ **saturation** saturación de oxígeno; ~ **uptake** consumo de oxígeno, capacidad aeróbica

oxygenation oxigenación

oxyhaemoglobin oxihemoglobina

oxymetazoline oximetazolina

oxymetholone oximetolona

oxymorphone oximorfona

oxymyoglobin oximioglobina

oxyphencyclimine oxifenciclimina

oxytetracycline oxitetraciclina

oxytocic oxitócico

oxytocin oxitocina, oxitócico; ~ **challenge test** prueba de provocación con oxitocina

ozone ozono; ~ **layer** capa de ozono, ozonosfera; ~ **therapy** ozonoterapia, terapia de ozono

ozonesphere capa de ozono, ozonosfera

P

p.r.n. cuándo lo necesite, según las necesidades

pacemaker marcapaso

pachipleuritis paquipleuritis

pachytene paquitena

pacifying demulcente, emoliente, calmante, que ablanda y relaja las zonas inflamadas o que ablanda la piel

package envase

packaging empaquetamiento

PaCO2 presión parcial del dióxido de carbono en la sangre arterial

paddy foot pie de inmersión, pie de trinchera

paediatric pediátrico

paediatrics pediatría

PAF factor activador de plaquetas

PAGE electroforesis en gel de poliacrilamida

Paget carcinoma enfermedad de Paget, cáncer de Paget, dermatitis papilar maligna, hiperostosis cortical deformante, osteítis deformante

Paget's disease enfermedad de Paget, cáncer de Paget, dermatitis papilar maligna, hiperostosis cortical deformante, osteítis deformante

pagophagia pagofagia

pain dolor, dolencia; ~ **clinic** centro de tratamiento del dolor; ~ **killer** calmante, analgésico, droga analgésica; ~ **management clinic** centro de tratamiento del dolor; ~ **reliever** calmante, analgésico, droga analgésica

painful doloroso, dolorido; ~ **hydronephrosis** hidronefrosis dolorosa; ~ **urination** disuria, emisión dolorosa de la orina

painkiller calmante, analgésico, droga analgésica

painless indoloro, sin dolor; ~ **hard tumor** cirro, quiste

painlessness indolencia

paint thinner disolvente de pintura

painter's syndrome encefalopatía tóxica crónica

paints pinturas

pair pareja, par; ~ **of chromosomes** par cromosómico, par de cromosomas

palatal palatino

palatine palatino; ~ **glands** glándulas palatinas; ~ **tonsil** amígdala faríngea, amígdala palatina

palev pálido

palindrome palíndromo

palindromic recidivante, palindrómico

palliative paliativo; ~ **care** tratamiento paliativo, paliativo, cuidado paliativo; ~ **surgery** cirugía paliativa; ~ **therapy** tratamiento paliativo, paliativo, cuidado paliativo; ~ **treatment** tratamiento paliativo, paliativo, cuidado paliativo

palm palma; ~ **of the hand** palma de la mano; ~ **-chin reflex** reflejo palmomentomano, reflejo palmomentoniano, reflejo palmomental

palmar palmar

palmomental reflex reflejo palmomentomano, reflejo palmomentoniano, reflejo palmomental

palmoplantar diffuse keratosis palmoplantar keratosisdifusa

palpable palpable

palpate, to palpar

palpebral palpebral

palpitation palpitación

palsy parálisis, paraplejía, perlesía, perlatico

panacea panacea, curalotodo

panaritium panadizo, uñero

Pancoast's syndrome síndrome de Pancoast; ~ **tumor** tumor de Pancoast, tumor del surco pulmonar

pancolectomy pancolectomía, colectomía

pancreas páncreas

pancreatectomy pancreatectomía

pancreatic pancreático; ~ **cancer** cáncer pancreático; ~ **carboxypeptidase** carboxipeptidasa; ~ **cyst** quiste pancreático,

quiste de páncreas; ~ **ductal carcinoma** carcinoma pancreatico ductal; ~ **elastase** elastasa pancreática; ~ **enzyme** enzima pancreática; ~ **function test** prueba de función pancreática; ~ **insufficiency** insuficiencia pancreática; ~ **kallikrein** calicreína hística; ~ **lipase** lipasa pancreática; ~ **pseudocyst** pseudoquiste pancreático; ~ **ribonuclease** ribonucleasa pancreática; ~ **RNase** ribonucleasa pancreática

pancreaticoduodenal pancreaticoduodenal; ~ **artery** arteria pancreaticoduodenal

pancreaticogastrostomy pancreatogastrostomía

pancreatitis pancreatitis, inflamación del páncreas

pancreatopeptidase elastasa pancreática

pancreatoptosis ptosis del páncreas

pancreozymin pancrozimina

pancytopenia pancitopenia

pandemic sub pandemia, adj pandémico

panel doctor médico autorizado, médico externo de hospital

panigau anquilostomiasis cutánea

panmyelopathy panmieloptisis, panmielopatía

panmyelophthisis panmieloptisis, panmielopatía

Panner disease síndrome de Panner, necrosis aséptica del cóndilo humeral; ~ **syndrome** síndrome de Panner, necrosis aséptica del cóndilo humeral

panniculitis paniculitis, reacción inflamatoria de la grasa debajo de la piel

panting jadeo, respiración superficial y rápida, hacer esfuerzos para respirar

pantoprazole pantoprazole

pantothenic acid ácido pantoténico; ~ **deficiency syndrome** síndrome de deficiencia de ácido pantoténico

PAP (prostatic acid phosphatase) fosfatasa ácida prostática

pap smear prueba de pap, prueba de Papanicolau

Pap test prueba de pap, prueba de Papanicolau

papain papaina

Papanicolaou stain tinción de Papanicolaou

papaver adormidera, amapola real, adormidera soporífera

papaveretum opio

papilla papila; **~ of the optic nerve** papila óptica; **~ pili** papila pilosa

papillary papilar; **~ adenocarcinoma** adenocarcinoma papilífero

papilledema papiledema, edema papilar, tumefacción del disco óptico, hinchazón de la papila óptica

papillitis papilitis, inflamación de una papila; **~** papilitis, inflamación o edema de la papila óptica

papillocarcinoma papillocarcinoma, epitelioma de la papila de Vater

papilloedema edema de la papila óptica, papiledema, edema papilar, tumefacción del disco óptico, hinchazón de la papila óptica

papillomavirus papilomavirus

papular urticaria prurigo simple, urticaria papular

papule pápula

papulosis papulosis; **~ atrophica maligna** papulosis atrófica maligna

para para; **~ ‑aminohippuric acid** aclaramiento del ácido para‑aminohipúrico; **~ ‑aminosalicylic acid** ácido p‑aminosalicílico; **~ anesthesia** paraanestesia; **~ ‑aortic** paraaórtico; **~ centesis** paracentesis, drenaje

paracetamol paracetamol

paradoxical paradójico, contradictorio; **~ aciduria** aciduria paradójica; **~ dysphagia** disfagia paradójica; **~ exophthalmos** exoftalmia paradójica; **~ respiration** respiración paradójica; **~ sleep** sueño REM, sueño paradójico; **~ thinking** pensamiento paradójico

paraesthesia parestesia, sensación de hormigueo, de pinchazos, paralgesia

paraffin bath baño de parafina

paraflexia pararreflexia

paraformaldehyde paste pasta de paraformaldehído

paragonimiasis paragonimiasis, infección por trematodos

parallel paralelo

parallelism paralelismo

paralysis parálisis, paraplejía, perlesía, perlatico; **~ of one side** hemiplejía

paralytic paralítico; **~ ileus** íleo paralítico

paralyze, to paralizar, inmovilizar

paramedic personal paramédico, paramédico

parameter parámetro, criterio

parametritis parametritis, parametría

parametrium mesométrio

paraneoplastic paraneoplásico; **~ neurologic syndrome** síndrome neurológico paraneoplásico

paranoia paranoia, delirio

paranoiac paranoide, paranoico

paraoxon paraoxón

paraphrenia parafrenia

paraphrenitis parafrenitis

paraplegia paraplejía

paraplegic parapléjico; **~** parapléjico

parasite parásito, parasitario

parasitic parasitario; **~ embolism** embolia parasitaria; **~ hemoptysis** paragonimiasis, infección por trematodos; **~ worm** parásito intestinal, gusano parásito, lombriz intestinal

parasitology parasitología

parasomnia parasomnia

parasympathetic parasimpático; **~ nervous system** sistema parasimpático nervioso; **~ paraganglia** paraganglios no cromafines, paraganglios parasimpáticos

parasympathicolytic parasimpaticolitico, parasimpatolítico

parasympathomimetic parasimpaticomimético

parathion paration

parathormone paratirina

parathyrin paratirina

parathyroid paratiroideo; **~ hormone** paratirina

paratid gland glándula parótida, parótida

paratyphoid paratifoideo

paratyphus vaccine vacuna anti‑paratífico

para‑urethritis periuretritis, parauretritis

paravenous paravenoso

paraventricular paraventricular

paravertebral paravertebval; **~ anesthesia** anestesia paravertebral; **~ blockade** bloqueo paravertebral; **~ infiltration** infiltración paravertebral

paravesical paravesical; **~ abscess** absceso paravesical; **~ hematoma** hematoma paravesical

paregoric paregórico

parenchyma parénquima

parenchymal parenquimatoso; ~ **exudate** exudado parenquimatoso

parenteral parentera; ~ **dyspepsia** dispepsia parenteral; ~ **feeding** nutrición parenteral; ~ **nutrition** nutrición parenteral

parents padres

paresis paresia, forma leve de parálisis; ~ **of adductors** paresia de los aductores

paresthesia parestesia, sensación de hormigueo, de pinchazos, paralgesia

paretic neurosyphilis neurosifilis, neurolúes

parietal parietal; ~ **fontanelle** fontanela parietal; ~ **pericardium** saco pericardio; ~ **pleurisy** pleuresia parietal

parkinsonism parkinsonismo

Parkinson's disease enfermedad de Parkinson, parálisis agitante; ~ **tremor** temblor de la enfermedad de Parkinson

paronychia paroniquia, inflamación de la uña

parotid lymph node ganglio linfático parotideo

parotiditis parotiditis, paperas, parotitis

parotitis parotiditis, paperas, parotitis

paroxysmal paroxístico

Parry's disease enfermedad de Basedow, bocio basedowificado

part parte

partaker participante

partial parcial; ~ **gastrectomy** gastrectomía parcial; ~ **hearing loss** hipoacusia, trastorno de la audición, sordera parcial; ~ **pressure** presión parcial; ~ **thromboplastin time** tiempo de tromboplastina parcial

partially completed medium medio semipreparado

participant participante

particle partícula, corpúsculo, parte elemental; ~ **counter** contador de partículas; ~ **counting immunoassay** inmunoanálisis particulométrico; ~ **radiation** radiaciones corpusculares

particular particular; ~ **quantity** magnitud particular

particularly particularmente, especialmente, sobre todo

partition tabique, partición, división; ~ **coefficient** coeficiente de reparto

partner pareja

parturition parto

paruteral parauréteral, paraurétrico

parvovirus parvovirus

pascal pascal

pass away, to morir; ~ **wind, to** arrojar flatos

passage paso, ductus, conducto, evacuación intestinal, introducción de un catéter

passive pasivo, no activo; ~ **anaphylaxis** anafilaxia pasiva; ~ **hemagglutination test** prueba de hemaglutinación pasiva; ~ **immunodiffusion test** prueba de inmunodifusión pasiva; ~ **smoking** tabaquismo pasivo, tabaquismo involuntario

passivity phenomenon síndrome de Clerambault-Kandinsky

passport pasaporte (m), documento de identidad

Pasteurella pestis pasteurella pestis; ~ **tularensis** pasteurella tularensis

pasteurellosis pasteurelosis

pastimes recreación, actividades recreativas, actividades de tiempo libre

pastoral care cuidado pastoral

patch parche; ~ **repair** reparación por escisión; ~ **test** test epicutáneo, prueba epicutánea

patchouli oil patchuli

patellar patelar; ~ **reflex** reflejo patelar; ~ **suture** sutura patelar

patellofemoral arthrosis artrosis patelofemoral

patent ductus Botalli conducto arterioso persistente

paternal inheritance herencia paterna

paternity test prueba de paternidad

pathlenght paso de luz

pathobiochemistry bioquímica clínica

pathogen patógeno

pathogenic propiedad patógena

pathologic patológico; ~ **entity** entidad patológica

pathological patológico, morboso; ~ **anatomy** anatomía patológica; ~ **laboratory** laboratorio de patología

pathologist patólogo

pathology patología, anatomía patológica; ~ **laboratory** laboratorio de patología

pathophysiology fisiopatología

pathopsychology psicopatología

patient paciente; ~ **advocate** defensor del

paciente; **~ care** atención médica en hospital;
~ compliance adhesión del paciente al
tratamiento; **~ dress** bata de hospital;
~ management manejo de casos,
administración de casos; **~ records**
expedientes, registros, registros médicos,
récords médicos, fichero médico; **~ transport**
transporte de pacientes

patient's discharge despido del hospital;
~ grievance procedure sistema de tramite de
quejas de pacientes

patulin patulina

paunch barriga, panza, vientre

pavulon pavulon

paw pata, zarpa

PCaP gene gen PCAP

peach durazno, melocotón

peak concentración máxima, pico de voltaje
transitorio; **~ expiratory flow rate** flujo
espiratorio máximo; **~ flow** flujo maximal;
~ level concentración máxima, pico de voltaje
transitorio; **~ metabolism** metabolismo
maximo

peanut cacahuete, maní

pear pera

pearl perla

pectase pectasa

pectin pectina; **~ esterase** pectasa

pectinate pectinato

pectoral pectoral; **~ muscle** músculo pectoral;
~ reflex reflejo costopectoral

pecularity idiosincrasia, alergia o sensibilidad
exagerada a un medicamento, peculiar a un
individuo

pedal podálico

Pedialyte pedialyte

pediatric pediátrico; **~ oncology** oncologia
pediatrica

pediatrician pediatra

pediatrics pediatría

pedicle pedículo; **~ of the allantois** cordón
amniótico, pedículo mesoabdominal

pediculosis pediculosis, infestación humana por
piojos; **~ pubis** pediculosis pubis

pediculus pedúnculos cerebelosos

pedigree árbol genealógico, estudio
genealógico, genealogía

pedodontics pedodoncia

pedological trait rasgo pedologico

pedology pedología

peduncle pedículo, petiolus, pedúnculo; **~ of
cerebellum** pedúnculos cerebelosos

peeling descamación, formación exagerada de
escamas en la piel

peer group grupo de comparación, grupo
comparable; **~ review** revisión por expertos

PEFR flujo espiratorio máximo

pellagra pelagra

pellet sedimento

pelvic pélvico; **~ exenteration** exenteración
pélvica; **~ fascia** aponeurosis pélvica; **~ floor**
piso pélvico, perineo, suelo pélvico; **~ girdle**
cinturón pélvico; **~ hematoma** hematoma
pélvico; **~ inflammatory disease** enfermedad
inflamatoria pélvica, debida a una infección
bacteriana, adnexitis; **~ mass** masa pelviana;
~ muscles musculatura pélvica;
~ presentation presentación de pie,
presentación pódalica, presentación pélvica;
~ scan escáner pelviano; **~ support** soporte
pélvico; **~ width** amplitud de la pelvis

pelvis pelvis, cadera

pemphigoid penfigoide

pemphigus pénfigo; **~ brasiliensis** pénfigo
brasileño; **~ erythematosus** pénfigo
eritematoso, síndrome de Senear-Usher;
~ foliaceus pénfigo foliáceo

penetrancy penetrancia

penetration penetración

penicillin penicilina; **~ G** bencilpenicilina;
~ scratch test prueba cutánea de la
penicilina; **~ V** fenoximetilpenicilina

penicillinase penicilinasa

penile fálico; **~ erection** erección; **~ implant**
androprótesis; **~ plastic induration** induración
plástica de los cuerpos cavernosos;
~ prosthesis androprótesis

penis miembro, pene, cosa

penlight linterna de bolsillo

pentagastrin pentagastrina; **~ test** prueba de la
pentagastrina

pentose pentosa; **~ phosphate pathway** via de
los pentosafosfatos

pentoxifylline pentoxifilina

pepper pimiento

pepsin pepsina

peptic péptico; ~ **ulcer** úlcera péptica, úlcera de estómago

peptide peptídico; ~ **hydrolase** hidrolasa peptídica; ~ **map** mapa peptídico

peptone broth caldo peptonado

perception percepción; ~ **disorder** distorsión de la percepción

perceptual de la percepción; ~ **distortion** distorsión de la percepción; ~ **disturbance** distorsión de la percepción

percolation percolación

percussion golpear, percusión

percutaneous percutáneo, a través de la piel intacta; ~ **catheter ablation** ablacion por cateter, ablación por radiofrecuencia, ablación eléctrica transvenosa; ~ **endoscopic gastrostomy** gastrostomía endoscopica percutánea; ~ **transluminal angioplasty** angioplastia transluminal percutanea; ~ **ultrasonic lithotripsy** litotripsia percutánea ultrasónica

perennial perenne, perpetuo, persistente

perfluorocarbon perfluorocarbono

perforated hymen himen perforado

perforation perforación, perforation, agujero, apertura

performance prestación, funcionamiento; ~ **characteristic** característica de funcionamiento; ~ **standard** norma de funcionamiento; ~ **status** estado general

perfusion perfusión; ~ **solution** solución de perfusión, soluciones para perfusión

perianal perianal; ~ **abscess** tlacotillo

periapex of a tooth región periapical de la dentadura

periappendicitis peritiflitis, periapendicitis

periarthritis periartritis

pericardial pericárdico; ~ **cavity** cavidad pericárdica; ~ **concretion** sínfisis pericárdica, concreción pericárdica; ~ **cyst** quiste pericárdico; ~ **effusion** derrame pericárdico; ~ **fluid** líquido pericárdico; ~ **murmur** roce pericárdico; ~ **sac** saco pericardio; ~ **scar** induración del pericardio; ~ **tap** pericardiocentesis, pericardiocentesis; ~ **window technique** pericardiostomía, técnica de ventana pericardica

pericardicentesis pericardiocentesis, pericardicentesis

pericardiocentesis pericardiocentesis, pericardicentesis

pericardiostomy pericardiostomía, técnica de ventana pericardica

pericarditis pericarditis, inflamación de la envoltura del corazón

pericardium pericardio

perichondrium pericondrio

peridontal splint surco dental primitivo, tablilla, gotiera, bruxismo, plana relajación, ferula oclusal

peridural peridural; ~ **anaesthesia** raquianestesia epidural, anestesia epidural; ~ **anesthesia** raquianestesia peridural; ~ **injection** inyección peridural

perimyelitis meningitis espinal, perimielitis

perinatal perinatal; ~ **medicine** perinatología; ~ **transmission** transmisión perinatal, transmisión vertical, transmisión maternofilial

perinatology perinatología

perineal perineal; ~ **fistula** fistula perineal; ~ **hernia** hernia isquiorrectal, la hernia perineal; ~ **hyperhidrosis** hiperhidrosis perineal

perineoplasty perineoplastia

period periodo

periodic cíclico, regular, repetido; ~ **abstinence** continencia periódica, método de Ogino; ~ **table of the elements** Tabla Periodica de los Elementos

periodontal periodontal; ~ **cyst** conducto periodontal; ~ **disease** enfermedad periodóntica, piorrea alveolar, parodontosis, periodontosis, enfermedad periodontal; ~ **pack** aposito periodontal; ~ **pocket** bolsa periodontal

periodontics parodontología

periodontitis periodontitis; ~ **simplex** periodontitis

periodontoclasia periodontoclasia, gingivopericementitis, paradontólisis

periodontology parodontología

periodontolysis periodontoclasia, gingivopericementitis, paradontólisis

periodontosis parodontosis

periods menstruación, regla

perioperative perioperativo

perioral perioral, situado alrededor de la boca
periorbital periorbitario; **~ hematoma** hematoma periorbitario
periosteum periostio
periostitis ossificans periostoma, periosteofito
peripheral distal, alejado, periférico; **~ blood flow** trastorno de la circulación periférica de la sangre; **~ blood lymphocyte** linfocito de sangre periférica; **~ motor neuron** neurona motora periférica; **~ nerve** nervio periférico; **~ nervous system** sistema nervioso periférico; **~ neuropathy** neuropatía periférica
peristalsis peristalsis
peristaltic peristáltico; **~ pumps** bombas de infusión implantables, bombas peristálticas
perithyphlitis peritiflitis, periapendicitis
peritoneal peritoneal; **~ carcinoma** carcinoma peritoneal; **~ cavity** cavidad peritoneal; **~ dialysis** diálisis peritoneal; **~ fluid** líquido peritoneal; **~ mesothelioma** mesotelioma peritoneal; **~ papillomatosis** papilomatosis; **~ puncture** peritoneocentesis; **~ recessus** fosa peritoneal
peritoneoscope peritoneoscopia
peritoneoscopy peritoneoscopia
peritoneum envoltura abdominal, peritoneo
peritonitis peritonitis, inflamación de la envoltura abdominal
periumbilical periumbilical
periurethral periuretral; **~ abscess** absceso periuretral
perivascular perivascular; **~ fibrous capsule** capsula fibrosa del higado, capsula fibrosa perivascularis
permanent permanente, permanente; **~ disability** incapacidad permanente
permeability permeabilidad
permeable permeable, poroso
permission permiso
permutation metabolismo, conjunto de reacciones bioquímicas dentro del organismo
pernicious dañino, nocivo, dañoso, pernicioso, desfavorable, peligroso, aniquilante; **~ anemia** anemia perniciosa; **~ hyperinsulinism** hiperinsulinismo espontáneo
pernio sabañón, congelación, pernio
peronial peroneo
peroral peroral, por boca

peroxidase peroxidasa; **~ activity** actividad peroxiddásica; **~ antibody test** prueba de anticuerpos de peroxidasa; **~ test** prueba de la peroxidasa
peroxisome peroxisoma, perixoma
peroxy benzoyl nitrate nitrato de peroxibenzoíllo
perphenazine perfenacina
persecution paranoia paranoia de persecución
persistent perenne, perpetuo, persistente, perseverante; **~ hyperbilirubinemia** hiperbilirrubinemia persistente; **~ pain** dolor persistente, dolor insistente; **~ recovery** curación definitiva
personal personal; **~ space** privacidad, espacio personal, derecho civil a la libertad contra intrusión en los asuntos
perspiration diaforesis, sudoración, transpiración, sudor
perspiratory glands glándulas sudoriparas, glándulas de transpiración
pertussis pertussis, tosferina, coqueluche
perversion perversión, desviación sexual
pervious permeable, poroso
pes calcaneus marcha sobre los talones; **~ valgus** pie valgo
pessary pesario
pet animal domesticado, mascota; **~ therapy** zooterapia
PET (positron-emission tomography) tomografía por emisión de positronos, TEP; **~ scan** tomografía por emisión de positronos, TEP
petechia petequia, puntos rojopurpúreos
pethidine meperidina; **~ hydrochloride** clorhidrato de petidina
petiole pedículo, petiolus, pedúnculo
petit mal epilepsia minor; **~ quartet** tetralogía del pequeño mal
petri dish plato de laboratório, cápsula de Petri, caja Petri
petrolatum petrolatum, vaselina en bruto
Pfeiffer's bacillus Haemophilus influenzae
PGD diagnóstico preimplantatorio
pH pH; **~ balance** pH de equilibrio; **~ equilibrium** pH de equilibrio; **~ -meter** peachímetro; **~ -metry** peachimetría
phacolysis facólisis

P

phage bacteriófago, fago; ~ **immunity** inmunidad a fagos; ~ **typing** tipificación con fagos

phagocyte fagocito

phagocytic fagocitario; ~ **anemia** anemia fagocitaria

phagocytosis fagocitosis

phalanges falanges

phallic fálico

phalloidine faloidina

phantom fantasma; ~ **limb syndrome** dolor fantasma, síndrome del miembro fantasma; ~ **pain** dolor fantasma, síndrome del miembro fantasma; ~ **pregnancy** seudociesis, seudoembarazo; ~ **sensation** dolor fantasma, síndrome del miembro fantasma; ~ **tumor** tumor fantasma, pseudotumor, tumor falso

pharmaceutical producto farmacéutico, farmaco; ~ **form** forma farmacéutica; ~ **industry** industria farmaceutica; ~ **services** servicios farmacéuticos

pharmaceutics ciencia farmacéutica, farmacia

pharmacist boticario, farmácia

pharmacodynamic action acción farmacodinámica

pharmacodynamics farmacodinamia

pharmacocinetics farmacocinética

pharmacological farmacológico; ~ **action** accion farmacologica; ~ **hypothermia** hipotermia farmacológica

pharmacology farmacologia

pharmacomania abuso de medicamentos

pharmacon fármaco, medicamento, medicina

pharmaco–toxicological protocol protocolo toxicofarmacológico

pharmacy farmacia, botica

pharmatoxicological tóxico–farmacológico

pharyngeal faríngeo; ~ **bursa** bolsa faríngea; ~ **cough** tos faríngea; ~ **exudate** exudado faríngeo; ~ **fornix** fórnix de la faringe; ~ **glands** glándulas faríngeas; ~ **stridor** estridor faríngeo; ~ **tonsil** amígdala faríngea, amígdala palatina

pharyngitis faringitis, inflamación de la garganta, inflamación de la faringe

pharynx faringe

phase fase; ~ **–contrast microscopy** microscopía de contraste de fases

phasmid fásmido

phenacetin fenacetina

phencyclidine fenciclidina

phenobarbital fenobarbital

phenobarbitone fenobarbital

phenolphthalein fenolftaleína, ~ **test** técnica de fenolftaleína

phenomenon fenómeno, manifestación, signo, síntoma

phenothiazine fenotiazina

phenotype fenotipo

phenotypic frequency frecuencia fenotípica

phenotypical fenotípico

phenoxybenzamine fenoxibenzamina

phenylalanine fenilalanina

phenylenediamine fenilenodiamina

phenylethylamine feniletilalamina

phenylpyruvic acid ácido fenilpirúvico

phenytoin fenitoina, Dilantin

pheochrome cromafin; ~ **cell** célula cromafin

pheochromocytoma feocromocitoma

pheromone feromona

Philadelphia chromosome cromosoma Filadelfia

phlebitis flebitis

phlebography flebografía

phlebosclerosis flebosclerosis

phlebotomist flebotomista

phlebotomy extracción de sangre, sangría; ~ **needle** aguja para extraer sangre

phlegm flema, esputo, pituita, mucus, moco, moquera

phlegmon flemón, inflamación difusa; ~ **of the chin** flemón del mentón, flemón del la barbilla

phobia fobia

phoniatry audiofonología

phosphate fosfato; ~ **acetyltransferase** fosfato-acetiltransferasa; ~ **buffer** tampón de fosfato

phosphatemia phosphatemia

phosphatidase fosfolipasa A2

phosphatides phospholipids, phosphatides

phosphatidylcholine fosfatidilcolina, lecitina

phospholipase fosfolipasa

phospholipid fosfolípido

phospholipids phospholipids, phosphatides

phosphonate fosfonato

phosphonecrosis necrosis fosfórica

phosphoproteins fosfoproteínas

phosphopyruvate carboxylase fosfoenolpiruvato-carboxicinasa, GTP

phosphoric acid ácido fosfórico

phosphorism intoxicación por fósforo, fosforismo

phosphorothioate fosforotioato

phosphoruria phosphaturia

phosphorus fósforo; ~ **poisoning** intoxicación por fósforo, fosforismo

phosphorylase fosforilasa; ~ **kinase** fosforilasa-cinasa

phosphorylation fosforilación

phosphotransacetylase fosfato-acetiltransferasa

phosphuria phosphaturia

photalgia fotalgia

photocautery fotocoagulación

photocell fotocélula

photocoagulation fotocoagulación

photodynamic fotodinámico; ~ **therapy** terapia fotodinámica, fototerapia

photometer espectrómetro

photometry espectrometría

photomultiplier fotomultiplicador

photophobia fotofobia, aversión a la luz

photosensitivity fotosensibilidad

photosensitization fotosensibilización

phototransduction fototransducción

phrenic frénico; ~ **nerve** nervio frénico, nervio motor del diafragma

phrenoglottic spasm laringismo, espasmo de la laringe, laringospasmo

phthirus pubis ladilla, phtirius pubis

phthisis caquexia, marasmo

physiatrics fisioterapia

physiatrist fisiatra

physiatry fisiatría

physic mental, relacionado con la mente

physical físico, corporal; ~ **ability** aptitud física, capacidad física; ~ **anthropology** somatología, antropología física; ~ **disability** discapacidad física, minusvalía, incapacidad;
~ **examination** reconocimiento físico, examen médico; ~ **exertion** esfuerza, movimiento;
~ **fitness** aptitud física, capacidad física;
~ **handicap** discapacidad física, minusvalía,

incapacidad; ~ **health** salud física;
~ **incapacity** discapacidad física, minusvalía, incapacidad; ~ **labor** esfuerzos físicos;
~ **stress** esfuerza, movimiento; ~ **therapist** fisioterapista, fisioterapeuta, kinesiólogo;
~ **therapy** fisioterapia; ~ **trauma** trauma, traumatismo

physician médico

physician's assistant médico asistente

physicochemical fisicoquímico

physiognomy fisonomía

physiologic fisiológico

physiological fisiológico, normal; ~ **plasticity** plasticidad fisiológica; ~ **saline solution** solución fisiológica; ~ **salt solución** fisiológica; ~ **variation** variación fisiológica

physiologist fisiólogo, fisiologista

physiology fisiología; ~ **of nutrition** fisiología de la nutrición; ~ **of reproduction** fisiología de la reproducción

physiopathology fisiopatología

physiotherapy fisioterapia

phytopharmaceutical product producto fitofarmacéutico, fitofármaco

phytotherapy fitoterapia, terapia herbaria, hierbas medicinales

pia mater piamadre

pian–bois espundia, leishmaniosis cutaneomucosa americana

pick one's nose, to meterse el dedo en la nariz, limpiarse la nariz con el dedo; ~ **-me-up** analéptico, medicamento de efecto estimulante en la psique

picornaviridae infection infección por picornaviridae

picornavirus picornavirus

PID enfermedad inflamatoria pélvica, debida a una infección bacteriana, adnexitis

pie pastel

pielography pielografía, urografía

Pierre Robin syndrome síndrome de Pierre Robin, síndrome de micrognatia-glosoptosis

pigeon breeder's lung pulmón de los criadores de aves

pigmentary ~ **mole** mola hidatídica, mola hidatidiforme, lentigo;
~ **retinopathy** retinopatía pigmentaria, retinitis pigmentaria; ~ **tumor** tumor

pigmentario
pigmentation pigmentación, depósito de materia colorante, coloración
piles hemorroides, almorranas
pill píldora, comprimido, pastilla; ~ **bottle** frasco medicinal
pillow almohada
pillowcase funda de almohada
pilocarpine pilocarpina; ~ **provocation** provocación con pilocarpina
piloerection piloerección, erección del pelo
pilomotor pilomotor; ~ **muscle** músculo piloerector, músculo erector del pelo; ~ **reaction** reflejo pilomotor; ~ **reflex** reflejo pilomotor
pilots' disease aeroastenia, aeroneurosis
pilous peludo, cabelludo, piloso
pimple grano, espinilla, granito, barro, nacido
pimply pustuloso
pinch, to pellizcar
pineal body epífisis; ~ **gland** glándula pineal, epífisis
pink rosa, rosado; ~ **disease** acrodinia, quiropodalgia; ~ **-eye** tracoma; ~ **finger** dedo meñique
pinocytosis pinocitosis
pinprick pinchazo
pinworm oxiuro, enterobius
piodermia piodermia, piodermitis
piperacillin piperacilina
piperazine adipate adipato de piperazina
piperonal piperonal
pipette pipeta, cuenta-gotas
piroplasmosis piroplasmosis, babesiasis, babesiosis
piss, to orinar, hacer pipí
pissing micción, acción de orinar
pit of the stomach boca del estómago
pituitary hipófisis, glandula pituitária; ~ **gland** hipófisis cerebral, cuerpo pituitario, glandula pituitaria; ~ **gonadotrophins** gonadotropina hipofisarias; ~ **hormone receptor** receptores de la hormona pituitaria; ~ **hormones** hormonas pituitarias
pityriasiform pitiriasiforme; ~ **eczematid** eccematide pitiriasiforme; ~ **seborrheic dermatitis** dermatitis pitiriasiforma seborreica
pityriasis pitiriasis, descamación de la piel en

pequeñas laminillas
pivampicillin pivampicilina
place sitio; ~ **of birth** lugar de nacimiento
placebo placebo
placenta placenta, secundinas; ~ **segundos**, placenta
placental placentario; ~ **failure** insuficiencia placentaria; ~ **incarceration** incarceración de la placenta; ~ **insufficiency** insuficiencia placentaria; ~ **lactogen** lactogenio placentario; ~ **septa** tabiques placentarios; ~ **stage** tercer periodo del trabajo de parto
planar chromatography cromatografía planar
plane joint articulación plana
planigraph tomógrafo
planning planificación, planeamiento, proyecto
plantar plantar; ~ **wart** verruga plantar
plasma plasma, líquido o fluido corporal; ~ **cell** plasmocito; ~ **cell myeloma** mieloma de célula plasmática; ~ **exchange** plasmaféresis, aféresis; ~ **expander** expansor plasmático; ~ **lemma** membrana plasmática, plasmalema; ~ **level** concentración plasmática; ~ **membrane** membrana plasmática, plasmalema; ~ **profile** perfil plasmático; ~ **protein** plasmaproteína, proteína del plasma; ~ **substitute** substitutivo del plasma
plasmablast plasmoblasto
plasmacyte plasmocito, célula plasmática, plasmocito
plasmacytoma mieloma múltiple, plasmocitoma, enfermedad de Kahler, enfermedad de Huppert, plasmacitoma, enfermedad de Bozzolo
plasmalogen synthase plasmalógeno-sintasa
plasmapheresis plasmaféresis, aféresis
plasmid plásmido, plásmide; ~ **vector** plásmido vector
plasmin fibrinolisina
plasminogen plasminógeno, precursor inactivo de la plasmina
plasmocyte plasmacito, célula plasmática, plasmocito
Plasmodium plasmodium malariae, parásito de la malaria, parásito concurrente
plaster emplasto; ~ **bandage** vendaje enyesado, férula de yeso; ~ **bandage splint** férula de vendas enyesadas, férula de yeso; ~ **cast (on a**

limb) enyesado; **~ of Paris** escayola, yeso; **~ splint** férula de yeso

plastic plástica; **~ surgeon** especialista en cirugía estética o cirugía plástica, cirujano plástico; **~ surgery** cirugía estética, cirugía plastica

plasticity plasticidad

plastosome mitocondria, mitocondria, plastosoma

platelet plaqueta; **~ activating factor** factor activador de plaquetas; **~ clumping** aglutinación de las plaquetas; **~ count** recuento de plaquetas

platispondilia platispondilia, aplanamiento de los cuerpos vertebrales

platyspondylia platispondilia, aplanamiento de los cuerpos vertebrales

plausibility verosimilitud

please por favor

pleomorphic pleomórfico

plethysmography pletismografía

pleura pleura

pleural pleural; **~ asbestosis** asbestosis pulmonar; **~ aspiration** punción pleural; **~ cough** tos pleural; **~ decortication** decortación pleural, pleurectomía; **~ effusion** derrame pleural, hidrotórax; **~ fluid** líquido pleural; **~ fremitus** frémito pleural; **~ needle biopsy** punción biopsia pleural; **~ plaque** placa pleural; **~ thickening** engrosamiento pleural, callosidad pleural

pleurectomy decortación pleural, pleurectomía

pleurisy pleuritis, pleuresía, hidrotórax, inflamación de la pleura

pleuritic callosity engrosamiento pleural, callosidad pleural

pleuritis pleuritis, pleuresía, hidrotórax, inflamación de la pleura

pleurodesis pleurodesis

pleuroperitoneal cavity cavidad pleuroperitoneal

pleuropyesis empiema empiema, piotórax, empiema pulmonar

plexus plexo

plica pliegue, reborde de tejido, plica

plication pliegue, reborde de tejido, plica

plicature pliegue, reborde de tejido, plica

plumbic anhydride lead dioxide, el óxido pulga, el anhidrido plúmbico, PbO2

plumbism gota saturnina, plumbismo, saturnismo crónico

PMN elastase elastasa de leucocito

PMS (premenstrual syndrome) distonía premenstrual, tensión premenstrual

pneumatic neumático; **~ disposal unit** aspirador limpiador

pneumoconiosis neumoconiosis

pneumocystis carinii pneumonia neumonía por pneumocystis carinii

pneumomediastinum neumomediastino

pneumonia pulmonía, neumonía

pneumonitis neumonitis, alveolitis

pneumopathy neumopatía, enfermedad del pulmón

podagra gota visceral

podiatrist podólogo

point mutation mutación puntual

poison toxina, veneno; **~ ivy** hiedra venenosa, zumeque venenoso; **~ , to** envenenar, atosigar

poisoning intoxicación, envenenamiento; **~ by mercury** hidrargirismo, hidrargirosis

poisonousness toxicidad

polarizing microscope microscopio de polarización

polarography polarografía

police policía

policitemia poliglobulia, policitemia

polio poliomielitis; **~ vaccine** vacuna contra la polio

poliomyelitis poliomielitis; **~ vaccine** vacuna contra la polio

pollen polen

pollution contaminación, polución; **~ of the biosphere** contaminación de la biosfera

polyacrylamide poliacrilamida; **~ gel** gel de poliacrilamida

polyarthritis poliartritis

polyclonal component componente policlonal

polycystic poliquístico; **~ kidney disease** poliquistosis renal, nefropatía poliquística, riñon poliquístico; **~ ovary syndrome** ovario poliquístico; **~ renal disease** nefropatía poliquística, riñon poliquístico, enfermedad renal poliquística

polycytemia poliglobulia, policitemia

polydactylism polidactilia

polydactyly polidactilia

polydeoxyribonucleotide synthase (ATP) DNA-ligasa (ATP)

polydipsia polidipsia

polygenes poligénes

polygenic inheritance herencia poligénica

polylinker poliligador

polymerase polimerasa; ~ catalytic center centro catalítico de la polimerasa; ~ chain reaction reacción de polimerización en cadena, reacción en cadena de la polimerasa

polymorphic polimórfico

polymorphism polimorfismo; ~ information content contenido informativo del polimorfismo; ~ rate frecuencia de polimorfismo

polymorphonuclear polimorfonuclear; ~ leukocyte leucocito polimorfonuclear

polymyxin polimixina

polyneuritis polineuritis

polyomavirus polyomavirus

polypeptide polipéptido; ~ chain cadena polipéptidica; ~ hormone hormona polipéptidica

polypharmacy polifarmacia

polyphosphorylase glucógeno-fosforilasa

polyribonucleotide nucleotidyltransferase polirribonucleótido-nucleotidiltransferasa

polytene chromosome cromosoma politénico

polytenic chromosome cromosoma politénico

polytherapy politerapia

polytoxicomania politoxicomania

polyunsaturated fatty acids poliinsaturados, ácidos grasos poliinsaturados

polyunsaturates poliinsaturados, ácidos grasos poliinsaturados

polyuria poliuria

polyvalent polivalente; ~ allergy alergia cruzada, alergia a sustancias emparentadas

polyvinyl alcohol alcohol polivinílico

pomphus ampolla, vesícula, vejiga, bullón, roncha

pontocerebellar angle syndrome síndrome del ángulo pontocerebeloso

pool mezcla; ~ therapy balneoterapia

poor pobre; ~ digestion malabsorción, trastorno

de la absorción intestinal de nutrientes; ~ prognosis pronóstico grave

poorly differentiated escasamente diferenciada; ~ differentiated cell célula escasamente diferenciada

pop, to tronar, crepitar

popliteal poplíteal; ~ fossa corva, poplíteal fossa, hueco poplíteo; ~ space corva, poplíteal fossa, hueco poplíteo

popping crujido, trueno, chasquido

population población

porcine bioprosthesis bioprótesis del corazón de cerdo

pores poros

pork puerco, cerdo; ~ tapeworm Tænia solium, tenia

porous permeable, poroso

porphobilinogen profobilinógeno

porphyria porfiria; ~ cutanea tarda porfiria cutánea tardía

porphyrin porfirina

portal system sistema porta

portly sobrepeso, pasado de peso, gordo, grueso, gordinflón, petacón, excesde peso

porto-caval anastomosis anastomosis porto-cava

port-wine stain mancha roja de nacimiento

position posición

positional cloning clonación posicional

positive positivo; ~ feedback retroalimentación psicológica; ~ intropic effect efecto positivo inotrópico; ~ predictive value valor predictivo de un resultado positivo

posology posología

post -post; ~ -catastrophe syndrome post-catastrophe syndrome; ~ -decompression shock choque post-descompresión; ~ - operative shock choque operatorio, sincope postoperatorio; ~ -poliomyelitis syndrome síndrome pos-poliomielitis; ~ -hepatitic cirrhosis cirrosis pos-hepatítica; ~ -coital test prueba de interacción moco-semen, prueba de inseminación; ~ -encephalitic Parkinson's disease enfermedad de Parkinson postencefálica

posterior posterior, situado detrás

posthumous póstumo

postmenopausal posmenopáusico

postmortem examination autopsia, necropsia, la autopsia médico-científica; ~ **lividity** livor mortis, prerigor

postnasal postnasal; ~ **catarrh** adenoiditis; ~ **drip** secreción crónica mucosa postnasal, goteo posnasal

postnatal posnatal, después del nacimiento; ~ **adaptation** adaptación postnatal

postnecrotic cirrhosis cirrosis posnecrótica

postoperative postoperatorio; ~ **angina** angina post-operativa; ~ **care** cuidados postoperatorios, tratamientos postoperatorios; ~ **hematuria** hematuria posoperatoria; ~ **ileus** íleo posoperatorio; ~ **pain** dolor posoperatorio; ~ **treatment** cuidados postoperatorios, tratamientos postoperatorios; ~ **wound infection** infección de herida operatoria

postpartum posparto, después del parto; ~ **amenorrhea** amenorrea posparto

postpoliomyelitis muscular atrophy síndrome pos-poliomielitis

postprandial posprandial, que se presenta después de una comida; ~ **hypoglycemia** hipoglucemia posprandial

postreplicative recombination repair reparación por recombinación posreplicativa

postsurgical posquirúrgico, postoperatorio

postsynaptic postsináptica
~ **dendrite** dendrita postsináptica;
~ **depolarization** despolarización postsináptica; ~ **inhibition** inhibición postsináptica

postsyncopal metabolic syndrome of bradycardia síndrome metabólico miocárdico de la bradicardia

posttraumatic postraumático, post-traumático

postural postural, relativo a la postura o posición; ~ **discomfort** malestar postural, postura incómoda

posture–related postural, relativo a la postura o posición

postvaccinal postvacunal; ~ **eczema** eccema postvacunal; ~ **fever** fiebre postvacunal; ~ **hepatitis** hepatitis por inoculacion, hepatitis serica; ~ **pseudokeloid** reacción vacunal queloide, pseudoqueloide postvacunal

potash óxido potásico

potassemia concentración de ion potasio en plasma/suero

potassium potasio; ~ **iodide** yoduro potásico; ~ **ion** ion potasio; ~ **nitrate** nitrato potásico; ~ **oxide** óxido potásico

potatoes papas

potatorum polyneuritis polineuritis alcohólica

potency potencia, poder, capacidad sexual, poder de un medicamento para producir los efectos, deseados, capacidad del embrión para desarrollarse

potential (adj) potencial, (sub) potencial; ~ **difference** diferencia de potencial

potentialization potencializción, potenciación

potentiation potencializción, potenciación

potentiometry potenciometría

poultice cataplasmo, compresa, emplasto, sinapismo

pour in, to infundir

powdered milk polvos lácteos

power density

PPI (proton pump inhibitor) agente inhibidor de la bomba de protones

practicability practicabilidad

practising medicine consultorio de medicina, consultorio médico, practica médica

prairie itch eccema de los graneros, prurito de los cereales

prebirth prenatal

precancerous precancerosa; ~ **cell** célula precancerosa; ~ **hyperkeratosis** hiperqueratosis precancerosa; ~ **state** estado precancerígeno

precautionary measures medidas de precaución

precipitation precipitación; ~ **test** prueba de la precipitación

precipitin precipitina; ~ **line** línea de precipitación

precision precisión; ~ **grasp** sujeción de precisión; ~ **grip** sujeción de precisión

preclinical preclínico; ~ **effect** efecto preclínico; ~ **stage** fase prodrómica, fase preclínica

precordial precordial, situado delante del corazón; ~ **protrusion** protrusión precordial, dilatación precordial

precursor precursor, que precede; ~ **product** producto precursor

prediastolic protodiastólico

predict, to predecir, pronosticar

predicted environmental concentration concentración ambiental prevista

predictive predictivo; ~ **medicine** medicina preventiva; ~ **value** valor predictivo

predictor predictor

predisposition predisposición, tendencia; ~ **to cancer** antecedente familiar de cáncer

prednisolone prednisolona

prednisone prednisona, dehidrocortisona

preeclampsia preeclampsia

preemies prematuros

pre-emphysematous lesion lesión preenfisematosa

Preferred Provider Organization Organización del seguro de salud

prefrontal cortex corteza prefrontal

pregnancy gestación, gravidez, embarazo; ~ **belt** faja de embarazada, faja de embarazo; ~ **chloasma** cloasma uterino; ~ **neuritis** neuritis gravídica; ~ **rate** índice de embarazo, porcentaje de embarazos; ~ **test** prueba de embarazo, análisis de embarazo

pregnant embarazada; ~ **woman** mujer embarazada

preimplantation genetic diagnosis diagnóstico preimplantatorio

Preisz-Nocard's bacillus Corynebacterium pseudotuberculosis

prekallikrein precalicreína

preliminary preliminar

preload precarga

premalignant premaligno

premarital prematrimonial, premarital; ~ **screening** analisis prematrimoniales, detección serológica premarital

premature prematuro; ~ **aging** progeria, infantilismo senil; ~ **baby** prematuro; ~ **baby unit** unidad de prematuros; ~ **birth** parto prematuro; ~ **delivery** parto prematuro; ~ **detachment of placenta** abruptio placentae; ~ **ejaculation** eyaculación precoz; ~ **heartbeat** contracción ventricular prematura; ~ **infant** prematuro; ~ **ovarian failure** insuficiencia ovárica prematura; ~ **ventricular contraction** contracción ventricular prematura

premed premedicación

premedication premedicación

premeditated suicide suicidio deliberado

premenstrual premenstrual; ~ **dystonia** distonía premenstrual, tensión premenstrual; ~ **hemorrhage** hemorragia premenstrual; ~ **syndrome** distonía premenstrual, tensión premenstrual

premessenger RNA RNA premensajero

premetrological variation variación premetrológica

premium prima de seguro

premonitory infarct infarto premonitorio

prenatal prenatal; ~ **belt** faja de embarazada, faja de embarazo; ~ **care** atención prenatal, asistencia prenatal; ~ **screening** detección prenatal

preoperative preoperatorio; ~ **autologous blood donation** autotransfusión preoperatoria; ~ **preparation** preparaciones preoperatorios

preparation preparado, medicamento confeccionado

prepatellar suture sutura patelar

prepuce prepucio, pliegue que cubre el pene o el clítoris

presbyatrics geriatría

presbyopia presbiopía, presbicia

prescribe, to recetar, prescribir

prescription prescripción; ~ **drugs** medicamento que se puede conseguir unicamente con receta; ~ **eyeglasses** anteojos con receta, lentes; ~ **for drugs** prescripción de drogas; ~ **medicine** medicamento que se puede conseguir unicamente con receta

present presente, actual (time), regalo

presentation presentación, presentación del feto respecto al cuello uterino

preservation integridad, conservación inalterada; ~ **medium** medio conservante

preservative agente conservante, conservador

preserved cadaver cadáver conservado en cera grasa (en adipocira)

pressoreceptor barorreceptor

pressure presión; ~ **flow** flujo por presión; ~ –

induced pain dolor por compresión; ~ **marking** jaspeado, marcas de presión; ~ **pain** dolor inducido por presión; ~ **sore** escara, úlcera por decúbito

presumptive presunto; ~ **diagnosis** diagnóstico provisorio

presymptomatic presintomático; ~ **genetic testing** tamizaje genética; ~ **screening** detección presintomática

presynaptic presináptico; ~ **facilitation** facilitación presináptica; ~ **membrane** membrana presináptica; ~ **neuron** neurona presináptica

prevalence prevalencia

prevention prevención

preventive preventivo; ~ **care** servicios sanitarios preventivos; ~ **measures** tratamiento preventivo; ~ **medical checkup** diagnóstico diagnóstico o preventivo, visita médica preventiva

previous previos

pre-zygotic exclusion exclusión precigótica

PRF prolactoliberina

priapism priapismo, erección anormal y persistente

prick, to pinchar

pricking pinchazo

prickle, to sentir hormigueo, sentir picazón; ~ **-cell** célula de Malpighi, célula espinosa; ~ **-cell layer** capa espinosa de la epidermis, capa de células espinosas

primary primario, principal, primero, al principio, originario; ~ **care** primeros auxilios; ~ **care physician** médico de atención primaria, médico principal; ~ **outbreak** foco primario, brote primario; ~ **standard** patrón primario

prime plasmid plásmido primero

primer cebador; ~ **extension** prolongación del cebador

primidone primidona

primosome primosoma

principal principal; ~ **component analysis** análisis de componentes principales

principle principio; ~ **of measurement** principio de medición; ~ **of relaxation oscillation** principio de la oscilación de relajamiento

printed form impreso, formulario

prion prión; ~ **disease** enfermedad de priones

prior anterior, previo; ~ **informed consent** consentimiento informado previo, consentimiento fundamentado previo, consentimiento consciente

privacy privacidad, espacio personal, derecho civil a la libertad contra intrusión en los asuntos

private privado; ~ **life** privacidad, espacio personal, derecho civil a la libertad contra intrusión en los asuntos; ~ **parts** vergüenzas, genitales

PRL prolactina

pro re nata cuándo lo necesite, según las necesidades

proangiotensin proangiotensina

probability verosimilitud

probacteriophage profago

probe sonda

probiotic probiótico; ~ **substance** sustancia probiótica

probit probit

problem problema

procaine procaína; ~ **esterase** carboxilesterasa

procedural memory memoria no declarativa, memoria implícita

procedure procedimiento, técnica

procedures manual manual de procedimientos

process proceso

processing metabolización

procrastinate, to postergar, procrastinar, postponer todo, andar con dilaciones

procreation procreación, reproducción

proctitis proctitis, inflamación del recto

proctologist proctólogo

proctology proctología

proctoscope proctoscopio, rectoscopio

prodromal prodrómico; ~ **stage** fase prodrómica, fase preclínica

prodrug profármaco

production producción, fabricación

productive productivo

proenzyme zimógeno, proenzima

professional professional; ~ **rehabilitation** rehabilitación funcional, reeducación funcional

profibrinogen profibrinolisina, plasminógeno

profibrinolysin profibrinolisina, plasminógeno

proficiency testing ensayo de aptitud

profound profundo; ~ **purulent blastomycosis** blastomicosis purulenta profunda

progeny descendencia, progenie, descendentes, progenitura

progeria progeria, infantilismo senil

progesterone progesterona

progestin progestina

progestogen progestógeno

prognosis prognosis, pronóstico, futuro

prognostic pronosticado, pronóstico

program programa

progranulocyte progranulocito

progressive progresivo, continuado, que avanza lentamente; ~ **hypertrophic glia cell** célula de neuroglía gigante; ~ **multifocal leukoencephalopathy** leucoencefalopatía multifocal progresiva; ~ **spinal amyotrophy** amiotrofia espinal progresiva

proinsulin proinsulina

projective proyectivo; ~ **test** test de proyección de la personalidad

prokaryote procariota, célula procariota

prokaryotic procarioto; ~ **cell** célula procariota, procariota

prolactin prolactina, hormona lactógena; ~ **-release-inhibiting factor** prolactostatina; ~ **-releasing factor** prolactoliberina

prolactinoma prolactinoma

prolapse prolapso, caída; ~ **of urethra** prolapso de la uretra

proliferation proliferación, multiplicación

proliferative proliferativo, prolífero

proline prolina

prolonged expiration espiración prolongada

prolymphocyte prolinfocito

promegakaryocyte promegacariocito

promegaloblast promegaloblasto

prominent prominente, saliente

promiscuous promiscuo

promonocyte promonocito

promoter promotor; ~ **screening vector** vector de detección de un promotor

pronase micolisina

pronation pronación

prone position posición en decúbito abdominal, postrado

pronormoblast pronormoblasto

proof-reading corrección de galeradas, corrección de pruebas (de imprenta)

propagation propagación

propanolol propanolol

properdin properdina; ~ **factor B** factor B de complemento

property propiedad

prophage profago

prophylactic profiláctico, preventivo; ~ **medical examination** diagnóstico diagnóstico o preventivo, visita médica preventiva

prophylaxis profilaxis, prevención

prophyria porfiria

propionibacterium bacteria propiónica, propionibacterium

propionic acid ácido propiónico

proplasmacyte proplasmocito

proportional proporcional

propranolol propranolol

proprietary patentado; ~ **medicinal product** especialidad medicinal; ~ **medicine** especialidad farmacéutica

proprioception propriocepción

proprioceptive propioceptivo; ~ **awareness** propriocepción; ~ **impulse** impulso propioceptivo; ~ **reflex** reflejo propioceptivo

proptosis exoftalmía, proptosis, propulsión del globo del ojo

propulsive propulsar, motor

proscar (drug) finasterida

prosopalgia tic doloroso, neuralgia del nervio trigémino, prosopalgia

prostaglandin prostaglandina; ~ **synthase** prostaglandina-endoperóxido-sintasa

prostate próstata; ~ **cancer** cáncer prostática; ~ **examination** reconocimiento de la próstata; ~ **gland** glandula prostática, próstata; ~ **infection** prostatitis, inflamación de la próstata; ~ **inflammation** prostatitis, inflamación de la próstata; ~ **specific antigen** antígeno específico de la próstata, AEP, antígeno específico prostático

prostatectomy prostatectomía total

prostatic prostático; ~ **acid phosphatase** fosfatasa ácida prostática; ~ **extirpation** prostatectomía total; ~ **fluid** líquido prostático

prostatism prostatismo

prostatitis prostatitis, inflamación de la próstata

prostetic group grupo prostético

prosthesis prótesis, miembro artificia

prosthetic dentistry laboratory taller de protesis dental

prostrate estar boca abajo, estar postrado, acostado boca abajo, prono

protaminase carboxipeptidasa B

protamine protamina; ~ **sulfate** sulfato de protamina; ~ **zinc insulin** insulina protamina de cin

protease proteasa, enzima que degrada proteínas; ~ **inhibitor** inibidor de la proteasa

protection segregación, prevención, protección

protective protector; ~ **breathing gear** máscara de protección respiratoria, mascarilla respiratoria, careta respiratoria; ~ **clothing** traje protector; ~ **immune response** respuesta de protección inmunitaria

protector protector

protein proteína; ~ **binding** unión a proteínas; ~ **characterization** caracterización de las proteínas; ~ **coat** envoltura proteica, cápside, revestimiento proteico; ~ **deficiency** carencia de proteínas, deficiencia proteica; ~ **denaturation** desnaturalización de proteínas; ~ **electrophoresis** electroforesis de proteínas; ~ **engineering** ingeniería de proteínas; ~ **kinase** proteína quinasa; ~ **messenger** mensajero proteínico; ~ **molecule** molécula proteica; ~ **sequencing system** sistema de secuenciación de proteínas; ~ **splicing** empalme de proteína, ayuste de proteínas; ~ **synthesis** biosíntesis de proteínas, síntesis proteica

proteinaceous proteináceo; ~ **infectious particle** prión; ~ **layer** capa de aleurona

proteinase proteasa; ~ **inhibitors** inhibidores de proteasas

proteinemia proteinemia, concentración de proteína en plasma, concentración de proteína en suero

protein proteína; ~ **caloric malnutrition** malnutrición proteico-calórica, carencia proteico-calórica; ~ **–glutamine g-glutamyltransferase** proteína-glutamina-g-glutamiltransferasa

proteinuria proteinuria, concentración de proteína en orina, excreción de proteína en orina

proteolysis proteólisis

proteolytic proteolítico; ~ **enzyme** enzima proteolítico, proteasa, enzima que degrada proteínas

proteomics proteómica

prothrombase factor Xa de la coagulación

prothrombin protrombina, factor II de la coagulación sanguínea; ~ **time** tiempo de protrombina

protirelin protirelina

protocol protocolo

protodiastolic protodiastólico; ~ **murmur** soplo protodiastólico

proton proton; ~ **microscope** microscopio protonico; ~ **pump** bomba de protones; ~ **pump blocker** agente inhibidor de la bomba de protones; ~ **pump inhibitor** agente inhibidor de la bomba de protones

proto–oncogene protooncogen, protooncogén

protoplasmatic protoplasmático; ~ **astrocyte** astrocito protoplasmático; ~ **poison** tóxico protoplasmático

protoporphyrin protoporfirina

prototroph prototrofo

protozoon protozoos, organismos unicelulares

protrude, to abultar, hinchar, abombar, sobresalir

protruding prominente, saliente; ~ **eyes** exoftalmía, proptosis, propulsión del globo del ojo

protrusion protrusión, bulto, comba, abultamiento; ~ **of the embryonic heart** protrusión precordial, dilatación precordial

provirus ADN retrovírico integrado, provirus

proximal proximal

prozone effect efecto prozona

PRPP synthetase ribosa-fosfato-pirofosfocinasa

PRR grado de repetición de impulsos

pruritic prurítico, hormigante, sarnoso, con picazón

pruritus prurito, escozor o picor, picazón, enfermedad de la piel caracterizada por picazón; ~ **hiemalis** dermatitis hiemalis, pruritis invernal

PSA (prostate specific antigen) antígeno específico de la próstata, AEP, antígeno específico prostático

psammoma psamoma; ~ **particles** cuerpos psamomatosos

Pschyrembel pregnancy sign seña Pschyrembel de embarazo

P-selectin selectina-P

pseudarthrosis seudoartrosis

pseudocast seudocilindro (urinario)

pseudocholinesterase pseudocolinesterase

pseudocowpox nódulo del ordenador

pseudocroup asma de Millar

pseudocyst pseudoquiste; ~ **of the pancreas** pseudoquiste pancreático

pseudoephedrine pseudoefedrina, un adrenérgico que actúa como vasoconstrictor y vasodilator

pseudogout condrocalcinosis

pseudohermaphroditism seudohermafroditismo

pseudomembrane seudomembrana

pseudomembranous seudomembranoso

pseudopregnancy seudociesis, seudoembarazo

pseudotumor seudotumor, tumor fantasma, tumor falso

psoralen psoraleno

psoriasiform eczematid eccemátide psoriasiforme

psoriasis psoriasis

psychiatric psiquiátrico, siquiátrico; ~ **emergency service** servicios psiquiátricos de urgencia; ~ **hospital** hospital psiquiátrico; ~ **nurse** enfermero psiquiátrico; ~ **patient** enfermo mental, pacente mental; ~ **social worker** asistente social del sector de psiquiatría; ~ **ward** servicio psiquiátrico

psychiatrist siquiatra, psiquiátra

psychiatry siquiatría

psychic mental, psíquico; ~ **deliquia** ausencias; ~ **distress** ansiedad psíquica, estrés psicológico; ~ **gaps** ausencias; ~ **healer** curandero, sanador; ~ **shock** choque psíquico, shock afectivo

psychoactive psicoactivo; ~ **drug** psicofármaco, agente psicotrópico

psychoanalytical psico-analítico

psychogalvanic response reflejo psicogalvanico

psychogenic psicógeno

psycholeptic psicoléptico

psychological psicológico, sicológico; ~ **diagnosis** diagnóstico sicológico; ~ **fatigue** fatiga mental, fatiga síquica; ~ **refractory period** periodo refractario psicológico; ~ **sexual dysfunctions** disfunciones sexuales psicológicas; ~ **stress** ansiedad psíquica, estrés psicológico

psychometric test prueba psicométrica

psychomotor psicomotor; ~ **activities** psicomotricidad, actividades de psicomotricidad; ~ **attack** acceso psicomotor; ~ **epilepsy** epilepsia psicomotora; ~ **hallucination** alucinación psicomotriz; ~ **impairment** deficiencia psicomotora

psychomotoricity psicomotricidad, actividades de psicomotricidad

psychophysics psicofísica

psychophysiology psicofisiología

psychosis psicosis

psychosocial psicosocial; ~ **deprivation** privación psíquica y social

psychosomatic psicosomático; ~ **constipation** estreñimiento psicosomático; ~ **diarrhea** diarrea síquica; ~ **illness** enfermedad psicosomática, trastorno psicofisiológico

psychotechnics psicotecnia, sicotecnia, psicotécnica

psychotechnology psicotecnia, sicotecnia, psicotécnica

psychotherapeutic psicoterapéutica

psychotherapy psicoterapia

psychotic psicopático, psicótico

psychotropic psicotrópico; ~ **drug** psicofármaco, agente psicotrópico; ~ **substances** sustancias psicotropas

pteroyl glutamic acid ácido folic, B9, folacin, folate

pterygium pterigión, carnosidad

pterygomaxillary fissure escotadura pterigomaxilar

PTH paratirina

ptomaine ptomaina, tomaína

ptosis ptosis

ptyalism ptialismo, sialorrea

puberty pubertad

pubescent pubescente

pubic púbico; ~ **bone** hueso púbico, pubis;
~ **bone index** índice del hueso ilíaco; ~ **hair**
vello, pelos, pelos púbicos; ~ **region** empeine
abdominal, ingle, verijas
pubis hueso púbico, pubis
Public Health Clinic Clínica de Salud Pública
publisher editor
pudendal canal conducto pudendo, conducto
de Alcock
pudgy sobrepeso, pasado de peso, gordo, grueso,
gordinflón, petacón, excesode peso
puerperal puerperal; ~ **abscess** sepsis puerperal,
eclampsia puerperal, absceso puerperal;
~ **eclampsia** sepsis puerperal, eclampsia
puerperal, absceso puerperal; ~ **infection**
sepsis puerperal, eclampsia puerperal, absceso
puerperal; ~ **sepsis** sepsis puerperal, eclampsia
puerperal, absceso puerperal
puerperium puerperio
puff abultamiento, inhalador, nebulizador
puffing resuello
puffy hinchado
pull a muscle, to desgarrarse un músculo, tener
un esguince; ~ , **to** jalar, tirar
pulled muscle músculo jalado; ~ **tendon**
desmectasia, tirón, tendon desgarrado
pulmonary pulmonar; ~ **alveoli** alvéolos
pulmonares; ~ **apoplexy** apoplejía
pulmonar; ~ **arterial hypertension**
hipertensión arterial pulmonar, hipertensión
pulmonar; ~ **artery** arteria pulmonar;
~ **asbestosis** asbestosis pleural; ~ **candidiasis**
candidiasis pulmonar; ~ **compliance**
complianza pulmonar; ~ **congestion**
congestión, muchedumbre; ~ **diffusion
capacity** capacidad de difusión pulmonar;
~ **dystonia** frenocardia; ~ **edema** edema
pulmonar; ~ **embolism** embolia pulmonar;
~ **emphysema** enfisema pulmonar; ~ **fibrosis**
fibrosis pulmonar; ~ **function test**
reconocimiento de la función pulmonar;
~ **hilum** hilio pulmonar; ~ **hypertension**
hipertensión arterial pulmonar, hipertensión
pulmonar; ~ **mechanics** mecánica pulmonar,
mecanica respiratoria; ~ **regurgitation** reflujo
en la válvula pulmonar del corazón,
insuficiencia de la válvula pulmonar; ~ **-renal
syndrome** estenosis de la válvula pulmonar,

síndrome de Goodpasture; ~ **rigidity** rigidez
pulmonar; ~ **sarcoidosis** sarcoidosis
pulmonar; ~ **scintigraphy** gammagrafía
pulmonar; ~ **semilunar valve** válvula
pulmonar, valva pulmonaria; ~ **trama** trama
pulmonar; ~ **trunk** arteria pulmonar;
~ **tuberculosis** tuberculosis pulmonar, tisis;
~ **valve** válvula pulmonar, valva pulmonaria;
~ **valvuloplasty** valvuloplastia, reparación
quirúrgica de la valvula cardiaca pulmonar;
~ **ventilation** ventilación pulmonar;
~ **window** ventana pulmonar
pulmonic pulmonar; ~ **valve** válvula pulmonar,
valva pulmonaria; ~ **valve stenosis** estenosis
de la válvula pulmonar, síndrome de
Goodpasture
pulsatile pulsátil; ~ **hematoma** hematoma
pulsátil
pulsation pulsación, latido rítmico
pulse pulso; ~ **oximetry** oximetría del pulso;
~ **rate** frecuencia de pulsaciones
pulvis Cosmi ungüento de Cosme
punch-drunk syndrome encefalopatía de los
boxeadores
punctate cataract catarata punteada, nube del
ojo
punctiform cataract catarata azul;
~ **hemorrhages** hemorragias puntiformes
puncture punción; ~ **of the bladder** punción de
la vejiga, punción vesical; ~ **syringe** jeringuilla
para punciones; ~ **wound** herida punzante,
punzada
puncture, to pinchar
pupil pupila, niña del ojo; ~ **dilation** dilatación
pupilar, midriasis
pupillary pupilar; ~ **constriction** miosis;
~ **dilation** dilatación pupilar, midriasis;
~ **reflex** reflejo pupilar
purgative purgativo
purification depuración, aclaramiento
purine purina; ~ **-pirimidine metabolism**
metabolismo de la purina-pirimidina
purinergic receptors receptores purinergicos
purity pureza
purpura púrpura
purslane verdolaga
Purtscher's disease angiopatía retiniana
traumática

purulent purulento, piógeno; ~ **arthritis** artritis supurada, artritis purulenta; ~ **exudate** exudado purulento; ~ **pleurisy** empiema empiema, piotórax, empiema pulmonar

pus pus

push, to empujar

pustular pustuloso

pustule pústula

pusy purulento, piógeno

put, to poner, meter, introducir, colocar; ~ **in quarantine**, to colocar em cuarentena; ~ **on make-up**, to maquillarse

PVA alcohol polivinílico

pyelitis pielitis, inflamación de pelvis renal

pyelonephritis pielonefritis

pyknosis picnosis

pyloric pilórico; ~ **antrum** antro pilórico; ~ **sphincter** esfínter pilórico

pylorospasm pilorospasmo

pylorus piloro, la salida del estómago

pyocin piocina; ~ **typing** piocinotipia

pyoderma piodermia, piodermitis

pyogenic purulento, piógeno; ~ **granuloma** granuloma piógeno; ~ **onychia** oniquia piógena; ~ **osteomyelitis** osteomyelitis piógena

pyorrhoea alveolaris parodontitis periodontoclasia, gingivopericementitis, paradontólisis

pyothorax empiema empiema, piotórax, empiema pulmonar

pyrazinamide pirizinamida

pyrexia pirexia, fiebre

pyridoxal piridoxal

pyridoxine piridoxina; ~ **dipalmitate** dipalmitato de piridoxina, piridoxina dipalmitato; ~ **hydrochloride** clorhidrato de piridoxina, piridoxina clorhidrato

pyrogenic pirógeno, que produce fiebre

pyrophosphoric acid ácido pirofosfórico

pyrosis pirosis, ardor de estómago

pyruvate piruvato; ~ **carboxylase** piruvato-carboxilasa; ~ **decarboxylase** piruvato-descarboxilasa; ~ **dehydrogenase** piruvato-deshidrogenasa; ~ **dehydrogenase complex** complejo piruvata deshidrogenasa; ~ **kinase** piruvato-cinasa; ~ **oxidase** piruvato-oxidasa

pyruvic acid ácido pirúvico

pzi insulina protamina de cinc

Q

qi qi, energía vital

q.i.d. cuatro veces al día

Qigong quigong

QRS complex complejo QRS, manifestación eléctrica de la contracción cardíaca

QT interval intervalo QT

Q-tip hisopo, escobillón

quack matasanos, farsante, charlatán

quack midwife rinconera

quackery charlatanería, curanderismo, curanderiá, charlatanismo

quacksalver healer merolico, curandero, sanador

qualitative cualitativo, relativo a la calidad, no cuantitativo; ~ **analysis** analisis cualitativo

qualitology cualitología

qualitometrics cualitometría

quality calidad; ~ **assessment** evaluación de la calidad; ~ **assurance** garantía de la calidad; ~ **audit** auditoría de la calidad; ~ **control** control de la calidad; ~ **management** gestión de la calidad; ~ **policy** política de la calidad

quanfication determinación

quantitative cuantitativo, que denota o expresa cantidad, relativo a la calidad, no cuantitativo; ~ **analysis** análisis cuantitativo

quantity magnitud

quarantine cuarentena; ~ **center** estación de cuarentena; ~ **station** local en cuarentena

quarter un cuarto

quaternary cuaternario

queasiness náusea, asco, basca, ganas de vomitar

Quellung test reacción de Quellung

question pregunta

questionable dudoso, discutible, cuestionable

Quetelet's index índice de Quetelet, índice de masa corporal

queuine queuina

quick-acting nitrate nitrato de acción rápida

quickened pulse rate aumento del ritmo cardíaco

quicksilver mercurio, azogue
quiescent quieto; ~ **plasma** plasma estable
Quincke disease edema angioneurótico, angioedema
quinidine quinidina
quinine quinina; ~ **exanthema** exantema quinino; ~ **intoxication** intoxicación por quinina; ~ **sulphate** sulfato de quinina
quinoline ácido quinolínico
quinolinic acid ácido quinolínico
quinolone quinolón, quinolona
quintary quintario; ~ **hyperparathyroidism** hiperparatiroidismo quintario
quiver, to tiritar

R

rabbit fever tularemia; ~ **ileal loop test** prueba del asa ileal en conejo
rabies rabia; ~ **virus** virus de la rabia
race raza, etnicidad
rachitic raquítico; ~ **eventration** eventración raquítica
rad dosis de radiación absorbida, rad
radial radial; ~ **immunodiffusion** inmunodifusión radial; ~ **keratotomy** queratotomía radial
radiant radiante; ~ **energy** energía radiante; ~ **excitance** excitancia radiante; ~ **flux** flujo radiante; ~ **intensity** intesidad radiante; ~ **power** potencia radiante
radiate, to expandarse
radiation radiación; ~ **absorbed dose** dosis de radiación absorbida, rad; ~ **creep** plastodeformación por radiación; ~ **embryopathy** embriopatía por radiaciones ionizantes; ~ **hazard** riesgo de irradiación; ~ **oncologist** radiooncólogo, radio-oncólogo; ~ **pneumonitis** neumonitis por radiación; ~ **sickness** síndrome agudo de las radiaciones, enfermedad producida por las radiaciones; ~ **therapy** radioterapia, terapia de radiación
radiculitis radiculitis
radiculopathy radiculopatía, avulsión del raíz de nervio
radio medical system sistema radiomédico

radioactive radioactivo; ~ **contamination** contaminación radioactiva; ~ **tagging** radiomarcado
radioactivity radioactividad
radioallergosorbent test prueba de radioalergosorbencia
radiocarpal joint articulación radio carpiana
radiodermatitis radiodermitis, dermatitis radiográfica
radiofrequency radiofrecuencia; ~ **catheter ablation** ablacion por cateter, ablación por radiofrecuencia, ablación eléctrica transvenosa; ~ **spectroscopy** espectroscopia por resonancia magnética nuclear
radiography radiografía
radioimmunoassay radioinmunoanálisis
radioimmunosorbent test prueba de radioinmunosorbencia
radioiodine yoduros radiactivos
radioisotope radisótopo, isótopo radiactivo; ~ **scanner** aparato de gamagrafía; ~ **scanning** gammagrafía
radiological radiológico; ~ **technologist** técnico de radiología
radiologist radiólogo
radiology radiología; ~ **technician** técnico de radiología; ~ **treatment plan** plan radioterapéutico
radiolucent radiotransparente
radioluminescence radioluminescencia
radionecrosis of the bone osteoradionecrosis
radionuclide radionucleido; ~ **activity** actividad radionucleido; ~ **imaging** cintigrafía
radiopharmaceutical radiofármaco
radioscopic apparatus fluoroscopio, aparato de radioscopia, roentgenoscopio
radiotherapy radioterapia, radiaciones, terapia de radiación
radiotransparent radiotransparente
radius radio
radon radón
rain lluvia
raised en relieve
raisins pasas
rambunctious intratable, indócil, malmandado
random esporádico; ~ **access** acceso aleatorio; ~ **access analyzer** analizador de acceso

R

directo; ~ **error** error aleatorio; ~ **priming** cebado aleatorio

randomization aleatorización, distribución al azar

randomized clinical trial ensayo clínico aleatorio; ~ **double-blind trial** prueba aleatoria en doble-ciego

range intervalo; ~ **of motion** amplitud de movimiento

ranitidine ranitidina

ranking clasificación

rape violación, estupro (de un menor de edad)

rapid rápida

raquianestesia anestesia epidural

rash salpullido, erupción de la piella, rash, exantema, roncha, verdugón

raspatory xister

rasping murmur ruido raspante

RAST prueba de radioalergosorbencia

rate índice, velocidad, ritmo; ~ **of conversion** velocidad de transformación; ~ **of reaction** velocidad de reacción; ~ **of sickness** morbididad, tasa de enfermos en una población

ratio razón; ~ **scale** escala racional

raucousness ronquera, afonia

Raynaud's phenomenon fenómeno de Raynaud

razor blade hojita de afeitar

RBC eritrocito; ~ **cast** cilindro hemático

RBE (relative biological effectiveness) eficacia biológica relativa, EBR

reabsorption reabsorción

reactant reactante

reaction at the infection limit reacción al límite de infección

reactivation reactivación

reactive reactivo; ~ **depression** trastornos de adaptación; ~ **leucocytosis** leucocitosis reactiva

reactivity reactividad

read, to leer

readability lectura mínima

reading lectura; ~ **frame** cuadro de lectura, marco de lectura; ~ **frameshift** desplazamiento del marco de lectura; ~ **glasses** anteojos para leer, gafas de lectura

readthrough translectura

readymade food preparados alimenticios

ready-to-use medium medio preparado

reagent reactivo; ~ **strip** tira reactiva

reagents kit equipo de reactivos

reagin regina

rebound de rebote; ~ **effect** rechazo, fenómeno de rebote; ~ **tenderness** hipersensibilidad al rebote

rebreathing reanimación, respiración

recalcitrant rebelde, acérrimo, persistente

receiver receptor

receptive aphasia afasia sensorial, afasia de Wernicke

receptor receptor

recessive recesivo; ~ **character** carácter recesivo; ~ **disease** enfermedad recesiva; ~ **gene** gen recesivo

recidivist recidivista

recipient receptor; ~ **cell** célula receptora

Recklinghausen disease enfermedad de Recklinghausen, osteítis fibroquística, osteítis paratiroidea

recognize, to reconocer

recombinant recombinante; ~ **DNA** ADN recombinante; ~ **vaccine** vacuna recombinante

recombination repair reparación por recombinación

recombinational hot-spot punto caliente de recombinación

recombinator recombinador

reconstitution reconstitución, regeneración lesionada

reconstructive reconstructivo; ~ **surgery** cirugía reconstructora, cirugía reconstructiva

reconvalescence convalecencia

recording thermometer termómetro registrador

recover, to recuperarse, restablecerse, sanarse

recovery curación, cura, restablecimiento, recuperación; ~ **period** tiempo de recuperación, periodo de recuperación; ~ **phase** convalecencia, fase de recuperación, etapa de recuperación; ~ **room** sala de recuperación; ~ **time** tiempo de recuperación, periodo de recuperación

recrudescence recrudecimiento

recrudescent recidivante, palindrómico; ~ **hepatitis** hepatitis recidivante

rectal rectal; ~ **examination** reconocimiento del recto; ~ **injection** irrigación colónica; ~ **sheath** vaina del recto

rectilinearity rectilinealidad, linealidad

rectosigmoidoscopy rectosigmoidoscopia

rectovaginal fistula fistula rectovaginal

rectovesical rectovesical

rectum recto, ampolla rectal

recuperate, to recuperarse, restablecerse, sanarse

recuperation restablecimiento, curación, recuperación, restitución

recurrence reincidencia, recidiva

recurrent recurrente; ~ **chancre** chancro recurrente; ~ **fever** fiebre americana, fiebre de picadura de garrapata

recurring recidivante, palindrómico; ~ **hepatitis** hepatitis recidivante

red rojo; ~ **blood cell** eritrocito, glóbulo rojo; ~ **blood cell count** recuento de los globulos rojos de la sangre; ~ **bone marrow** médula roja; ~ **striated muscles** músculos esqueléticos

reddened enrojecido, rojizo

reddish enrojecido, rojizo

redness enrojecimiento

redox oxidorreducción, oxidación-reducción

reduced libido libido disminuida

reductase reductasa

reduction reducción

redundant DNA secuencia repetitiva de ADN

Reed–Sternberg cells célula de Reed-Sternberg

re–education reeducación física, rehabilitación, reinserción en la vida activa

Reese syndrome síndrome de Reese

refer a patient, to referir un paciente

reference referencia; ~ **delusion** paranoico sensitivo; ~ **distribution** distribución de referencia; ~ **electrode** electrodo de referencia; ~ **individual** individuo de referencia; ~ **laboratory** laboratorio de referencia; ~ **limit** límite de referencia; ~ **material** material de referencia; ~ **method** método de referencia; ~ **population** población de referencia; ~ **procedure** procedimiento de referencia; ~ **range** intervalo de referencia; ~ **sample** muestra de referencia; ~ **value** valor de referencaia

referral remisión de pacientes; ~ **base** banco de referencias; ~ **database** base de datos referencial; ~ **service** servicio de referencias, centro de orientación

refined petroleum jelly vaselina purificada

reflectance spectrometry espectrometría de reflectancia

reflection factor factor de reflexión

reflective refletor, reflectora

reflex reflejo

reflexive relation relación reflexiva

reflexology reflexología

reflux reflujo, flujo de retorno

refractive index índice de refracción

refractometry refractometría

refractory refractario, rebelde; ~ **period** periodo refractario neurológico

regain to consciousness, to volver en sí conocimiento

regeneration reconstitución, regeneración

region región, parte del cuerpo

regional local, regional, no general; ~ **enteritis** enfermedad de Crohn, ileitis regional, enteritis regional; ~ **ileitis** enfermedad de Crohn, ileitis regional, enteritis regional

registered nurse enfermera titulada

regression regresión

regular cíclico, regular, repetido

regularly regularmente

regulation regulación

regulator gene gen regulador

regulon regulón

regurgitation regurgitación, reflujo del contenido de un órgano hueco

rehabilitation reeducación física, rehabilitación, reinserción en la vida activa

rehabilitative medicine reeducación física, rehabilitación, reinserción en la vida activa

rehydrating of plasma reconstitución, regeneración lesionada

rehydration rehidratación

reinfection reinfección

rejuvenate, to rejuvenecer

relapse recaída, recidiva; ~ **rate** tasa de reincidencias, proporción de reincidentes; ~ , **to recaer**

relapsing recidivante; ~ **fever** borreliosis, infección por borrelia; ~ **ophthalmoplegia** diplejía facial congénita, síndrome de Moebius

relative relativa; ~ **atomic mass** masa atómica relativa; ~ **density** densidad relativa; ~ **error** error relativo; ~ **inaccuracy** inexactitud relativa; ~ **molecular mass** masa molecular relativa; ~ **quantity** magnitud relativa

relatives parientes

relax, to relajarse

relaxant relajante

relaxation relajación; ~ **therapy** terapia de relajación

relaxing demulcente, emoliente, calmante, que ablanda y relaja las zonas inflamadas o que ablanda la piel

release liberación; ~ **factor** factor de terminación; ~ **of the active component** liberación del compuesto activo

Relenza zanamivir, Relenza

relevant relevante, sobresaliente, importante

reliability fiabilidad

relief alivio, aligeramiento, remedio, desahogo

relieving posture postura antálgica

religious religioso; ~ **intolerance** intolerancia religiosa

REM sleep sueño REM, sueño paradójico

remembering anamnesis

remission periodo de remisión, remisión de los síntomas; ~ **remisión**

remittent fever fiebre a remitir

remote assistance for surgeons asistencia quirúrgica a distancia

removal eliminación. extracción, extirpación, extirpación quirúrgica

remove, to quitar

renal renal; ~ **calculus** cálculos renales; ~ **clearance** depuración renal; ~ **cluster** glomérulo; ~ **colic** cólico de riñón, cólico renal, cólico nefrítico; ~ **cysts** quistes renales; ~ **disease** nefropatía, enfermedad del riñón; ~ **function test** prueba para la función renal; ~ **glycosuria** glucosuria renal; ~ **hemorrhage** nefrorragia, hemorragia renal; ~ **incision** nefrotomía; ~ **insufficiency** insuficiencia renal; ~ **osteodystrophy** osteodistrofia renal; ~ **suture** nefrorrafia, nefropexia; ~ **tubular acidosis** acidosis tubular renal; ~ **tubule** túbulo renal; ~ **ultrasound** ecografía renal

renaturation renaturalización

renewal recambio, turnover (inglés)

renin renina

renovascular renovascular

REO virus Reovirus, Reoviridae

reoccurrence recaída, reincidencia

reovirus Reovirus, Reoviridae

repeat repetición

repeatability repetibilidad

repetitive repetidor; ~ **DNA fragment** fragmento de ADN repetitivo; ~ **DNA sequence** secuencia repetitiva de ADN

replacement vector vector por sustitución

repletion llenado, repleción; ~ **of the bladder** llenado vesical

replication replicación, duplicación; ~ **fork** horquilla de replicación

replicon replicón; ~ **fusion** fusión de replicones

report informe

reporter gene gen indicador

representational difference analysis análisis de diferencias representativas

repress, to reprimir, represar

repression represión

reproducibility reproducibilidad

reproduction procreación, reproducción

reproductive reproductivo; ~ **health** salud en materia de procreación, salud reproductiva; ~ **organs** genitales; ~ **physiology** fisiología de la reproducción

requesting doctor médico solicitante

required evaporation evaporación requerida

research investigación, descubrimiento; ~ , **to** pesquisar, buscar, escudriñar, examinar, indagar, investigar

resection resección

reservoir reservorio, depósito

residence time periodo de permanencia

residential home for the elderly casa de reposo

residual residual; ~ **functional capacity** capacidad funcional restante

residue residuos, huellas

resistance aguante, resistencia, endurecimiento, induración; ~ **cardiography** cardiografía de impedancia; ~ **transfer factor** plásmido de resistencia

resistant resistente

resistivity resistividad

resolution resolución

resorption resorción, absorción de agua y de solutos por células vivas
respiration respiración
respirator respirador, aparato respiratorio
respiratory respiratorio; ~ **acidosis** acidosis respiratoria; ~ **alkalosis** alcalosis respiratoria; ~ **anaphylaxis** anafilaxia respiratoria; ~ **arrest** insuficiencia respiratoria, paro respiratorio; ~ **failure** insuficiencia respiratoria, paro respiratorio; ~ **impairment** insuficiencia respiratoria, paro respiratorio; ~ **infection** infección respiratoria; ~ **mask** máscara de protección respiratoria, mascarilla respiratoria, careta respiratoria; ~ **mechanics** mecánica pulmonar, mecánica respiratoria; ~ **medicine** neumología; ~ **syncytial virus** virus respiratorio sincitial; ~ **system** vías respiratorias, sistema respiratorio; ~ **therapy** terapéutica inalatoria, toxicología respiratoria; ~ **toxicology** toxicología inalatoria, toxicología respiratoria
respond, to responder, contestar
rest tiempo libre, descanso; ~ **home** casa de reposo; ~, **to** descansar
restless legs piernas inquietas, sensación de hormigueo en la profundidad de ambas piernas
restorative surgery cirugía plástica
restrain, to reprimir, represar
restraint sujeción, restricción física, inmobilización; ~ **system** sistema de retención, sistema de sujeción
restrict, to restringir, limitar
restricted transduction transducción restringida
restriction restricción; ~ **endonuclease** endonucleasa de restricción; ~ **enzyme** enzima de restricción; ~ **mapping** cartografía de restricción; ~ **site** centro de restricción
result hallazgo, resultado, observacion; ~ **of microbiological analysis** resultado del análisis microbiológico
resuscitate, to resucitar, reanimar
resuscitation resucitación, reanimación, restablecimiento de la vida de un sujeto aparentemente muerto; ~ **mask** máscara para reanimación; ~ **medium** medio de reanimación
retard atraso, retraso, demora; ~, **to** atrasar, impedir, retrasar
retardation retardo, retraso

retention sujeción, restricción física, inmobilización, absorción, captación, retención
reticular reticular; ~ **dermis** dermis reticular; ~ **fibers** fibras reticulares; ~ **network** red de fibras reticulares
reticulocyte reticulocito
retina retina
retinal retinal; ~ **atrophy** atrofia de la retina; ~ **detachment** desprendimiento de retina; ~ **dysplasia** displasia retiniana; ~ **ganglion cells** celulas del ganglio retiniano; ~ **glioma** retinoblastoma, ~ **image** imagen retiniana; ~ **neovascularization** neovascularización retiniana; ~ **vein occlusion** oclusión de la vena retiniana
retinoblastoma retinoblastoma
retinoic acid ácido retinoico, tretinoína
retinol retinol; ~ **–binding protein** proteína enlazante de retinol
retinopathy retinopatía, enfermedad no inflamatoria de la retina
retinoscope oftalmoscopio, esquiascopio
retinyl palmitate palmitato de retinilo
retraction retracción, encogimiento o reducción de un órgano o tejido
retractor retractor
retriever vector vector recuperador
retroactive retroactivo
retrobulbar retrobulbar, detrás del bulbo raquídeo, detrás del globo ocular; ~ **neuritis** neuritis óptica retrobulbar
retrocortine prednisona, dehidrocortisona
retrograde retrógrado, que va hacia atrás, que degenera, deteriora
retroperitoneal retroperitoneal; ~ **connective tissue** tejido conjuntivo retroperitoneal; ~ **sarcoma** sarcoma retroperitoneal
retroposon retrotransposón
retrosternal retrosternal, detrás del esternón
Retrovir AZT, cidovudina, azidotimidina, Retrovir
retroviral retrovírico; ~ **drug** antirretroviral, gente anti-retrovírico, fármaco anti-retrovírico; ~ **infection** infección causada por retrovirus
retrovirus retrovirus; ~ **of simian origin** retrovirus de origen símico
Rett syndrome síndrome de Rett
return vuelta (f); ~ **flow** reflujo, flujo de

retorno; ~ , **to** volver

reuptake reabsorción

revaccination inyección secundaria, revacunación, inyección de refuerzo

revaluation reevaluación, revalorización

reverse inverso, opuesto; ~ **osmosis** ósmosis inversa; ~ **transcriptase** retrotranscriptasa, DNA-polimerasa dirigida por RNA

reversible reversible, que puede desaparecer totalmente al suprimirse la causa; ~ **inhibitors** inhibidores reversibles

reversion reversión

revive, to resucitar, reanimar

revulsive revulsivo, contrairritante, que provoca una irritación que tiene el propósito de aliviar alguna otra

Reye's syndrome síndrome de Reye

Rh factor factor Rh

rhabdomyolysis rabdomiolisis

rhabdomyosarcoma rabdomiosarcoma

rhagade rágade, fisura, grieta o escara lineal de la piel

rheograph reógrafo

rheumatic reumático; ~ **arteritis** arteritis reumática; ~ **fever** fiebre reumática; ~ **heart disease** cardiopatía reumática; ~ **nodules** nódulos reumáticos; ~ **pericarditis** pericarditis reumática

rheumaticy reumatoide, que se asemeja al reumatismo

rheumatism reumatismo

rheumatoid reumatoide, que se asemeja al reumatismo; ~ **arthritis** artritis reumatoide; ~ **factor** factor reumatoideo

rheumatology reumatología

rhinitis rinitis, inflamación de la mucosa nasal

rhinolith litiasis nasal

rhinopharyngitis rinofaringitis, inflamación de la mucosa nasal y de la faringe

rhinoplasty rinoplastia, cirugía plástica de la nariz

rhinorrhea rinorrea, secreción intensa de moco nasal

rhinoscope concoscopio, espéculo nasal, rinoscopio

rhinosporidiosis rinosporidiosis

rhinosporidium rhinosporidium

rhinovirus rinovirus

rhizotomy rizotomía

rhodopsin rodopsina

rhomboid fossa fosa romboidea

rhonchus roncus, ronquido, onido asmático

rhythm ritmo; ~ **method** continencia periódica, método de Ogino

rhytidectomy ritidoplastia, ritidectomia

rhytidoplasty ritidoplastia, ritidectomia

RIA radioinmunoanálisis

rib costilla; ~ **cage** caja torácica

ribavirin ribavirín

riboflavin riboflavina

ribonucleic acid ácido ribonucleico

ribonucleoprotein ribonucleoproteína

riboprobe ribosonda

ribose ribosa

ribosomal ribosómico; ~ **ribonucleic acid** ácido ribonucleico ribosómico; ~ **RNA** RNA ribosómico

ribosome ribosoma; ~ **-bindig site** centro de unión al ribosoma

ribozyme ribozima

rice arroz

ricin ricina, ricino

rickets raquitismo; ~ rickettsia, tipo de microorganismos

Riedel's thyroiditis estruma de Riedel, tumor férreo

rifampicin rifampicina

Rift Valley fever fiebre del Valle del Rift

right a la derecha; ~ **-handed** derecho; ~ **- hander** diestro; ~ **to the** a la derecha

rigid rígido; ~ **cataplexy** rigidez cataléptica; ~ **laryngoscope** laringoscopio rígido

rigidity rigidez, envaramiento

rigor mortis rigor mortis

ring anillo; ~ **finger** dedo anillo, dedo anular; ~ **vaccination** vacunación de urgencia, vacunación de emergencia

Ringer's solution solución de Ringer

ringing in my ears un zumbido en los oídos

ring-test ensayo del anillo de Bang, prueba del anillo

ringworm tiña, una enfermedad de la piel producido por hongos; ~ **of the scalp** tiña tonsurante

risk riesgo; ~ **factor** factor de riesgo

risky arriesgado, aventurado, peligroso

RIST prueba de radioinmunosorbencia
ritalin metilfenidato
river blindness oncocercosis, una forma filariasis en America Central y del Sur y en África
RNA ARN; **~ –directed DNA polymerase** DNA-polimerasa dirigida por ARN; **~ –polymerase** ARN-polimerasa; **~ processing** maduración del ARN
RNase ribonucleasa pancreática
robotry automática
robustness robustez
ROC curve [en semiología] curva de rendimiento diagnóstico
Rocky Mountain spotted fever Fiebre maculosa de las Montañas Rocosas
rolling circle círculo rodador
room temperature temperatura ambiente
root raíz; **~ canal** canal en la raíz; **~ canal plugger** obturador de canalización
ropinirole ropinirol
Rorschach test psicodiagnóstico de Rorschach
Rosenthal's syndrome síndrome de Melkersson-Rosenthal
rotational frequency frecuencia rotacional
rotator cuff rotador del hombro, manguito del rotador; **~ cuff tendinitis** tendinopatía del hombro, tendinitis del hombro
rough áspero
round redondo; **~ about** aproximado
rounded swollen abotagado, hinchado, hipatado, turgente
routine rutina (f); **~ examination** examen sistemático; **~ screening** detección sistemática; **~ vaccination** vacunación sistemática
routinely rutinariamente, usualmente
royal real; **~ jelly** jalea real (de las abejas)
rash salpullido, rash, exantema, roncha, verdugón
rub frotación; **~ one's eyes, to** frotarse los ojos; **~ , to** frotar, esfregar, refregar
rubbing frotamiento, fricción; **~ alcohol** alcohol isopropílico, alcohol alcanforado
rubella rubéola, sarampión alemán, sarampión de los tres días
rugine xister, raspador
rumbling tummy borborigmo, gorgoteo en el vientre
rumination rumiación, mericismo
run serie; **~ –down** agotado, debilitado, quemado, cançado; **~ off** prueba de transcripción (no iniciada); **~ on** prueba de transcripción (iniciada)
runaway plasmid plásmido autorreplicable
rupture rotura, hernia, desgarro de tejidos o de un órgano; **~ of a ligament** desgarro de un ligamento; **~ of a tendon** rotura de un tendón; **~ of a muscle** distensión muscular
ruptured aneurysm aneurisma roto

S

Sabouraud agar agar de Sabouraud
saccharimeter glucómetro
saccharin sacarina
saccoradiculography sacoradiculografía
saccule sáculo
Sachs bacillus Clostridium septicum
sacroiliac arthritis artritis sacro-ilíaca; **~ joint** articulación sacroilíaca
sacrolumbar sacrolumbar; **~ transition area** zona de unión sacrolumbar
sacrum hueso sacro, sacro; **~ block of the pelvis** bloque del sacro de la pelvis
saddle block anesthesia anestesia en silla de montar
safe inocuo
safety seguridad, inocuidad; **~ belt** cinturón de seguridad; **~ –in-use evaluation of additives** evaluación de la seguridad en la utilización de los aditivos
safranin safranina
sagittal sagital; **~ axis** eje sagital; **~ plane** plano sagital
salbutamol salbutamol
salicylate salicilato; **~ derivative** derivado de salicilato
salicylic acid ácido salicílico
salicylism salicismo, abuso crónico de medicamentos que contienen salicilatos
saline salino, salado, de la naturaleza de las sales, que contiene sales; **~ infusion** perfusión de cloruro de sodio

saliva saliva; ~ trap recogida de saliva

salivary salival; ~ amylase amilasa salival;
~ calculi litiasis salival; ~ fistula fistula de las
glandulas salivales; ~ glands glandulas
salivales

salivation salivación, secreción de saliva

salmonella salmonela; ~ typhimurium
Salmonella typhimurium; ~ –shigella agar
agar para Salmonella y Shigella

salmonellosis salmonelosis

Salozapyrin salazopirina

salpingitis salpingitis, inflamación de la trompa
uterina, inflamación de la trompa auditiva

salpingolysis salpingólisis

salpingo–oophoritis salpingo-ovaritis, salpingo-
ooforitis

salt sal; ~ exsiccosis exicosis por falta de sal;
~ –free diet dieta sin sal; ~ tolerance test
prueba de tolerancia a la sal

salty salado, salado, de la naturaleza de las sales,
que contiene sales

saluric salurético, que induce la eliminación de
sal por la urina

salve for wounds ungüento para heridas,
pomada para heridas

same lo mismo

sample muestra, especimen; ~ excision biopsia

sampler muestreador

sampling muestreo

sanatorium sanatorio

sandwich sándwich; ~ immunoassay
inmunoanálisis en sándwich

sanitary sanitario; ~ authorities servicio
sanitario; ~ napkin toalla sanitaria, compresa
higiénica

saphenous safena; ~ artery arteria safena;
~ vein vena safena

saponins saponinas

saprophyte saprofito, microorganismo que vive
a expensas de materias orgánicas en
descomposición, parásito que no causa
enfermedad

sarcoidosis sarcoidosis, enfermedad de
Schaumann, sarcoide de Boeck

sarcolemma sarcolema

sarcolysine melfalan

sarcoma sarcoma, tumor maligno; ~ of the
testicle sarcoma testicular

sarcoptes scabiei sarcoptes scabiei

sarcosine sarcosina

sartorius muscle músculo sartorio

satellitism test prueba del satelitismo

saturated saturado; ~ chloroform–air mixture
mezcla saturada de cloroformo y aire; ~ fatty
acids ácidos grasos saturados

saturation saturación; ~ fraction fracción
saturante

Saturday sábado

saturnine saturnino; ~ encephalopathy
encefalopatía saturnina; ~ polyglobulism
poliglobulia saturnina

sausage salchicha

saw palmetto saw palmetto, serenoa repens

scab on a wound postilla, costra

scabbed tinoso, sarnoso

scabies escabiosis; ~ sarna

scaffolding andamiaje

scalding hot water agua de escaldado

scale balanza, escala

scaling of the skin pitiriasis, descamación de la
piel en pequeñas laminillas

scalp cuero cabelludo, casco de la cabeza

scalpel bisturí

scaly escamoso, que tiene escamas; ~ skin
ictiosis, trastorno de la piel que la hace seca y
escamosa

scan, to explorar, hacer un imagen diagnóstica

scanning exploración; ~ electron microscope
microscopía electrónica de barrido,
microscopía de exploración electrónica

scaphoid escafoideo; ~ bone escafoides del
tarso, escafoides del carpo; ~ fossa fosa
escafoidea

scapula omóplato, escápula, paleta

scapulohumeral periarthritis periartritis
escapulo-humeral

scar cicatriz; ~ tissue tejido cicatrizal, un cicatriz

scarlatina fiebre escarlatina

scarlatinal angina angina escarlatinosa

scarlet fever fiebre escarlatina

scarred cicatrizado

scarring cicatrización

scatter diseminación, siembra, dispersión de la
infección

scavenger cell fagocito

scented aromático, de buen olor

Scheuermann's disease enfermedade de Scheuermann, una anomalia esquelética consistente en cifosis

schistosome dermatitis dermatitis de esquistosoma, anquilostomiasis

schistosomiasis bilharziosis, esquistosomiasis

schizophrenia esquizofrenia, locura de desdoblamiento

schizophrenic esquizofrenico; **~ psychosis** psicosis esquizofrenica

Schmitz's bacillus Shigella dysenteriae de tipo 2

Schmorl's bacillus Fusobacterium necrophorum

school escuela

Schottmüller's bacillus Salmonella schottmuelleri

Schriddes' disease eritroblastosis fetal

Schwann's sheath neurolema, neurilema, células de Schwann

sciatic nerve nervio ciático

sciatica ciática, dolor que se irradia de la espalda a las extremidades inferiores

scientific cientifico; **~ breakthrough** avance científico

scintigram cintigrama, escintilograma

scintigraphy cintigrafia; **~ of the lung** gammagrafía pulmonar

scintillation centelleo; **~ counter** contador de centelleo; **~ detector** detector de centelleo; **~ index** índice de centelleo

scintillator contador de centelleo

scissors tijeras

sclera esclerótica, blanco de los ojos

sclerocystic ovaries ovario poliquístico

sclerodactyly esclerodactilia, acrosclerosis

scleroderma dermatosclerosis, esclerodermia

sclerosing esclerosante; **~ cholangitis** colangitis obliterante primaria; **~ osteomyelitis** osteomielitis esclerosante

sclerosis esclerosis, induración o dureza

sclerotherapy escleroterapia

sclerotic endurecimiento en forma de tumor (en la piel), esclerótico

scoliosis escoliosis

scorpion escorpión

scotoma escotoma, pérdida de la facultad visual en zonas bien circunscritas del campo visual

scrape, to escariar (la piel); **~ mark** chafado,

estregadura; **~ –off layer** capa de extracción; **~ one's knee, to** arañarse la rodilla

scratch arañazo, rasguño; **~ , to** arrañar

scratchy ronco; **~ throat** ronquera, afonia

screening cribado, tamizaje, detección precoz, diagnóstico diagnóstico o preventivo; **~ mammogram** mamografía tomada en programa de detección selectiva

scrotal hernia hernia escrotal

scrotum escroto

scrub itch trombidiosis; **~ mark** chafado, estregadura; **~ , to** raspar, fregar, afretar

scurvy escorbuto

seasonal estacional; **~ affective disorder** trastorno afectivo estacional

sebaceous sebáceo; **~ acne** acné sebácea; **~ adenoma** adenoma sebáceo; **~ glands** glándula sebácea; **~ matter** sebo cutáneo, la secreción sebácea cutánea, el tejido graso cutáneo

seborrhea seborrea, excreción excesiva de sustancia grasa

seborrheic seborreico; **~ dermatitis** dermatitis seborreica; **~ keratosis** queratosis seborreica

second segundo

secondary secundario, siguiente, dependiente, de 2 orden; **~ care** atención secundaria de salud; **~ hypogonadism** hipogonadismo secundario; **~ infection** infección secundaria, superinfección; **~ malnutrition** malnutrición secundaria; **~ standard** patrón secundario

second–hand smoking tabaquismo pasivo, tabaquismo involuntario

secretin secretina

secretion secreción, flujo, excreción

secretory secretor, secretora; **~ mucosa** mucosas secretorias; **~ phase** fase de secreción

sedation sedación

sedative calmante, sedante; **~** sedante, calmante, tranquilizante, ansiolítico, medicamento contra la ansiedad

sedentary sedentario, que se sienta habitualmente, de hábitos inactivos, relativo a la posición sentada

sediment sedimento, precipitación de un sólido en un sistema líquido

sedimentation sedimentación, asentamiento de partículas sólidas de una solución en el fondo

 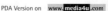

del envase; ~ **coefficient** coeficiente de sedimentación; ~ **of the blood** sedimentación sanguínea; ~ **velocity** eritrosedimentación
see, to ver; ~ **spots, to** ver puntos luminosos
segment segmento, parte de un organismo u órgano
segmented gamma-scanning barrido segmentado con rayos gamma; ~ **neutrophil** neutrofilocito segmentado
segregation segregación, prevención, protección
Seidlitz salt sal de Epsom, sal de Selditz
seizure convulsiones, acceso; ~ **of narcotics** confiscación de estupefacientes, incautación de heroína
selection elección, selección; ~ **of sex by genetic manipulation** elección del sexo por manipulación genética
selective selectivo; ~ **acces** acceso selectivo; ~ **enrichment medium** medio de enriquecimiento selectivo; ~ **isolation medium** medio de aislamiento selectivo; ~ **serotonin reuptake inhibitor** inhibidor selectivo de la reabsorción de serotonina
selenite broth caldo con selenita
selenium selenio
self-cloning autoclonación; ~ **-employed** independiente; ~ **-esteem** autoestima; ~ **-help** autoayuda; ~ **-help center** centro para autoayuda; ~ **-image** autoimagen; ~ **-medication** automedicación; ~ **-mutilation** automutilación, autolesión; ~ **-replication** autorreplicación; ~ **-splicing** autoeliminación de intrones; ~ **-worth** autoestima
sella turcic silla turca
SEM (scanning electron microscopy) microscopía de exploración electrónica, microscopía electrónica de barrido
semeiologic value valor semiológico
semeiology semiología
semen semen, esperma; ~ **evaluation** contrastación del esperma, conservación del esperma; ~ **storage** almacenado del esperma, conservación del esperma
semiconductor detector detector semiconductor
semi-conservative DNA replication replicación semiconservativa del ADN

seminal seminal; ~ **fluid** semen, esperma; ~ **plasma** plasma seminal; ~ **vesicle** vesícula seminal; ~ **vesiculitis** espermatocistitis
semi-occlusive dressing aposito semi-oclusivo
semiquantitative semicuantitativo
semisynthetic semisintético, producido por manipulación química de sustancias naturales
Senear-Usher disease pénfigo eritematoso, síndrome de Senear-Usher
senescence envejecimiento, vejez
senile senil; ~ **angioma** angioma senil; ~ **dementia** demencia senil; ~ **keratosis** queratosis senil, queratosis actínicas; ~ **lentigo** lentigo de vejez; ~ **nanism** progeria, infantilismo senil
senility senilidad, ancianidad, vejez
sensation percepción, sensación; ~ **of panic** sensación de panico; ~ **of pressure** sensación de presión
sense sentido, sensación; ~ **codon** codón traducible; ~ **of inferiority** complejo de inferioridad; ~ **of panic** sensación de panico; ~ **of smell** olfacción, olfato, sentido olfativo; ~ **of taste** gusto, sentido gustativo, sentido del gusto; ~ **of touch** sentido del tacto; ~ **strand** cadena homosentido
sensible sensato, sabio
sensitive sensible; ~ **nerve root** raíz sensitiva; ~ **paranoiac** paranoico sensitivo; ~ **to ampicillin** sensible a la ampicilina
sensitivity límite de detección, sensibilidad; ~ **test** prueba de sensibilidad; ~ **to vibrations** sensibilidad a la vibración; ~ **training** entrenamiento de la sensibilidad, educación de la sensibilidad
sensitization sensibilización, administración de un antígeno para inducir una respuesta inmunitaria
sensor sensor
sensorineural hearing loss sordera sensorineural, sordera de percepción, sordera neurosensorial, hipoacusia neurosensorial
sensory sensorial, perteneciente o relativo a las sensaciones; ~ **alexia** alexia sensorial; ~ **aphasia** afasia sensorial, afasia de Wernicke; ~ **apraxia** apraxia sensorial; ~ **awareness** examen mediante los sentidos; ~ **deprivation** privación sensorial; ~ **evaluation** análisis

organoléptico, análisis sensorial, prueba de degustación; **~ fatigue** fatiga sensorial; **~ hairs** cilios sensoriales; **~ nerves** nervios sensoriales; **~ neuron** neurona sensorial; **~ organ** órgano de los sentidos; **~ receptor** receptor sensorial

sentinel de guardia; **~ animal** animal testigo; **~ health event** vigilancia de guardia; **~ lymph node** ganglio linfático centinela; **~ surveillance** vigilancia de guardia

separation desprendimiento, separación, disociación; **~ anxiety** miedo al abandono

separator separador

sepsis sepsis, septicemia

septal abscess absceso del tabique nasal

September septiembre

septic séptico, contaminado por gérmenes; **~ abortion** aborto séptico, aborto infectado; **~ angina** angina séptica; **~ arthritis** artritis séptica; **~ bursitis** bursitis séptica; **~ embolism** embolia séptica; **~ ileus** íleo séptico; **~ infarct** infarto infectado; **~ iritis** iritis séptica; **~ shock** choque séptico

septicemia sepsis, septicemia, intoxicación de la sangre por microorganismos

septum septum, tabique de separación; **~ lucidum** septum pellucidum; **~ pellucidum** septum pellucidum

sequel secuela, complicación

sequela secuela, complicación

sequencing secuenciación; **~ of human genome** secuenciación del genoma humano; **~ primer linker** esplínquer

sequential secuencial; **~ acces** acceso secuencial; **~ immunoassay** inmunoanálisis secuencial

sequestra secuestro, fragmento de tejido muerto separado del tejido sano

sequestrum secuestro, fragmento de tejido muerto separado del tejido sano

Sereny test prueba de Sereny

series serie

serine serina

serious serio, grave

sermorelin sermorelina

seroconversion seroconversión (f), cambio de una prueba serológica de negativa a positiva

serodiagnosis serodiagnóstico

serological serológico, perteneciente o relativo al estudio de la inmunidad a través del suero; **~ exam** prueba serológica, ensayo serológico; **~ test** prueba serológica, ensayo serológico; **~ typing** serotipificación

serology serología

serotonin serotonina; **~ antagonist** fármaco antiserotoninérgico; **~ receptor** receptor de serotonina; **~ uptake inhibitor** inhibidor de la absorción de serotonina, inhibidor de la captación de serotonina

serotype serotipo

serotyping tipificación serológica, serotipificación

serous seroso; **~ erythrocytic cholinesterase** colinesterasa del suero; **~ exudate** exudado seroso; **~ osteomyelitis** osteomielitis serosa

serum suero, un líquido cristalino e incoloro; **~ globulin** seroglobulina; **~ glucose level** suero del nivel de glucosa; **~ level** concentración sérica

set of chromosomes cariotipo

setback revés, contrariedad, fracaso

seven siete

seventeen diecisiete

seventh séptimo

seventy setenta

severe severo; **~ constipation** entablazón, estreñimiento severo; **~ pain** dolor recio, punzada, dolor fuerte

severity gravedad

sewage aguas residuales

sex sexo; **~ chromosomes** gonosomas, cromosomas sexuales; **~ chromosome disorders** trastornos de los cromosomas sexuales; **~ hormone-binding globulin** globulina enlazante de las hormonas sexuales; **~ -linked** ligado al sexo; **~ organs** genitales, partes (nobles, ocultas, privadas)

sexology sexología

sexual sexual; **~ ability** poder sexual, capacidad sexual, potencia; **~ behavior** comportamiento sexual; **~ hygiene** higiene sexual; **~ preference** inclinación sexual, preferencia sexual; **~ promiscuity** promiscuidad sexual; **~ violence** violencia sexual

sexuality sexualidad

sexually sexual; **~ transmitted** venéreo,

perteneciente o relativo al contacto sexual o transmitido por él; ~ **transmitted disease** enfermedad de transmisión sexual

SGOT aspartato-aminotransferasa

SGPT alanina-aminotransferasa

shaft (of bone) cuerpo, diáfisis

shake, to agitar, temblar, estremecerse, tiritar

shakiness temblor intencional, temblor que aparece al intentar efectuar un movimiento voluntario coordinado

shall poder, deber

shame verguenza

sharp agudo; ~ **pain** dolor recio, punzada, dolor fuerte

sharpness acuidad, agudeza

shave, to afeitarse

shaving afeitado; ~ **brush** brocha de afeitar; ~ **cream** crema de afeitar; ~ **soap** jabón de afeitar

she ella

sheaf of fibers haz de fibras, cordón, tracto

shearing fracture fractura por torsión

sheathing involucro, vaina

sheet sábana

Shiga-Kruse's bacillus Shigella dysenteriae tipo 1

shigellosis disentería amebiana, shigellosis

shin canilla; ~ **bone** tibia, espinilla

shingles zona, herpes zoster

shirk, to fingirse enfermo, hacerse el enfermo

shiver, to temblar, estremecerse, tiritar, temblequear

shivering escalofríos; ~ **attack** escalofríos incontrolables, el tiriton, el malestar en que tiembla mucho

shivers escalofríos, fríos

shock shock, choque, susto, espanto; ~ **lung** síndrome de insuficiencia respiratoria del adulto

shooting up consumidor de drogas por vía intravenosa, drogadicto que se administra la droga por vía intravenosa

short corto, breve; ~ **time ago** hace poco

shortage deficiencia, defecto, falta

shortly after birth perinatal, que ocurre inmediatamente antes o después del nacimiento

shortness of breath respiración entrecortada,

falta de hálito, estar sin aire, desalentado

short corto, bajo, chaparro; ~ **-sighted** miopía, vista corta; ~ **-tempered** irritable, quisquilloso, susceptible, colérico, irascible, arrebatadizo, gruñon; ~ **-term** duración breve, de corto plazo, temporario

shot inyección

shotgun cloning clonación al azar; ~ **method of cloning** clonación en perdigonada

shots vacunas

shoulder hombro; ~ **blade** escápula, omóplato, paleta; ~ **girdle** cintura escapular; ~ **tendon inflammation** tendinitis del hombro

show, to indicar, visualizar

shower baño de ducha; ~ **cubicle** cabina de ducha

shrink, to achicar, encogerse

shrinkage of neurons degeneración de las neuronas, decadencia neural

shunt anastomosis, abocamiento; ~ **blood** sangre corticocircuitada

shut-down state estado de desconexión parcial

shuttle vector vector transportador

sialic acids ácidos sialicos

sialorrhoea ptialismo, sialorrea

siblings hermanos, hijos o hijas de los mismos padres

sicca-syndrome síndrome de Sjoegren

siccative desecante, secante

sick enfermo

sickening repugnante, repulsivo

sickle cell anemia anemia falciforme, drepanocitosis

sickly decrépito, desvaído, endeble, vetusto, enfermizo; ~ **child** niño enfermizo, niño delicado; ~ **smell** olor empalagoso, hediondez, fetidez

sickness insurance seguro de enfermedad

side effect efecto colateral, efecto no deseado de una medida terapéutica o medicina

sideremia concentración de hierro (II+III) en plasma/suero

siderosis siderosis

sideway lateral, alejado del centro o de la línea media

siemens siémens

sievert siévert

sight vista

sigmoid sigmoide, de forma similar a las letra S; **~ colon** sigma iliaca, el colon sigmoideo

sign fenómeno, manifestación, signo, síntoma

signal señal

signature firma

significant significativo, que tiene importancia

signs signos

silencer lentificador

silent mutation mutación imperceptible

silhouette silueta

silica gel gel de sílice, sílice gelatinosa

silicon silicio; **~ breast implant** implante mamario de silicona; **~ ointment** pomada de silicona

silicosis silicosis

silicotuberculosis silicotuberculosis

silver plata; **~ bromide–iodide** bromoyoduro de plata; **~ iodide** yoduro de plata

simian fissure cisura simiesca, cisura perpendicular externa

similar análogo, de acción parecida

simple simple; **~ fracture** fractura cerrada, fractura simple; **~ strand DNA** DNA monocatenario

simulation simulación

simulator simulador

simultaneous simultáneo, que se hace o ocurre al mismo tiempo

simvastatin sinvastatina

sinapism sinapismo, cataplasma

single soltero; **~ -acting** simple efecto; **~ chain** cadena sencilla; **~ -drug–treatment** monoterapia, terapia con sólo un medicamento; **~ hit** impacto único; **~ site mutation** mutación puntual; **~ -stranded DNA** ADN de cadena sencilla

singultus singulto, hipo

sinoatrial node nudo sinoauricular, nudo excitomotor

sinus seno; **~ tachycardia** taquicardia sinusal

sinusal sinusal, relativo o perteneciente a una bolsa o una cavidad, en particular a la cámara superior del corazón; **~ osteoma** osteoma sinusal

sinusitis sinusitis, inflamación de una bolsa o una cavidad en el cránio

Sippy diet dieta de Sippy; **~ treatment** tratamiento de Sippy

siriasis golpe de calor, siriasis, insolación, asoleada, solanera

sismotherapy sismoterapia

sisomicin sisomicina

sister hermana; **~ -in-law** cuñada

sit down, to tomar asiento, sentarse

site-directed mutagenesis mutagénesis específica puntual, mutagénesis sitio dirigida; **~ -specific mutation** mutación en un punto específico; **~ -specific recombination** recombinación específica de sitio; **~ -specific treatment** tratamientos localizados específicos

sitting sedentario, de hábitos inactivos, que se sienta habitualmente, relativo a la posición sentada

situation anxiety miedo mórbido

six seis

sixteen dieciséis

sixth sexto

sixty sesenta

sizing column columna de exclusión molecular

Sjögren's syndrome síndrome de Sjoegren, síndrome de Sjoegren

skeletal esquelético, perteneciente o relativo al esqueleto; **~ balance** equilibro esquelético, un resumen del estado del esqueleto; **~ muscle** músculo esquelético; **~ muscle myosin** miosinas de músculo esquelético; **~ scintigraphy** escintigrafía ósea

skeleton esqueleto

skewing distorsión

skiascope oftalmoscopio, esquiascopio

skid resistant antiderrape, antipatinante, antideslizante, antirresbaladizo

skin piel; **~ atrophy** atrofia cutánea; **~ biopsy** biopsia cutánea; **~ cancer** cáncer de la piel, cáncer cutáneo, epitelioma; **~ carcinoma** cáncer de la piel, cáncer cutáneo, epitelioma; **~ color** pigmentación, depósito de materia colorante, coloración; **~ coloring** pigmentación, depósito de materia colorante, coloración; **~ detaching** escoriación dérmica, despegamiento cutáneo; **~ disease** dermopatía, enfermedad de la piel; **~ fibroblast** fibroblasto de la piel; **~ flap** colgajo cutáneo; **~ graft** injerto de la piel, borde dérmico; **~ inflammation** dermatitis, inflamación de la piel; **~ irritation** irritación cutánea; ~ **lesions** lamparones; ~ **melanoma** melanoma, cáncer melánico; ~ **pocket** bolsilla de piel; ~ **rash** exantema; ~ **reflex** reflejo cutáneo; ~ **temperature** temperatura cutánea, temperatura de la piel; ~ **testing** test epicutáneo, prueba epicutánea

skinny magro

skull cráneo, calavera

slant agar culture cultivo inclinado

SLE lupus eritematoso sistémico, lupus eritematoso diseminado, enfermedad de Biett, el lupus eritomasodiscoide

sleep sueño; ~ **apnea syndrome** síndrome de la apnea del sueño, síndrome de apnea del sueño; ~ **disorder** trastorno del sueño; ~ **epilepsy** narcolepsia; ~ **-inducing** soporífico, que causa o induce al sueño o sopor; ~ , **to** estar dormido, dormir

sleepiness somnolencia, modorra, sonolencia

sleeping pill píldora de dormir, pastilla que induce sueño; ~ **sickness** enfermedad del sueño

sleepless insomne, sin dormir

sleeplessness insomnio, incapacidad para dormir, vigilia anormal

sleep-walking sonambulismo, andar en sueños

sleepy sueño

slide portaobjetos, diapositiva; ~ **agglutination test** prueba de la aglutinación en portaobjetos

sliding hernia hernia por deslizamiento

slight ligero, pequeño; ~ **deafness** hipoacusia, disminución de la audición; ~ **pain** dolor ligero, dolor leve

slimming pérdida de peso, el adelgazamiento

slimy con pituita

sling cabestrillo, banda, lazo

slipped disc disco herniado, disco protruído

slippery resbaladizo, lúbrico, resbaloso

slot ranura; ~ **blot** transferencia en ranura

slow despacio, lento; ~ **breathing** bradipnea, respiración lenta; ~ **down, to** atrasar, impedir, retrasar; ~ **release agent** agente de liberación controlada, agente de liberación retardada; ~ ~ **release form** forma farmacéutica de liberación retardada

sluggishness bradiquinesia, lentitud anormal de los movimientos

slurred speech mal articulado

small pequeño, chico, poco, apenas (adv); ~ **intestine** intestino delgado, intestino pequeño

smallpox viruela; ~ **vaccine** vacuna de viruela

smarting sensation escozor, escocimiento, dolor ardiente

smear frotis

smell olor, olfato; ~ **of sweat** sobaquina, olor corporal, olor fétido asociado con la transpiración rancia; ~ , **to** oler

smelling salts sal revulsiva, sal inglesa

Smith syndrome síndrome de Smith

smoke humo; ~ **inhalation** inhalación de humos; ~ , **to** fumar

smokeless tobacco tabaco sin humo, tabaco sin combustión

smokers' leukoplakia leucoplasia del fumador

smoking tabaquismo, uso de tabaco

smooth liso; ~ **muscle** músculo liso, el músculo de contracción involuntaria

snack bocadillo

snake serpiente, culebra; ~ **bite** mordedura de serpiente; ~ **venom** veneno de serpiente

snapping hip cadera de resorte

sneeze estornudo; ~ , **to** estornudar

snore, to roncar, roncando

snoring ronquido

snot mucus, moco, moquera

snout hocico

snow nieve

snuffling gangoso, násico, nasalizado

so así que (adv), por eso (conj); ~ **so** más o menos

soaking maceración, hinchazón o ablandamiento por contacto con líquidos

soap jabón

soapy jabonoso

sober no embriagado, sobrio; ~ **up, to** recuperar la sobriedad, quitarse la merluza, espabilar la borrachera

sobriety serenidad

social social; ~ **adjustment** adaptación social; ~ **facilitation** facilitación social; ~ **gerontology** gerontología social; ~ **interaction** relaciones humanas, relaciones interpersonales; ~ **medicine** medicina social; ~ **psychologist** psicología social, psicología evolutiva; ~ **skills** capacidad por contacto, aptitud comunicativa; ~ **therapist** socioterapeuta; ~ **worker** asistente social

sodas refrescos, gaseosas, sodas

sodium sodio; ~ **chloride** sal de sodio, sal comun; ~ **cyclamate** ciclamato sódico; ~ **fluoride** fluoruro de sodio; ~ **hydrogen carbonate** hidrogenocarbonato, carbonato ácido de sodio; ~ **hydroxide** lejía de sosa, sosa líquida, hidróxido sódico líquido, NaOH; ~ **iodide** yoduro de sodio; ~ **ion** ion sodio; ~ **lactate** lactato sódico, el lactato de sodio, E325; ~ **lye** lejía sódica; ~ **pump** bomba de sodio, mecanismo teórico que explicaria el flujo de sangre en un vaso durante una transfusión; ~ **saccharine** sacarina sódica; ~ **sulfate** sulfato sódico

soft fláccido, laxo, flojo, blando, débil; ~ **drink** refresco; ~ **palate** paladar suave, paladar blando; ~ **tissue** tejido blando; ~ **tissue** parte blanda

soften, to suavizar, ablandar

soiled sucio, sucia; ~ **dressing** aposito usado, las vendas usadas

solace alivio, aligeramiento, remedio, desahogo

solar solar; ~ **cheilitis** queeilitis solar; ~ **dermatitis** quemadura del sol, eritema solar; ~ **keratosis** queratosis solar, queratosis senil; ~ **plexus** plexo solar

sole of the foot planta del pie

solid masivo, grande, amplio, macizo; ~ **culture medium** medio de cultivo sólido

solitary solitario; ~ **plasmacytoma** plasmocitoma solitário

solubility solubilidad; ~ **product** producto de solubilidad

solubilizer agente de solubilización

solution liquor, líquido, ~ solución, preparado líquido que contiene una o varias sustancias químicas solubles, relajación o preparación

solvation solvatación

solvent disolvente, solvente; ~ **syndrome** encefalopatía tóxica crónica

solvents disolventes

somatic somático, corporal; ~ **cell** célula somática; ~ **gene mutation** mutación genica somática; ~ **gene therapy** terápia genética de células somaticas

somatization somatización

somatoliberin somatoliberina

somatology somatología, antropología física

somatomedin somatomedina

somatomotor activity actividad somatomotriz; ~ **adaptive response** respuesta adaptiva somatomotriz

somatorelin somatorelina

somatostatin somatostatina, una hormona que inhibe el factor estimulante de la liberación de somatotropina de la hipófisis anterior

somatotrophin somatotropina, hormona del crecimiento

somatotropin receptors receptores de somatotropina; ~ **-releasing factor** somatoliberina

some algún, algunos

something algo

somnambulism sonambulismo, andar en sueños

somnipathy trastorno del sueño

somnolence somnolencia, modorra, sonolencia

son hijo

Sonne-Duval's bacillus Shigella sonnei

soon pronto

soothing demulcente, emoliente, calmante, que ablanda y relaja las zonas inflamadas o que ablanda la piel; ~ **lotion** emoliente, que ablanda la piel

soporific soporífico, píldora de dormir, pastilla que induce sueño

sorbic acid ácido sórbico

sorbitol sorbitol

sordes saburra

sore doloroso, dolorido, llaga; ~ **bottom** proctitis, inflamación del recto; ~ **breasts** mastitis, inflamación de la glándula mamaria; ~ **muscles** agujetas; ~ **throat** faringitis, inflamación de la garganta, inflamación de la faringe, dolor de garganta, laringitis, inflamación de la laringe

sorting separación, clasificación

souffle soplo, abultamiento

sound sleep sueño profundo

soup sopa

sour agrio

southern blot transferencia southern

space intervalo, porción de espacio o de tiempo entre dos cosas; ~ **medicine** medicina espacial, aeroespacial; ~ **sense** sentido del espacio

S

spacer espaciador; ~ **DNA** DNA espaciador;
~ **RNA** RNA espaciador
span grip sujeción de una pelota
Spanish español
spare time tiempo libre, descanso
sparganosis esparganosis
spasm convulsión, espasmo; ~ **of the larynx**
laringismo, espasmo de la laringe
spasmodic espasmódico, perteneciente o
relativo al espasmo o de su naturaleza;
~ **diathesis** diatesis espasmódica; ~ **hiccup**
singulto espasmódico; ~ **laryngitis** asma de
Millar; ~ **pain** calambres
spasmolygmus singulto espasmódico
spasmolytic espasmolítico, medicamento que
sirve para resolver los espasmos
spasmus nutans corea de la cabeza
spastic espástico, que hace referencia a la
espasticidad o a los espasmos; ~ **aphonia**
afonía espasmódica, afonía espástica; ~ **colon**
colon irritable, colon inestable; ~ **cough** tos
espasmódica; ~ **ileus** íleo espástico
spasticity espasticidad, aumento de la
resistencia muscular frente a los movimientos
pasivos
spatial espacial; ~ **aptitude** aptitud espacial,
sentido del espacio; ~ **disorientation**
desorientación espacial; ~ **orientation**
orientación espacial; ~ **relations** relaciones
espaciales
spaying ovariectomía, ooforectomía,
ovariotomía normal, castración
speak, to hablar
specialist especialista
specialty especialidad
species especie, un preparado terapéutico
specific específico, determinado, propio y
característico de una especie o de una
enfermedad; ~ **activity** actividad específica;
~ **conductance** conductancia específica;
~ **heat capacity** capacidad térmica específica;
~ **volume** volumen específico
specification especificación
specificity especificidad
specimen muestra, especimen
spectinomycin espectinomicina
spectral bandwidth anchura de banda espectral
spectrometer espectrómetro

spectrometry espectrometría
spectrophotometer espectrómetro
spectrophotometry espectrometría
spectroscopy espectroscopia
spectrum espectro, zona de actividad de un
antibiótico
specular reflectance reflectancia especular
speculum espéculo
speech habla; ~ **audiometry** audiometría vocal,
audiometría de la palabra; ~ **defects**
alteraciones del habla, trastornos del lenguaje;
~ **disorders** defectos de dicción, alteraciones
del habla, trastornos del lenguaje;
~ **pathologist** terapeuta de dicción,
logopedista, logopeda; ~ **pathology**
audiofonología, logopedia; ~ **therapist**
logoterapeuta médico, ortofonista, terapeuta
de dicción; ~ **therapy** tratamiento ortofónico,
logoterapia, fonoaudiología
speed velocidad; ~ **up, to** catalizar, acelerar
sperm esperma; ~ **donor** donante de espermas;
~ **duct** conducto deferente; ~ **-killing**
contraceptive espermicida, producto que
extermina los espermatozoide
spermacidal jelly jalea espermaticida, gelatina
vaginal
spermacide espermicida
spermatocele espermatocele
spermatogenesis espermatogénesis, proceso de
formación de los espermatozoides
spermatozoid espermatozoide
spermicidal foam espuma espermaticida
spermicide espermicida, producto que
extermina los espermatozoides
spermidine espermidina
sphenoid bone hueso biforme
sphenoidal process of the palatine bone
apófisis esfenoidal del hueso palatino
sphincter esfinter, músculo de cierre
sphincterotomy esfincterotomía
sphingomyelin esfingomielina;
~ **phosphodiesterase** esfingomielina
fosfodiesterasa
sphingomyelinase deficiency disease
enfermedad de Niemann, enfermedad de
Niemann-Pick, esfingolipidosis,
esfingomielinasa
sphygmomanometer esfigmomanómetro,

tensiometro

sphyrectomy esfirectomía, escisión del martillo

spica bandage vendaje en espiga

spicy picante

spider araña; **~ bite** aracnidismo; **~ nevus** araña vascular

spike concentración máxima, pico de voltaje transitorio

spina bifida espina bífida; **~ bifida occulta** disrafia oculta

spinach espinaca

spinal espinal, relativo a la columna vertebral; **~ anesthesia** anestesia espinal, raquianaestesia; **~ column** columna vertebral; **~ commissure** comisura espinal; **~ cord** médula espinal, médula dorsal; **~ dura mater** duramadre espinal; **~ dysraphism** disrafia; **~ fluid** líquido espinal; **~ fusion** fusión espinal; **~ ganglion** ganglio espinal; **~ meningitis** meningitis espinal, perimielitis; **~ nerve plexuses** plexos de los nervios raquidianos; **~ nerves** nervios raquídeos; **~ neurasthenia** neurastenia espinal; **~ osteoarthritis** artrosis osteofítica raquídea; **~ osteophytosis** osteofitosis osteofitosis vertebral, síndrome de Barré-Liéou; **~ reflexotherapy** reflexoterapia; **~ scoliosis** escoliosis de la columna vertebral; **~ tap** punción lumbar

spindle huso; **~ fiber** fibra fusiforme, huso mitótico; **~ inhibitor** inhibidor de huso mitótico

spine espina dorsal

spinobulbar muscular atrophy trastornos musculares atróficos, miotonía atrófical la enfermedad de Steiner

spinocerebellar ataxia type 3 enfermedad de Machado-Joseph

spinous espinoso; **~ foot** pie espinoso; **~ layer of epidermis** capa espinosa de la epidermis, capa de células espinosas; **~ process** apófisis espinosa de la vértebra

spiral fracture fractura por torsión

spiramycin espiramicina

spirits bebidas alcohólicas

spiritual healer curandero, sanador

spirochete espiroqueta

spirometer espirómetro

spirometry espirometría

spit, to escupir

spleen bazo; **~ enlargement** agrandamiento del bazo, esplenomegalia; **~ infection** esplenitis

splenomegaly agrandamiento del bazo, esplenomegalia

spliceosome espliceosoma

splicing eliminación de intrones; **~ site** zona de unión exón-intrón

splinker esplínquer

splint férula, tablilla; **~ , to** entablillar, colocar férula

splinter astigón, esquirla, astilla

split fisura, grieta, brecha, raňura; **~ gene** gen discontinuo

spoiled food comida podrida

spondylitis espondilitis, inflamación de las vértebras

spondylosyndesis fusión espinal

spondylotherapy spondylotherapy, vertebroterapia

sponge bath baño de asiento

spongiform encephalopathy encefalopatía espongiforme

spongy esponjoso

spontaneous espontaneo; **~ abortion** mal parto, mala cama, aborto; **~ recovery** recuperación espontanea; **~ remission** remisión espontánea

sporadic esporádico; **~ hemophilia** hemofilia esporádica

spore espora

sporicide esporicida

sporotrichosis esporotricosis

sporozoite esporozoíto

sports deporte; **~ medicine** medicina esportiva

spots manchas

spotting manchas de sangre

spouse cónyuge

sprain esguince, dislocación, torcedura, torsión; **~ one's ankle, to** esguinzarse el tobillo

sprained ankle esguince de tobillo

spray spray (inglés), pulverizador, atomizador; **~ dispenser** inhalador, nebulizador

spread by metastasis, to metastatizar

spreading difusión, dispersión

spring primavera

springy elástico, saltarín, flojo

spur espolón

spurious aneurysm aneurisma falso;
~ **claudication** pseudoclaudicación

sputum esputo, flema, gargajos; ~ **induction** esputo inducido

squamous escamoso, que tiene escamas; ~ **cell** célula escamosa; ~ **cell carcinoma** carcinoma de células escamosas

square cuadrado

squat, to estar en cuclillas, ponerse en cuclillas, sentarse en cuclillas, acuclillarse

squint estrabismo, bizco, desviación de un ojo de su dirección normal; ~, **to** mirar de ojo entrecerrado, fruncir la vista

SS agar agar SS

ssDNA DNA monocatenario

S-shaped sigmoide, de forma similar a las letra S

St. Anthony's fire erisipela; ~ **John's wort** hipérico

stab culture cultivo por picadura; ~, **to** apuñalar; ~ **wound** cuchillada, cortadura profunda, inciso, herida por arma blanca

stabbing pain punzadas

stability estabilidad

stabilization estabilización, creación de un estado estable

staff plantilla, personal

stagger, to tambalear, titubear

staggered cut corte en bisel

staggering gait marcha inestable

staging estadiaje, estadificación

stagnation of blood flow hemostasia primaria, hemostasis

stain tinción; ~, **to** manchar, macular

staining coloración, mancha

stairs escaleras

stamina aguante, resistencia, endurecimiento, induración

stammer, to balbucear

stammering tartamudez, pselismo

stanch, to restañar la sangre, detener una hemorragia

stand puesto; ~ **up, to** levantarse

standard patrón, norma, estándar; ~ **deviation** desviación típica; ~ **dosing** dosis normal; ~ **uptake value** valor de captación estándar, suv

standardize, to estandarizar, comparar con un

estándar, establecer patrones o estándares

standardized estandarizado; ~ **exercise tolerance test** ensayo de tolerancia al ejercicio normalizado; ~ **genetic assay** técnica genética estandarizada

stand-by state estado de reposo

staphylococcal estafilocócico; ~ **enterotoxin** enterotoxina estafilocócica; ~ **skin infections** infecciones cutaneas estafilocócicas

staphylococcus estafilococo; ~ **pneumonia** neumonia estafilocócica; ~ **aureus** estafilococo dorado; ~ **aureus toxin** toxina de staphylococus aureus

staphyloma estafiloma

staphylotoxin toxina estafilocócica

staple grapa para sutura

starch almidón; ~ **hydrolysis test** prueba de la hidrólisis del almidón

Starr-Edwards valv prótesis de Starr-Edwards, una válvula cardiaca artificial

start codon codón de iniciación; ~, **to** empezar; ~ **-up time** periodo de arranque

startle reaction sobresalto, reacción ante la sorpresa

starvation inanición, mala nutrición, desnutrición, subalimentación

starve to death, to morir de hambre

stasis estasis, estancamiento de sangre u otro líquido en una parte del organismo, estado de equilibrio entre fuerzas opuestas; ~ **dermatitis** dermatitis estásica

state estado, situación; ~ **-certified psychologist** psicólogo diplomado; ~ **of mind** estado de animo, estado mental; ~ **of the art** estado actual

statement of dose posología

statins estatinas, inhibidores de la HMG-CoA reductasa

stationary phase fase estacionaria

statistic estadístico

statistical estadístico; ~ **questionnaire** cuestionario estadístico

statistics estadística

status estado, condición, situación, crisis o punto culminante; ~ **asthmaticus** estado asmático, crisis asmática aguda

statutory rape violación de menores

stay, to seguir

STD (sexual transmitted diseases) enfermedad de transmisión sexual

steady constante, ininterrumpido, regular; ~ **state** estado de equilibrio, una situación en que una variable no cambia

steam sterilization esterilización por vapor

steatonecrosis necrosis grasa, esteatonecrosis

steatorrhea esteatorrea, cantidad excesiva de grasas en las heces

steatosis esteatosis, acumulación excesiva de glóbulos grasos en los tejidos

Steers replicator replicador de Steers

Steinert's disease distrofia miotónica de Steinert, enfermedad de Steinert, miotonía atrófica, distrofia miotónica

stem bromelain bromelaina de tronco; ~ **cell** célula madre, célula puripotencial

stenosis estenosis, estrechamiento de un conducto; ~ **of aortic valve** estenosis aórtico; ~ **of the coronary artery** estenosis arterial coronaria; ~ **of the pulmonary valve** estenosis de la válvula pulmonar, síndrome de Goodpasture

stereopsis estereopsis

stereoscopic estereoscópico; ~ **depth perception** percepción de la profundidad con la visión estereoscópica; ~ **vision** estereopsis

stereotaxis estereotaxia

stereotypy estereotipia; ~ **of movements** movimientos estereotipados

sterile estéril; ~ **abscess** absceso estéril; ~ **clothing** ropas esterilizadas; ~ **environment** ambiente estéril; ~ **room** cuarto estéril, el cuarto aséptico

sterility esterilidad

sterilization esterilización, procedimiento que hace incapaz a un individuo para reproducción, eliminación completa de microorganismos

sterilize, to desinfectar, esterilizar

Sternberg chloromyelosarcomatosis cloromielosarcomatosis de Sternberg

sternoclavicular joint articulación esternoclavicular

sternocleidomastoid artery arteria esternocleidomastoidea

sternum esternón, hueso del pecho

steroid esteroida, esteroide, tipo de compuesto químico

steroidal esteroideo; ~ **anti-inflammatory drugs (SAID)** fármacos antiinflamatorios esteroideos

stertor estertor, respiración anhelosa

stertorous respiration estertor, respiración anhelosa

stethoscope estetoscopio

stick palo; ~ **one's tongue out, to** sacar la lengua; ~ , **to** pinchar

sticking adhesión, fijación, unión anormal de tejidos u órganos

sticky pegajoso; ~ **end** extremo cohesivo; ~ **tape** cinta adhesiva

stiffen, to entumecer, entorpecer, envarar, ponerse tieso

stiffness rigidez, envaramiento; ~ **of neck** rigidez de la nuca; ~ **of the shoulder** rigidez del hombro

still pues, todavía, tranquilo

stillbirth muerte fetal, nacido muerto

stimulant estimulante, un agente que produce estimulación

stimulants, to take doparse

stimulate, to activar, estimular, acelerar, reactivar

stimulation excitación, estimulación

stimulon estimulón

sting picadura

stinging pain escozor, escocimiento, dolor ardiente

stink fetidez; ~ , **to** heder

stirrup estribo

stitch punto; ~ **up a wound** suturar una herida

stitches puntos de sutura

stiumulator adyuvante, sustancia que contribuye a la acción de otra, sustancia añadida a una vacuna que refuerza su efecto

stock existencias, reserva

stockinet vendaje tubular, stockinette

stoichiometric number número estequiométrico

stoma estoma, una apertura artificial de un órgano interno en la superficie del cuerpo

stomach abdomen, vientre, estómago; ~ **ache** dolor de vientre; ~ **acidity** acidez gástrica; ~ **cancer** cáncer gástrico, cáncer de estómago; ~ **lining** mucosa gástrica, revestimiento del estómago; ~ **ulcer** úlcera de estómago, úlcera péptica

stomata estomas

stomatitis estomatitis (f), inflamación de la mucosa oral

stomatological estomatológico, perteneciente o relativo a la rama de la medicina que se ocupa de la boca y sus enfermedades

stomatology estomatología

stomion estomio

stone cálculo, piedra

stool deposición, defecación, las heces, excrementos; ~ **culture** cultivo de la defecación, coprocultivo; ~ **sample** prueba de heces

stop parada, alto, descanso, pausa; ~ **codon** codón de terminación, codón de paro, codón terminador; ~ **smoking, to** cesar el uso de tabaco

stopping inhibición, atenuación, supresión o bloqueo de una función o reacción

storage almacenamiento

stout sobrepeso, pasado de peso, gordo, grueso, gordinflón, petacón, excesode peso

stove estufa

strabismus estrabismo, bizco, desviación de un ojo de su dirección normal

straddle, to montar a horcajadas, ahorajarse, cabalgar

straighten up, to enderezarse, estirar, extenderse

strain cepa; ~ **a muscle, to** desgarrarse un músculo, tener un esguince; ~ **fracture** fractura por arrancamiento; ~ **trauma** traumatismo por esfuerzo

strained tendon desmectasia, tirón, tendon desgarrado

strait jacket camisa de fuerza

strand cadena; ~ **of DNA** cadena de ADN

strange object cuerpo extraño

strangulated encarcerado, estrangulado; ~ **hernia** hernia estrangulada

strangulation estrangulación; ~ **ileus** íleo por estrangulamiento

strangury estranguria

stratification estratificación

stratigraph tomógrafo

stratum filamentosum capa espinosa de la epidermis, capa de células espinosas; ~ **granulosum** capa queratohialina, capa granulosa de la epidermis; ~ **spinosum epidermidis** capa espinosa de la epidermis, capa de células espinosas

strawberry fresa

streaks of blood rayas de sangre

street calle

strength intensidad, grado de fuerza o tensión

strenuous activity esfuerzo, actividad fuerte

streptococcal estreptocócico; ~ **throat infection** infección estreptocócica de la garganta

streptococcus streptococcus; ~ **species** especie de estreptococos

Streptococcus pyogenes estreptococo piogénico

streptokinase estreptoquinasa

streptomycin estreptomicina

stress fatiga mental, estrés; ~ **headache** cefalgia tensional; ~ **incontinence** incontinencia de esfuerzo, incontinencia por estrés; ~ **test** prueba de ejercicio

stressed out padeciendo de estrés

stressful estresante, lleno de tensión nerviosa

stressor factor de estrés, cosa estresante

stretch marks estrías, veteaduras, vetas, rayas, líneas; ~ **, to** estirarse

stretcher camilla, parihuelas; ~ **cart** camilla con ruedas, portacama rodante, parihuelas

stretching dilatación, ensanchamiento, agrandamiento o expansión de un órgano hueco

stria vascularis estria vascular

striae estrías, rayas, líneas, pequeñas cicatrizes del estiramiento de la piel; ~ **atrophicae** estrías, veteaduras, vetas; ~ **cutis distensae** estrías, veteaduras, vetas

striated estriado; ~ **muscle** músculo estriado, músculo de contracción voluntaria; ~ **muscle fiber** fibras musculares estriadas

strict estricto, rigoroso

stricture estrechez

stricturotomy estricturotomia

stridor estridor, ruidos respiratorios

stringency rigor

strobila estrobilo

stroke apoplejía, ictus, accidente

cerebrovascular agudo, ataque cerebral;
~ **center** unidades de ictus; ~ **volume** volumen sistólico

stroma of the iris estroma del iris

stromal estromal; ~ **adenomyosis** adenomiosis, endometriosis uterina; ~ **cell** célula estromal, una célula grande con proyecciones que existe en la médula ósea

strong fuero

Strong's bacillus Shigella flexneri

strongyloidiasis estrongiloidiasis

strophulus prurigo simple, urticaria papular

structural estructural; ~ **anomaly** malformación estructural

struma estruma, bocio, engrosamiento del tiroides

strumous bubo bubón estrumoso

Stuart factor factor X de la coagulación; ~ **transport medium** medio de transporte de Stuart

stump muñón

stupidity estupidez, bobería, burrada

stupor estupor, pérdida parcial o casi completa de la conciencia

Sturge–Weber syndrome angiomatosis encefalotrigeminal, angiomatosis meningo-oculo-faciale

stutter tartamudez, pselismo; ~ **, to** tartamudear, balbucear, gaguear

stuttering goteo de orina; ~ tartamudez, pselismo

sty (on eyelid) perilla (del ojo), orzuelo (del ojo)

styptic hemostático

styptics hemostáticos

subacute subagudo, un poco agudo

subarachnoid subaracnoideo; ~ **anaesthesia** anestesia espinal, raquianaestesia; ~ **space** espacio subaracnoideo

subcapital humerus fracture fractura condilar del húmero

subcapsular subcapsular, que está situado o que ocurre debajo de una cápsula

subcellular microsurgery microcirugía subcelular; ~ **organelle** orgánulo subcelular, organito

subchondral subcondral; ~ **cysts** quistes oseos

subclavian artery arteria subclavicular

subclinical subclínico, que transcurre sin

manifestar síntomas; ~ **spontaneous abortion** aborto espontáneo subclínico

subconjunctival subconjuntival, que está situado o que ocurre debajo de la conjuntiva; ~ **apoplexy** apoplejía subconjuntival

subcutaneous subcutáneo, que está situado o que sucede por debajo de la piel; ~ **cellular tissue** tejido celular subcutáneo; ~ **cellulitis** celulitis subcutánea; ~ **injection** inyección subcutanea; ~ **wire suture** sutura profunda con hilo metalico

subdural subdural; ~ **hematoma** hematoma subdural; ~ **hygroma** higroma subdural; ~ **space** espacio subdural

subepithelial subepitelial; ~ **connective tissue** tejido conjuntivo subepitelial

subfacial herniation hernia subfactorial, herniación cerebral

subjective subjetivo

sublingual sublingual, referido o situado debajo de la lengua

subluxation subluxación

submaxillary lymph node ganglio linfático submaxilar

sub-micron particle partícula submicrónica

suboccipital suboccipital; ~ **injection** inyección suboccipital; ~ **plexus** plexo venoso suboccipital; ~ **trigeminal rhizotomy** operación de Dandy

subperiosteal subperióstico; ~ **abscess** absceso subperióstico; ~ **fracture** fractura subperiostática, a fratura subperiósseo; ~ **hematoma** hematoma subperióstico

subscapular subescapular

subset subgrupo, subconjunto

subspecies subespecie

substance sustancia, agente; ~ **abuse** abuso de substancias toxicas o de medicamentos, los trastornos relacionados con sustancias; ~ **concentration** concentración de sustancia; ~ **content** contenido de sustancia; ~ **flow rate** caudal de sustancia; ~ **fraction** fracción de sustancia; ~ **rate** caudal de sustancia

substantia alba sustancia blanca

substernal goiter bocio subesternal

substitute sustituto; ~ **blood product** sustituto de la sangre, sustitutivo de la sangre, substituto sanguineo

substitution sustitución

substrate sustrato, base, sustancia básica

subsystem subgrupo, subconjunto

subtalar subastragalina

subthalamic subtalámico; ~ **decussation** decusación subtalámica de Forel; ~ **nuclei** núcleos hipotalámicos

subtherapeutic subterapéutico; ~ **level** concentración subterapéutica

subtilisin subtilisina

suckle, to lactar, amamantar, dar pecho

suckling lactante, bebé

suction succión, aspiración; ~ **-pipe** bomba de vacío, aspirador, eyector; ~ **tube** canula de aspiracion

sudden abrupto, repentino, brusco; ~ **attacks** a modo de ataques; ~ **cardiac death** muerte cardiaca repentina; ~ **infant death syndrome** Síndrome de Muerte Infantil Súbita (SIMS), muerte súbita del lactante

suddenly (adj) súbito; ~ **(adv)** de repente

Sudeck's atrophy algodistrofia

suffering from... aquejado de ...

suffocate, to sofocar, ahogar, sofocar

suffuse, to infundir

sugar azúcar

suicidal suicido; ~ **ideation** ideas suicidas; ~ **tendencies** tendencias suicidas

suicide suicidio; ~ **gene** gen suicida

suitable respiratory equipment equipo respiratorio adecuado

sulbactam sulbactam

sulci surcos

sulcus fisura, hendedura, cisura, surco

sulfadiazine sulfadiacina

sulfamethazine sulfadimidina

sulfamethoxazole sulfamethoxazol

sulfasalazine salazopirina

sulfatase arilsulfatasa

sulfation factor somatomedina

sulfinic acids ácidos sulfínicos

sulfite reductase hemoprotein hemoproteína de sulfito reductasa

sulfoacid ácido sulfónico

sulfonamides sulfonamidas

sulfonilamide sulfanilamida

sulfur azufre, alcrebite; ~ **dioxide** dioxido de azufre; ~ **granule** gránulo de azufre

(Actinomyces)

sulindac sulindac, un agente antiinflamatorio

sulph hemoglobin sulfahemoglobina

sulphite lye lignosulfito; ~ **waste liquor** lejías residuales al sulfito

sulphur azufre, alcrebite

sulphuric acid ácido sulfúrico

summer verano

sun sol

sunburn quemadura del sol, eritema solar

Sunday domingo

sunstroke insolación, asoleada, solanera

supercilium ceja

supercoil superhélice

supercoiled DNA DNA superhelicoidal

superficial superficial; ~ **punctuate keratitis** keratitis puntiforme superficial

supergene supergén

superhelical turn vuelta superhelicoidal

superhelix superhélice

superinfection superinfección

superior articulación radiocubital superior

superstitious supersticioso

supervision supervisión

supination supinación

supine supino

supple elástico, saltarín, flojo

supplement suplemento

suppository supositorio, calilla, calía

suppress, to suprimir

suppressing supresión

suppressor T cell linfocito T supresor, célula T supresora

suppuration supuración, formación de pus

suppurative supurado; ~ **cholecystitise** colecistitis supurada; ~ **pleurisy** empiema, piotórax, empiema pulmonar

suprapatellar bursa bolsa suprapatelar

suprapiriform hernia hernia suprapiramidal

suprarenal suprarrenal; ~ **cortex** corteza suprarrenal, corteza adrenal; ~ **glands** glándulas adrenales, glándulas suprarrenales, suprarrenales

supraventricular supraventricular, por encima o en la parte superior de una pequeña cavidad

supurative supurativo

surdity sordera, deterioro de la capacidad auditiva

surface superficie; **~ anesthesia** analgesia de superficie; **~ antigen of hepatitis B** HBsAg, antígeno de superficie de la hepatitis-B; **~ tension** tensión superficial

surfactant (agente) tensoactivo

surgeon cirujano; **~ gloves** guantes cirúrgicos, guantes estériles; **~ gown** vestimenta para quirófano; **~ report** informe del cirujano, relato operatorio

surgery cirugía

surgical quirúrgico; **~ abdomen** abdomen agudo; **~ catgut** catgut quirúrgico; **~ diathermy** electrocoagulación; **~ dressing** venda, vendaje, envoltura; **~ excision** abscisión quirúrgica; **~ gauze** gasa; **~ gloves** guantes cirúrgicos, guantes estériles; **~ intervention** intervención quirúrgica; **~ journal** registro de las operaciones; **~ mask** máscara protectora; **~ mesh** malla para cirugía; **~ preparation** preparación para cirugía; **~ removal** escisión, extirpación; **~ robotics** robótica quirúrgica, robótica médica; **~ shock** choque operatorio, síncope postoperatorio

surrepressive superrepresivo; **~ mutation** mutación superrepresiva

surrogate genetics mutagénesis inversa; **~ marker** marcador indirecto; **~ mother** madre subrogada, madre portadora, la madre de alquiler

surrounding envolvente; **~ soft tissue** tejido blando rodeando

susceptible irritable, quisquilloso, susceptible, colérico, irascible, arrebatadizo, sensitivo; **~ to ampicillin** sensible a la ampicilina

suspenders tirantes

suspension suspensión

sustained release drug fármaco a difusión regulada, fármaco de liberación controlada

sutural dehiscence suturas soltando, dehiscencia de las suturas

suture clip grapa

suv valor de captación estándar, suv

swab hisopo, escobillón; **~ holder** herramienta para manejar tampones

swallow, to tragar, deglutir

swallowing ingestión, toma, deglución; **~ reflex** reflejo de deglutir

sweat sudor; **~ glands** glándulas sudoríparas, glándulas de transpiración, glándulas apocrinas; **~ ,** to sudar

sweating transpiración, sudación, sudor, sudoración

sweaty face hiperhidrosis facial

sweet dulce

Sweet's syndrome síndrome de Sweet, dermatosis neutrofílica febril aguda

swell, to hinchar

swelling tumefacción, hinchamiento, hinchazón; **~ due to infection** tumefacción infecciosa; **~ of the foot** hinchazón del pie, tumefacción del pie

swine fever peste porcina; **~ fever vaccine** vacuna anti-peste

swollen hinchado; **~ abdomen** abdomen hinchado, vientre hinchado; **~ belly** abdomen hinchado, vientre hinchado; **~ bladder** distensión vesical; **~ lymph glands** linfadenopatía, tumefacción de uno o más ganglios linfáticos; **~ lymph nodes** agrandamiento de los nódulos linfáticos, aumento de los ganglios linfáticos; **~ optical disk** papiledema, edema papilar, tumefacción del disco óptico, hinchazón de la papila óptica

swoon soponcio, patatús, síncope

sycosis of the beard tiña de la barba, sicosis de la barba

symmetric simétrico

sympathetic simpático; **~ friend** amigo comprensivo; **~ hypertension** hipertensión simpática; **~ nervous system** sistema nervioso simpático; **~ trunk** tronco simpático

sympathico-vasal attack acceso simpatico-vascular

sympatholytic agents simpatolíticos

sympathomimetic simpaticomimético; **~ drug** fármaco simpaticomimético

symptom síntoma

symptomatic sintomático, perteneciente a los síntomas; **~ anemia** anemia sintomática; **~ arthritis** artritis sintomática; **~ bronchitis** bronquitis sintomática; **~ dysmenorrhea** dismenorrea sintomática; **~ hemoglobinuria** hemoglobinuria sintomática; **~ hydrocele** hidrocele sintomático; **~ impotence** impotencia sintomática

symptomatology sintomatología, síntomas combinadas de una enfermedad

symptom–free carrier portador asintomático

symptomless carrier portador asintomático

synaptic sináptico, que pertenece o afecta a la zona de contacto entre dos neuronas; ~ **transmission** transmisión sináptica

synaptonemal complex complejo sinaptonémico

syncope síncope, desmayo, desvanecimiento

syncytium sincitio

syndrome síndrome, conjunto de síntomas

synergetic sinérgico -ica

synergism sinergia

synergistic sinérgético

synergy sinergia; ~ **test** prueba de la sinergia

synovial sinovial; ~ **biopsy** biopsia sinovial, punción biopsia sinovial; ~ **bursa** bolsa sinovial; ~ **chondromatosis** condromatosis sinovial; ~ **fluid** líquido sinovial; ~ **fold** pliegue sinovial; ~ **hernia** hernia sinovial; ~ **joint** diartrosis, articulación sinovial; ~ **membrane** membrana sinovial; ~ **needle biopsy** punción biopsia sinovial

synovitis sinovitis, inflamación de una membrana sinovial

synovium membrana sinovial

synthesis síntesis

synthetase sintasa

synthetic sintético; ~ **enzyme analogue** enzima sintética; ~ **hormone** hormona sintética

syphilis sífilis

syphilis–related luético, sifilítico

syphilitic sifilítico; ~ **abscess** úlcera sifilítica; ~ **induration** induración de Hunter, induración sifilítica

syringe jeringa

syrup jarabe; ~ **of ipecac** jarabe de ipecacuana

system sistema; ~ **of measurement** sistema de medición

systematic sistemático; ~ **error** error sistemático

systemic sistémico, que afecta al cuerpo en una forma total; ~ **amyloidosis** amiloidosis sistémica; ~ **exposure** exposición general; ~ **fungal infection** micosis profunda; ~ **immunodeficiency** inmunodeficiencia sistémica; ~ **lupus erythematosus** lupus eritematoso sistémico, lupus eritematoso diseminado, enfermedad de Biett, el lupus eritematosodiscoide; ~ **mycosis** micosis profunda; ~ **weakness** achaque, debilidad

systolic sistólico; ~ **blood pressure** presión arterial sistólico; ~ **click** chasquido sistólico; ~ **murmur** soplo cardíaco sistólico, soplo sistólico; ~ **volume** volumen sistólico

T

T3 triiodotironina

T4 tiroxina; ~ **cell** célula T4, linfocito T4, linfocito coadyuvante, linfocito colaborador

tabes dorsalis tabes dorsal, ataxia locomotriz progresiva

tabetic dissociation disociación tabética

table mesa; ~ **of contents** contenido (de un documento); ~ **salt** sal de sodio, sal comun; ~ **spoon** cucharada

tablet píldora, comprimido, pastilla

tachyarrhythmia taquiarritmia, forma rápida e irregular del ritmo cardíaco

tachycardia taquicardia, aceleración de la frecuencia cardíaca

tachyphylaxis taquifilaxia, efecto decreciente de un medicamento

tactile táctil; ~ **perception** sentido del tacto; ~ **sense** sentido del tacto

tag, to marcar

tagged atom átomo marcado

tail cola, rabo; ~ **of epididymis** cola del epidídimo

tailbone colita, rabadilla, hueso coccígeo

take, to llevar(se), tomar, coger, agarrar, robar; ~ **a deep breath, to** respirar profundo, respirar hondo; ~ **a misstep, to** pisar en falso, pisar mal; ~ **a pill, to** tomar una píldora; ~ **care of, to** cuidar a; ~ **measurements, to** efectuar medidas; ~ **your pulse, to** tomar el pulso

talcum talco; ~ **powder** polvo de talco

talkative hablador, loquaz, parlanchín

talocalcanean joint articulación calcaneoastragalina

talonavicular joint articulación talonavicular

tamoxifen tamoxifén

tampon tampón higiénico; ~ **plugger** herramienta para manejar tampones
tandem tándem; ~ **repeat** repetición en tándem
tangible palpable
tanner's disease pigeonnau, l'ulcération chromique
tannic acid ácido tánico
tanning broncear, bronceado por el sol
tantalum tántalo
tapeworm tenia, solitaria, cestodo
tapping golpear, percusión
tardive tardío; ~ **dyskinesia** discinesia tardía
target diana; ~ **value** valor asignado
tarry stool defecación sanguinolenta, sangre en el excremento, la hematozequia
tarsal tarso; ~ **acne** acné tarsi; ~ **joint** articulación tarsiana
tartar cálculo dental, sarro dental
tartaric acid ácido tartárico
taste gusto; ~ **buds** bulbos gustatorios, papilas del gusto; ~ **test** análisis organoléptico
tat gene gen trans-activador
tattoo tatuaje
taxonomy taxonomía
Tay-Sachs disease enfermedad de Tay-Sachs
T-cell linfocito T
T-dependent antigen antígeno timodependente
TDM monitorización farmacoterapéutica
tea té (con leche); ~ **tree oil** aceite de arbol de te
teach, to enseñar
teaching hospital for midwifery escuela de obstetricia para comadronas
teaspoon cucharadita
technique técnica
teenage adolescencia; ~ **pregnancy** embarazo en adolescencia
teeth dientes
teicoplanin teicoplanina
telangiectasia telangiectasia, dilatación de vasos terminales todo en la cara
telangiectic glioma glioma telangiectásico
Telematics Systems Sistemas telemáticos, asistencia sanitaria

telemedicine telemedicina, telediagnóstico
telephone teléfono; ~ **number** número de teléfono
tell, to decir
tellurite reduction test prueba de reducción de la telurita
temperate phage fago atenuado
temperature temperatura
template molde
temple templo, sien
temporal temporal; ~ **arteritis** arteritis temporal; ~ **lobe** lóbulo temporal; ~ **operculum** opérculo temporal; ~ **resolution** resolución temporal, tiempo de resolución
temporary duración breve, de corto plazo, temporario, transitorio, pasajero; ~ **amnesia** amnesia lacunar; ~ **disability** incapacidad temporaria, discapacidad temporaria
temporomandibular joint articulación temporomaxilar, articulación temporomandibular
ten diez
tendency tendencia, disposición, predisposición
tendinitis tendinitis (f), inflamación de un tendón
tendon tendón
tendosynovitis tendovaginitis
tenesmus tenesmo, deseo doloroso e ineficaz de orinar o defecar
Tenon capsule cápsula de Tenon
tenophony roce pericárdico
tenosynovitis tenosinovitis (f), inflamación de un tendón y de su vaina
TENS (transcutaneous electrical nerve stimulation) estimulación eléctrica transcutánea de nervios
tense tenso; ~ **up, to** ponerse tenso
tensioactive tensioactivo, que ejerce efecto sobre tensión superficial
tension tensión, tono, potencial eléctrico, presión; ~ **headache** cefalgia tensional; ~ **pneumothorax** neumotórax de tensión
tensor tympani músculo del martillo, el músculo tensor del tímpano
tenth décimo, diez (in dates); ~ **cranial nerve** nervio vago
tentorial hernia hernia tentorial
tepid tibio

teratogen teratógeno

teratogenic teratogénico, que genera malformaciones; ~ **effects** efectos teratógenos

teratogenicity teratogenicidad

teratological teratológico; ~ **dislocation of the hip** luxación teratológica de la cadera

teratoma teratoma, un tumor constituido por diversos tipos de tejido

terbinafine terbinafina

terbutaline terbutaline

term período, trimestre, término; ~ **of pregnancy** término del embarazo

terminal final, último, postrero; ~ **care** centro de cuidados paliativos, asistencia emocional del morubundo; ~ **renal disease** enfermedad renal en etapa fina

terminator terminador

test prueba, análisis; ~ **insemination** inseminación de prueba; ~ **on animals** experimentación con animales

testectomy orquidectomía, orquiectomía

testicle testículo, gonada masculina

testicular testicular, perteneciente o relativo a los testículos; ~ **adenocarcinoma** adenocarcinoma testicular; ~ **aplasia** aplasia testicular; ~ **artery** arteria espermática; ~ **biopsy** biopsia testicular; ~ **cancer** cáncer de testículo, neoplasia maligna de los testículos; ~ **cyst** quistes testiculares; ~ **ectopy** ectopia testicular; ~ **insufficiency** insuficiencia testicular; ~ **pain** orquialgia; ~ **teratoma** teratoma testicular

testing pruebas; ~ **laboratory** laboratorio de ensayo; ~ **of drugs** control de medicamentos; ~ **strip** tira reactiva

testis testículo, gonada masculina

testosterone testosterona; ~ **patch** parche transdermico de testosterona; ~ **propionate** propionato de testosterona

tetanus tétano(s); ~ **immunoglobulin** inmunoglobulina antitetánica; ~ **shot** vacuna antitetánica; ~ **toxoid** toxoide tetánico; ~ **vaccine** vacuna antitetánica

tetany tetania

tetracycline tetraciclina

tetrahydrofolate dehydrogenase dihidrofolato-reductasa

tetrazolium tolerance tolerancia al tetrazolio

Texas mange eccema de los graneros, prurito de los cereales

thalamus tálamo, masa importante de núcleos grises

thalassemia anemia mediterránea, talasemia

thalidomide talidomina

thallium talio; ~ **bromoiodide** bromoyoduro de talio; ~ **scan** escintigrafia al talio

than que

thanatology tanatologia

thanks gracias

that (far) aquel, aquella; ~ **(near)** eso, esa, eso, este, esta, -o, que

Thayer–Martin agar agar de Thayer-Martin

THC (tetrahydrocannabinol) tetrahidrocannabinol, THC

the el, la, los, las

thebaine tebaina, paramorfina

theca cell célula tecal; ~ **tumor** tecoma, tumor de las células tecales

thecoma tecoma, tumor de las células tecales

their sus

them a ellos, -as

theophylline teofilina

theoretical teórico

theory hipótesis, suposición

therapeutic terapéutico, que sirve para la curación; ~ **drug monitoring** farmacoterapéutica; ~ **index** índice terapéutico; ~ **level** concentración terapéutica; ~ **protocol** protocolo terapéutico; ~ **range** intervalo terapéutico

therapist terapeuta

therapy terapia, tratamiento terapéutico

there ahí, allí

thermal térmico, que hace referencia al calor o a la temperatura; ~ **conductivity detector** detector de conductividad térmica; ~ **stress** incomodidad térmica, malestar por causa del frio/del calor

thermic test prueba calórica

thermocautery termocauterio

thermocoagulation termocoagulación

thermodynamic temperature temperatura termodinámica

thermography termografía

thermolabile antigens antígenos capsulares

thermolysin termolisina

thermometer termómetro

thermoregulation termorregulación, regulación del calor o de la temperatura

thermosensitive termosensible; **~ mutation** mutación termosensible

these estos, -as

they ellos, -as

thiabendazole tiabendazol, un antihelmíntico

thiamin tiamina; **~ hydrochloride** clorhidrato de tiamina; **~ mononitrate** mononitrato de tiamina

thiaminase tiaminasa

thiamine tiamina

thiamphenicol tiamfenicol

thick grueso

thickening engrosamiento

thigh muslo

thimerosal timerosal, un antiinfeccioso

thin delgado; **~ tube** cánula, tubo que se introduce en el organismo; **~ -layer chromatography** cromatografía en capa fina; **~ -skinned** irritable, quisquilloso, susceptible, colérico, irascible, arrebatadizo, gruñon

thing pene, cosa, objeto

think, to pensar

thinking disorder alteracion del razonamiento, trastorno mental

thiocyanic acid ácido tiociánico

thioflavine tioflavina

thioglucosidase tioglucosidasa

thioglycolate broth caldo con tioglicolato

third tercero; **~ degree burn wounds** quemadura de tercer grado; **~ part** un tercio

thirst sed

thirteen trece

thirty treinta

this este, esta; **~ week** esta semana

Thomsen disease ataxia muscular de Thomsen, miotonia congénita

thoracentesis toracocentesis

thoracic torácico, perteneciente o relativo al tórax o que lo afecta; **~ aorta** aorta torácica; **~ cavity** cavidad torácico; **~ gas volume** volumen de gaz intratorácico; **~ vertebrae** vértebras dorsales

thoracocentesis toracocentesis

thoracolumbar toracolumbar

thoracotomy toracotomía, punzamiento del

tórax

thorax pecho, tórax

those (far) aquellos, -as; **~ (near)** esos, -as

though aunque, bien que

thought pensamiento, idea, intención; **~ disorder** alteracion del razonamiento, trastorno mental

thousand mil

three tres; **~ hundred** trecientos

threonine treonina

threshold umbral; **~ of consciousness** umbral de consciencia; **~ of pain** umbral del dolor, tolerancia del dolor

throat garganta, tragadero; **~ culture** cultivo de la garganta

throb, to retachar, pulsar, latir

throbbing headache dolor de cabeza punzante; **~ hematoma** hematoma pulsátil; **~ pain** palpitaciones

thrombasthenia trombastenia

thrombectomy trombectomia

thrombin trombina; **~ time** tiempo de trombina

thromboangiitis obliterans tromboangitis obliterante, la enfermedad de Buerger

thrombocyte plaqueta; **~** trombocito, plaqueta

thrombocytopenia trombocitopenia, disminución del número de plaquetas en la sangre

thrombocytosis trombocitosis (f), aumento exagerado de las plaquetas en la sangre

thromboembolism tromboembolismo

thrombokinase factor Xa de la coagulación, trombocinasa

thrombolysis trombólisis

thrombolytic trombolítico, que disuelve o desintegra un trombo

thrombophlebitis tromboflebitis, inflamación de una vena

thromboplastin protrombinasa, factor xa, tromboplastina, trombocinasa

thrombosis trombosis

thromboxane tromboxano; **~ synthase** tromboxano-A-sintasa

thrombus trombo, tapón de sangre en el sistema circulatorio

through a través de; **~ the skin** percutáneo, a través de la piel intacta

throw up, to estar nauseado, vomitar, tener

náuseas

thrush candidiasis, algodoncillo, afta, infección por un hongo del género candida

thumb pulgar

Thursday jueves

thylakoid tilacoide

thymic tímica; ~ **asthma** laringismo, espasmo de la laringe, laringospasmo; ~ **hormone** hormona del timo, hormona tímica; ~ **tissue** tejido tímico

thymidine timidina, desoxitimidina; ~ **kinase** timidina-cinasa

thymin timin

thyrocalcitonin tirocalcitonina, calcitonina

thyroglobin tiroglobina

thyroid tiroides, glándula tiroidea; ~ **-blocking agent** bloqueador de hormonas tiroideas; ~ **cancer** cáncer de tiroides; ~ **dysfunction** disfunción tiroidea; ~ **enlargement** estruma, bocio, engrosamiento del tiroides; ~ **functioning** funcionamiento de la tiroides; ~ **gland** glándula tiroidea; ~ **hormones** hormonas tiroideas; ~ **scan** gammagrafía tiroidea; ~ **-stimulating hormone** tirotropina, TSH

thyroliberin tiroliberina

thyropexin tiropexina

thyrostatic tirostático, sustancia que inhiben la biosíntesis y/o la secreción de hormonas tiroideas

thyrotoxicosis tirotoxicosis, conjunto de síntomas debido a un exceso de hormonas tiroideas

thyrotrophin tirotropina

thyrotropin-releasing factor tiroliberina

thyroxine tiroxina; ~ **5-deiodinase** tiroxina-desiodinasa; ~ **binding globulin** globulina enlazante de la tiroxina

tibia tibia, espinilla

tic tic, movimiento involuntario que se produce repetidamente; ~ **douloureux** tic doloroso, neuralgia del nervio trigémino, prosopalgia

ticarcillin ticarcilina

tick garrapata, caparra; ~ **-bite fever** fiebre americana, fiebre de picadura de garrapata; ~ **-borne disease** enfermedad transmitida por garrapata; ~ **fever** piroplasmosis, babesiasis, babesiosis

tickle, to cosquillas, cosquillear

tidal volume volumen de ventilación pulmonar

tightness tirantez, sensación de estrechez

tilt table mesa basculante

time tiempo, hora; ~ **cluster** agrupación temporal; ~ **off** tiempo libre, descanso

timed-release drug fármaco a difusión regulada, fármaco de liberación controlada

tincture tintura; ~ **of iodine** tintura de yodo

tinea tiña, una enfermedad de la piel producido por hongos; ~ **barbae** tiña de la barba, sicosis de la barba; ~ **pedis** tiña podal, infección superficial crónica con hongos de la piel del pie

tingle, to sentir hormigueo, sentir picazón

tingling parestesia, hormigueos, pinchazos

tinidazole tinidazol

tinnitus tinitus, tintineo, zumbido de oído, zumbidos, ruido de aleteo

tired agotado, debilitado, quemado, cansado

tiredness cansancio

tissue tejido; ~ **acidosis** acidosis tisular; ~ **antithromboplastin** antitromboplastina tisular; ~ **compatibility** histocompatibilidad; ~ **fluid** líquido tisular; ~ **polypeptide antigen** antígeno polipeptídico hístico; ~ **regeneration** neogénesis, regeneración; ~ **repair** regeneración, reconstitución; ~ **replacement** sustitución de tejidos; ~ **specific expression** expresión tisular específica; ~ **specimen** muestra de tejido; ~ **therapy** terapia tisular; ~ **thromboplastin** tromboplastina tisular; ~ **transplantation** terapia tisular

titanium dioxide dióxido de titanio

titration valoración

titre título, valor, grado, proporción

T lymphocyte linfocito T

TMN staging system sistema TNM de estadiaje

to a, para; ~ **be menstruating** tener la visita, tener la menstruación; ~ **have intense sexual appetites** ser de naturaleza fuerte; ~ **the left** a la izquierda; ~ **the right** a la derecha

tobacco tabaco; ~ **smoking** tabaquismo; ~ **use** tabaquismo

tobramycin tobramicina

tocopherol tocoferol, antioxidante

today hoy

toe dedo del pie

toilet aseo, servicio, baño, privada, inodoro, baño; **~ paper** papel de excusado, papel higiénico; **~ soap** jabón de tocador; **~ training** adiestramiento en el uso de excusados

tolbutamide tolbutamida

tolerability tolerabilidad

tolerance tolerancia, capacidad de soportar dosis elevadas de una droga tóxica; **~ test** prueba de tolerancia; **~ to stress** tolerancia al estrés

tolnaftate tolnaftato, un antifúngico sintético

tomographic scanner rastreador, ecógrafo

tomography tomografía, radiografía de una sección del cuerpo o de un órgano

tomorrow mañana

tone tensión, tono, potencial eléctrico, presión

toner astringente, que produce sequedad en la piel

tongue lengua; **~ blade** depresor de lengua; **~ depressor** sujetalengua

tonic tónico, que produce y restablece el tono normal, que se caracteriza por tensión continua

tonsil amígdala, angina, tonsila

tonsillar tonsilar

tonsillitis amigdalitis, tonsilitis, inflamación de una amígdala/angina

tooth diente; **~ ache** dolor de muelas, dolor de dientes, dentalgia; **~ brush** cepillo de dientes; **~ decay** caries; **~ erosion** erosión dentaria

toothpaste pasta dentífrica

tophus tofo, depósito de urato que se produce en caso de gota

topical tópico, local, restringido, no general; **~ availability** disponibilidad tópica; **~ corticosteroid** corticosteroide tópico

torn desgarro; **~ ligament** desgarro ligamentoso

torsade de pointes torsade de pointes (french)

torsion esguince, dislocación, torcedura, torsión; **~ dystonia** distonía muscular deformante; **~ of the testicle** torsión testicular

torticollis tortícolis, cuello torcido

torulosis criptococosis

torus uretericus pliegue interuretera

total total, absoluto; **~ aphasia** afasia completa; **~ blood** sangre

touch contacto, tacto; **~ , to** palpar

touchy irritable, quisquilloso, susceptible, colérico, irascible, arrebatadizo, sensitivo

tourniquet torniquete

towards en dirección

town localidad

toxemia toxemia, intoxicación de la sangre

toxic tóxico, venenoso; **~ epidermal necrolysis** necrólisis epidérmioca tóxica; **~ gas** gas tóxico; **~ hemolytic anemia** anemia hemolítica tóxica; **~ hepatitis** hepatitis tóxica; **~ level** concentración tóxica

toxicity toxicidad; **~ test** test de toxicidad, ensayo de toxicidad

toxicologic toxicológico, perteneciente o relativo a la ciencia que estudia los venenos

toxicological toxicológico, perteneciente o relativo a la ciencia que estudia los venenos

toxicology toxicología

toxicomania toxicomanía, dependencia de una droga, drogadicción

toxin toxina, veneno

toxoid anatoxina, toxoide

toxoplasma toxoplasma

toxoplasmatic chorioretinitis coriorretinitis por toxoplasma

toxoplasmosis toxoplasmosis

toxoplasmotic adenopathy adenopatía toxoplasmódica

t-PA (tissue-type plasminogen activator) activador hístico del plasminógeno, activador tisular del plasminógeno, activador de tejido plasminógeno

trabecula trabécula

trabecular trabecular; **~ adenoma** adenoma trabecular; **~ carcinoma** carcinoma trabecular, el carcinoma de célula de Merkel; **~ vein** vena trabecular

trace residual; **~ analysis** análisis de oligoelementos; **~ element** oligoelemento, elemento traza

traceability trazabilidad

tracer trazador; **~ atom** atomo marcado

traces huellas

trachea tráquea

tracheal traqueal; **~ cannula** cánula de traqueotomia; **~ swab** hisopo traqueal

tracheitis traqueítis, inflamación de la tráquea

trachelectomy traquelectomía
trachelitis cervicitis, inflamación del cuello del útero
tracheomalacia traqueomalacia, desgaste de la tráquea
tracheotomy traqueotomia
trachoma tracoma
tract haz de fibras, cordón, tracto
traction tratamiento por extensión, tracción; ~ **apparatus** aparato de tracción; ~ **device** aparato de tracción
trade sample muestra comercial; ~ **-off** solución de compromiso, equilibrio entre dos cosas, compensación recíproca, solución transaccional
traffic accident accidente de tráfico
trailer sequence secuencia remolque
training adiestramiento, aprendizaje
tranquilizer sedante, calmante, el sedativo
trans-acting responsive sequence secuencia de nucleótidos TAR, secuencia receptora en trans, secuencia TAR; ~ **fatty acid** ácido graso trans
transactivator gene gen trans-activador
transaminasa transaminasa, tipo de enzima
transaminasemia concentración de alanina-aminotransferasa en plasma
transcript transcrito, transcripto; ~ **mapping** cartografía del transcrito
transcription transcripción; ~ **factor** factor de transcripción; ~ **initiation site** sitio de iniciación de la transcripción
transcutaneous transcutáneo, a través de la piel intacta
transdermal transdérmico, que pasa a través de la piel; ~ **patch** parche transdermico
transducer transductor
transducing phage fago transductor
transfer transferencia, conducción, paso de un síntoma o una enfermedad de una parte hacia otra; ~ **factor** factor de transferencia; ~ **ribonucleic acid** ácido ribonucleico transferente; ~ **RNA** RNA de transferencia; ~ , **to** trasladar
transferability transferibilidad
transferase transferasa
transferrin transferrina
transformant transformado
transformation transformación, cambio de

forma o estructura
transfusion transfusión; ~ **of liquids** infusión
transgenetics transgenética
transgenic transgénico -ica; ~ **animal** animal transgénico, un animal modificado genéticamente; ~ **organism** organismo transgénico, organismo geneticamente modificado
transgressive segregation segregación transgresiva
transhepatic percutaneous cholangiography colangiografía percutanea transhepática
transient transitorio, pasajero; ~ **amnesia** amnesia lacunar; ~ **blindness** amaurosis fugax; ~ **ischemic attack** accidente isquémico transitorio, ataque de isquémia transitoria
transition transición; ~ **mutation** mutación transicional; ~ **tumor** tumor de transición
transitional lombosacral vertebra vértebra lumbar transicional
transitory transitorio, pasajero
transketolase transcetolasa
translation traducción
translational feedback regulation retrorregulación traduccional
translator traductor
translocation translocación; ~ **multivalent** multivalente de translocación; ~ **of chromosomes** transbordación de cromosomas
translucence transparencia, translucidez
transmissible trasmisible; ~ **mutations** mutaciones trasmisibles; ~ **spongiform encephalopathy** encefalopatía espongiforme transmisible, EET
transmission transmisión, transferencia; ~ **factor** factor de transmisión; ~ **of infection** transmisión de infección
transmittance transmitancia
transparency transparencia, translucidez
transparent transparente
transparietal liver biopsy biopsia hepática transparietal por aspiración
transpeptidase transpeptidasa
transpiration transpiración; ~ **efficiency** rendimiento de la transpiración
transplacental transplacentario
transplanation trasplante
transplant trasplante; ~ **bank** banco de órganos

transponible transponible

transport transporte; **~ medium** medio de transporte; **~ number** número de transporte; **~ protein** proteína transportadora

transposable element elemento transponible

transposition transposition

transposon transposón

transrectal transrectal; **~ ultrasound** ultrasonido transrectal

transthoracic transtorácico; **~ echography** ecografía torácica; **~ pressure** presión transtorácica

transtyretin transtiretina

transudate trasudado

transurethral transuretral, que conduce a través de la uretra o la atraviesa

trans-vaginal ultrasound ultrasonido transvaginal

transvalvular hernia hérnia trasvalvular

transversal transversal; **~ comparison** comparación transversal

transverse transverso; **~ colon** colon transverso; **~ diameter** diámetro transverso

trapezius muscle músculo trapecio

trash desechos

trauma lesión, daño, desperfecto, traumatismo, herida, lastimadura, trauma

traumatic traumático, perteneciente o relativo a un trauma o traumatismo, o causado por él; **~ arthritis** artritis traumática; **~ fever** fiebre traumática; **~ glycosuria** glucosuria de origen traumático; **~ neurosis** post-catastrophe syndrome; **~ retinal angiopathy** angiopatía retiniana traumática

traumatology traumatología

treat, to tratar; **~ with medicine, to** medicinar, curar, medicamentar, medicar, sanar

treating irradiated individuals tratamiento de personas irradiadas; **~ physician** médico adscrito, médico tratante, médico que atiende, médico curante

treatment tratamiento; **~ plan** plan terapéutico

tremble to temblar, estremecerse, tiritar, temblequear

tremor temblor; **~ of hands** temblor de las manos

trench foot pie de inmersión, pie de trinchera; **~ mouth** gingivitis necrótica, gingivitis ulcerosa

trend tendencia, disposición, predisposición

trepanation craniotomía, trepanación

tretinoin ácido retinoico, tretinoina

TRF tiroliberina

triamcinolone acetonide acetónido de triamcinolona

triazine triazina

triceps muscle músculo tríceps

trichinella larvae triquina

trichinosis triquinosis

trichloromethane cloroformo, triclorometano

trichomoniasis tricomoniasis

trickling instilación, administración de un líquido gota a gota

tricuspid valve válvula tricúspide

tricyclic tricíclico, constituido por tres anillos enlazados entre sí; **~ antidepressant** antidepresivo tricíclico; **~ compound** compuesto tricíclico

tridihexethyl chloride cloruro de tridihexetil

triethanolamine trolamina

trifacial nerve nervio trigémino

triflupromazine triflupromazina

trigeminal trigémino; **~ nerve** nervio trigémino; **~ neuralgia** tic doloroso, neuralgia del nervio trigémino, la prosopalgia

trigger factor causante; **~ zone** zona resorte, zona de excitabilidad aumentada

triglyceride triglicérido; **~ lipase** triacilglicerol-lipasa

triglyceridemia concentración de triglicérido en plasma/suero

triiodothyronine triiodotironina

trimeprazine trimepracina

trimethoprim trimetoprima

trimming glycosidase glucosidasa scindidora

triple triple, el triple, tres veces

trismus trismo, imposibilidad de apertura total de la boca

trisomic trisómico

trivalent trivalente, que se une con tres átomos de hidrógeno o los sustituye

trombidiasis trombidiosis

trophic trófico, nutritivo

trophism trofismo, vitalidad

trophoblast trofoblasto, capa externa de células del blastocisto

trophozoite

trophozoite trofozoito

tropical tropical; ~ **area** zona tropical; ~ **sprue** enfermedad celíaca

troponin T troponina T

trouble problema, dificultad, molestia

true verdadero; ~ **aneurysm** aneurisma verdadero; ~ **negative** negativo verdadero; ~ **positive** positivo verdadero; ~ **ribs** costillas verdaderas; ~ **value** valor verdadero

trueness veracidad

trypanosome tripanosoma, un especie de protozoo parasito

trypsin tripsina; ~ **inhibitors** inhibidores de tripsina

trypsinogen tripsinogeno; ~ **kinase** aspergilopepsina I

trypticase soy broth caldo con tripticasa de soja

tryptophan triptófano

tsetse fly mosca tsétsé

TSG (tumor suppressor gene) gen supresor de tumor

TSH tirotropina, TSH

tubal tubarico; ~ **abortion** aborto tubárico; ~ **ligature** ligadura de trompas, ligadura tubarica; ~ **obstruction** obstrucción tubaria; ~ **occlusion** oclusión tubarica

tube tubo; ~ **agglutination test** prueba de aglutinación en tubo; ~ **feeding** alimentación por sonda

tubercle tubérculo

tubercular tubercular, tísico

tuberculin tuberculina; ~ **patch test** prueba de la tuberculina

tuberculosis tuberculosis; ~ **vaccine** vacuna contra la tuberculosis

tuberculostatic tuberculostático, medicamento que inhibe el crecimiento del bacilo de la tuberculosis

tuberculous tuberculoso; ~ **abscess** absceso tuberculoso

tuberosity tuberosidad

tuberous tuberoso; ~ **angioma** angioma tuberoso; ~ **chorditis** corditis tuberosa; ~ **sclerosis** enfermedad de Bourneville, esclerosis cerebral tuberosa, epiloia

tubular tubular, que tiene forma de tubo; ~ **gauze** vendaje tubular, stockinette; ~ **necrosis** nefropatía tubular, necrosis tubular; ~ **obstruction** obstrucción tubular

tubulin tubulina

Tuesday martes

tuft of hair mata de pelo

tularemia tularemia

tumefaction tumefacción, hinchamiento

tummy barriga, panza, vientre; ~ **ache** dolor de vientre, dolor de estómago

tumor tumor, neoplasia, neoplasma; ~ **marker** marcador tumoral; ~ **necrosis factor** factor de necrosis tumoral; ~ **nodule** nódulo tumoral; ~ **suppressor gene** gen oncosupresor; ~ **virus** virus oncogénico, oncovirus

tumorigenic tumorigénico, cancerígeno, carcinogénico, oncogénico

tumorous tumoroso; ~ **involution** involución tumorosa

tumour tumor, neoplasma

tunica túnica; ~ **adventitia** túnica adventicia; ~ **externa** túnica adventicia; ~ **intima** túnica intima

tuning fork diapasón

tunneling tunelización

turbidimetric immunoassay inmunoanálisis turbidimétrico

turbidimetry turbidimetría, nefelometría

turbinate turbinado; ~ **bone** cornete; ~ **cell** célula turbinado

turnaround cambio de rumbo, giro radical, plazo; ~ **time** tiempo de entrega, tiempo de respuesta

Turner's syndrome síndrome de Turner

turning pale blanqueamiento; ~ **red-faced** eritema emotivo, rubor, ruborícese

turnover recambio, turnover (inglés)

turpentine terementina, aguarrás

tussive syncope síncope provocado por la tos

tweezers hierros, pinzas, tenacillas

twelve doce

twenty veinte

twice dos veces; ~ **a day** dos veces al día

twist esguince, dislocación, torcedura, torsión

twisted ankle esguince de tobillo

twisting esguince, dislocación, torcedura, torsión; ~ **number** número de vueltas helicoidales

twitch fasciculación, fibrilación; ~ , **to** crisparse

two dos; ~ **-dimensional** bidimensional; ~ **-horned** bicórneo; ~ **hundred** doscientos; ~ **-phase** difásico, que ocurre en dos fases; ~ **-sided** bilateral, que tiene dos lados, relativo a dos lados

tylectomy tumorectomia, mastectomia segmental

tympanic timpánico; ~ **crest** cresta timpánica; ~ **membrane** tímpano

tympanocentesis miringotomía

tympanogram timpanograma

tympanomastoid fissure cisura timpanomastoidea

tympanotomy miringotomía

type tipo; ~ **I diabetes** diabetes mellitus dependiente de insulina, diabetes de tipo I; ~ **II diabetes** diabetes que no es dependiente de insulina, diabetes de tipo II

typhoid tifoidea; ~ **fever** fiebre tifoidea, tifus abdominal

typhus tifus, tifo

typing tipificación

tyrosine tirosina; ~ **decarboxylase** tirosina descarboxilasa; ~ **kinase** tirosina quinasa

U

ubiquitin ubiquitina

ubiquitous ubiquo

ulcer ulcus (latín), úlcera

ulceration ulceración, proceso de formación de una úlcera

ulcerative ulcerante; ~ **colitis** colitis ulcerosa; ~ **gastritis** gastritis ulcerante; ~ **gingivitis** gingivitis necrótica, gingivitis ulcerosa

ulcerogenic ulcerógeno, que produce úlceras

ulcus cruris úlcera crural

ulna cúbito

ulnar cubital; ~ **nerve compression syndrome** síndrome de compresión del nervio ulnar

ultracentrifugation ultracentrifugación

ultracentrifuge ultracentrifugadora

ultrafiltration ultrafiltración

ultrasensitive con una gran detectabilidad

ultrasonic ultrasónico; ~ **lancet** lanceta ultrasónica; ~ **therapy** terapia por ultrasonido

ultrasonogram sonograma

ultrasonography ultrasonografía

ultrasound ultrasonido; ~ **examination** diagnóstico por ultrasonido, exploración ecográfica; ~ **scanning** ultrasonografía

ultrastructure ultraestructura

ultraviolet B radiation radiación ultravioleta B

umbilical umbilical; ~ **artery** arteria umbilical; ~ **cord** cordón umbilical; ~ **duct** conducto vitelino; ~ **hernia** hernia umbilical; ~ **region** región umbilical

umbilicus ombligo

unbearable insoportable, insufrible, inaguantable; ~ **pain** dolor insoportable

unbound no unido

unbuckle, to desabrocharse

uncarthrosis uncartrosis

uncertainty incertidumbre

uncle tío

unconscious inconsciente

unconsciousness falta de conocimiento, insensibilidad

uncooperative cooperativo, nada servicial, poco dispuesto a ayudar

under bajo, debajo de

underarm odor sobaquina, olor corporal, olor fétido asociado con la transpiración rancia

undercooked insuficientemente cocinado

underpants calzón, los calzoncillos

undershirt camiseta

understand, to entender

understanding comprensión

underwear ropa interior, lencería

underweight bajo peso, magro

undescended testicle criptorquidea, testículo no descendido

undifferentiated indiferenciado; ~ **epithelioma** epitelioma indiferenciado; ~ **leukemia** leucemia indiferenciada

undress, to desvestirse, desnudarse

uneasiness incomodidad, molestias, malestar

unfavorable dañino, nocivo, dañoso, pernicioso, desfavorable

unguis uña

unhealthy mórbido, malsano

unhurt ileso, incólume

U

unified unificado; ~ **atomic mass unit** unidad de masa atómica unificada

uniform homogéneo, uniforme, de la misma clase, de la misma especie, de estructura totalmente igual

unilateral unilateral, situado en un solo lado o que afecta un solo lado; ~ **compound pitting** punteado compuesto unilateralmente; ~ **subluxation** subluxación unilateral

unique único; ~ **number** número único

unit unidad; ~ **dose** dosis única

unlucky infausto

unprofessional antiprofesional, poco profesional

unruly intratable, indócil, malmandado

unsanitary insalubre, antihigiénico

unsaturated fatty acids ácidos grasos no saturados

unskilled midwife rinconera

unstable lábil, inestable, fácilmente modificable o alterable, inconstante; ~ **angina** angina inestable

unsteady gait tambaleos en la marcha, marcha inestable, inseguridad al andar

untwisting enzyme DNA-topoisomerasa

unusual atípico, irregular, que difiere de lo normal, anormal, inhabitual

unwanted pregnancy embarazo no deseado

unwinding protein proteína desenrolladora

unzip, to desabrocharse

up arriba; ~ **mutation** mutación aceleradora

u-plasminogen activator activador del u-plasminógeno

upon encima de

upper superior; ~ **abdomen pain** epigastralgia, dolor alrededor del estómago; ~ **airways** vías aerodigestivas; ~ **extremity** extremidad superior; ~ **lip** labio superior; ~ **motor neuron** neurona superior, neurona cortical; ~ **respiratory tract** tracto respiratorio superior; ~ **respiratory tract infection** infección de las vías respiratorias; ~ **urinary tract** as vías urinarias altas

upset distraído, irritado; ~ **stomach** estómago revuelto, gastritis

upstream río arriba

uptake absorción, captación, retención; ~ **of radionuclides** captación de radionucleidas

uracil uracilo, base nitrogenada pirimidínica que constituye el ARN

uranoschisis paladar hendido, boquinete, labio cucho

urate urato; ~ **oxidase** urato-oxidasa

urea urea; ~ **hydrolysis test** prueba de hidrólisis de la urea

urease ureasa

uremia uremia, acumulación de urea en la sangre

uremic urémico; ~ **colitis** colitis urémica; ~ **dyspnoea** disnea urémica

ureter uréter

ureteral ureteral; ~ **cancer** cáncer ureteral; ~ **catheter** catéter ureteral, sonda ureteral; ~ **diverticulum** divertículo ureteral; ~ **duplication** duplicidad verdadera; ~ **dystopia** distopia ureteral; ~ **fistula** fístula ureteral; ~ **resection** resección ureteral

ureteric fold pliegue interureteral

uretero-enteric anastomosis anastomosis ureteroentérica

ureteropyelography pielografía, urografía

urethra uretra, atraviesa, caño

urethral uretral; ~ **cancer** carcinoma ureteral; ~ **carcinoma** carcinoma uretral; ~ **exudate** exudado uretral; ~ **meatus** hoyito del chi; ~ **polyp** pólipo uretral

urethritis uretritis

urgency urgencia

uric úrico; ~ **acid** ácido úrico

uricemia concentración de urato en plasma

uricosuric uricosúrico, agente que promueve la secreción urinaria de ácido úrico

uridine uridina

urinal bacín, botella, orinal

urinalysis análisis de orina

urinary urinario; ~ **bladder** vejiga urinaria; ~ **calculus** cálculo urinario, cistolito, cálculo de la vejiga; ~ **cast** cilindro urinario; ~ **catheter** catéter, tubo urinario; ~ **discomfort** molestia al orinar; ~ **dribbling** goteo de orina; ~ **incontinence** incontinencia urinaria, incapacidad de control de la orina; ~ **infection** infección urinaria; ~ **output** diuresis, gasto urinario; ~ **plasminogen**

activator activador plasminógeno urinario;
~ **sediment** sedimento urinario;
~ **stone** cálculo urinario; ~ **tract** vías urinarias; ~ **tract disease** enfermedad de las vías urinarias;
~ **tract infection** infección urinaria; ~ **tract x-ray** urografía, radiografía del aparato urinario

urinate, to orinar, hacer pipí

urination micción (f), acción de orinar

urine orina; ~ **bottle** bacín, botella, orinal;
~ **culture** cultivo de la urina; ~ **degradation** degradación de la urea; ~ **retention** retención de orina; ~ **sample** muestra de orina, prueba de orina; ~ **sediment** sedimento urinario;
~ **specimen** prueba de orina; ~ **test** análisis de orina

uriniferous tubules tubulos uriníferos

urobilinogen urobilinógeno

urodynamic urodinámico; ~ **examination** exploración urodinámica

urogenital urogenital, referente a los órganos urinarios y sexuales; ~ **candidiasis** candidiasis urogenital, moniliasis

urography urografía, radiografía del aparato urinario

urokinase uroquinasa, una enzima producida en el riñón que es un activador del sistema fibrinolítico; ~ **-type plasminogen activator** activador plasminógeno urinario

urolith cálculo urinario

urologist urólogo

urology urología

uropoiesis uropoyesis

uroporphyrin uroporfirina

uroporphyrinogen–III synthase uroporfirinógeno–III-sintasa

urticaria habones, urticaria

urushiol urusiol

us nos

use uso; ~ **, to** usar, utilizar

usual acostumbrado, habitual

usually usualmente

uterine uterino; ~ **abrasion** curetaje, legrado uterino; ~ **colic** cólico uterino; ~ **contraction** contracción uterina; ~ **curettage** curetaje, legrado uterino; ~ **dilator** dilatador uterino;
~ **endometriosis** adenomiosis, endometriosis

uterina; ~ **fibroma** fibroma uterino; ~ **flexion** flexión del útero; ~ **hyperkinesia** hipercinesia uterina; ~ **leiomyoma** leiomioma, mioma uterino, tumor benigno y frecuente del músculo uterino; ~ **lining** pared uterina; ~ **rupture** rotura uterina

uterus útero, matriz

utricle utrículo

uvea úvea del ojo

uveitis uveítis, inflamación de la túnica vascular del ojo

uvula campanilla, úvula

V

vaccinate, to inocular, vacunar

vaccination vacunación, inmunización;
~ **keloid** reacción vacunal queloide, pseudoqueloide postvacunal

vaccine vacuna

vaccinia vacuna

vacuant laxante, un medicamento contra el estreñimiento

vacuolation vacuolación

vacuole vacuola

vagal vagal, perteneciente o relativo al nervio vago, décimo nervio craneal

vagina vagina

vaginal vaginal, que afecta a la vagina;
~ **atresia** atresia vaginal; ~ **canal** conducto vaginal; ~ **candidiasis** candidiasis vaginal;
~ **contents** contenido vaginal; ~ **discharge** flúor albus, flujo blanco, pérdidas blancas, excreción vaginal; ~ **douche** aplicación de duchas; ~ **dryness** sequedad vaginal;
~ **hematoma** hematoma vaginal; ~ **insert** óvulo vaginal; ~ **jelly** gelatina vaginal, jalea espermicida; ~ **ovule** óvulo vaginal; ~ **plexus** plexo vaginal; ~ **ring** anillo vaginal;
~ **secretion** secreción vaginal; ~ **spasm** vaginismo; ~ **speculum** espéculo de Barnes, espéculo vaginal; ~ **suppository** óvulo vaginal; ~ **tablet** comprimido vaginal

vaginismus vaginismo

vaginitis vaginitis, colpitis, una infección

vaginal

vaginomycosis micosis vaginal

vaginoperitoneal hydrocele hidrocele vaginoperitoneal

vagolytic vagolítico

vagotomy vagotomía

vagotonia vagotonía, excitabilidad aumentada del nervio vago

vague illness malestar (m)

vagus nerve nervio vago, par cranial esencial para el lenguaje y la deglución

valerian opoponaco, valeriana; ~ **herb tea** infusión de valeriana

validity validez

valine valina

Valium Valium

valproic acid ácido valproico

Valsalva's maneuver maniobra de Valsalva

value valor

valvular valvular; ~ **aneurysm** aneurisma valvular; ~ **pneumothorax** neumotórax valvular; ~ **regurgitation** insuficiencia de la válvula pulmonar, insuficiencia pulmonar

valvule válvula

van de Kamer test determinación de lípido en heces

vancomycin vancomicina

vaporizer evaporador, nebulizador

variability variabilidad

variable variable; ~ **gene** gen variable

variance variancia

variation variación, modificación de propiedades

varicella varicela, viruela loca; ~ **vaccine** vacuna contra la varicela; ~ **-zoster virus** virus varicella-zóster, herpesvirus 3 humano, virus de la varicela

varicelliform diphtheria difteria variceliforme

varicosclerosation tratamiento esclerosante de las varices

varicose veins varices

varicosity varicosidad, venas varicosas

varix varix, varices

varus foot pie varo

vas deferens conducto deferente

vascular vascular, referido a los vasos sanguíneos; ~ **collagen disease** estenosis de la válvula pulmonar, síndrome de Goodpasture; ~ **doppler** Doppler vascular; ~ **goiter** estruma aneurismática; ~ **mole** masa sanguínea; ~ **prosthesis** prótesis arterial, prótesis vascular; ~ **spider** araña vascular; ~ **system** sistema vascular; ~ **volume** volumen sanguíneo

vascularization vascularización

vasculitis vasculitis, inflamación de los vasos sanguíneos

vasectomy vasectomía

vaseline vaselina

vasoactive vasoactivo, que ejerce un efecto sobre el calibre de los vasos sanguíneos

vasoconstriction vasoconstricción, estrechamiento de los vasos sanguíneos

vasoconstrictive agents vasoconstrictores

vasoconstrictors vasoconstrictores

vasodilatation vasodilatación, dilatación de los vasos sanguíneos; ~ **murmur** soplo de expulsión

vasodilator vasodilatador directo

vasofunctional hematuria hematuria angioneurótica, hematuria vasofuncional

vasomotor vasomotor, que afecta al calibre de los vasos; ~ **ataxia** ataxia vasomotriz; ~ **rhinitis** rinitis vasomotora

vasoparalysis vasoparálisis, vasoplegia

vasopressin vasopresina; ~ **-resistant diabetes** diabetes insipida nefrogenica

vasopressor vasopresor, agente que estimula la contracción del tejido muscular de los capilares y las arterias

vasovagal syncope crisis sincopal, síndrome de Gowers

vector vector

vectorcardiogram vectocardiograma

vegetables verduras

vegetative vegetativo, que funciona de manera involuntaria o inconsciente; ~ **reflex** reflejo vegetativo

vehicle vehículo, transportador, (farma) excipiente

vein vena; ~ **x-ray** flebografía, radiografía de una o más venas

velocity velocidad

velopharyngeal insufficiency insuficiencia velofaringea, insuficiencia palatofaringea

vena cava veina cava; ~ **compression syndrome** síndrome de compresión de la cava inferior; ~ **infundibulum** infundíbulo de la veina cava

venereal venéreo; ~ **bubo** bubón venéreo; ~ **disease** enfermedad venérea; ~ **lymphogranuloma** linfogranuloma venéreo, linfopatía venérea

veno–arterial shunting shuntado venoso

venography flebografía radiológica, venografía

venombin venombina A

venous venoso, perteneciente o relativo a las venas, que está provisto de venas; ~ **admixture** shuntado venoso; ~ **blood** sangre venosa, sangre desoxigenada; ~ **congestion** congestión venosa; ~ **doppler** Doppler venoso; ~ **hyperemia** hiperemia venosa; ~ **occlusion** oclusión venosa; ~ **return** retorno venoso

ventilation ventilación, aireación por la respiración; ~ **pneumonitis** fiebre de las humidificadoras

ventilator respirador, aparato respiratorio

ventral ventral, relativo al vientre, delante de un punto de referencia

ventricle (of heart) ventrículo (cardiaco)

ventricular ventricular, perteneciente o relativo a una pequeña cavidad; ~ **depolarization** despolarización ventricular; ~ **fibrillation** fibrilación atrial; ~ **flutter** flúter ventricular; ~ **pressure** presión ventricular; ~ **response** respuesat ventricular; ~ **rhythm** ritmo idioventricular; ~ **septal defect** comunicación interventricular

ventriculogram ventriculografia

ventriculography ventriculografia

Verneuil's disease hidrosadenitis supurativa

verruca vulgaris mesquino, verruga común

versus contra

vertebra vértebra

vertebrae vértebras

vertebral vertebral, perteneciente o relativo a las vértebras; ~ **artery** arteria vertebral; ~ **column** columna vertebral

vertebrosternal ribs costillas verdaderas

vertical vertical

vertigo mareos, mal de altura, soroche, vértigo

very muy; ~ **well** muy bien

vesanic dementia delirio onírico, demencia vesánica, onirismo

vesical vesical; ~ **atrophy** atrofia de la vejiga; ~ **distension** distensión vesical; ~ **paralysis** parálisis de la vejiga

vesicle ampolla, vesícula, vejiga, bullón, roncha; ~ **syringe** jeringuilla para irrigación

vesico–uterine vesicouterino; ~ **fistula** fístula vesicouterina; ~ **ligaments** ligamentos vesicouterinos

vesicovaginal vesicovaginal; ~ **fistula** fístula vesicovaginal; ~ **interposition of the uterus** interposición vesicovaginal del útero

vesicular vesicular, en forma de vesícula o ampolla, con formación de vesículas o ampollas; ~ **enanthema** enantema vesicular; ~ **endometriosis** endometriosis vesical; ~ **mole** mola hidatídica, mola hidatidiforme, lentigo; ~ **stomatitis** estomatitis vesicular

vestibular vestibular, perteneciente o relativo a un vestíbulo o que se dirige a él; ~ **ataxia** ataxia vestibular; ~ **nerve** nervio vesticular; ~ **neuritis** neuritis vestibular

vestibulocochlear nerve nervio estatoacústico

vestigial rudimentario, vestigial

veterinarian veterinario

veterinary veterinario; ~ **medicine** medicina veterinaria

viable viable; ~ **aerobic bacteria** bacterias aerobias viables; ~ **embryo** embrión viable

vial ampolla, vial

vibrator aparato de vibromasaje, máquina eléctrica de masaje, vibrador

vibratory–massage device aparato de vibromasaje, máquina eléctrica de masaje, vibrador

victim victima; ~ **of a disaster** siniestrado, accidentado; ~ **of an accident** siniestrado, accidentado

video surgery video-cirugía

Vienna paste pasta de Viena

vif gene (virion infectivity factor gene) gen vif

vigilance vigilia, estado de alerta o de observación

villous velloso; ~ **arthritis** artritis vellosa; ~ **carcinoma** carcinoma velloso

vinca alkaloids alcaloides de la vinca

V

Vincent's bacillus Fusobacterium fusiforme; ~ **gingivitis** gingivitis necrótica, gingivitis ulcerosa

vinegar vinagre

vinorelbine vinorelbina

violent violento, fuerte; ~ **death** muerte violenta; ~ **hemoptysis** hemoptisis severa

viper víbora

virago virago, hombruna

viral viral, perteneciente o relativo a los virus, causado por ellos; ~ **DNA** ADN vírico; ~ **hepatitis** hepatitis vírica, hepatitis infecciosa; ~ **meningitis** meningitis aséptica, meningitis viral; ~ **oncogene** oncogén vírico; ~ **particle** virión; ~ **pneumonia** neumonía viral

Viramune Viramune

viremia viremia

virgin virgen

virile viril, masculino, varonil

virilism virilismo, masculinidad

virilization virilización, masculinización

virion virión; ~ **protein** proteína del virión

viroid viroide

virological virológico; ~ **examination** examen virológico

virology virología; ~ **laboratory** laboratorio de virología; ~ **workup** examen virológico

virulence virulencia

virulent virulento; ~ **bacteria** bacterias virulentas; ~ **bacteriophages** bacteriófagos virulentos; ~ **strain** cepa virulenta

virus virus; ~ **free** exento de virus; ~ **suspension** suspensión de virus

visceral visceral, perteneciente o relativo a una víscera; ~ **pleura** pleura visceral

visceroptosis visceroptosis abdominal

viscid mucus flema, esputo, pituita

viscosity viscosidad, grado de fluidez de las sustancias en estado líquido o gaseoso

visible manifiesto, ostensible, evidente, visible

vision visión; ~ **chart** cuadro de agudeza visual, tabla oftálmica; ~ **problems** problemas de visión; ~ **test** examen de la vista

visual visual, relativo a la visión; ~ **acuity** agudeza visual; ~ **cortex** corteza viaula; ~ **disturbance** trastorno visual; ~ **memory** memoria visual

visually visualmente; ~ **evoked potentials** potenciales evocados visuales; ~ **impaired** cierta medida, ciego; ~ **impaired person** discapacitado de la vista

vital vital; ~ **bodily functions** principales funciones corporales; ~ **capacity** capacidad vital; ~ **energy** qi, energía vital; ~ **organ** órgano vital; ~ **signs** signos vitales; ~ **statistics** estadísticas vitales, estadística relativa al estado civil

vitality vitalidad

vitamin vitamina; ~ **A** retinol; ~ **B1** tiamina, vitamina B1; ~ **B9** vitamina B9, ácido folic, folacin, folate; ~ **B12** cobalamina, vitamina B12, cianocobalamina, hidroxocobalamina; ~ **C** vitamina C, ácido ascorbico; ~ **D (calciferol)** vitamina D (calciferol); ~ **D2** ercalciol, vitamina D2; ~ **D3** colecalciferol, vitamina D3; ~ **deficiency symptoms** síntomas carenciales, mal carencial, enfermedad por carencia de vitaminas; ~ **E** tocoferol; ~ **H** biotina, vitamina H

vitelline vitelino; ~ **duct** conducto vitelino; ~ **membrane** membrana vitelina

vitiligo vitíligo

vitrectomy vitrectomía

vitreous vítreo, cristalino; ~ **humor** cuerpo vítreo, humor vítreo

VLDL cholesterol colesterol de lipoproteínas de muy baja densidad, colesterol de VLDL

vocal vocal; ~ **audiometry** audiometría vocal, audiometría de la palabra; ~ **cords** cuerdas vocales; ~ **fremitus** vibraciones vocales

vocational vocacional; ~ **counseling** orientación profesional, consejería profesional; ~ **rehabilitation** rehabilitación vocacional; ~ **retraining** rehabilitación profesional

voice voz; ~ **therapy** terapia de la voz

voicebox laringe

volar palmar

volatile volátil; ~ **fatty acid** ácido graso volátil

Vollmer's test prueba de la tuberculina

volt volt

voltage-gated potassium channels canales de potasio con entrada de voltaje

volume volumen; ~ **deficiency collapse** shock hipovolémico; ~ **fraction** fracción de volumen

volumetric flask matraz aforado; **~ pipet** pipeta aforada

volumetry volumetría

volumic volúmico -ica; **~ mass** masa volúmica

voluntary voluntario, voluntaria; **~ muscle** músculo estriado, músculo de contracción voluntaria

volunteer voluntario, voluntaria

vomit, to estar nauseado, vomitar, tener náuseas

vomiting emesis, vómito; **~ blood** hematemesis, vómitos de sangre; **~ reflex** reflejo de vómitar

vomitus emesis, vómito

von Recklinghausen's disease neurofibromatosis, polifibromatosis neurocutánea pigmentaria, enfermedad de Recklinghausen, osteítis fibroquística

vortex vórtice; **~ mix** mezcla vorticial

vulva vulva

vulval vulvar, perteneciente o relativo a los órganos sexuales externos de la mujer

vulvitis vulvitis

vulvovaginal candidiasis candidiasis vulvovaginal, vulvovaginitis por Candida

vulvovaginitis vulvovaginitis

W

waist cintura

waiting list lista de espera

waking dream state delirio onírico, demencia vesánica, onirismo

walk, to caminar; **~-in clinic** clínica sin cita previa; **~ on tiptoes, to** caminar de puntillas

walker andador, andadera

walking on one's heels marcha sobre los talones; **~ stick** bordón

wall pared; **~ of the intestine** pared intestinal; **~ of the stomach** pared del estomago

wan decaído, apático

warble tumor barro de tabano, miasis furunculoide

ward sala, pabellón; **~ for infectious diseases** sala de enfermos infecciosos

warfarin cumafeno, warfarin

warm up, to precalentarse, aflojarse, entrar en calor

warming pad almohada eléctrica, cojín eléctrico

wash irrigación (f), riego o aporte sanguíneo; **~, to** raspar, fregar, afretar

washcloth paño para lavarse, manopla

washing irrigación, riego o aporte sanguíneo; **~ out** elutriación, decantación, aplicación de duchas

wasp avispa

waste desechos; **~ passage** cloaca, parte posterior de los intestinos del embrión

wastewater aguas residuales

wasting atrofia; **~ away** caquexia, adelgazamiento extremo, debilitación general; **~ paralysis** atrofia muscular; **~ syndrome** caquexia busulfánica

water agua; **~ –borne disease** enfermedad de transmisión hídrica, la enfermedad hídrica; **~ closet** baño, inodoro; **~ jet** chorro de água (en una alberca); **~ pills** píldoras para sacar el agua; **~ retention** retención hídrica; **~ sparkling** agua con gaz

watery acuoso, diluído, que contiene agua

watt watt

wave onda

wavelength longitud de onda

wavenumber número de onda

wax bath baño de parafina

waxy céreo; **~ cast** cilindro céreo; **~ liver** hígado amiloideo, hígado cireo

WBC leucocito; **~ cast** cilindro leucocitario; **~ count** concentración de leucocitos en sangre, medida de la concentración de leucocitos; **~ differential count** recuento diferencial leucocitario, fórmula leucocitaria

we nosotros, -as

weak débil

weaken, to atenuar, reducir

weakened agotado, debilitado, quemado, cançado

weakness astenia, cansancio físico intenso, debilidad corporal general, falta de fuerza

weaning destete

wearable defibrillator desfibrilador llevadero

weariness lasitud, debilidad, cansancio, agotamiento, laxitud

weather tiempo

weave, to tambalear, titubear

wedge-shaped piramidal, cuneiforme

Wednesday miércoles

week semana

Weeks bacillus Haemophilus influenzae

weeping ear otorrea, derrame que tiene lugar por la oreja

Wegener's granulomatosis granulomatosis de Wegener

weight peso; ~ **gain, to** engordar, aumentar de peso; ~ **lifting** levantamiento de pesos/pesas; ~ **loss** enflaquecimiento, pérdida de peso

weightlessness ingravidez

Weil's disease enfermedad de Weil, leptospirosis

Welch-Frankel's bacillus Clostridium perfringens

welder's eyes ojos de soldador; ~ **lung** siderosis

welfare bienestar; ~ **state** estado benefactor, estado asistencial

well bien; ~ **-being** bienestar; ~ **differentiated cell** célula bien diferenciada; ~ **-muscled** bien musculado, muscular

wellness salud, sanidad, salubridad, buena salud, buen estado

welt verdugo, patacón, verdugón, roncha

Werner's syndrome sindrome de Werner

Wernicke's encephalopathy encefalopatía alcohólica

West Nile fever virus virus del Nilo occidental

western blot transferencia western

wet mojado; ~ **nurse** nodriza

wettability humectabilidad, mojabilidad

what qué

wheat trigo

wheelchair silla de ruedas

wheeled stretcher camilla con ruedas, portacama rodante, parihuelas

wheeze, to resollar, respirar con dificultad, silbar el pecho

wheezing roncus, sonido asmático, respiración sibilante

when cuando

where donde

which qué

while durante

whiner llorón, gimoteador, llorona

whiplash cuello lastimado, golpe de conejo, lesión del latigazo

Whipple's disease enfermedad de Whipple; ~ **operation** duodenopancreatectomía

whirlpool bath bañera de hidromasaje, baño de remolino

whistling roncus, sonido asmático, respiración sibilante

white caucasiano, blanco; ~ **blood cell** glóbulo blanco, leucocito; ~ **blood cell count** recuento de los glóbulos blancos de la sangre; ~ **matter** substancia blanca; ~ **matter of the cerebellum** substancia blanca del cerebro; ~ **poppy** adormidera, amapola real, adormidera soporífera

whitish blanquecino, blancuzco

whitlow panadizo

Whitmore's bacillus Pseudomonas pseudomallei

who quién

WHO (World Health Organization) Organización Mundial de la Salud, OMS

whole intacto; ~ **blood** sangre total, sangre íntegra, sangre pura, sangre entera, sangre completa; ~ **body scanner** rastreador del cuerpo entero

wholeness integridad, conservación inalterada

whooping cough pertussis, tos ferina, coqueluche

why por qué

Widal test prueba de Widal

wide ancho, extenso, vasto; ~ **eyes** dilatación pupilar, midriasis

widely distributed difundido, disperso, extendido

widow viuda

widowed viudo

widower viudo

width anchura

wife esposa

Wilkins-Chalgren agar agar de Wilkins-Chalgren

willingness to pay disponibilidad a pagar

Wilson's disease enfermedad de Wilson, degeneración hepatolenticular

wind meteorismo, presencia de gas en el vientre o intestino

window period período ventana, etapa de latencia

windpipe tráquea

wine vino

wink, to destellar, parpadear, pestañear

winter invierno; ~ **blues** trastorno afectivo estacional; ~ **itch** dermatitis hiemalis, pruritis invernal

wipe, to secarse, enjugar, resecar, desecar, enjugar, limpearse

wire alambre, cable; ~ **mesh stent** malla metálica stent, prótesis intraventricular

wisdom sabiduría; ~ **tooth** muela del juício

wise sabio

witch doctor merolico, curandero, sanador

with con; ~ **me** conmigo

withdraw, to retirar

withdrawal supresión

within dentro de; ~**run imprecision** imprecisión intraserial; ~**subject biological variation** variación biológica intraindividual, variabilidad biológica intraindividual

Wolff–Parkinson–White syndrome síndome de Wolff-Parkinson-White

woman mujer; ~ **'s period** regla

womb útero, matriz; ~ **neck** cervix uterino, cuello uterino

women's panties bragas, braguitas, pantimediás; ~ **underwear** bragas, braguitas, pantimediás

wonky eyes nistagmo ocular, nistagmo

woozy mareado, aturdido, ligeramente indispuesto, delirante; ~ **, to be** estar mareado, sentirse desfalleciente

work, to trabajar; ~ **out, to** hacer ejercicios; ~ **posture** postura en el trabajo; ~**related disability** incapacidad profesional, discapacidad laboral, invalidez profesional; ~ **up, to** elaborar

worker trabajador; ~ **in a factory** trabajador en una fábrica

workers' compensation indemnización por accidente laboral, indemnización por accidente de trabajo; ~ **compensation insurance** seguro de accidentes del trabajo, indemnización de accidentes del trabajo; ~ **compensation offset** descuento (compensado) por compensación de trabajadores

workout entrenamiento, ejercicio

workplace lugar de trabajo; ~ **hazard** peligro en el lugar de trabajo

workshop seminario, taller

workup elaboración de una séria de pruebas médicas

worm lombriz, gusano

wormwood ajenjo, lombriz de la madera

worn out sin fuerzas, agotado, debilitado, decrépito, desvaído, endeble, vetusto

worry aprensión, preocupación

worse peor

worsening agravamiento, empeoramiento, exacerbación

wound lesión, daño, desperfecto, traumatismo, herida, lastimadura; ~ **closure** cierre de una herida; ~ **parasite** parásito facultativo; ~ **suture** sutura; ~ **swab** hisopo para tomar muestras; ~ **, to** herir, lastimar

wreak havoc, to causar estragos, destrozar

wrenching pain tirones

Wright stain tinción de Wright

wrinkled arrugado, surcado de arrugas

Wrisberg's cartilage cartílago cuneiforme, cartílago de Wrisberg

wrist muñeca, carpo; ~ **bones** huesos del carpo; ~ **joint** carpo, articulación de la muñeca, articulación radio carpiana; ~ **luxation** luxación de la muñeca, luxación radiocarpiana

write, to escribir

writhing number número de vueltas superhelicoidales

X

xanthin xantina

xanthine oxidase xantina-oxidasa

xanthoma xantoma (m), tumoración benigna

xanthomatosis corneae xantomatosis de la córnea, distrofia adiposa de la córnea

xanthopsia xantopsia, visión amarillenta

X-autosome translocation translocación de X-autosomas

xenobiotic xenobiótico; ~ **compound** compuesto xenobiótico; ~ **substance** sustancia xenobiótica, compuesto xenobiótico

xenodiagnosis xenodiagnóstico

xenogenic xenogénico, heterógeno
xenon xenón; ~ **effect** efecto xenón;
~ **poisoning** envenenamiento por el xenón
xenotransplant injerto heterólogo,
xenotrasplante, heteroimplante
xeroderma xerodermia
xerophthalmia xeroftalmía, sequedad del globo
ocular
xerostomia xerostomía
xerotic keratitis queratitis xerótica
x-ray radiografía, rayos x; ~ **dermatitis**
radiodermitis, dermatitis radiográfica;
~ **pelvimetry** pelvimetría radiográfica
X-scanning exploración longitudinal
xylometazoline xilometazolina
xylose xilosa
xyster xister, raspador

Y

YAC (yeast artificial chromosom) cromosoma
artificial de levadura
yawn, to bostezar
year año
yeast levadura; ~ **extract** extracto de levadura
yellow amarillo; ~ **cartilage** cartílago elástico;
~ **fever** fiebre amarilla; ~ **vision** xantopsia,
visión amarillenta
yellowish complexion tinte ictérico, tinte
amarillento
Yersinia pestis pasteurella pestis
yes sí
yesterday ayer
yogurt yogur
you tú (sg), usted / Vd. (s, formal), vosotros (mp),
-as (fp) (fam), ustedes / Vds. (p, formal)
young joven
your tu (fam), vuestro (ms), -a (fs), su (formal),
tus (fam), vuestros (mp), -as (fp), sus (formal)
youth juventud; ~ **counseling center** centro de
orientación de la juventud
Y-scanning exploración transversal
yttrium itrio, un elemento químico

Z

zalcitabine zalzitabina, didesoxicitidina
zanamivir zanamivir
zeaxanthin zeaxantina, E161h
Zenker's crystals cristales asmáticos de
Charcot-Leyden
zero cero; ~ **gravity** ingravidez
zeta potential potencial zeta
zidovudine AZT, cidovudina, zidovudina,
azidotimidina
Ziehl-Neelsen stain tinción de Ziehl-Neelsen
ZIFT (zygote intrafallopian transfer)
transferencia intratubaria de zigotos
zinc zinc; ~ **chills** fiebre del fundidor de cinc;
~ **disease** fiebre del fundidor de cinc; ~ ~
finger dedo de zinc; ~ **fume fever** fiebre del
fundidor de cinc; ~ **oxide** óxido de cinc;
~ **oxide paste** pomada de óxido de cinc;
~ **sulphate** sulfato de cinc
zip code zona postal, código postal, C.P.
zoledronic acid ácido zoledrónico
zoonosis zoonosis, enfermedades transmitidas
por algunos animales al ser humano
zootechnical zootécnico; ~ **additive** aditivo
zootécnico; ~ **treatment** tratamiento
zootécnico
zootherapy zooterapia
zwitterion ión anfótero, amfoion, ion dipolar,
ion híbrido
zygoma hueso malar
zygomatic cigomático; ~ **arch** arco cigomático;
~ **bone** pómulo, hueso malar
zygote zigoto, cigoto, óvulo fecundado;
~ **intrafallopian transfer** transferencia
intratubaria de zigotos
zygotene cigotena, anfiteno
zygotic zigótico; ~ **induction** inducción zigótica
zymogen zimógeno
zymogenic bacteria zimógenos, cimógenos
zymotic zimótico

Spanish – English
Dictionary

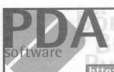

A

a to, by; **~ dentro** into; **~ desde** from; **~ él** him; **~ ellos, –as** them; **~ la derecha** right, to the right; **~ la izquierda** left, to the left; **~ medianoche** at midnight; **~ mediodía** at noon; **~ mí** me; **~ través** de through; **~ través** across

abajo down

abdomen *m* abdomen, gut; **~ m agudo** acute abdomen, surgical abdomen; **~ m hinchado** swollen abdomen, swollen belly

abdominal *adj* abdominal, gut-related

abdominoplastia *f* abdominoplasty, abdominal panniculectomy, cosmetic surgery of the abdomen

abducción *f* abduction; **~ f forzada** forced abduction

abductor *m* abductor

abeja *f* bee

aberración *f* aberration; **~ f cromosómica** chromosomal aberration, chromosome aberration, mutation of chromosome

aberrante *adj* aberrant, irregular, abnormal

abetalipoproteinemia *f* abetalipoproteinemia

abierto *adj* open

abiogénesis *f* abiogenesis, spontaneous generation

abiotrofia *f* abiotrophy

ablación *f* ablation, extirpation, the removal of an organ by surgery; **~ del vítreo** ablation of vitreum; **~ f por cateter** radiofrequency catheter ablation, transvenous electric ablation, catheter ablation, percutaneous catheter ablation; **~ f por radiofrecuencia** radiofrequency catheter ablation, transvenous electric ablation, catheter ablation, percutaneous catheter ablation

ablandar *v* to soften

abocamiento *m* bypass, shunt

abogar mediate, to

abombar *v* to bulge, protrude

abordaje *m* incision

aborto *m* abortion, miscarriage; **~ m espontáneo** sub-clinical spontaneous abortion; **~ m espontáneo subclínico** sub-clinical spontaneous abortion; **~ m habitual** habitual abortion, three or more consecutive spontaneous abortions; **~ m incipiente** incipient abortion; **~ m infectado** septic abortion; **~ m provocado** induced abortion, therapeutic abortion; **~ m séptico** septic abortion; **~ m tubárico** tubal abortion

abotagado *adj* distended, rounded swollen, bloated

abrasión *f* abrasion, graze, curettage, decortication, scraping off; **~ f corneal** abrasion of the cornea, corneal abrasion

abrazaderas *f pl* braces (limbs), band clasp

abreacción *f* abreaction

abreboca *m* gag, bite block, mouth prop, rubber mouth-gag

abril *m* April

abruptio *m* **placentae** premature detachment of placenta, abruptio placentae

abrupto *adj* abrupt, sudden

absceso *m* abscess; **~ m cerebral** brain abscess, cerebral abscess; **~ m estéril** sterile abscess; **~ m intraperitoneal** peritoneal abscess, encysted peritonitis; **~ m nefrítico** nephritic abscess; **~ m paravesical** paravesical abscess; **~ m periuretral** periurethral abscess; **~ m puerperal** puerperal sepsis, puerperal infection, puerperal eclampsia, puerperal abscess; **~ m subperióstico** subperiosteal abscess

abscisión *f* excision, abscision; **~ f quirúrgica** surgical excision, surgical abscision

absorbancia *f* absorbance, extinction, optical density; **~ f decimal** decadic absorbance; **~ f linéica** lineic absorbance

absorbencia *f* absorbency

absorción *f* uptake, absorption, retention; **~ f gastrointestinal** gastrointestinal absorption

absortividad *f* absorptivity; **~ f decimal molar** molar decadic absorptivity

abstinencia *f* abstinence, going without, refraining, drug withdrawal

abuela *f* grandmother

abuelo *m* grandfather

abulia *f* abulia, debilitation of the will, bewilderment

abultamiento *m* puff, bulge, protrusion

abultar v to bulge, to protrude

abusar v to injure, to harm, to abuse, to hurt

abuso m abuse; ~ m **de alcohol** alcohol abuse, alcoholism; ~ m **de fármacos** drug use, drug consumption, drug abuse; ~ m **de medicamentos** pharmacomania, abusive taking of drugs

abusos m pl **perpetrados contra los niños** child abuse

acalasia f achalasia; ~ f **del esofago** esophageal achalasia, constriction of the lower portion of the esophagus, cardiospasm

acalenturado adj feverish

acantocitosis f acanthocytosis

acariasis f acariasis, infestation with or disease caused by mites

ácaro adj mite

ácaros m pl **de la sarna** mange mites

acatafasia f agrammatism, acataphasia

acatarrarse v to catch a cold

acatisia f achatisia, cathisophobia, an urge to move about and an inability to sit still

acceso m attack, access, seizure, convulsions; ~ m **aleatorio** random acces; ~ m **cortical** cortical attack; ~ m **psicomotor** psychomotor attack; ~ m **secuencial** sequential acces; ~ m **selectivo** selective acces

accidentado m victim of a disaster, victim of an accident, casualty

accidental adj accidental

accidente m accident; ~ m **cerebrovascular agudo** apoplexy, stroke, cerebrovascular accident; ~ m **de trabajo** accident at work; ~ m **de tráfico** traffic accident; ~ **isquémico transitorio** m ischemic attack, mini-stroke, small stroke

acción f action; ~ f **alucinógena** hallucinatory action; ~ f **cito-tóxica** cytotoxic effect; ~ f **de orinar** micturition, urination; ~ f **farmacológica** pharmacological action

acciones f pl **por daños y perjuicios** claim for damages, claim for compensation

acedías f pl heartburn, pyrosis, cardialgia, pain in the heart area

acefalia f acephalia, acephaly

aceite m oil; ~ m **alcanforado** camphor oil, camphorated oil; ~ m **de almendra** almond oil; ~ m **de inmersión** immersion oil; ~ m **de**

ricino castor oil; ~ m **mineral** mineral oil

aceitoso adj oily, greasy

aceleración f acceleration; ~ f **del pulso** increase in the pulse rate

acelerador m **lineal de partículas** linear accelerator

acelerar v to accelerate; ~ v **una reacción química** to catalyse, to speed up (a cemical reaction)

acenocumarol m nicoumalone

acérrimo adj persistent

acetábulo m acetabulum

acetato-cinasa f acetate kinase

acetazolamida f acetazolamide

acetil f **cisteína** acetyl cysteine

acetilación f acetylation

acetilcoenzima A m acetylcoenzyme A, coenzyme A

acetilcolina f acetylcholine

acetilcolinesterasa f acetylcholinesterase, cholinesterase, true cholinesterase

acetoacetato m acetoacetato

acetona f acetone; ~ f **de ayuno** inanition acetone from fasting

acetónido m acetonide

acetonuria f ketonuria, acetonuria

acezar v to gasp, to have trouble breathing

achaque m systemic weakness

achicar v to shrink

aciclovir m acyclovir

acidez f acidity; ~ f **gástrica** stomach acidity, gastric acid secretion; ~ f **reactiva** acid rebound

acidificación f acidifying, acidification

ácido m acid; ~ m **acetilsalicílico** aspirin, acetylsalicylic acid; ~ m **acetoacético** acetoacetic acid; ~ m **aminobutírico** aminobutyric acid; ~ m **aminolevulínico** aminolevulinic acid; ~ m **ascórbico** ascorbic acid, ascorbate, vitamin C; ~ m **barbitúrico** barbituric acid; ~ m **biliar** bile acid; ~ m **butanoico** butyric acid, butanoic acid, ethylacetic acid; ~ m **butírico** butyric acid, butanoic acid, ethylacetic acid; ~ m **cianhídrico** hydrogen cyanide, hydrocyanic acid, HCN; ~ m **cítrico** citric acid; ~ m **clavulánico** clavulanic acid; ~ m **clorhídrico** hydrochloric acid, muriatic

acid; ~ *m* **cólico** cholic acid;
~ *m* **desoxirribonucleico** deoxyribonucleic acid; ~ *m* **etileno diaminado tetracético** ethylene diamine tetraacetic acid;
~ *m* **fenilpirúvico** phenylpyruvic acid;
~ *m* **fólico** folic acid, pteroyl glutamic acid, folacin, vitamin B9; ~ *m* **fosfórico** phosphoric acid; ~ *m* **gástrico** gastric acid;
~ *m* **glucurónico** glucuronic acid;
~ *m* **glutámico** glutamic acid; ~ *m* **graso** fatty acid; ~ *m* **láctico** lactic acid, lactic acids, E270;
~ *m* **litocólico** litocholic acid;
~ *m* **mefenámico** mefenamic acid;
~ *m* **nalidíxico** nalidixic acid; ~ *m* **nicotínico** niacin, nicotinic acid, a B-complex vitamin;
~ *m* **nucleico** nucleic acid; ~ *m* **orgánico** organic acid; ~ *m* **oxolínico** oxolinic acid;
~ *m* **p-aminosalicílico** para-aminosalicylic acid, PASA; ~ *m* **pantoténico** pantothenic acid; ~ *m* **pirofosfórico** pyrophosphoric acid; ~ *m* **pirúvico** pyruvic acid;
~ *m* **propiónico** propionic acid, methylacetic acid;
~ *m* **quinolínico** quinolinic acid, quinoline;
~ *m* **retinoico** retinoic acid, vitamin A acid, tretinoin; ~ *m* **ribonucleico** ribonucleic acid;
~ *m* **salicílico** salicylic acid; ~ *m* **sórbico** sorbic acid; ~ *m* **sulfúrico** sulfoacid;
~ *m* **sulfúrico** sulfuric acid; ~ *m* **tánico** tannic acid, tannin; ~ *m* **tartárico** tartaric acid;
~ *m* **tiocínico** thiocyanic acid, sulfocyanic acid; ~ *m* **úrico** uric acid; ~ *m* **valproico** valproic acid

ácidorresistente *adj* acid-fast
ácidos *m pl* acids; ~ *m pl* **grasos insaturados** non-saturated fatty acids; ~ *m pl* **grasos no esterificados** free fatty acids; ~ *m pl* **grasos no saturados** unsaturated fatty acids;
~ *m pl* **grasos saturados** saturated fatty acids, saturates; ~ *m pl* **grasos volátiles** volatile fatty acids; ~ *m pl* **lácticos** lactic acids, lactic acids; ~ *m pl* **neuramínicos** neuraminic acids;
~ *m pl* **siálicos** sialic acids, derivatives of neuraminic acid; ~ *m pl* **sulfínicos** sulfinic acids

acidosis *f* acidosis, high blood acidity;
~ *f* **compensada** compensated acidosis;
~ *f* **diabética** diabetic acidosis;
~ *f* **hematógena** hematogene acidose;
~ *f* **hiperclorémica** hyperchloremic acidosis;
~ *f* **láctica** lactic acidosis, buildup of lactic acid in the body; ~ *f* **metabólica** metabolic acidosis; ~ *f* **respiratoria** respiratory acidosis;
~ *f* **tubular renal** renal tubular acidosis
acidótico *adj* acidotic
aciduria *f* aciduria, an acid urine;
~ *f* **paradójica** paradoxical aciduria
acil-CoA-deshidrogenasa *f* acyl dehydrogenase
acinesia *f* akinesia, lack of movement
acinetobacter *m* acinetobacter, herella
aclaramiento *m* purification, clearance; ~ *m* **del ácido para-aminohipúrico** para-aminohippuric acid clearance
aclasia *f* aclasis; ~ *f* **diafisaria** diaphyseal aclasis, multiplex exostosis
aclimatización *f* acclimatization, adaptation
aclorhidria *f* achlorhydria, anachlorhydria, anacidity
acné *f* acne, blackheads, pimples; ~ *f* **brómica** bromide acne, a symptom of brominism;
~ *f* **clórica** chloracne; ~ *f* **infecciosa** infectious acne; ~ *f* **necrótica** necrotic acne, necrotic granuloma, acne necrotica miliaris;
~ *f* **rosácea** acne rosacea, facial erythrosis;
~ *f* **sebácea** sebaceous acne; ~ *f* **tarsi** tarsal acne, tarsis acne
acomodación *f* accommodation, adjustment
acompañante *adj* associated, concomitant, accessory
acondrodisplasia *f* chondrodystrophy, achondrodysplasia
acoplamiento *m* connecting, coupling
acostado *adj* reclining, lying down; ~ **boca abajo** lying prone, face down, prostrate;
~ **boca arriba** lying face up
acostarse *v* to lie down
acostumbrado *adj* habitual, usual
acrania *f* acrania, born with no cranium
acreditación *f* accreditation
acrementación *f* accretion
acrocianosis *f* acrocyanosis, blueness
acrodermatitis *f* enteropathic acrodermatitis;
~ **enteropática** enteropathic acrodermatitis

acrodinia f acrodynia, pink disease, Feer's disease
acromatopsia f achromatopsia, total color blindness
acromegalia f acromegaly; ~ **precoz** early acromegaly, somatotropin hypersecretion syndrome
acromioclavicular adj acromio-clavicular
acromión m acromion
acroosteolisis f acro-osteolysis; ~ **f profesional** occupational acro-osteolysis; ~ **f progresiva** neuropathic osseous atrophy, neurotrophic osseous atrophy, neurogenic arco-osteolysis
acrosclerosis f sclerodactyly, acroscleroderma
acrosoma m acrosome
ACTH f ACTH, adrenocorticotropic hormone
actina f actin
actinodermatitis f actinodermatitis, actinodermatosis
actinomicetos m pl actinomyces
actinomicosis f actinomycosis; ~ **cutánea** dermal actinomycosis
activación f activation; ~ **f de la célula huésped** activated host cell
activador m activator; ~ **m hístico del plasminógeno** tissue-type plasminogen activator, t-PA, TPA; ~ **m plasminógeno urinario** urinary plasminogen activator, urokinase-type plasminogen activator; ~ **m tisular del plasminógeno** tissue-type plasminogen activator, t-PA, TPA
activar v to activate, to stimulate
actividad f activity; ~ **f anticolinesterásica** anticholinesterase activity; ~ **f bioquímica** biochemical activity; ~ **f catalítica** catalytic activity; ~ **f de colinesterasa** cholinesterase activity; ~ **f de psicomotricidad** psychic & motor functions, psychomotoricity, psychomotor activities; ~ **f eléctrica del cerebro** electrical activity of the brain; ~ **f enzimática** enzymatic activity, enzyme activity; ~ **f epigenética** epigenetic environment; ~ **f específica** specific activity; ~ **f iónica** ionic activity; ~ **f peroxidásica** peroxidase activity; ~ **f radionucleida** radionuclide activity
actividades f pl **de tiempo libre** pastimes, leisure activities, hobbies, recreational activities; ~ **f pl recreativas** pastimes, leisure activities, hobbies, recreational activities
activo adj active
actual (time) present, current
acuerdos m pl **de Helsinki** Helsinki accord, Helsinki declaration, Helsinki Agreement
acuidad f acuity, sharpness
acumulación f accumulation, build-up
acumulativo adj cumulative, increasing
acuoso adj aqueous, watery, diluted
acupresión f acupressure, pressure point massage
acupuntura f acupuncture
acústico adj acoustic
acústica f **médica** medical acoustics
adaptación f accommodation, adjustment, adaptation; ~ **f enzimática** enzymatic adaptation; ~ **f funcional** functional adaptation; ~ **f genética** genetic adaptation; ~ **f postnatal** postnatal adaptation, postnatal growing functions; ~ **f social** social adjustment, social adaptation
adecuado adj adequate, homologous
adelgazamiento m emaciation, extreme leanness; ~ **m extremo** cachexia, wasting away
adelgazar v to lose weight
adenilato-ciclasa f adenylylcyclase
adenina f adenine
adenitis f adenitis, gland inflammation; ~ **f mesentérica** mesenteric lymphadenitis, mesenteric adenitis
adenocarcinoma m adenomatoid carcinoma; ~ **m papilífero** papillary adenocarcinoma; ~ **m testicular** testicular adenocarcinoma
adenoepitelioma m adenomatous carcinoma, adenoepithelioma
adenofibroma m adenofibroma, fibro-adenoma
adenoiditis f naso-pharyngeal catarrh, postnasal catarrh
adenoma m adenoma, non-cancerous tumor of glandular tissue; ~ **m basófilo** basophil adenoma; ~ **m cortical** cortical adenoma; ~ **m eosinófilo** eosinophilic adenoma, eosinophil adenoma; ~ **m fibroso** adenofibroma, fibroadenoma; ~ **m sebáceo** sebaceous adenoma; ~ **m trabecular** trabecular adenoma

adenomatosis f adenomatosis; ~ f **endocrina** endocrine adenomatosis

adenomiosis f stromal adenomyosis, adenomyoma of the uterus, uterine endometriosis

adenopatía f adenopathy, a general term for glandular disease; ~ f **toxoplasmódica** toxoplasmotic adenopathy

adenosina f adenosine; ~ f **monofosfato** adenosine monophosphate, AMP; ~ f **monofosfato cíclico** cAMP, cyclic adenosine monophosphate; ~ **–desaminasa** f adenosine deaminase; ~ **–trifosfatasa** f adenosinetriphosphatase, ATPase

adenotomía f lymphadenectomy, adenotomy

adenovirus m adenovirus; ~ m **humano** human adenovirus

adherencia f adhesion; ~ f **de la fimbria** fimbrial adhesion

adhesión f adhesion, sticking; ~ f **del paciente al tratamiento** compliance, following doctor's orders

adicción f bad habit, addiction, craving; ~ f **a la heroína** heroin addiction; ~ f **a las drogas** drug addiction, toxicomania

adicional adj additional

adicto adj addicted; ~ m **a drogas** drug addict

adiestramiento m training; ~ m **de la memoria** memory training

adipato m **de piperazina** piperazine adipate, veterinary anthelmintic

aditivo m additive, add-on; ~ m **alimentario antioxidante** antioxidant food additive; ~ m **zootécnico** zootechnical additive

administración f administration; ~ f **cruzada de un placebo** crossover administration of placebo; ~ f **de casos** case management, patient management

administrar v to administer

admisión f admission; ~ f **en un hospital** admission to hospital, hospitalization

admisiones f pl, **tasa de** index of admissions to hospital, admission rate

ADN m deoxyribonucleic acid, DNA; ~ m **de doble cadena** double-stranded DNA; ~ m **de enlace** linker DNA, adaptor DNA; ~ m **de**

unión linker DNA, adaptor DNA; ~ m **mitocondrial** mitochondrial DNA; ~ **polimerasa** f DNA polymerase, reverse transcriptase; ~ m **recombinante** recombinant DNA; ~ m **retrovírico integrado** integrated retroviral DNA, provirus; ~ m **vírico** viral DNA

adolescente m/f adolescent, juvenile, young, teenager

adormecerse v to fall asleep

adormecimiento m numbness, obnubilation; ~ m **en los pies** numbness of feet

adormidera f opium poppy, white poppy, papaver; ~ f **soporífera** opium poppy, white poppy, papaver

adrenalectomía f adrenalectomy, surgical removal of the adrenal gland

adrenalina f epinephrine, adrenalin(e)

adrenérgico adj adrenergic, acting like adrenaline

adrenodoxina f adrenodoxin

adrenolítico f adrenolytic, adrenaline inhibitor, adrenaline-blocking

adriamicina f adriamycin, doxorubicin

adsorción f adsorption, sticking to a surface

aducción f adduction

adulto m adult, grownup

adverso adj adverse, harmful

adyuvante m adjuvant, stiumulator

AEP m prostate specific antigen, PSA

aeroastenia f aerasthenia, pilots' disease

aerobio m aerobic, with oxygen

aeroespacial space medicine, aerospace medicine

aerofagia f aerophagy, air swallowing

aerogénico adj aerogenic

aeroneurosis f aerasthenia, pilots' disease

aerosol m aerosol, spray

aerotitis f aerosinusitis, sinus pain due to changing atmospheric pressures

aerotolerante adj aerotolerant

afasia f aphasia, difficulty in speaking or complete lack of speach; ~ f **completa** global aphasia, total aphasia, expressive-receptive aphasia; ~ f **de Broca** motor aphasia, expressive aphasia, ataxic motor aphasia, Broca's aphasia; ~ f **de Wernicke** sensory aphasia, amnesic aphasia, receptive aphasia; ~ f **motora** motor aphasia, expressive aphasia,

ataxic motor aphasia, Broca's aphasia;
~ f **sensorial** sensory aphasia, amnesic aphasia,
receptive aphasia
afección f affection, fondness, condition,
sickness, disorder; ~ f **cardiaca** cardiac
disorder
afectado adj affected
afectivo adj affective, emotional
afeitarse v to shave
aféresis f plasmapheresis, plasma exchange
a-fetoproteína f a-fetoprotein
afiebrado adj feverish
afijo m appendix
afinidad f affinity, attraction
aflatoxina f aflatoxin
aflicción f distress, affliction
aflojarse v limber up, to, warm up, to buckle at
the knees
afonía f aphonia, loss of voice, hoarseness,
scratchy throat, raucousness; ~ f **espasmódica**
spastic aphonia; ~ f **espástica** spastic aphonia
AFP f alpha-fetoprtein, AFP
afretar v to scrub, to wash, to clean
afta f canker sore (in the mouth), aphthous
ulcer
afuera out, outside
agacharse v to lean forward, to bend over
agalactia f agalactia, not producing milk
a-galactosidasa f melibiase
agammaglobulinemia f gamma-globulinemia,
type of immune deficiency
agar m agar; ~ m **de MacConkey** MacConkey
agar; ~ m **de Sabouraud** Sabouraud agar;
~ m **de Thayer-Martin** Thayer-Martin agar;
~ m **de Wilkins-Chalgren** Wilkins-Chalgren
agar; ~ m **nutritivo** nutrient agar; ~ m **sangre**
blood agar; ~ m **SS** SS agar
agarosa f agarose
agente m substance, agent; ~ m **adventicio**
adventitious agent; ~ m **alquilante** alkylating
agent; ~ m **bloqueante ganglionar** ganglionic
blocking agent; ~ m **bloqueante**
neuromuscular neuromuscular blocking
agent, neuromuscular blocker;
~ m **carcinógeno** carcinogen;
~ m **conservante** preservative;
~ m **de liberación controlada** slow release agent;
~ m **de liberación retardada** slow release

agent; ~ m **de solubilización** solubilizer,
solubilizing agent; ~ m **despolarizante**
neuromuscular muscle relaxant, neuromuscular
depolarizing agent; ~ m **intercalable**
intercalating agent; ~ m **psicotrópico**
psychoactive drugs, psychotropic drug;
~ m **tensoactivo** surfactant
agitación f agitation
agitado adj agitated, worked up, nervous, hyper
agitar v to shiver, to tremble, to shake
aglomerado m agglomerate
aglutinación f agglutination; ~ f **de las**
plaquetas blood platelet aggregation, platelet
clumping
aglutinina f agglutinin, agglutinating
antibody; ~ f **heterogenética** heterogenic
agglutinin
agonía f agony, extreme pain
agonista m agonist, substance that acts like
another substance
agorafobia f agoraphobia, fear of open places
agosto m August
agotado adj exhausted, run-down, weakened,
tired, dragging, worn out
agotamiento m weariness, depletion,
exhaustion, burnout, lassitude, fatigue;
~ m **psíquico** burnout, exhaustion, inability to
cope
agramatismo m agrammatism, acataphasia
agrandamiento m dilatation, stretching,
expansion; ~ m **de los nódulos linfáticos**
swollen lymph nodes, enlarged lymph nodes;
~ m **del bazo** enlargement of the spleen,
splenomegaly
agranulocitosis f agranulocytosis, bone marrow
failure
agravamiento m aggravation, exacerbation,
worsening
agregación f aggregation, joining;
~ f **eritrocítica** intravascular erythrocyte
aggregation, intravascular agglutination
agresividad f aggressiveness
agrio adj sour
agrupación f cluster, concentration;
~ f **temporal** cluster
agua m water; ~ m **activada** activated water;
~ m **caliente** hot water; ~ m **con gas**
sparkling water; ~ m **hirviente** boiling water,

scalding hot water; ~ **m oxigenada** H2O2, hydrogen peroxide; ~ **m tibia** lukewarm water

aguantar v **la respiración** to hold your breath

aguante m endurance, stamina

aguarrás m turpentine, a concrete oleoresin obtained from pine trees

aguas f pl **residuales** wastewater, sewage

agudeza f acuity, sharpness; ~ f **visual** visual acuity

agudo adj acute, sharp, severe, harsh

aguja f needle; ~ f **hipodérmica** hypodermic needle; ~ f **para extraer sangre** phlebotomy needle

agujero m hole, foramen; ~ **m obturador** obturator foramen; ~ **m intervertebral** intervertebral foramen

agujeta f charley horse

agujetas f pl sore muscles

ahí there

ahogamiento m drowning

ahogar v to suffocate, to choke, to asphyxiate

ahogarse v to drown

ahora now

ahorcadura f death by hanging

AINE m pl NSAIDs, non-steroidal anti-inflammatory drugs

aire m air

aireación f **por la respiración** breathing

aislar v to isolate

ajenjo m wormwood, absinthe

ajuste m accommodation, adjustment; ~ **m quiropráctico** chiropractic adjustment

alanina f alanine; ~ **-aminotransferasa** f alanine transaminase; ~ f **transaminasa** alanine transaminasa

al atardecer in the evening

al azar accidental, by chance

albaricoque m apricot

albendazol m albendazole

albúmina f albumin

albuminuria f albuminuria, albumin in the urine

alcalino adj alkaline

alcaloide m alkaloid, bitter plant poison; ~ m **de ipecacuana** ipecac, an emetic

alcaloides m pl alkaloids; ~ m pl **de la vinca** vinca alkaloids, periwinkle alkaloids; ~ m pl **del ergot** ergot alkaloids; ~ m pl **del opio** opium alkaloids

alcalosis f alkalosis, high blood alkalinity; ~ f **de altitud** altitude alkalosis; ~ f **metabólica** metabolic alkalosis; ~ f **respiratoria** respiratory alkalosis

alcohol m alcohol; ~ m **absoluto** absolute alcohol; ~ m **alcanforado** rubbing alcohol, isopropyl alcohol; ~ m **bencílico** benzylalcohol; ~ m **butílico** butylalcohol; ~ m **deshidrogenasa** alcohol dehydrogenase; ~ m **isopropílico** rubbing alcohol, isopropyl alcohol, C3H8O; ~ m **metílico** methanol, methyl alcohol; ~ m **polivinílico** polyvinyl alcohol, PVA

alcohólico m alcoholic, person with drinking problem, drunkard

alcoholismo m alcohol abuse, alcoholism

alcohol-oxidasa f alcohol oxidase

alcohómetro m alcoholometer

al contado cash

alcrebite m sulfur, sulphur

aldehído-deshidrogenasa f aldehyde dehydrogenase

aldilla f crotch, pubic region, groin

aldolasa f aldolase

aldosterona f aldosterone

aleatorización f randomization

alejado adj distal, peripheral

alelo m allele

alelotipo m allelotype

alendronato m alendronate

alérgeno m allergen, substance causing allergy; ~ m **de contacto** contact allergen; ~ m **respiratorio** airborne allergen, respiratory system sensitizer, inhalational allergen

alergia f allergy, allergic reaction, allergic response; ~ f **cruzada** cross-allergy, multi-allergy, polyvalent allergy

alérgico adj allergic

alergista f allergist, immuno-allergist

alergología f allergology

alergólogo m allergist, immuno-allergist

alerta f alert

aletargado adj lethargic

aleteo m **del corazón** flutter

alexia f alexia; ~ f **motora** cortical alexia, motor alexia; ~ f **sensorial** sensory alexia

alferecía f an undefined nervous condition, febrile convulsions in children

algas *f pl* algae

algesia *f* algesia, increased sensitivity to pain

algia *f* algia, pain

algo something

algodistrofia *f* Sudeck's atrophy, Sudeck's disease; ~ *f* simpática reflex sympathetic dystrophy syndrome, complex regional sympathetic dystrophy

algodón *m* cotton; ~ *m* hidrófilo absorbent cotton

algodoncillo *m* thrush, candidiasis, thrush, Candida mycosis

algofobia *f* algophobia, abnormal and persistent fear of pain

algoritmo *m* algorithm

alguien anybody

algún any

ALH *m* human leukocyte antigen, HLA antigen system

alheña *f* henna

alholva *f* fenugreek, herb with medicinal properties

alicuota *adj* aliquot

alienación *f* alienation, depersonalization, a dream-like feeling

aligeramiento *m* relief, solace, balm, comfort

alimentación *f* food; ~ *f* en exceso overeating; ~ *f* por sonda gastrogavage, tube feeding, feeding by a stomach tube, gavage

alimentario *adj* alimentary, food-related, digestion-related

alimento *m* nutrient, nutrition, food

alimentos *m pl* food; ~ *m pl* orgánicos organic food; ~ *m pl* para diabéticos diabetic foods; ~ *m pl* saludables health food

alinfocitosis *f* alymphocytosis

aliviarse *v* to give birth, to deliver a baby, to get better

alivio *m* relief, solace, balm, comfort

al lado beside

almacenado *m* del esperma semen storage

almacenamiento *m* storage

almidón *m* starch

almohada *f* pillow, cushion; ~ *f* eléctrica heating pad, warming pad

almorragia *f* nosebleed, nasal hemorrhage, bloody nose

almorranas *f pl* hemorrhoids, piles

almuerzo *m* lunch

aloanticuerpo *m* alloantibody, isoantibody

aloe *m* aloe vera, succulent medicinal herb; ~ vera *m* aloe vera, succulent medicinal herb

aloenzima *f* allozyme, variant of an enzyme

alogénico *adj* homologous, allogenic, allogeneic

aloinjerto *m* allograft, allogenic graft, allogenic transplant, homologous graft

alopatía *f* allopathy (as opposed to homeopathy)

alopecia *f* alopecia, baldness, loss of hair

alopurinol *m* allopurinol sodium

alpha1–antitripsina *f* alpha1-antitrypsin

alpha2–antiplasmina *f* alpha2-antiplasmin

alpha–amilasa *f* alpha-amylase; ~ – fetoproteína *f* alpha-fetoprotein, AFP

al primer paso on the first pass

al principio primary, first, main

alquilato *m* alkylate

alquitrán *m* de hulla coal tar

alteración *f* disorder, alteration, change; ~ *f* de la conciencia altered consciousness; ~ *f* de la función cognitiva cognitive function; ~ *f* del juicio impaired judgement, alteration in judgement, deficient judgement; ~ *f* del razonamiento thought disorder, thinking disorder, disturbance in the mental process; ~ *f* neurológica neurological disorder

alteraciones *f pl* alterations, changes; ~ *f pl* del habla speech disorders, speech defects; ~ *f pl* del ritmo cardíaco cardiac arrythmia

alternar *v* to alternate

alternativo *adj* alternative

altitud *f* height

alto *adj* high; ~ *adj* en colesterol high cholesterol

alucinación *f* hallucination; ~ *f* psicomotriz psychomotor hallucination

alumbrar *v* to give birth, to deliver a baby

aluminio *m* aluminum, aluminium

alveolitis *f* alveolitis, alveolar inflammation, pneumonitis; ~ *f* alérgica extrínseca hypersensitivity pneumonitis, extrinsic allergic alveolitis

alveolo *m* alveolus

alveolos *m pl* pulmonares pulmonary alveoli

ama *f* de casa housewife

amalgama *f* amalgam; ~ *f* dental amalgam

filling

amamantamiento *m* breast feeding, nursing a baby, lactation, milk production

amamantar *v* to lactate, to nurse, to suckle, to breast feed a baby

amanita *f* amanita, a poisonous fungus

amantadina *f* amantidine

amapola *f* real opium poppy, white poppy, papaver

amargo *adj* bitter

amarillo *adj* yellow

amasamiento *m* kneading

amasar *v* to knead

amaurosis *f* amaurosis, blindness, being blinded; ~ *f* fugax amaurosis fugax, transient blindness due to retinal ischemia

ambiente *m* environment; ~ *m* emocional affective climate, emotional climate; ~ *m* estéril sterile environment

ambliopía *f* amblyopia, lazy eye (syndrome)

ambos both

ambulancia *f* ambulance

ambulante *adj* ambulant, outpatient, ambulatory

ambulatorio *adj* ambulant, outpatient, ambulatory

ambulatorio *m* outpatient, ambulatory patient

ameba *f* ameba, amoeba

amebiasis *f* amebiasis; ~ *f* cutánea cutaneous amebiasis; ~ *f* hepática hepatic amebiasis, amebic liver abscess; ~ *f* intestinal intestinal amebiasis

amenorrea *f* amenorrhoea, lack of menstruation, lack of periods; ~ *f* posparto postpartum amenorrhea

amfoion *m* hybrid ion, zwitterion, amphoteric ion, zwitter ion, dipolar ion

amiba *f* ameba, amoeba

amibiasis *f* hepática hepatic amebic abscess

amicrobiosis *f* amicrobiosis; ~ *f* intestinal intestinal amicrobiosis

amiga *f* friend (female)

amígdala *f* tonsil; ~ *f* faríngea palatine tonsil, pharyngeal tonsil; ~ *f* palatina palatine tonsil, pharyngeal tonsil

amigdalitis *f* tonsillitis

amigo *m* friend (male); ~ *m* comprensivo sympathetic friend

amikacina *f* amikacin

amilasa *f* amylase; ~ *f* salival salivary amylase

amiloide *m* amyloid

amiloidosis *f* amyloidosis, deposition of amyloid, amyloid degeneration; ~ *f* conjuntiva amyloidosis of the conjunctiva; ~ *f* sistémica systemic amyloidosis

amina *f* amine, organic compound containing nitrogen; ~ ~oxidasa (cuprífera) *f* diamine oxidase

aminas *f pl* biógenas biogenic amines

aminoácido *m* amino acid; ~ *m* esencial essential amino acid

aminoaciduria *f* amino-aciduria

aminoglicósido *m* aminoglycoside

amiotonía *f* amyotonia

amiotrofia *f* amyotrophy, atrophy of muscle tissue; ~ *f* espinal progresiva progressive spinal amyotrophy

amitriptilina *f* amitriptyline

amlodipino *m* amlodipine

amnesia *f* amnesia, memory loss, loss of memory; ~ *f* lacunar temporary amnesia, transient amnesia

amniocéntesis *f* amniocentesis

amnios *m* amnion

amnioscopia *f* amnioscopy

amniotomía *f* amniotomy, artificial rupture of the amniotic sac

amodorrado *adj* sleepy, drowsy

amoniaco *m* ammonia

amonio *m* ammonium

amortiguador *m* buffer

amoxicilina *f* amoxicillin

AMP *m* cíclico cAMP, cyclic adenosine monophosphate; ~ ~desaminasa *f* myoadenylate deaminase

ampere *f* ampere

amperimetría *f* amperometry

ampicilina *f* ampicillin

amplia infiltración *f* ample infiltration

amplificación *f* amplification; ~ *f* de DNA DNA amplification; ~ *f* genetica gene amplification

amplímero *m* amplimer

amplio *adj* massive, solid

amplio *m* espectro broad spectrum

amplitud f amplitude, width; ~ f **de la pelvis** amplitude of pelvis, pelvic width; ~ f **de movimiento** range of motion; ~ f **ecológica** ecological amplitude/scope, ecological impact

ampolla f ampule, vial, blister, small sealed flask, small bottle, bulla, bleb, pomphus, cartridge; ~ f **febril** fever blister; ~ f **rectal** rectal blister

amputación f amputation; ~ f **de un dedo** amputation of a finger; ~ f **del brazo** amputation of upper arm

amputado m amputee

amputar v to amputate

anabolismo m anabolism, body-building

anacidez f anacidity, achlorhydria, anachlorhydria

anaclorhidria f anachlorhydria, achlorhydria, anacidity

anacrotismo m anacrotic pulse

anacusia f anacusis, nerve deafness

añadido adj additional

añadir v to add

anaerobio adj anaerobic, without oxygen; ~ **exigente** fastidious anaerobe; ~ m **facultativo** facultative anaerobe; ~ adj **obligado** obligate anaerobe

anaerogénico adj anaerogenic

anafiláctico adj anaphylactic; ~ m anaphylactic shock, anaphylaxis, acute hypersensitivity reaction

anafilactógeno m **respiratorio** airborne allergen, respiratory system sensitizer, inhalational allergen

anafilactoxina f anaphylatoxin

anafilaxia f anaphylaxis; ~ f **activa** active anaphylaxis; ~ f **cutánea pasiva** cutaneous anaphylaxis, PCA; ~ f **heteróloga** heterologous anaphylaxis; ~ f **homóloga** homologous anaphylaxis; ~ f **invertida** inverse anaphylaxis; ~ f **pasiva** passive anaphylaxis; ~ f **respiratoria** respiratory anaphylaxis

anafilotoxina f anaphylatoxin

anal adj anal

analéptico m analeptic, pick-me-up

analgésico m analgesic, pain killer, pain reliever; ~ m **antipirético** antipyretic analgesic

analgésicos m pl analgesics; ~ m pl **no opioides** non-narcotic analgesics; ~ m pl **opioides** narcotic analgesics

análisis m test, analysis, decomposition, analytical test, laboratory test; ~ m **clínico** clinical analysis; ~ m **coste–efectividad** cost-benefit analysis; ~ m **cromosómico** chromosome analysis; ~ m **cualitativo** qualitative analysis; ~ m **cuantitativo** quantitative analysis; ~ m **de alergia** allergy test; ~ m **de componentes principales** principal component analysis; ~ m **de diferencias representativas** representational difference analysis; ~ m **de embarazo** pregnancy test; ~ m **del sangre** blood test; ~ m **de oligoelementos** trace analysis; ~ m **de orina** urinalysis, urine test; ~ **prematrimoniales** m pl premarital screening, serological screening before marriage; ~ m **químico** chemical analysis

analítico adj analytical

analito m analyte, substance to analyze

analizado m analyte, substance to analyze; ~ m **de acceso directo** random access analyzer

analizador m analyser

analogía f affinity, attraction

análogo adj analogous, similar, identical

análogo m analog, analogue; ~ m **de los nucleósidos** nucleoside analog, nucleoside analogue

anamnesis f anamnesis, remembering, recalling, recollection

anastomosis f anastomosis, bypass, shunt, connection between two vessels or tubes; ~ f **crural** crural anastomosis; ~ f **porto–cava** porto-caval anastomosis, portocaval shunt; ~ f **ureteroentérica** uretero-enteric anastomosis

anatomía f anatomy; ~ f **patológica** pathology, morbid anatomy, anatomical pathology, anatomic pathology

anatómico adj anatomical, pertaining to the body, body-related

anatomopatólogo m pathologist, anatomo-pathologist

anatoxina f anatoxin, toxoid

anchura f width

ancianidad f senility, old age

anciano m elderly person

andador m, **–a** f walker

andadura f gait

andamiaje m scaffolding

andar v to walk, to go; ~ v **con dilaciones** procrastinate, to; ~ v **en sueños** somnambulism, sleep-walking

andrógeno adj masculine, male, androgenic

andrógeno m androgen, androgenic hormone

androginismo m androgyny, masculin pseudo-hermaphroditism

andrógino adj androgynous, androgenous

andropausia f andropause, male climacterium, male menopause

androprótesis f penile prosthesis, penile implant

androstenodiona m androstenedione

anejo m anejo

anemia f anemia; ~ f **aplástica** pancytopenia, aplastic anemia; ~ f **con agranulocitosis** anemia associated with agranulocytosis; ~ f **con neutropenia** anemia associated with neutropenia; ~ f **de Fanconi** Fanconi's anemia, Fanconi's pancytopenia, Fanconi's panmyelopathy, Fanconi's refractory anemia; ~ f **fagocitaria** phagocytic anemia; ~ f **falciforme** sickle cell anemia, an inherited blood disorder characterized by chronic anemia; ~ f **ferropénica** iron-deficiency anemia, hypoferric anemia; ~ f **hemolítica** hemolytic anemia; ~ f **hemolítica autoinmune** hemolytic autoimmune anemia, autoimmune hemolytic anemia; ~ f **hemolítica tóxica** toxic hemolytic anemia; ~ f **hipocrómica** hypochromic anemia; ~ f **infantil** infantile anemia; ~ f **infecciosa** infectious anemia; ~ f **mediterránea** thalassemia, Mediterranean anemia; ~ f **microcítica** microcytic anemia; ~ f **nutricional** nutritional anemia; ~ f **perniciosa** pernicious anemia; ~ f **por carencia de hierro** iron-deficiency anemia, hypoferric anemia; ~ f **por déficit de ácido fólico** folic acid deficiency anemia, nutritional macrocytic anemia; ~ f **por plomo** anemia due to lead exposure; ~ f **saturnina** lead poisoning anemia, lead poisoning dyscrasia; ~ f **sintomática** symptomatic anemia

anémico adj ferriprive, anemic, iron-deficient

anergia f anergia, inactivity

anestesia f anesthesia, deadening of sensation; ~ f **basal** basal narcosis; ~ f **de superficie** surface anesthesia; ~ f **en silla de montar** saddle block anesthesia; ~ f **endostal** endosteal anesthesia; ~ f **epidural** epidural anaesthesia, peridural anaesthesia, caudal anesthesia, raquianesthesia; ~ f **espinal** spinal anesthesia, subarachnoid anaesthesia; ~ f **general** general anesthesia; ~ f **local** local anesthesia; ~ f **obstétrica** obstetrical anesthesia; ~ f **paravertebral** paravertebral anesthesia; ~ f **por inhalación** inhalation anesthesia

anestesiar v to anesthetize, to numb up

anestésico adj anesthetic, m drug to deaden sensation

anestesista m anesthesiologist

aneuploidía f aneuploidy

aneurina f thiamine, vitamin B1, aneurin

aneurisma m aneurysm, swelling in artery wall; ~ m **abdominal** abdominal aneurysm; ~ m **aórtico** aortic aneurysm; ~ m **cerebral** cerebral aneurysm, brain aneurysm; ~ m **congénito** congenital aneurysm; ~ m **disecante** dissecting aneurysm, aortic dissection; ~ m **exógeno** exogenous aneurysm; ~ m **falso** false aneurysm, spurious aneurysm; ~ m **herniario** hernial aneurysm; ~ m **intracraneal** intracranial aneurysm, cerebral aneurysm; ~ m **micótico** mycotic aneurysm; ~ m **orbital** orbital aneurysm; ~ m **roto** ruptured aneurysm; ~ m **sacular** berry aneurysm; ~ m **valvular** valvular aneurysm; ~ m **verdadero** true aneurysm

aneusoploidía f aneuploidization

anexitis f adnexitis, Pelvic Inflammatory Disease

anexo m adnex

anfetamina f amphetamine

anfiartrosis f cartilaginous joint, amphiarthrosis

anfíteno m zygotene

anfolito m ampholytoid, ampholyte, ampholytic agent

anfotericina B f amphotericin B

anfotérico adj amphoterous, amphoteric

anfótero adj amphoterous, amphoteric

Angelica f archangelica Angelica archangelica, angelica root

angiítis f angitis, inflammation of a blood

vessel; ~ f alérgica allergic angiitis, hypersensitivity angiitis

angina f sore throat, pharyngitis, angina; ~ f aguda acute tonsillitis; ~ f de decúbito angina decubitus, decubitus angina; ~ f de pecho angina pectoris, angina in the chest; ~ f escarlatinosa scarlatinal angina; ~ f folicular follicular tonsillitis, lacunar tonsillitis; ~ f herpética herpes pharyngis, angina herpetica, vesicular pharyngitis; ~ f inestable unstable angina; ~ f lacunar lacunar tonsillitis; ~ f monocítica infectious mononucleosis, glandular fever, monocytic angina, monocuclear leukocytosis, Epstein-Barr disease; ~ f necrótica necrotic angina; ~ f péctoris angina pectoris, angina in the chest; ~ f post-operativa postoperative angina; ~ f séptica septic angina; ~ f tóxica toxic tonsillitis

anginoso adj anginal, angina-related

angiodermatitis f pruriginosa disseminated pruritic angiodermatitis

angioedema m angioneurotic edema, Quincke disease, angioedema, skin blistering

angiografía f angiography

angioma m angioma; ~ m capilar hipertrófico hypertrophic capillary angioma; ~ m cavernoso cavernous angioma; ~ m cerebral encephalic angioma; ~ m de la piel angiomyoma of the skin, red birthmark; ~ m senil senile angioma; ~ m serpiginoso infectious angioma; ~ m tuberoso tuberous angioma; ~ m venoso racemoso venous racemose angioma

angiomatosis f angiomatosis; ~ f encefalotrigeminal Sturge-Weber syndrome, encephalotrigeminal angiomatosis; ~ f meningo-oculo-faciale Sturge-Weber syndrome, encephalotrigeminal angiomatosis

angioneurótico adj angioneurotic

angiopatía f angiopathy; ~ f capilar capillaropathy; ~ f retiniana traumática traumatic retinal angiopathy, angiopathia retinae traumatica

angioplastia f angioplasty; ~ f con balón balloon angioplasty; ~ f coronaria coronary angioplasty; ~ f de balon balloon angioplasty; ~ f por láser laser angioplasty; ~ f transluminal percutanea percutaneous transluminal angioplasty;

angioqueratoma m angiokeratoma

angiosarcoma m angiosarcoma; ~ m hepatítico angiosarcoma of the liver; ~ m mixomatoso myxomatous angiosarcoma

angiotensina f angiotensin

ángulo m angle; ~ m de divergencia divergence range, divergence angle

angustia f heartache, emotional devastation, mental anguish, mental distress, psychic distress; ~ f cardíaca heart palpitation, cardiac palpitation, heart throb

anhídrido m plúmbico lead dioxide, plumbic anhydride

anhidro adj anhydrous, without water

anhidrosis f anhydrosis, loss of the ability to sweat

anillo m ring; ~ m crural femoral ring, crural ring; ~ m vaginal vaginal ring

animal m animal; ~ m domesticado pet, domesticated animal; ~ m testigo sentinel animal, control animal; ~ m transgénico transgenic animal, a genetically modified animal

aniónico adj anionic, with a negative charge

aniquilante adj pernicious, malignant, fatal, harmful

anisocoria f anisocoria, different sized pupils

anisoiconia f aniseikonia, aniseiconia

anisol m anisole, methoxybenzene

anistreplasa f anistreplase, anisoylated plasminogen streptokinase activator complex

ano m anal orifice, anus

año m year

anodoncia f anodontia

anogenital adj anogenital, anus and genital-related

anomalía f anomaly, abnormality, deviation; ~ f cromosómica chromosomal abnormality; ~ f de la personalidad lack of sense of personal worth, feelings of inadequacy; ~ f del arco aórtico aortic arch syndrome; ~ f del citoplasma cytoplasmic abnormality, anomaly of the cytoplasm; ~ f neuroquímica neurochemical abnormality

anómalo *adj* aberrant, irregular, abnormal, anomalous

anorectal *adj* anorectal, pertaining to the anus and rectum

anoréctico *adj* anorexiant, appetite suppressant, appetite depressant, anorectic agent

anorexia *f* anorexia, lack of appetite

anoréxico *adj* anorexic, anorexiant

anorexígeno *m* anorexiant, appetite suppressant, appetite depressant, anorectic agent

anormal *adj* abnormal, anomalous, aberrant, irregular, atypical, unusual

anosmia *f* anosmia, lack of sense of smell

anovular *adj* anovulatory, without producing an egg

anoxia *f* anoxia, total lack of oxygen

anquilosis *f* ankylosis, fusion of bones across a joint; ~ *f* **fibrosa** fibrous ankylosis; ~ *f* **ósea** osseous ankylosis, bony ankylosis

anquilostomiasis *f* ankylostomiasis, hookworm anemia; ~ *f* **cutánea** cutaneous ankylostomiasis, panigau (a Brazilian name), hookworm, ground itch

ansiedad *f* anxiety, vague sensation of uneasiness; ~ *f* **generalizada** generalized anxiety; ~ *f* **inducida por la castración** fear of castration; ~ *f* **psíquica** psychic distress, mental anguish, psychological stress, emotional stress

ansiolítico *m* anxiolytic, tranquilizer, psychotropic drug, sedative

ansioso *adj* anxious

antagónico *adj* hostile, antagonistic

antagonista *m* antagonist, antagonist (muscle), substance tending to nullify effects of another; ~ *m* **adrenérgico** adrenergic antagonists, adrenergic blocking agents, adrenergic blockers, adrenolytic drugs; ~ *m* **de la aldosterona** aldosterone antagonist; ~ *m* **de la dopamina** dopamine antagonist, antidopaminergic agent, dopamine receptor blocking agent; ~ *m* **del calcio** calcium antagonist; ~ *m* **de los opiáceos** opiate antagonist; ~ *m* **de hormonas** hormone antagonist opioid antagonist

anteayer day before yesterday

antebrazo *m* forearm

antecedente *m* antecedent, precursor, forerunner, medical history; ~ *m* **familiar de cáncer** family history of cancer, predisposition to cancer

anteojos *m pl* eyeglasses, eyewear; ~ *m pl* **con receta** prescription eyeglasses, eyewear; ~ *m pl* **para leer** reading glasses

anterógrado *adj* anterograde, moving forward

antes (de) before

antiácido *adj* antiacid, *m* antacid, indigestion remedy

antiadrenérgico *adj* antiadrenergic

antialérgico *adj* antiallergic, allergy relief

antiamebiano *adj* amebicide

antianticuerpo *m* anti-antibody

antiarrítmico *m* antiarrhythmic, irregular heartbeat drug

antiarrugas *f pl* wrinkle

antiasmático *m* antiasthmatic, asthma drug, asthma medication

antibacteriano *m* antibacterial, bacteria-destroying

antibiograma *m* antibiogram, antibiotic sensitivity test

antibioterapia *f* antibiotherapy, treatment with antibiotics

antibiótico *adj* antibiotic

antibiótico *m* antibiotic; ~ *m* **betalactámico** beta-lactam antibiotic

anticoagulante *m* anticoagulant, substance that prevents blood clotting; ~ *m* **lúpico** lupus anticoagulant

anticodón *m* anticodon

anticolinérgico *m* anticholinergic, agent blocking the parasympathetic nerves

anticomplementario *adj* anticomplementary

anticoncepción *f* contraception

anticonceptivo *m* contraceptive

anticonvulsivo *m* anticonvulsant, substance to stop convulsions

anticuerpo *m* antibody; ~ *m* **antimicrosómico** antimicrosomal antibody; ~ *m* **antimitocondrial** antimitochondrial antibody; ~ *m* **antinuclear** antinuclear antibody, ANA; ~ *m* **circulante** circulating antibody; ~ *m* **contra el núcleo** antibody anti-core; ~ *m* **fluorescente antitreponémico** FTA; ~ *m* **gástrico** gastric cytoplasmic antibody; ~ *m* **monoclonal** monoclonal antibody, mca

anticuerpos *m pl* antibodies; ~ *m pl* **antihepatitis** hepatitis antibodies; ~ *m pl* **antitisulares** antitissue antibodies; ~ *m pl* **que presentan reacciones cruzadas** cross-reactive antibodies

antidepresivo *m* antidepressant, anti-depressant drug; ~ *m* **tricíclico** tricyclic antidepressant, tricyclic compound

antiderrape *adj* anti-skid, nonslip, non-skid, skid resistant

antideslizante *adj* anti-skid, nonslip, non-skid, skid resistant

antidiabético *m* antidiabetic, diabetes drug

antidifusor *m* **de rejilla móvi** Bucky diaphragm, mobile antiscatter grid, reciprocating Bucky frame

antidiurético *m* antidiuretic, substance to slow urine formation

antidopaminérgico *m* antidopaminergic

antídoto *m* antidote

antiemético *adj* antiemetic, substance to stop nausea or vomiting

antiepiléptico *adj* antiepileptic, epilepsy drug, anticonvulsant

antiespumante *adj* antifoaming agent, antifoam agent, foam inhibitor, foam suppressant

antiestreptolisina *f* antistreptolysin

antiestrogénico *adj* antioestrogenic, estrogen suppressant

antiestrogénico *m* antiestrogen drug, estrogen suppressant

antifebril *adj* antifebrile, antithermic

antifibrinolisina *f* antiplasmin, antifibrinolysin

antifibrinolítico *adj* antifibrinolytic, drug to stop breakdown of blood clots

antifúngico *m* antifungal

antígeno *m* antigen, foreign substance; ~ *m* **carbohidratado** carbohydrated antigen; ~ *m* **carcinoembrionario** carcinoembryonic antigen, CEA; ~ *m* **CD8** CD8 antigen; ~ *m* **de histocompatibilidad** major histocompatibility antigen; ~ *m* **de superficie de la hepatitis-B** hepatitis B surface antigen, surface antigen of hepatitis B; ~ *m* **específico prostático** prostate specific antigen, PSA; ~ *m* **extraño** foreign antigen; ~ *m* **leucocitario humano** human leukocyte antigen, HLA antigen system; ~ *m* **MC** MC antigen; ~ *m* **nuclear de la hepatitis B** hepatitis B core antigen; ~ *m* **nuclear extraíble** extractable nuclear antigen, ENA; ~ *m* **oncofetal** oncofetal antigen; ~ *m* **polipeptídico hístico** tissue polypeptide antigen; ~ *m* **timodependiente** T-dependent antigen, thymus dependent antigen; ~ *m* **VIH** HIV antigen

antígenos *m* antigens; ~ *m pl* **capsulares** thermolabile antigens; ~ *m pl* **HLA** HLA-antigens, human leukocyte antigens

antiglobulina *f* antiglobulin, anti-human globulin immune serum, Coombs' reagent, Coombs serum

antihelmíntico *m* anthelmintic, anti-worm medication

antihipertensivo *m* antihypertensive, high blood pressure drug

antihistamínico *m* antihistamine

antiinfeccioso *adj* antiinfective, disinfection

antiinflamatorio *m* anti-inflammatory, substance to reduce swelling

antimetabolito *m* antimetabolite

antimicobacteriano *adj* antimycobacterial

antimicótico *m* antimycotic, antifungal, fungal treatment

antimicrobiano *adj* antimicrobial, substance to kill microorganisms

antimicrobiano *m* antimicrobial, substance to kill microorganisms

antimitótico *m* antimitotic, anti-cancer drug

antineoplásico *m* antineoplastic, anti-cancer drug

antioxidante *m* antioxidant, substance to stop decay

antiparasitario *adj* antiparasitic

antipatinante *adj* anti-skid, nonslip, non-skid, skid resistant

antipirético *m* antipyretic, fever treatment

antiplasmina *f* antiplasmin, antifibrinolysin

antiprofesional *adj* unprofessional, contrary to professional ethics

antiproliferativo *adj* antiproliferative, substance to stop spread

antipruriginoso *m* antipruritic, itch treatment

antipsicótico *adj* neuroleptic, antipsychotic

antipsicótico *m* antipsychotic, neuroleptic, major tranquilizer

antirresbaladizo *adj* anti-skid, nonslip, non-skid, skid resistant

antirretroviral *m* antiretroviral agent, retroviral drug

antiséptico *m* antiseptic, desinfectant

antispasmódico *m* antispasmodic, spasm treatment drug

antisuero *m* immune serum, antiserum, therapeutic serum

antitérmico *adj* antifebrile, antithermic

antiterminación *f* antitermination

antitorsión *f* detorsion

antitoxina *f* antitoxin, vaccine

antitripsina *f* antitrypsin

antitrombina *f* antithrombin

antitromboplastina *f* antithromboplastin; ~ *f* tisular tissue antithromboplastin

antitrombótico *m* antithrombotic, an agent limiting or restricting blood coagulation

antitumorígeno *m* antitumor, anti-cancer drug, antineoplastic, counteracting tumor formation

antitusivo *m* cough suppressant, antitussive

antiviral *m* antiviral, antiviral drug

antivírico *adj* antiviral, antiviral drug

antojos *m pl de* craving for something

antracosis *f* black lung disease, coal workers' pneumoconiosis, miners' black lung, colliers' anthracosis

ántrax *m* anthrax

antro *m* antrum; ~ *m* **pilórico** antrum pyloricum, pyloric antrum

antropología *f* anthropology; ~ *f* **física** somatology, physical anthropology; ~ *f* **médica** medical anthropology

antropometría *f* anthropometry

antroposofía *f* anthroposophy

anuria *f* anuria, anuresis, complete suppresion of urine production by the kidneys

aorta *f* aorta; ~ *f* **torácica** thoracic aorta

aortografía *f* aortography

apaciqua *adj* obtundent, soothing, which dulls the pain

aparato *m* gadget, contrivance, apparatus, device; ~ *m* **craniocervical de ortodoncia** headgear, headcap, (in orthodontic treatment); ~ *m* **de gamagrafía** radioisotope scanner; ~ *m* **de oxígeno para reanimación** oxygen resuscitation apparatus; ~ *m* **de oxigenoterapia** oxygen resuscitation apparatus; ~ *m* **de radioscopía** fluoroscope, radioscopic apparatus; ~ *m* **de reanimación manual** manual resuscitation appliance; ~ *m* **de respiración artificial** oxygen resuscitation apparatus; ~ *m* **de tracción** traction apparatus, traction device; ~ *m* **digestivo** gastrointestinal tract, alimentary canal; ~ *m* **electromédico** electromedical equipment, electromedical device; ~ *m* **estimulador del ventrículo cardiaco** left ventricular assist device, LVAD; ~ *m* **locomotor** musculoskeletal system, locomotor system; ~ *m* **médico implantable activo** implantable medical device; ~ *m* **ortodóncico** orthodontic appliance; ~ *m* **ortodóncico funcional** functional orthodontic appliance; ~ *m* **para enderezar los dedo** traction appliance for straightening the fingers; ~ *m* **para masaje** massage apparatus, massaging device; ~ *m* **para sordos** hearing apparatus

apareamiento *m* mating; ~ *m* **de bases** base pairing; ~ *m* **génico** gene coupling

aparejo *m* gadget, contrivance, apparatus, device

apatía *f* apathy, lack of feeling or emotion, indiference

apático *adj* maudlin, lackadaisical, apathetic

apectomía *f* apicoectomy, apiectomy

apellido *m* last name

apenas *adv* little, small

apéndice *m* appendix

apendicitis *f* appendicitis

apertura *f* perforation

apetito *m* appetite

apical *adj* apical, near the apex

apicectomía *f* apicoectomy, apiectomy

apirético *adj* afrebrile, no fever

aplasia *f* aplasia, lack of development of an organ; ~ *f* **testicular** testicular aplasia; ~ *f* **vesical** aplasia of the urinary bladder

aplicación f application; ~ f **de duchas** elutriation, washing out, vaginal douche, washing out the vagina; ~ f **matemática** mapping

apnea f apnea, cessation of breathing

apófisis f apophysis, process of a bone; ~ f **coracoides** coracoid process; ~ f **mastoides** mastoid process

apolipoproteína f apolipoprotein

apomorfina f apomorphine

aponeurosis f aponeurosis; ~ f **abdominal** abdominal fascia, abdominal aponeurosis; ~ f **pélvica** pelvic fascia, Cruveilhier fascia; ~ f **perineal profunda** Camper ligament

apoplejía f apoplexy, stroke, cerebrovascular accident; ~ f **pulmonaria** pulmonary apoplexy, pulmonic apoplexy

apoptosis f apoptosis, programmed cell death

apósito m dressing, gauze, pad, bandage; ~ m **contentivo** elastic bandage, Ace bandage; ~ m **de gasa** gauze dressing; ~ m **líquido** liquid dressing for a wound, liquid bandage; ~ m **periodontal** periodontal pack, surgical pack; ~ m **semi-oclusivo** semi-occlusive dressing, occlusive bandage

apoyar v to assist, to help, to aid

apraxia f apraxia; ~ f **ideomotora** ideomotor apraxia, ideokinetic apraxia; ~ f **sensorial** sensory apraxia; ~ f **vesical** apraxia of urinary bladder

apreciar v to observe

aprensión f concern, apprehension, worry

apretar v **el puño** to make a fist, to clench one's fist

apropiado adj adequate

aprotinina f aprotinin

aproximadamente adv approximately, about

aproximado adj approximate, round (about)

aptitud f aptitude, capacity, ability; ~ f **comunicativa** social skills, interpersonal skills, the ability to establish social contacts; ~ f **espacial** spatial aptitude, space sense; ~ f **física** physical fitness, physical ability

apuñalar v to stab

aquejado de complaining of ...

aquel m, **aquella** f that (far)

aquellos m pl, **-as** fp those (far)

aquí here

arabinosa f arabinose

arabinósido m arabinoside; ~ m **de citosina** cytarabine arabinoside

aracnidismo m arachnidism, spider bite

aracnoide adj arachnoid

aracnoiditis f arachnoiditis, inflammation of the arachnoid membrane

araña f spider; ~ f **vascular** vascular spider, nevus arachnoides; ~ f **viuda negra** black widow spider

arañarse v to scrape; ~ v **la rodilla** to scrape one's knee

arañazo m scratch

arbitrar v to mediate

árbol m tree; ~ m **bronquial** bronchial tree; ~ m **genealógico** pedigree, genealogy

arbovirus m arbovirus

arca f armpit

archivos m pl **del fichero médico** computerized records, patient records online, computer files on patients

arco m arch; ~ m **cigomático** zygomatic arch

ardor m burning (sensation); ~ m **de estómago** heartburn, pyrosis, cardialgia, pain in the heart area

aréico adj areic

arenilla f urinary gravel

arginasa f arginase, arginine amidinase

arilsulfatasa f arylsulfatase, sulfatase

arinencefalia f alobar holoprosencephaly

armadura f **de implantación dental** dental-implant framework

armario m cupboard

ARN-polimerasa f RNA-polymerase, RNA transcriptase

arodillarse v kneel, to

aromático adj aromatic, scented

arañar v to scratch, to scrape, to abrade

arrastrarse v to crawl

arrebato m seizure, convulsions

arriba adv above, up

arriesgado adj risky, dangerous

arritmia f arrhythmia, irregular heartbeat; ~ f **cardiaca** cardiac arrhythmia

arritmogénico adj arrhythmogenic, causing abnormal heartbeat

arrojar v **flatos** to fart, to pass wind, to cut one, to break wind

arroz m rice
arrugado adj wrinkled, wrinkly
arsénico m arsenic
arte m **médico** art of healing, healing arts
arteria f artery; ~ f **basilar** basilar artery;
~ f **braquial** brachial artery; ~ f **carótida**
carotid artery, principal artery of the neck & head; ~ f **del cráneo** carotid artery, principal artery of the neck & head; ~ f **facial** facial artery; ~ f **femoral** femoral artery;
~ f **ileocólica** ileocolic artery; ~ f **pulmonar**
pulmonary trunk, pulmonary artery;
~ f **subclavicular** subclavian artery;
~ f **umbilical** umbilical artery; ~ f **vertebral**
vertebral artery, paired arteries which supply the muscles of the neck, spinal cord and cerebellum
arterial adj arterial, pertaining to the arteries, artery-related
arteriografía f arteriography, angiography of arteries
arteriola f arteriole
arteriolar adj arteriolar, arteriole-related
arteriopatía f **oclusiva** occlusive arterial disease
arteriosclerosis f arteriosclerosis, hardening of the arteries
arteriovenoso adj arteriovenous, artery and vein-related
arteritis f arteritis; ~ f **de células gigantes**
giant cell arteritis, temporal arteritis, systemic vasculitis; ~ f **necrosante** necrotizing arteritis; ~ f **reumática** rheumatic arteritis;
~ f **temporal** temporal arteritis; ~ f **viral**
viral arteritis
articulación f articulation, verbal articulation, knuckle; ~ f **acromioclavicular**
acromioclavicular joint; ~ f **atlantoaxial**
atlantoaxial joint, atlanto-axial joint;
~ f **carpiana** carpal joint; ~ f **cotiloidea** ball-and-socket joint, hip joint; ~ f **cubital** elbow joint; ~ f **de la muñeca** carpus, wrist joint;
~ f **esternoclavicular** sternoclavicular joint;
~ f **plana** plane joint, gliding joint; ~ f **radio carpiana** radiocarpal joint, wrist joint;
~ f **sacroilíaca** sacroiliac joint, sacro-iliac articulation; ~ f **sinovial** synovial joint;
~ f **tarsiana** tarsal joint;
~ f **temporomandibular** jaw joint, mandibular

joint, TMJ, temporomandibular joint
articulaciones (pl f) principales major joints
articular adj articular, joint-related
artificial adj artificial, factitious
artilugion m gadget, contrivance, apparatus, device
artopatía f neuropathic arthropathy;
~ f **neuropática** neuropathic arthropathy
artralgia f arthralgia, pain in a joint
artritis f arthritis, joint illness;
~ f **alcaptonúrica** alkaptonuric arthritis;
~ f **alérgica** allergic arthritis; ~ f **amiloidea**
amyloid arthritis; ~ f **hemofílica** hemophilic arthritis; ~ f **purulenta** purulent arthritis;
~ f **reumatoide** rheumatoid arthritis, atrophic arthritis, chronic inflammatory arthritis;
~ f **sacro-ilíaca** sacroiliac arthritis;
~ f **séptica** septic arthritis; ~ f **sintomática**
symptomatic arthritis; ~ f **supurada** purulent arthritis; ~ f **temporomaxilar** arthritis in the temporomandibular joint; ~ f **traumática**
traumatic arthritis; ~ f **vellosa** villous arthritis
artrocentesis f arthrocentesis, joint aspiration, puncture of a joint
artrodesis f arthrodesis, arthrokleisis
artrogriposis f arthrogryposis
artropatía f arthropathy, joint disease;
~ f **menopáusica** ovariprival arthropathy;
~ f **neurotrófica** neurotrophic arthropathy
artroplastia f arthroplasty, surgical repair of a joint; ~ f **de la cadera** hip replacement
artrópodo m arthropod
artroscopía f arthroscopy
artrosis f arthrosis, joint disease; ~ f **de la rodilla** gonarthrosis; ~ f **deformante**
hypertrophic degenerative arthrosis; ~ f **del codo** osteoarthritis of the elbow;
~ f **osteofítica raquídea** spinal osteoarthritis;
~ f **patelofemoral** patellofemoral arthrosis
asa f loop; ~ f **calibrada** calibrated loop
asado m barbecue
asas f pl **intestinales** intestinal loops
asbestosis f asbestosis; ~ f **pleural** pulmonary asbestosis; ~ f **pulmonar** pleural asbestosis
ascárid m Ascaris, ascarid, a roundworm
ascitis f ascites, abdominal dropsy, hydroperitonea, peritoneal dropsy
asco m nausea, queasiness, feeling sick, feeling

nauseated
ascorbato m ascorbate, ascorbic acid
aseo m bathroom, toilet
asepsia f asepsis, cleanliness, absence of infectious microorganisms
aséptico adj aseptic, free of germs, clean
asertividad f assertiveness, insistent, self-assured, or demanding behavior
asesor m adviser; ~ **dietético** dietician, nutritionist, an expert in nutrition
asesoramiento m counseling; ~ **matrimonial** marriage counseling, relationship counseling; ~ **m para grupos** group counseling
asfixia f asphyxia, suffocating; ~ **f intrauterina** intra-uterine asphyxia
así que adv so
asilo m nursing home
asimbolia f del dolor pain asymbolia
asimétrico adj asymmetric
asimilar v to assimilate
asintomático adj asymptomatic, without symptoms
asistencia f assistance, help, care; ~ f a **domicilio** home nursing care; ~ f **de hospital integrado** f integrated health care, managed care; ~ f **emocional del morbundo** hospice care, terminal care; ~ f **médica** health care, medical care, healthcare services; ~ f **médica a domicilio** home health care, home health service; ~ f **prenatal** prenatal care; ~ f **sanitaria** health care, medical care, healthcare services; ~ f **social** income support, aid to dependant families, financial aid
asistente m/f attendant, assistant; ~ f **de enfermería** nurse's aide, nursing assistant; ~ **m de médico** medical assistant, doctor's assistant; ~ **m médico social** medical social worker; ~ **m social** social worker, social case worker
asistir v assist, to, help, to, aid, to, be present, to, attend, to
asistolia f asystole, cardiac arrest
asma f asthma, bronchospasm, bronchial asthma; ~ m **bronquial extrínseca** extrinsic asthma; ~ m **de Millar** pseudocroup, Millar's asthma, catarrhal croup, spasmodic laryngitis
asmático adj asthmatic
asociación f association, combination

asoleada f heliosis
asparragina f asparagine
asparraginasa f asparaginase
aspartamo m aspartame, a low-calorie sweetener
aspartato m aspartate; ~ **–aminotransferasa** f SGOT
aspergilopepsina f trypsinogen kinase; ~ f proteinase B
aspergilosis f aspergillosis
áspero adj rough
aspiración f suction, aspiration; ~ f **de gases** inhalation, aspiration of gases, breathing in
aspirador m exhaust fan, exhauster, suction-pipe, ventilator; ~ **m central de basuras** central vacuum cleaner system, pneumatic disposal unit, cleaning aspirator; ~ **m de polvo** dust eliminator, dust separator, dust collector, ventilator; ~ **m limpiador** pneumatic disposal unit; ~ **m mecánico** mechanical aspirator; ~ **m ultrasónico** Cavitron ultrasonic surgical aspirator
aspirar v inhale, to, breathe in, to
aspirina f aspirin, acetylsalicylic acid
asta f de Ammon hippocampus, Ammon's horn
astenia f asthenia, weakness, loss of strength, debilitation; ~ f **neurocirculatoria** effort syndrome, neurocirculatory asthenia, cardiac neurosis, DaCosta's disease, DaCosta's syndrome
astenopía f eyestrain, asthenopia; ~ f **conjuntival** conjunctival asthenopia; ~ f **muscular** motor asthenopia, muscular asthenopia
astigmatismo m astigmatism; ~ m **corneal** corneal astigmatism; ~ m **hiperópico** hyperopic astigmatism; ~ m **miópico** myopic astigmatism; ~ m **mixto** mixed astigmatism
astigón m splinter
astillas f pl de hueso bone chips, bone fragments
astrágalo m ankle bone, malleolus
astringente adj astringent, toner
astringir v to bind, to constrict, to contract
astrocito m astrocyte; ~ m **protoplasmático** protoplasmatic astrocyte
astrocitoma m astrocytoma; ~ m **cerebelar** cerebellar astrocytoma

astrocitos *m pl* neuroglial cells, macroglia, astroglia, astrocytes

astroglia *f* neuroglial cells, macroglia, astroglia, astrocytes

atamoxef moxalactam

ataque *m* attack, convulsion, seizure, hysteric fit, insult, have a fit, to, to throw a fit, to; ~ *m* **cardíaco** myocardial infarction, heart attack; ~ *m* **cerebral** apoplexy, stroke, cerebrovascular accident; ~ *m* **de isquemia en el cerebro** ischemic stroke (in the brain); ~ *m* **de isquémia transitoria** ischemic attack, mini-stroke, small stroke, ~ *m* **del corazón** heart attack; ~ *m* **isquémico** ischemic seizure, ischemic attack

ataxia *f* ataxia, lack of coordination, unsteady gait; ~ *f* **telangiectasia** Louis-Bar syndrome, ataxia-telangiectasia, Boder-Sedgwick syndrome; ~ *f* **vasomotriz** vasomotor ataxia; ~ *f* **vestibular** vestibular ataxia

atelectasia *f* atelectasis, partial or complete collapse of the lung; ~ *f* **fetal congénita** congenital fetal atelectasis

atención *f* attention, care, courtesy; ~ *f* **ambulatoria** outpatient clinic, ambulatory care, outpatient treatment, outpatient care; ~ *f* **domiciliaria** home health care, home health service; ~ *f* **médica** health care, medical care, healthcare services; ~ *f* **prenatal** prenatal care

atenciones *f pl* **a largo plazo** long-term care

atendimiento *m* treatment, consultation; ~ *m* **ambulatorio** outpatient treatment, outpatient consultation

atento *adj* observant, attentive

atenuación *f* inhibition, stopping

atenuado *adj* attenuated

atenuancia *f* attenuance; ~ *f* **decimal** decadic attenuantion

atenuar *v* to attenuate, to reduce, to weaken

ateroma *m* atheroma, encysted tumor

ateromatosis *f* atheromatosis, thickening of the arteries

aterosclerosis *f* atherosclerosis

atetosis *f* athetosis, slow, writhing movements especially of the hands

atípico *adj* atypical, unusual, abnormal, irregular

atlantoaxial *adj* atlantoaxial

atomizador *m* atomizer, nebulizer, spray dispenser, spray

átomo *m* atom; ~ *m* **marcado** tracer atom, labeled atom, tagged atom, radioactive and traceable atom

atonía *f* atony, lack of muscle tone

atónico *adj* atonic

atopia *f* atopy, hereditary allergic hypersensitivity

atópico *adj* atopic

atópico *m* allergic reaction, allergic response

atosigar *v* poison, to

atóxico *adj* atoxic, non-poisonous, non-toxic

atrabiliario *adj* irritable, cranky, touchy, short-tempered, in a bad mood

atragantarse *v* to choke on food

atrapamiento *m* entrapment, trapping; ~ *m* **neural** nerve entrapment, compression neuropathy, compression syndrome

atrasar *v* to retard, to slow down, to delay

atraso *m* delay, retard; ~ *m* **mental** mentally retarded

atraviesa *f* urethra

atrazina *f* atrazine

atresia *f* atresia, absence or closure of a natural passage of the body; ~ *f* **del intestino delgado** atresia of the small intestine; ~ *f* **vaginal** vaginal atresia

atrial *adj* atrial

atrio *m* atrium

atrioventricular *adj* atrioventricular, pertaining to both an atrium and a ventricle of the heart

atrofia *f* atrophy, wasting away, wasting; ~ *f* **cardíaca** cardiac atrophy; ~ *f* **cerebral** cerebral atrophy; ~ *f* **cutánea** skin atrophy; ~ *f* **de la retina** retinal atrophy; ~ *f* **del nervio óptico** atrophy of the optic nerve, optic atrophy; ~ *f* **dérmica neurogénica** dermatophy; ~ *f* **muscular** wasting paralysis, muscular atrophy; ~ *f* **óptica** atrophy of the optic nerve, optic atrophy; ~ *f* **por inactividad** inactivity atrophy, atrophy of disuse; ~ *f* **por inanición** inanition atrophy

atropina *f* atropine, a parasympatholytic agent

aturdido *adj* light-headed, dizzy, woozy, lightheadedness

audición *f* hearing

audífono m hearing aid, auditory apparatus hearing apparatus, auditory prosthesis, otophone

audiofonología f speech pathology, phoniatry

audiometría f audiometry; ~ f de la palabra vocal audiometry, speech audiometry; ~ f electroencefalográfica evoked response audiometry, cortical audiometry; ~ f por potenciales evocados evoked response audiometry, cortical audiometry; ~ f vocal vocal audiometry, speech audiometry

auditivo adj auditory, related to hearing

auditoría f de la calidad quality audit

aumento m increase; ~ m de los ganglios linfáticos swollen lymph nodes, enlarged lymph nodes; ~ m del ritmo cardiaco quickened pulse rate, increased heart rate; ~ m del tamaño del corazón cardiomegaly, enlargement of the heart; ~ m del tamaño del hígado hepatomegaly, liver enlargement

aunque though, although

aura f aura, warning sensation preceding an epileptic seizure

aural adj aural

auricular adj auricular, pertaining to the ear

auscultación f auscultation, listening with a stethoscope

ausencia f absence (seizure), mild epilepsy

ausencias f pl psychic gaps, absences, psychic deliquia

autismo m autism

autoaglomeración f autoagglomeration

autoaglutinina f autoagglutinin

autoanalizador m automated analyzer

autoanticuerpo m autoantibody

autoantígeno m autoantigen

autoayuda f self-help, mutual help

autoclave m autoclave

autoclonación f self-cloning

autodesvalorización f feelings of worthlessness, feelings of inadequacy, lack of self-esteem

autoeliminación f de intrones self-splicing

autoestima f self-esteem, self-worth, self-respect

autoexploración f de la mama breast self-examination

autoimagen m self-image

autoinmune adj autoimmune, immune response against the body's own tissues

autolesión f self-mutilation, automutilation

autolobectomía f autolobectomy

automática adj automatic

automatismo m automatism, aimless and indirected behaviour; ~ m cardiaco automatism of the heart, cardiac automatism

automatización f automation

automedicación f self-medication

automutilación f self-mutilation, automutilation

autónomo adj autonomic, functionally independent, autonomous

autoplastia f autoplasty, autologous graft, autograft

autopsia f autopsy, necropsy, post mortem, postmortem examination; ~ f médico-científica postmortem examination

autorización f authorization

autorradiografía f autoradiography, autoradiograph

autorreplicación f self-replication

autosoma m autosome, euchromosome

autosómico adj autosomal

autotopoagnosia f autotopoagnosia

autotransfusión f autologous transfusion, autohemotransfusion; ~ f preoperatoria preoperative autologous blood donation

autotrasplante m autologous transplantation

autótrofo adj autotroph

auxiliar m helper; ~ m de médico medical assistant, doctor's assistant

avance m advance, breakthrough; ~ m científico scientific breakthrough

avascular adj avascular

aventado adj flatulent

aventurado adj risky, dangerous

avidez f avidity, eagerness; ~ f de un antisuero antiserum avidity

avispa f wasp

axila f armpit

ayer yesterday

ayuda f help, assistance; ~ f a los ancianos elder care, care of the elderly; ~ f humanitaria humanitarian assistance, humanitarian aid

ayudante m assistant; ~ m de médico medical assistant, doctor's assistant; ~ m técnico

médico assistant medical technician
ayudar v to assist, to help, to aid
ayunar v to fast
azatioprina f azathioprine
azidotimidina f AZT, Retrovir, zidovudine, azidothymidine
azitromicina f azithromycin
azlocilina f azlocillin
azogue m Hg, mercury, quicksilver
azoospermia f azoospermia, lack of spermatozoa in semen
azotemia f azotemia, renal failure, excess of nitrogenous compounds in the blood
AZT AZT, Retrovir, zidovudine, azidothymidine
azucar m sugar; ~ **m de uva** glucose, dextrose, grape sugar; ~ **m invertido** invert sugar
azufre m sulfur, sulphur
azul adj blue

B

babaza f froth in mouth
babesiasis f piroplasmosis, tick fever, babesiosis, Babesia infection
babesiosis f piroplasmosis, tick fever, babesiosis, Babesia infection
Bacillus m **acidophilus** lactobacillus acidophilus; ~ **m anthracis** Davaine's bacillus
bacilo m bacillus; ~ **m anaerobio** anaerobic rod; ~ **m grampositivo** gram positive rod; ~ **m gramnegativo** gram-negative rod; ~ **m no esporulado** nonsporeforming bacillus
bacín m urine bottle, urinal
bacinilla f bedpan
bacteria f bacterium; ~ **coliformes** coliform bacteria, coliform organism, bacterium coli; ~ **f de la lepra** leprosy bacterium, mycobacterium leprae; ~ **f propiónica** propionibacterium
bacteriano adj bacterial
bacterias f pl bacteria (pl); ~ **f pl aerobias viables** viable aerobic bacteria; ~ **f pl anaerobias** anaerobic bacteria; ~ **f pl Leptospira** leptospira bacteria; ~ **f pl virulentas** virulent bacteria
bactericida adj bactericidal; ~ **m** bactericide,

anti-bacteria drug
bacteriemia f bacteriemia, bacteria in the blood, bacteriotoxemia
bacteriófago m phage, bacteriophage; ~ **m anticolérico** choleraphage; ~ **m lamda** phage lambda; ~ **m virulento** virulent bacteriophage
bacteriología f bacteriology
bacteriológico adj bacteriological, relating to the study of bacteria
bacterioproteínas f pl bacterioproteins
bacteriostático adj bacteriostatic, antibiotic
bacteriuria f bacteriuria, bacteria in urine
bagazosis f bagassosis, sugar cane lung
baja f medical certificate
bajar v to lower, to get down
bajo adj low, prp under; ~ **la línea cero** negative; ~ adj **volumen plasmático** low plasma volume
balance m balance; ~ **m de nitrógeno** nitrogen balance, nitrogen equilibrium
balanitis f balanitis
balanza f scale
balazo m gunshot
balbucear v to stutter, to stammer
balistocardiografía f ballistocardiography
balneoterapia f pool therapy, hydrotherapy, balneotherapy
balón m balloon; ~ **m gástrico** gastric balloon, gastric bubble, Ballobes balloon
banco m bank; ~ **m de datos** data base; ~ **m de órganos** organ bank, transplant bank; ~ **m de referencias** referral bank
banda f band, sling (for arm)
bandeo m **cromosómico** chromosome banding
bañera f bathtub; ~ **f de hidromasaje** whirlpool bath, jacuzzi, hot tub
baño m toilet, lavatory, water closet, bathroom; ~ **m de asiento** sponge bath; ~ **m de ducha** shower; ~ **m de parafina** paraffin bath, wax bath; ~ **m de remolino** whirlpool bath, jacuzzi, hot tub
barba f beard, chin
barbilla f beard, chin
barbiturato m barbiturate
bario m barium
barorreceptor m baroreceptor, pressoreceptor
barorreflejo m baroreflex

B

barotitis f **media** aerosinusitis, sinus pain due to changing atmospheric pressures

barotraumatismo m barotrauma; ~ m **del oído** barotitis, aero-otitis media, aviator's ear

barrera f barrier; ~ f **hematoencefálica** blood-brain barrier, blood brain barrier

barrido m **segmentado con rayos gamma** segmented gamma-scanning

barriga f belly, stomach, paunch, tummy

barro m boil, furuncle, bump, swelling, bruise; ~ m **de tabano** warble tumor; ~ m **terapéutico** medicinal mud, healing mudpack, fangotherapy, mud packs; ~ m **termal** medicinal mud, healing mudpack, fangotherapy, mud packs

bartolinitis f bartholinitis

basal adj basal, normal

basaloma m basal cell carcinoma, basaloma

basca f náusea, queasiness, feeling sick, feeling nauseated

base f substrate, substance on which an enzyme act; ~ f **de ácido nucleico** nucleic base, nucleotide base; ~ f **nucleotídica** nucleic base, nucleotide base

basín m bedpan

basófilo m basophilocyte, basophil, basophil leucocyte, basophilic cell

basofilocito m basophilocyte, basophil, basophil leucocyte, basophilic cell

bastante adj lots, lots (of), a lot

bastón m cane, walking stick

bata f dressing gown, bathrobe, white coat

bata f **de hospital** hospital gown, laboratory coat, lab coat, white coat

bazo m spleen; ~ m **amiloideo** amyloid spleen

bebé m baby

beber v to drink

bebida f drink; ~ f pl **alcohólica** alcoholic drink, spirit

behaviorismo m behaviorism

bencilpenicilina f penicillin G

beneficio m benefit; ~ m **de incapacidad** disability benefit; ~ m **médico suplementario** major medical benefit, major medical expense insurance

benigno adj benign, non-malignant

benzaldehído m benzaldehyde, benzoic aldehyde

benzodiazepina f benzodiazepine

béquico m cough suppressant, antitussive

beriliosis f beryllium disease

betabloqueador m betablocker, beta blocker, beta-antagonist

betabloqueante m betablocker, beta blocker, beta-antagonist

betaendorfina f endorphin, a neuropeptide

beta-lactamasa f beta-lactamase

betalactámico m beta-lactam antibiotic

betametasona f betamethasone

betamimético m betamimetic

betaoxidación f beta-oxidation

biberón m baby bottle, nursing bottle, infants' feeding bottle

biblioteca f library; ~ f **genómica** genomic library

bicapa f **lipídica** lipid bilayer, double lipid layer

bicarbonato m bicarbonate

bíceps m musculus biceps brachii, biceps

bicicleta f bicycle; ~ f **ergométrica** ergometric bicycle, stationary bicycle, exercise bicycle

bicórneo adj bicornuate, two-horned

bien adv good, fine; ~ **musculado** adj well-muscled, muscular; ~ **que** though, although

bienestar m well-being, welfare

bifásico adj biphasic, two-phase

bifosfonato m biphosphonate

bifurcación f bifurcation, branch

bigeminismo m bigeminy, bigemina, pulsus bigeminus

bigote m mustache, moustache

biguanida f biguanide

bilateral adj bilateral, two-sided

bilharziosis f schistosomiasis, bilharziasis

biliar adj biliary, bile-related

bilirrubina f bilirubin; ~ f **esterificada** direct bilirubin; ~ f **no esterificada** indirect bilirubin

bilis f bile, gall, gall bladder disease, cholecystitis

biocatalizador m biocatalyst

biocenosis f biocenosis, biotic community

biodegradable adj biodegradable

biodegradación f biodegradation, biodegrading

biodisponibilidad f bioavailability, effectiveness

bioelectrónica f bioelectronics

bioenergía f bioenergy

bioensayo m bioassay, biological testing

bioequivalencia f bioequivalence

bioequivalente *m* bioequivalent
bioética *f* bioethics
biofeedback *m* biofeedback
bioflavenoide *m* bioflavenoid
bioingeniería *f* bioengineering, biomedical engineering
biología *f* biology; ~ *f* **celular** cell biology, cytobiology; ~ *f* **clínica** clinical biology; ~ *f* **médica** clinical biology; ~ *f* **molecular** molecular biology
biológico *adj* biological
bioluminiscencia *f* bioluminescence
biomaterial *m* biomaterial
biomecánica *f* biomechanics
biomedicina *f* biomedicine
biomédico *adj* biomedical
biometría *f* biometrics, biometry, the statistical analysis of biological observations and phenomena
biometría ocular ocular biometry
biomicroscopia *f* biomicroscopy
biomicroscopio *m* biomicroscope, a microscope with a rectangular light source
biónica *f* bionics
biopelícula *f* biofilm
bioprótesis *f* bioprosthesis; ~ *f* **aórtica** aortic bioprosthesis; ~ *f* **del corazón de cerdo** bioprosthesis, valve from a pig's heart, heterograft bioprosthesis
biopsia *f* biopsy, sample excision; ~ *f* **con aguja** needle biopsy, aspiration biopsy; ~ *f* **cutánea** skin biopsy; ~ *f* **de médula ósea** bone marrow biopsy
bioquímica *f* biological chemistry, biochemistry; ~ *f* **clínica** clinical biochemistry, pathobiochemistry, chemical pathology
bioquímico *adj* biochemical
bioretroalimentación *f* biofeedback
biorritmo *m* biorhythm
bioseguridad *f* biosafety
biosensor *m* biosensor
biósfera *f* biosphere
biosíntesis *f* biosynthesis; ~ *f* **de aminoácidos** biosynthesis of amino acids; ~ *f* **de proteínas** protein synthesis
biotécnica *f* biotechnology
biotecnología *f* biotechnology
biótico *f* biotic

biotina *f* biotin, vitamine H
biotipificación *f* biotyping
biotipo *m* biotype; ~ *m* **ginecoide** gynecoid biotype
biotipología *f* biotypology
biotoxicología *f* biotoxicology
biotransformación *f* biotransformation, chemical changes
bisinosis *f* byssinosis
bisturí *m* scalpel; ~ *m* **electrónico** electrotome; ~ *m* **láser** laser scalpel
bizco *m* squint, strabismus
bizcocho *m* pie, cake
b-lactamasa *f* cephalosporinase
blanco *adj* caucasian, white
blando *adj* flaccid, flabby, soft
blanqueador *m* bleach
blanqueamiento *m* turning pale, blanching, going pallid
blanquecino *adj* whitish, off-white in color
blanquillo *m* egg white
blastema *m* blastema; ~ *m* **nefrógeno** nephrogenic blastema
blastocito *m* blastocyte, blastocyst, blastula, embryonic tissue formed before implantation
blastomero *m* blastomere
blastomicosis *f* blastomycosis; ~ *f* **fistulosa glútea** fistulous gluteal blastomycosis; ~ *f* **norteamericana** Gilchrist disease, North American blastomycosis; ~ *f* **por glenospora** glenosporosis; ~ *f* **purulenta profunda** profound purulent blastomycosis
blastoporo *m* gastrula, an embryonic stage of animal development
blástula *m* blastocyte, blastocyst, blastula, embryonic tissue formed before implantation
blefarelosis *f* blepharelosis
blefaritis *f* blepharitis, eyelid inflammation; ~ *f* **eritematosa** erythematous blepharitis; ~ *f* **folicular** follicular blepharitis; ~ *f* **oleosa** greasy blepharitis, blepharitis oleosa
blefaroadenitis *f* blepharo-adenitis
blefarocalasia *f* blepharochalasis, ptosis atrophica
blefaroconjuntivitis *f* blepharoconjunctivitis
blefaromelasma *m* melasma, blepharomelasma, blotchy skin
blefaroplastía *f* blepharoplasty

blenorragia f blennorrhagia, gonorrhea, clap, gonorrhoea

blíster m blister pack

bloque m block

bloqueador m blocker, blocking agent, antagonist; ~ m **adrenérgico** adrenergic antagonist, adrenergic blocking agent, adrenergic blocker, adrenolytic drug; ~ m **del sol** sunscreen

bloqueo m blockage, block, blocking, obstruction; ~ m **de entrada** entry exclusion; ~ m **del tronco simpático** blockage of sympathetic trunk, denervation of the sympathetic trunk, ~ m **intraventricular** intraventricular block; ~ m **nervioso** nerve bloc; ~ m **paravertebral** paravertebral blockade

bobería f stupidity

boca f mouth; ~ f **arriba** to lie face up, to lie on your back; ~ f **del estómago** pit of the stomach, cardial sphincter

bocadillo m snack

bocado m **de Adán** Adam's apple, laryngeal prominence

bochornos m pl hot flashes

bocio m struma, goiter, thyroid enlargement; ~ m **basedowificado** Parry's disease, Basedow's disease; ~ m **coloideo** colloid goiter, adenoma gelatinosum; ~ m **endémico** endemic goiter; ~ m **quístico** cystic goiter; ~ m **subesternal** substernal goiter, intrathoracic goiter

bola f lump; ~ f **de pelo** hairball

bolsa f bag; ~ f **de agua caliente** hot water bottle, hot pack; ~ f **de aguas** amniotic sac; ~ f **de colostomía** colostomy bag; ~ f **de hielo** ice pack; ~ f **sinovial** synovial bursa; ~ f **sinovial subcutánea** subcutaneous synovial bursa

bolsilla f **de piel** skin pocket

bolos m bolus

bomba f bomb, pump; ~ f **de calcio** calcium pump, calcium ATPase; ~ f **de infusión implantable** implantable infusion pump; ~ f **de protones** proton pump, H+/K+-ATPase; ~ f **de sodio** sodium pump, a molecular mechanism by which sodium ions are actively transported across a plasma membrane; ~ f **de vacío** exhaust fan, exhauster, suction-pipe,

ventilator, suction pump; ~ f **peristáltica** peristaltic pump

boquinete m cleft palate, uranoschisis

borborigmo m borborygmus, rumbling tummy, growling tummy

borde m edge, brim, border; ~ m **de la célula** cell border; ~ m **dérmico** skin graft, epidermal graft

bordón m cane, walking stick

borracho adj inebriated, drunk

borramiento m cervical effacement of the cervix

borrego m lamb

Borrelia f **burgdorferi** Borrelia burgdorferi

borreliosis f borreliosis, borrelia infection, relapsing fever, recurrent fever, spirillum fever

bostezar v to yawn

botánica f botany; ~ f **farmacéutica** pharmaceutical botany

botella f bottle

botica f pharmacy, drug store

boticario m druggist, pharmacist, chemist

botiquín m **de emergencia para quemaduras** emergency kit for burns

botiquín m **de urgencia** first aid kit, first aid chest

botones m pl bellboy, bellhop; ~ m pl **de aceite** oil acne, oily pimples

botriocefalosis f bothriocephalosis

botulismo m botulism

bóveda f hard palate, roof of the mouth; ~ f **del cráneo** cranial vault, calvaria

bradicardia f bradycardia, slow heartbeat

bradicinina f bradikinin

bradipnea f bradypnea, slow breathing

bradiquinesia f bradykinesia, sluggishness

panal descartable m disposable diaper

bragas f pl women's panties, women's underwear

braguero m back brace, back support; ~ m **inguinal** inguinal truss, hernia truss; ~ m **para hernia** hernial truss, hernia bandage

braguitas f pl women's panties, women's underwear

brazo m arm; ~ m **artificial** upper arm prosthesis, artificial arm

brecha f fissure, crack, split

breve adj short

brocha f **de afeitar** shaving brush

bromelaína f **de tronco** stem bromelain, bromelain

bromhidrosis f bromhidrosis, foul-smelling sweat

brominismo m brominism, bromine cachexia

bromismo m brominism, bromine cachexia

bromo m bromine

bromocriptina f bromocriptine

bromoyoduro m bromoiodide; ~ m **de plata** silver bromoiodide; ~ m **de talio** thallium bromoiodide

bronceado m tanned, brown

broncoblastomicosis f bronchoblastomycosis

broncoconstricción f bronchoconstriction, constriction of air passages

broncodilatación f bronchodilatation, dilated state of a bronchus, widening of the airways, broncholysis

broncodilatador m bronchodilator, a drug to help breathing

broncoectasia f bronchiectasia; ~ **atelectásica congénita** atelectatic congenital bronchiectasia

broncoespasmo m bronchospasm, bronchial asthma

broncofonía f bronchophony; ~ f **afónica** f aphonic bronchophony

broncógeno adj bronchogenic

broncografía f bronchography, an x-ray of the bronchial tree after injecting a contrast medium

broncolisis f bronchodilatation, dilated state of a bronchus, widening of the airways, broncholysis

bronconeumonía f bronchopneumonia, bronchial pneumonia; ~ f **diseminada** disseminated bronchopneumonia

bronconeumopatía f **crónica obstructiva** COPD, chronic obstructive pulmonary disease

broncopulmonar adj bronchopulmonary, chest-related

broncoscopio m bronchoscope, endoscopic examination or surgery of the bronchi

bronquial adj bronchial

bronquiectasia f bronchiectasis, widening of the airways

bronquio m bronchus

bronquiolitis f bronchiolitis; ~ f **obliterante** obliterating bronchiolitis, bronchiolitis obliterans; ~ f **obliterante congénita** congenital obliterating bronchiolitis

bronquitis f bronchitis; ~ f **asmática** asthmatic bronchitis, chronic obstructive bronchitis; ~ f **crónica** chronic bronchitis; ~ f **infecciosa** infectious bronchitis; ~ f **necrótica** necrotic bronchitis; ~ f **obstructiva** obstructive bronchitis; ~ f **obstructiva crónica** asthmatic bronchitis, chronic obstructive bronchitis; ~ f **sintomática** symptomatic bronchitis

brote m outbreak; ~ m **de un diente** teething, dentition; ~ m **primario** primary outbreak

brucelosis f brucellosis (a disease of cattle)

brusco adj abrupt, sudden

bruxismo m night guard, mouth guard, biteguard, occlusal splint, peridontal splint, dental prosthesis

bruxomanía f grinding one's teeth, bruxism

bubas f pl inflamed lymph nodes, buboes (in the armpit)

bubón m buboes, swollen lymph nodes; ~ m **estrumoso** strumous bubo; ~ m **maligno** malignant bubo; ~ m **venéreo** venereal bubo

bucal adj buccal, mouth or cheek-related

bucofaríngeo adj buccopharyngeal, pertaining to the mouth and pharynx

buen adj **estado** wellness, being well

buena adj **salud** health, wellness, being well

bueno m good, fine

buffer m buffer

bulbar adj bulbar, bulbous, bulb-related

bulbo m bulb; ~ m **del vestíbulo** bulb of vestible; ~ m **gustatorio** taste bud; ~ m **olfatorio** olfactory bulb; ~ m **raquídeo** myelencephalon, medulla oblongata

bulimia f bulimia

bullar adj blistered, bullous

bullón m blister, bulla, bleb, pomphus

bulto m bulge, protrusion, lump

bunio m bunion

burrada f stupidity

bursitis f bursitis; ~ f **aséptica** aseptic bursitis, inflammation of a bursa not caused by infection; ~ f **séptica** septic bursitis

buscar v to research, to investigate, to examine

búsqueda f search; ~ f **de factores de riesgo** screening for risk factors; ~ f **de sangre oculta en las deposiciones** fecal occult blood test, hemoccult test

butirato m butyrate

by-pass m bypass
~ m **coronario** coronary bypass surgery

C

C.P. zip code, postal code

cabalgar v to straddle, to have one leg on each side

cabello m hair

cabelludo adj hairy, pilous

cabestrillo m sling (for arm)

cabeza f head; ~ f **corta** caput breve, the short head of biceps femoris muscle; ~ f **del fémur** head of the femur, femoral head; ~ f **del húmero** capitulum of humerus, head of the humerus; ~ f **del músculo** head of a muscle, caput musculi

cabina f booth, cab; ~ f **de ducha** shower cubicle, shower stall

cacahuete m peanut

cachete m cheek

cada all; ~ **(hora et.)** every; ~ **(uno, una)** each

cadáver m dead body, cadaver, corpse

cadena f strand; ~ f **adelantada** leading strand; ~ f **alimentaria** food chain; ~ f **antisentido** antisense strand; ~ f **de ADN** strand of DNA; ~ f **de custodia** chain of custody; ~ f **discontínua** lagging strand; ~ f **doble** double strand; ~ f **hidrocarbonada** hydrocarbon chain; ~ f **homosentido** sense strand

cadera f hip, pelvis, coxa; ~ f **de resorte** clicking hip, snapping hip

caderinas f pl cadherins, liver cell adhesion molecules

cadmio m cadmium

caduceo m caduceus

café m coffee; ~ m **con leche** coffee with milk; ~ m **descafeinado** decaffeinated coffee

cafeína f caffein

caída f fall, prolapse; ~ f **de cabello** loss of hair

caja f **de urgencia** first aid kit, first aid chest; ~ f **Petri** petri dish; ~ f **torácica** rib cage

calacio m chalazion

calambre m charley horse; ~ m **en la pantorilla** cramp in the calf; ~ m **muscular** muscle cramp, muscle spasm

calambres m pl spasmodic (cramplike) pain; ~ m pl **en el vientre** colic, cramps, abdominal pain

calavera f skull, cranium

calcáneo m heel bone, calcaneum

calcaneodinia f pain in the heel, calcaneodynia

calcar m calcar; ~ m **femoral** femoral calcar, calcar femoral

calcariavis f calcar avis

calcemia f calcemia, excess blood calcium

calcidiol m calcidiol

calcifediol m calcifediol

calciferol m calciferol

calcificación f calcification, calcinosis; ~ f **valvular del corazón** calcification of the cardiac valve

calcinosis f calcification, calcinosis

calcio m calcium

calcioantagonista m calcium antagonist

calciohidrógenocarbonato m calcium hydrogen carbonate

calciol f vitamin D3

calcitonina f calcitonin, thyrocalcitonin

calcitriol m calcitriol

calciuria f calciuria, calcium in the urine

cálculo m stone, calculus; ~ m **biliar** gallstone, biliary calculus, biliary concretion; ~ m **de fosfato de calcio** calcium phosphate calculus, calcium phosphate crystals; ~ m **de la vejiga** urinary calculus, urinary calculus disease; ~ m **dental** dental calculus, tartar, dental plaque; ~ m **intradiverticular** diverticular concretion; ~ m **intrahepático** hepatolith; ~ m **renal** nephrolith, kidney stone; ~ m **urinario** urinary stone, urolith, urinary calculus, urinary calculus disease; ~ m **vesical** calculus vesicalis, bladder calculi, bladder stone

caldo m broth; ~ m **con selenita** selenite broth; ~ m **con tetrationato** tetrathionate broth; ~ m **con tioglicolato** thioglycolate broth; ~ m **con tripticasa de soya** trypticase soy broth; ~ *m* **de enriquecimiento** enrichment culture; ~ *m* **nutritivo** nutrient broth; ~ *m* **peptonado** peptone broth

calendario *m* calendar; ~ *m* **menstrual** menstrual calendar

caléndula *f* officinalis calendula officinalis, marigold

calentarse *v* to get hot, to become hot

calentura *f* fever; ~ *f* **roja** breakbone fever, dengue

calía *f* suppository

calibración *f* calibration

calibrador *m* calibrator

calicreína *f* **hística** glandular kallikrein, kidney kallikrein, pancreatic kallikrein, tissue kallikrein

calicreína *f* **plasmática** kininogenin, serum kallikrein, plasma kallikrein

calidad *f* quality

caliente *adj* hot

calilla *f* suppository

calle *f* street

callo *m* corn, clavus; ~ *m* **cartilaginoso** chondral callus

callosidad *f* callosity, callouses; ~ *f* **pleural** pleural thickening, pleuritic callosity

calloso *adj* callous, hardened

calmante *adj* sedative, soothing, relaxing, pacifying

calmante *m* sedative, tranquilizer, pain killer, analgesic, pain reliever, painkiller

calmarse *v* to calm down

calomel calomel, mercurous chloride, dimercury dichloride, white powder containing mercury

calomelano *m* pl calomel, mercurous chloride, dimercury dichloride

calor *m* heat

calores *m* pl hot flashes

caloría *f* calorie

calostro *m* colostrum

calostrorrea *f* colostrorrhea

calpaina *f* calpain, a cysteine proteinase found in many tissues

calusterona *f* calusterone

calvaria *f* cranial vault, calvaria

calvicie *f* baldness

calvo *adj* bald

calzado *m* footwear

calzón *m* underpants

calzoncillos *m* pl underpants

cama *f* bed; ~ *f* **de hospital** hospital bed; ~ *f* **del injerto óseo** bone chip bed

cámara *f* chamber; ~ *f* **anaerobia** anaerobic chamber; ~ *f* **de ionización** ionization chamber; ~ *f* **de recuento** counting chamber; ~ *f* **frigorífica** cold room

cambio *m* change, shift; ~ *m* **antigénico** antigenic shift; ~ *m* **genómico** genetic change, genomic change

cambrillón *m* **detorción del pie** detorsion arch-support (for the foot), arch-support device

camilla *f* stretcher, litter; ~ *f* **con ruedas** gurney, stretcher cart, wheeled stretcher

caminar *v* to walk; *v* **de puntillas** to walk on tiptoes

camisa *f* shirt, jacket; ~ *f* **de fuerza** strait jacket

camiseta *f* undershirt, T-shirt

camisón *m* gown

campanilla *f* uvula

campilobacter *m* campylobacter coli

canal *m* channel; ~ *m* **biliar** bile duct, biliary duct; ~ *m* **carpiano** carpal tunnel of the wrist; ~ *m* **del parto** birth canal; ~ *m* **en la raíz** root canal (dentist); ~ *m* **lagrimal** tear duct, lacrimal duct

cáncanos *m* pl louse (singular), lice (plural)

cáncer *m* carcinoma, cancer; ~ *m* **broncopulmonar** lung cancer; ~ *m* **cavernoso** cavernous cancer; ~ *m* **cutáneo** skin cancer, malignant epithelioma, skin carcinoma; ~ *m* **de estómago** gastric cancer, stomach cancer, gastric carcinoma; ~ *m* **de hígado** cancer of the liver, hepatoma; ~ *m* **de la piel** skin cancer, malignant epithelioma, skin carcinoma; ~ *m* **de mama** breast cancer, mamma carcinoma; ~ *m* **de Paget** Paget's disease, Paget carcinoma; ~ *m* **de pulmón** lung cancer; ~ *m* **de testículo** testicular cancer; ~ *m* **de tiroides** thyroid cancer; ~ *m* **del anexo** adnexal cancer; ~ *m* **del cuello del útero** cervix, cervical cancer; ~ *m* **del esófago** esophageal cancer, cancer of the esophagus, esophageal neoplasm; ~ *m* **dendrítico de mama** dendritic carcinoma of the mamma; ~ *m* **digestivo** digestive Karposi's sarcoma; ~ *m* **gástrico** gastric cancer,

stomach cancer, gastric carcinoma;
~ *m* **hepatocelular** hepatocellular cancer, hepatocellular carcinoma, primary liver cancer; ~ *m* **inducido por el amianto** asbestos-induced cancer; ~ *m* **inducido por virus** cancer induced by a virus; ~ *m* **invasivo** expanding cancer; ~ *m* **mamario** breast cancer, mamma carcinoma; ~ *m* **melánico** malignant melanoma, naevo-carcinoma, melanoblastoma, skin melanoma, skin cancer; ~ *m* **neuroendocrino** neuroendocrine cancer, neuroendocrine carcinoma; ~ *m* **pancreático** pancreatic cancer; ~ *m* **prostática** prostate cancer, carcinoma of the prostate; ~ *m* **ureteral** ureteral cancer

cancerígeno *adj* carcinogenic, oncogenic, cancer-causing, tumorigenic

canceroso *adj* cancerous

candela *f* candela

candida *f* candida

candidiasis *f* candidiasis, thrush, Candida mycosis, moniliasis

candidiasis *f* candidiasis; ~ *f* **oral** oral candidiasis, oral thrush; ~ *f* **pulmonar** pulmonary candidiasis; ~ *f* **urogenital** urogenital candidiasis, urogenital candidosis; ~ *f* **vaginal** vaginal candidiasis, vulvovaginal candidiasis, vaginal yeast infection; ~ *f* **vulvovaginal** vaginal candidiasis, vulvovaginal candidiasis, vaginal yeast infection

canijo *adj* frail, delicate, weak, infirm

canilla *f* shin

cannabis *f* cannabis, hashish

caño *m* urethra

cansado *adj* run-down, weakened, tired, dragging, worn out

cansancio *m* lassitude, weariness, fatigue, tiredness, exhaustion, burnout, inability to cope; ~ *m* **de los ojos** eyestrain, asthenopia

cantidad *f* amount; ~ *f* **de sustancia** amount of substance

cánula *f* cannula, thin tube; ~ *f* **buca** buccal nozzle, buccal cannula; ~ *f* **de aspiracion** suction tube; ~ *f* **de traqueotomía** tracheal cannula

cansado *adj* run-down, weakened, tired, dragging, worn out

capa *f* coat, layer, cloak, cape; ~ *f* **de extracción** excised layer; ~ *f* **de ozono** ozone layer; ~ *f* **espinosa de la epidermis** prickle-cell layer, spinous layer of epidermis, stratum spinosum epidermidis, stratum filamentosum; ~ *f* **granulosa de la epidermis** granular layer of epidermis, keratohyaline layer, stratum granulosum; ~ *f* **leucocitaria** buffy coat, crusta phlogistica; ~ *f* **queratohialina** granular layer of epidermis, keratohyaline layer, stratum granulosum

capacidad *f* capacity; ~ *f* **aeróbica** oxygen uptake, oxygen absorbtion, oxygen capacity; ~ *f* **de difusión pulmonar** pulmonary diffusion capacity; ~ *f* **enlazante** binding capacity; ~ *f* **física** physical fitness, physical ability; ~ *f* **funcional restante** residual functional capacity; ~ *f* **hospitalar** hospital capacity; ~ *f* **por contacto** social skills, interpersonal skills, the ability to establish social contacts; ~ *f* **sexual** potency, sexual ability; ~ *f* **tamponadora** buffer capacity; ~ *f* **térmica** heat capacity; ~ *f* **térmica específica** specific heat capacity; ~ *f* **térmica molar** molar heat capacity; ~ *f* **vital** lung capacity, vital capacity

capacitación *f* empowerment

capacitancia *f* capacitance; ~ *f* **eléctrica** electric capacitance

caparra *f* tick

capilar *adj* capillary

capiloropatía *f* capillaropathy

capítulo *m* **humera** capitulum of humerus, head of humerus

capnofílico *adj* capnophilic

caprolactama *m* caprolactam

capsaicina *f* capsaicin

cápsida *f* capsid, protein coat

cápsula *f* capsule; ~ *f* **de Petri** petri dish; ~ *f* **de Tenon** fascia bulbi, Tenon capsule; ~ *f* **fibrosa del higado** fibrous capsule of liver, hepatobiliary capsule; ~ *f* **fibrosa perivascularis** perivascular fibrous capsule

capsulectomía *f* capsulectomy

capsulitis *f* capsulitis; ~ *f* **adhesiva** adhesive capsulitis

captación *f* uptake, absorbing, retention; ~ *f* **de radionucleidas** uptake of radionuclides

captopril *m* captopril

capuchón *m* top, cap, hood; ~ *m* **cervical** cervical cap, diaphragm, diaphragm pessary; ~ *m* **en bóveda** cervical cap, diaphragm, diaphragm pessary

caquexia *f* cachexia, wasting away, marasmus, phthisis; ~ *f* **endocrina** endocrine cachexia; ~ *f* **ictérica** icterophthisis

cara *f* face; ~ *f* **de corte** cutting face, section

carabina *f* **molecular** molecular chaperone, chaperone protein

carácter *m* character

característica *f* character trait, characteristic

característico *adj* classic, characteristic

caracterización *f* characterization

carbamazepina *f* carbamazepine

carbamoil *m* carbamoyl

carbamoil-fosfato-sintasa *f* CPS

carbazole *m* carbazole

carbenicilina *f* carbenicillin

carbinol *m* methanol, methyl alcohol

carbohidrato *m* carbohydrate

carbohidratos *m pl* carbohydrates

carbón *m* carbon; ~ *m* **activado** activated carbon, activated charcoal

carbonato *m* carbonate; ~ *m* **ácido de amonio** hydrogen carbonate; ~ *m* **ácido de sodio** sodium hydrogen carbonate, hydrogen carbonate; ~ **–deshidratasa** *f* carbonate dehydratase

carbono *m* carbon

carboxihemoglobina *f* carboxyhemoglobin

carboxilesterasa *f* carboxylesterase

carboxipeptidasa *f* carboxypeptidase

carbunco *m* carbuncle; ~ *m* **contagioso** malignant carbuncle, contagious carbuncle

carcinogénico *adj* carcinogenic, cancer-causing; ~ *m* **no genotóxico** non-genotoxic carcinogen

carcinoide *m* carcinoid

carcinoma *m* carcinoma, cancer; ~ *m* **adenoide quístico** cylindroma, adenocystic carcinoma; ~ *m* **basaloide** basaloid carcinoma; ~ *m* **basocelular** basal cell carcinoma, basaloma; ~ *m* **de célula de Merkel** trabecular carcinoma, Merkel cell carcinoma; ~ *m* **de células escamosas** squamous cell carcinoma; ~ *m* **de los anejos** adnexal

carcinoma; ~ *m* **ductal in situ** intraductal noninfiltrating carcinoma; ~ *m* **exofítico** exophytic tumor, exophytic carcinoma; ~ *m* **hepatocelular** hepatocellular carcinoma; ~ *m* **intracanicular no infiltrante** ductal carcinoma in situ, intraductal noninfiltrating carcinoma; ~ *m* **invasivo** invasive carcinoma, expanding cancer, invasive cancer; ~ *m* **neuroendocrino** neuroendocrine cancer, neuroendocrine carcinoma; ~ *m* **osteoide** osteoid carcinoma, osteoplastic cancer; ~ *m* **pancreatico ductal** pancreatic ductal carcinoma; ~ *m* **peritoneal** peritoneal carcinoma; ~ *m* **trabecular** trabecular carcinoma, Merkel cell carcinoma; ~ *m* **uretral** urethral carcinoma, urethral cancer; ~ *m* **velloso** villous carcinoma

cardenal *m* bruise, bruising, contusion, ecchymosis

cardíaco *adj* cardiac

cardialgia *f* heartburn, pyrosis, cardialgia, pain in the heart area

cardias *m* cardial sphincter; ~ *m* **móvil** mobile cardia

cardiogénico *adj* cardiogenic

cardiografía *f* cardiography; ~ *f* **de impedancia** cardiography, type of impedance plethysmography

cardiología *f* cardiology

cardiológico *adj* cardiological

cardiomegalia *f* cardiomegaly, enlargement of the heart; ~ *f* **glucógena** cardiomegaly

cardiomiopatía *f* cardiomyopathy

cardiopatía *f* cardiopathy, heart disease; ~ *f* **congénita** congenital heart defect; ~ *f* **congénita cianotica** cyanotic congenital heart disease; ~ *f* **coronaria** coronary heart disease; ~ *f* **micótica** mycotic cardiopathy; ~ *f* **reumática** rheumatic heart disease, rheumatic carditis

cardiopulmonar *adj* cardiopulmonary

cardiorrespiratorio *adj* cardiorespiratory, heart and lung-related

cardioselectivo *adj* cardioselective, affecting the heart mostly

cardioespasmo *m* cardiospasm, esophageal achalasia

cardiotomia *f* cardiotomy

cardiotónico adj cardiotonic

cardiotoxicidad f cardiotoxicity

cardiotóxico adj cardiotoxic, poisonous to the heart

cardiovascular adj cardiovascular, heart and blood vessel-related

cardioversión f cardioversion

carencia f lack, shortage, scarcity; ~ f de actividad anergia, inactivity; ~ f de hierro deficiency; ~ f de proteínas protein deficiency; ~ f intelectual loss of intelligence, disintegration of intelligence, mental deterioration

careta f mask; ~ f de oxígeno oxygen mask; ~ f respiratoria respiratory mask, breathing apparatus

carga f charge; ~ f axial axial loading; ~ f eléctrica electric charge; ~ f electrostática electrostatic charge; ~ f genética genetic load

caries f dental caries, tooth decay, cavity (dental); ~ f dental aguda acute caries; ~ f negra black caries

carina f de la tráquea carina tracheae

cariocinesis f karyokinesis

cariólisis f karyolysis

cariología f cariology, the study and understanding of tooth decay

carioplasma m nucleoplasm, nucleoplasma

cariotipo m karyotipe, caryotype, set of chromosomes; ~ m electroforético electrophoretic karyotipe

carminativos m pl carminatives, antiflatulents

carne f meat; ~ f de vaca beef

carnosidad f fleshy growth, pterygium

carotenoide f carotenoid

carótida f carotid

carpo adj carpal; ~ m carpus, wrist joint, wrist

carrito m trolley, cart; ~ m de medicamentos medicine cart, medicine wagon

cartilaginoso adj cartilaginous, chondral

cartílago m cartilage; ~ m elástico yellow cartilage, elastic cartilage; ~ m intervertebral intervertebral disk

cartilagcartografía f mapping

cartografía f mapping; ~ f cerebral brain mapping; ~ f de restricción restriction mapping; ~ f del transcrito transcript

mapping; ~ f genética genetic mapping

casa f house; ~ f de convalecencia convalescent home, sanatorium; ~ f de crianza foster home; ~ f de reposo rest home, residential home for the elderly

casado adj married

casco m de la cabeza scalp

caseína f casein

casete f cassette

casmodia f convulsive yawn

caso m case; ~ m crónico chronic case, patient suffering from a chronic disease; ~ m limítrofe borderline case

caspa f dandruff

casquete m cervical cervical cap, diaphragm, diaphragm pessary

castañetear m de dientes chattering of teeth

castillete m ortodontico headgear, headcap (in orthodontic treatment)

castración f castration, neutering, ovariectomy, oophorectomy, excision of an ovary, spaying; ~ f química chemical castration

casuística f casuistics, recording & study of cases of disease

catabolismo m catabolism

cataforesis f cataphoresis

catalasa f catalase

catalepsia f catalepsy, sustained physical immobility; ~ f cerebelosa cerebellar catalepsy

catalizador m catalyst; ~ m bioquímico biochemical catalyst

catalizar v to catalyse

catamnesis f catamnesis, follow-up

cataplasma m cataplasm; ~ m emoliente emollient poultice; ~ m ocular eye compress, ocular cataplasm

cataplasmo m medicated compress, poultice; ~ m de mostaza poultice, sinapism, mustard plaster

cataplejía f cataplexy

cataplexia f cataplexy

catarata f cataract; ~ f azul blue-dot cataract, punctiform cataract; ~ f capsulolenticular capsular cataract; ~ f en flor de tornasol chalcosis of lens; ~ f incipiente incipient cataract; ~ f punteada punctate cataract; ~ f sanguínea bloody cataract, cruent cataract

catarro m cold, catarrh, head cold,

nasopharyngitis; ~ *m* **de pecho** bronchitis
catarsis *f* catharsis
catártico *adj* cathartic
catatonía *f* catatonia, a phase of schizophrenia
catatónico *adj* catatonic
catecolamina *f* catecholamine, CA
catepsina *f* cathepsin
catéter *m* catheter, urinary catheter;
~ *m* **balón** balloon catheter; ~ *m* **balón de Fogarty** Fogarty balloon catheter; ~ *m* **de intubación** endotracheal tube, intubation catheter; ~ *m* **flotante de arteria pulmonar** balloon-flotation pulmonary artery catheter; ~ *m* **ureteral** ureteral catheter
cateterismo *m* catheterization, fitting a (urine) bag; ~ *m* **cardíaco** catheterization; ~ *m* **de la papila duodenal** catheterization of the duodenal papilla; ~ *m* **permanente** indwelling catheter
catexis *f* quirúrgico surgical catgut
catgut *m* **quirúrgico** surgical catgut
catión *m* cation
catorce *adj* fourteen
caucásico *adj* caucasian, white
caudal *adj* caudal, towards the tail, nearer the tail; ~ *m* **catalítico** catalytic flow rate, catalytic rate; ~ *m* **de actividad catalítica** catalytic activity flow rate, catalytic activity rate; ~ *m* **de filtración glomerular** glomerular filtration rate, GFR; ~ *m* **de masa** mass rate; ~ *m* **de número** number flow rate; ~ *m* **de sustancia** substance flow rate, substance rate; ~ *m* **de volumen** volume flow rate
caumestesia *f* caumesthesia, a subjective heat sensation of uncomfortably high temperature
causa *f* factor, cause; ~ *f* **de una enfermedad** etiology, cause of a disease
causal *adj* causal, causative
causalidad *f* causation
causar *v* to cause, to make; ~ *v* **estragos** to wreak havoc
causativo *adj* causal, causative
cáustico *adj* caustic, corrosive
cauterio *m* cautery
cauterización *f* cauterization; ~ *f* **dentinaria** dentine cauterization
caverna *f* cave, cavern; ~ *f pl* **del cuerpo esponjoso** venous spaces of corpus

spongiosum
cavidad *f* cavity, hollow; ~ *f* **abdominal** abdominal cavity; ~ *f* **alantoidea** allantoic cavity; ~ *f* **bucal** buccal cavity; ~ *f* **de Meckel** Meckel's cavity; ~ *f* **del septum pellucidum** cavity of septum lucidum, Arantius ventricle; ~ *f* **intracelular** intercellular cavity; ~ *f* **pericárdica** pericardial cavity; ~ *f* **peritoneal** peritoneal cavity; ~ *f* **pleuroperitoneal** pleuroperitoneal cavity; ~ *f* **torácico** thoracic cavity
cebado *m* **aleatorio** random priming
cebador *m* primer
cecolostomía *f* cecocolostomy
cecostomía *f* cecostomy
cecropina *f* cecropin, inducible antibacterial protein
cefaclor *m* cefaclor
cefadroxilo *m* cefadroxil
cefalalgia *f* cephalalgia, headache, cephalea; ~ *f* **histamínica** cluster headache, Horton's headache, histaminic headache, neuralgic migraine
cefalea *f* migraine; ~ *f* **incapacitadora** debilitating migraine, severe headache; ~ *f* **indurativa** nodular headache, cephalea nodularis; ~ *f* **nodular** nodular headache, cephalea nodularis; ~ *f* **postejercicio** exertional headache
cefalexina *f* cephalexin, cefalexin
cefalgia *f* headache; ~ *f* **tensional** tension headache, stress headahe
cefaloglicina *f* cephaloglycin (a cephalosporin antibiotic)
cefaloridina *f* cefaloridine, cephaloridine
cefalosporina *f* cephalosporin
cefalotina *f* cephalothin, a cephalosporin antibiotic
cefamandol *m* cefamandole
cefazolina *f* cefazolin
cefixima *f* cefixime
cefmenoxima *f* cefmenoxime
cefmetazol *m* cefmetazole
cefonicido *m* cefonicid
cefoperazona *f* cefoperazone
cefotaxima *f* cefotaxime
cefotetano *m* cefotetan
cefoxitina *f* cefoxitin

cefradina f cefradine, cephradine

cefsulodina f cefsulodin

ceftazidima f ceftazidime

ceftizoxima f ceftizoxime

ceftriaxona f ceftriaxone

cefuroxima f cefuroxime

ceguera f amaurosis, blindness, being blinded; ~ f **diurna** hemeralopia, day blindness; ~ f **nocturna** night blindness, nocturnal amblyopia, hemeralopia

ceja f eyebrow, supercilium

celoniquia f koilonychia, thin, brittle fingernails

celos m pl mórbidos morbid jealousy

célula f cell; ~ f **anfitriona** host cell; ~ f **asesina natural** natural killer, natural killer cell, NK cell; ~ f **basal** basal cell; ~ f **bien diferenciada** well differentiated cell; ~ f **cebada** adipose cell, lipocyte, fat cell; ~ f **citotóxica natural** natural killer, natural killer cell, NK cell; ~ f **cromafin** chromaffin cell, pheochrome cell; ~ f **del ganglio retiniano** retinal ganglion cell; ~ f **dentrítica** dentritic cell; ~ f **de Malpighi** prickle-cell, malpighian cell; ~ f **de Mast** mastocyte, connective tissue cell, mast cell; ~ f **de memoria** memory cell; ~ f pl **de Reed-Sternberg** Reed-Sternberg cell; ~ f **endotelial** endothelial cell; ~ f **escamosa** squamous cell, squamous epithelial cell, a flat, thin cell found in the outer layer of the skin; ~ f **escasamente diferenciada** poorly differentiated cell; ~ f **espinosa** prickle-cell, malpighian cell; ~ f **estromal** stromal cell, a large, well-like cell in the bone marrow; ~ f **eucariota** eukcaryotic cell, eukcaryote; ~ f **híbrida** hybrid cell; ~ f **huésped** host cell; ~ f pl **intersticial de Leydig** interstitial cels of the testicle; ~ f **madre** stem cell; ~ f **madre embrionaria** embryonic stem cell; ~ f **madre hematopoyética** hematopoietic stem cell; ~ f **mesenquimal** mesenchymal cell; ~ f **mieloide** myeloid cell, myeloid tissue; ~ f **nula** null cell; ~ f **oligodendroglial** oligodendrocyte, oligodendroglia; ~ f **plasmática** plasmacyte, plasmocyte; ~ f **precancerosa** precancerous cell; ~ f **presentadora de antígeno** antigen-presenting cell; ~ f **procariota** prokaryotic cell,

prokaryote; ~ f **receptora** recipient cell; ~ f **somática** somatic cell; ~ f **T asesina** killer T cell, cytotoxic T lymphocyte, cytotoxic T cell; ~ f **T citotóxica** T lymphocyte, cytotoxic T cell; ~ f **T supresora** suppressor T lymphocyte; ~ f **T4** helper lymphocyte, helper cell, T4 cell; ~ f **turbinado** turbinate cell

celulasa f cellulase

celulitis f cellulite (fat cells), cellulitis, inflammation of connective tissue; ~ f **orbitaria** orbital cellulitis periophthalmitis; ~ f **subcutánea** subcutaneous cellulitis

centelleo m scintillation

centímetro m centimeter; ~ m **cúbico** cubic centimeter

centimorgan m centimorgan, a unit of distance measured between two genes

central adj central

centrífuga f centrifuge; ~ f **el hemolizado** centrifuged hemolisate

centrifugación f centrifugation

centrifugadora f centrifuge

centriolo m centriole, the self-replicating, short, fibrous, rod-shaped organelle of animal cells

centro m centre; ~ m **aceptor** acceptor site, entry site; ~ m **activo** active site; ~ m **ambulatorio** outpatient clinic, ambulatory care, outpatient treatment, outpatient care; ~ m **catalítico** catalytic centre; ~ m **comunitario de salud** community health center, community health care, community health services; ~ m **de cuidados paliativos** hospice care, terminal care; ~ m **de mutación** mutation site; ~ m **de orientación** referral service, information service; ~ m **de orientación de la juventud** youth counseling center; ~ m **de planificación familiar** family planning clinic; ~ m **de restricción** restriction site; ~ m **de tratamiento del dolor** pain clinic, pain management clinic; ~ m **de unión** binding site; ~ m **donador** donor site; ~ m **germinal** germinal center; ~ m **iniciador** initiator site; ~ m **para autoayuda** self-help center

centrómero m centromere, kinetochore

centrosoma f centrosome

cepa f strain; ~ f **heterocigota** heterozygous

strain; ~ f **homeopática** homeopathic stock;
~ f **microbiana** microbial strain;
~ f **neurotrópica** neurotropic strain;
~ f **virulenta** virulent strain (of an infectious organism)

cepillarse v to brush; ~ v **los dientes** to brush one's teeth

cepillo m **de dientes** tooth brush; ~ m **para dentadura** dental-plate brush; ~ m **para el pelo** hair brush

ceramidasa f ceramidase

cerdo m pork

cerebelo m cerebellum

cerebeloso adj cerebellar

cerebral adj cerebral

cerebro m brain, cerebrum

cerebrósido–sulfatasa f cerebroside-sulfatase

cerebrospinal adj cerebrospinal, pertaining to the brain and spinal cord

cerebrovascular adj cerebrovascular

cero m zero

cerrado adj closed

cerrar v to close, to shut; ~ v **la mano** to make a fist, to clench one's fist

certificable adj certifiable, to be reported

ceruloplasmina f ceruloplasmin, ferroxidase

cerumen m cerumen, earwax

cerveza f beer; ~ f **medicinal** medicinal beer

cervical adj cervical, pertaining to the neck of the uterus

cervicitis f cervicitis, trachelitis

cervix m cervix; ~ m **insuficiente** incompetent cervix, insufficiency of the cervix;
~ m **uterino** cervix (uteri), neck of the uterus, womb neck

cesar v to stop; ~ v **el uso de tabaco** to stop smoking, to quit smoking

cesárea f Caesarean section, C-section, Caesarean

cestodo m cestode, tapeworm

cetoacidosis f ketoacidosis; ~ f **diabética** diabetic ketoacidosis, severe, out-of-control diabetes that needs emergency treatment

cetohexocinasa f ketohexokinase

cetonuria f ketonuria, acetonuria

chabacano m apricot

chafado m scrape mark, scrub mark, scuff mark

chalazion m chalazion

chalazodermia f dermatolysis, cutis laxa, chalazodermia, loose skin, dermatochalasis

chamorro m calf

chancro m chancre; ~ m **de Hunter** Hunter chancre, hard chancre; ~ m **duro** Hunter chancre, hard chancre; ~ m **recurrente** chancre

chanza f mumps

chaperona f chaperone

chaperonina f chaperonine

charlatán m quack, charlatan, fraud

charlatanería f charlatanry, charlatanism, quackery, fraudulence, deceit

charlatanismo m quackery, fraudulence, charlatanry, deceit

chasquido m click (valve), clicking, popping;
~ m **de una articulación** clicking, popping of a joint; ~ m **sistólico** click, mesosystolic click

chata f bedpan

chemonucleolisis f chemonucleolysis

cheposa f humpbacked

cheque m check

chequeo m **médico** check-up, general physical examination

chichi f nipple

chichón m lump, boil, furuncle, bump, swelling, bruise; ~ m **en la cabeza** boil, furuncle, bump, swelling, bruise

chico adj little, small

chocar v to jar, to jolt, to bump, to jostle

chochero m medical practitioner in Mexico

choque m shock, accident (crash);
~ m **eléctrico** electric shock; ~ m **hemolítico** hemolysis shock; ~ m **insulínico** insulin shock, severe condition that exists when the level of blood glucose drops quickly. ~ m **operatorio** post-operative shock, surgical shock;
~ m **post–descompresión** post-decompression shock, post-decompression syndrome;
~ m **psíquico** psychic shock, mental shock, emotional shock; ~ m **séptico** septic shock, bacteriemic shock; ~ m **térmico** heat shock

choquezuela f kneecap, patella

chorro m blennorrhagia, gonorrhea, clap, gonorrhoea; ~ m **de agua** jet of water (in pool), water jet

chueco adj crooked

cianocobalamina f cobalamin, vitamin B12,

cyanocobalamin

cianosis f cyanosis, bluish discoloration of skin and mucous membranes

cianotica adj cyanotic, bluish

ciantoato m cyanthoate

cianuro m cyanide; ~ m **de hidrógeno** hydrogen cyanide, hydrocyanic acid, HCN

ciática f sciatica

cibernética f cybernetics

cíbrido m cybrid

cicatriz f scar; ~ f **elevada** cheloid, keloid, an elevated, irregular scar

cicatrización f cicatrization, scarring

cicatrizado adj scarred, scarring, cicatrizing

ciclamato m cyclamate; ~ m **sódico** cyclamate

ciclazocina f cyclazocine

cíclico adj cyclic, periodic, regular

ciclo m cycle; ~ m **cardíaco** cardiac cycle; ~ m **menstrual** menstrual bleeding pattern, menstrual cycle

ciclofosfamida f cyclophosphamide

ciclooxigenasa f COX, cyclooxygenase

ciclopentano m cyclopentane

ciclopentolato m cyclopentolate

cicloplejía f cycloplegia, eye muscle paralysis

ciclopléjico m cycloplegic, a drug that paralyzes the ciliary muscle

ciclopropano m cyclopropane, a flammable gaseous saturated used as a general anesthetic

ciclosporiasis f cyclosporiasis, traveler's disease, an infection with a parasitic protozoa called Cyclospora

ciclosporina f ciclosporin

cicuta f hemlock; ~ f **acuatica** cowbane, cicuta virosa; ~ f **virosa** cicuta virosa

CID disseminated intravascular coagulation, DIC

cidovudina f AZT, Retrovir, zidovudine, azidothymidine

ciego adj blind; ~ m visually impaired, partially sighted, legally blind

cien adj hundred

ciencia f science; ~ **farmacéutica** pharmaceutics; ~ **médica** medical science

cierre m occlusion, momentary closure, bite, closing; ~ m **de una herida** wound closure, closing the wound

cifosis f kyphosis, cyphosis

cigarillo m cigarette; ~ m **con poco contenido de alquitrán** low-tar cigarette

cigotena f zygotene

cigoto m zygote, fertilized ovum

cilindro m cast; ~ m **bacteriano** bacterial cast; ~ m **céreo** waxy cast; ~ m **hemático** RBC cast; ~ m **leucocitario** WBC cast; ~ m **sanguíneo** erythrocyte cast; ~ m **urinario** urinary cast

cilindroma m cylindroma, adenocystic carcinoma

cilindruria f cylindruria

cilios m pl **sensoriales** sensory hairs

cimógenos zymogenic bacteria

cinanquia f sore throat, pharyngitis, angina

cinco adj five

cincuenta adj fifty

cinesiterapia f movement therapy, kinesiatrics, movement-cure, kinesitherapy

cinestesia f kinesthesis, kinesthetic memory, sensation of movement, proprioception

cinética f kinetics, theory of motion, mechanics

cinético adj kinetic, motion-related

cinetocoro m centromere, kinetochore

cinta f tape, ribbon; ~ f **adhesiva** adhesive tape, sticky tape; ~ f **para medir** measuring tape

cintigrafía f radionuclide imaging, scintigraphy

cintigrama m scintigram; ~ m **óseo** bone scan

cintura f waist, lower back, lumbar region; ~ f **escapular** shoulder girdle

cinturón m belt, girdle, sash; ~ m **de seguridad** safety belt (in a vehicle), shoulder belt; ~ m **pélvico** pelvic girdle

cinureninasa f kynureninase

ciprofloxacino m ciprofloxacin

ciproheptadina f cyclopheptadine, Periactin, Cyprohept

circulación f circulation; ~ f **de sangre** circulation (of blood); ~ f **periférica de la sangre** peripheral blood flow

círculo m circle; ~ m **rodador** rolling circle

circumferencia f circumference

circuncisión f circumcision, the surgical removal of end of the prepuce of the penis; ~ f **de la mujer** female circumcision

cirro m painless hard tumor, cyst

cirrosis f granular induration, cirrhosis; ~ f **atrófica** atrophic cirrhosis; ~ f **biliar** biliary liver cirrhosis, xanthomatous cirrhosis; ~ **f cardíaca** cardiac cirrhosis; ~ **f del hígado** cirrhosis, liver disease; ~ **f hepática** cirrhosis of the liver; ~ **f pos-hepática** hepatitic cirrhosis; ~ **f posnecrótica** postnecrotic cirrhosis; ~ **f renal** cirrhosis of the kidney

cirugía f surgery; ~ **f colorectal** colorectal surgery, colon and rectal surgery, proctology; ~ **f con láser** laser surgery; ~ **f conservadora de la mama** breast-conserving surgery; ~ **f de derivación coronaria** coronary bypass operation/surgery; ~ **f de la bóveda craneal** calvarial plastic surgery, surgery of the cranial vault; ~ **f de reconstrucción de la cabeza femoral** plastic surgery on the femoral head; ~ **f de urgencia** emergency surgery, emergency operation; ~ **f en los ojos** lasix, eye surgery to correct myopia; ~ **f endoscópica** endoscopic surgery, endosurgery; ~ **f estética** cosmetic surgery, plastic surgery, aesthetic surgery; ~ **f informatizada** computer-assisted surgical intervention; ~ **f invasiva** invasive surgery; ~ **f laparoscópica** laparoscopic surgery; ~ **f muco-gingival** mucogingival surgery; ~ **f paliativa** palliative surgery; ~ **f plástica** cosmetic surgery, plastic surgery, aesthetic surgery; ~ **f plástica de la nariz** cosmetic surgery of the nose, rhinoplasty; ~ **f por colgajo cutáneo** plastic surgery by a flap method; ~ **f reconstructiva** reconstructive surgery; ~ **f conservadora** conservative surgery

cirujano m surgeon; ~ **m ortopedista** orthopedic surgeon; ~ **m plástico** plastic surgeon

cisplatino m cisplatin

cistectomía f cystectomy, excision of the urinary bladder

cisteína f cysteine

cisterna f cisterna

cisticercosis f cysticercosis, infection with cysticerci

cistina f cystine

cistinosis f cystinosis, cystine storage disease

cistinuria f homozygous cystinuria

cistitis f cystitis, inflammation of the bladder; ~ **f química** chemical cystitis

cisto m cyst

cistoide adj cystoid

cistolithiasis f cystolithiasis, the presence of a vesical calculus

cistolito m urinary calculus, urinary calculus disease

cistometría f cystometry, manometry of the bladder

cistoscopia f cystoscopy, bladder examination, endoscopic examination of the urinary bladder

cistoscopio m cystoscope; ~ **m aspirador** evacuation cystoscope; ~ **m de irrigación** irrigation cystoscope; ~ **m ureteral** ureter cystoscope

cistotomía f cystotomy

cistrón m cistron

cisura f fissure, groove, sulcus; ~ **f vesicointestinal** fissura vesico-intestinalis

citarabina f cytarabine

citidina f cytidine

citobiología f vCell biology, cytobiology

citocinesis f cytokinesis

citocromo m cytochrome; ~ **–oxidasa** f cytochrome oxidase

citodiagnóstico m **exfoliativo** exfoliative cytodiagnosis

citogenética f cytogenetics

citología f cytology; ~ **f exfoliativa** cytodiagnosis, exfoliative cytology; ~ **f vaginal** cervical-vaginal swab

citomegalovirus m cytomegalovirus, herpes virus 5

citometría f cytometry; ~ **f de flujo** flow cytometry

citopatología f cytopathology

citoplasma m cytoplasm, main part of a cell's contents

citoquímica f cytochemistry

citoquina f cytokine; ~ **f neurotóxica** neurotoxic cytokine

citosina f cytosine, component of nucleic acid

citostático adj cytostatic

citotóxico adj cytotoxic

citrato m citrate

citrulina f citrulline

ciudad f city

clamidia f chlamydia; ~ **f trachomatis** chlamydia trachomatis

clamidospora f chlamydospore

claritromicina *f* clarithromycin
claro *adj* light
clase *f* kind, type
clásico *adj* classic
clasificación *f* classification, sorting, classifying, ranking
claudicación *f* claudication, limping, lameness
claustro *m* claustrum
clave *f* code, key, password; **~ f genética** genetic code
clavícula *f* collarbone, clavicle
clavos *m pl* **ortopédicos** bone pins, bone nails
cleptolagnia *f* kleptolagnia
clima *m* climate, atmosphere; **~ m afectivo** affective climate, emotional climate
climaterio *m* climacterium, menopause
clindamicina *f* clindamycin
clínica *f* hospital, clinic; **~ f ambulatoria** outpatient clinic, ambulatory care, outpatient treatment, outpatient care; **~ f de maternidad** maternity clinic; **~ f de odontólogo** dental clinic
clínicamente muerto *m* brain dead
clínico *adj* clinical; **~ m clinician**
clinomanía *f* extreme sleepiness, morbid sleepiness, clinomania
clitoral *adj* clitoral, clitoris-related
clitorídeo *adj* clitoral, clitoris-related
clítoris *m* clitoris
cloaca *f* waste passage, cloaca
cloasma *m* chloasma; **~ m colemico** cholemic chloasma; **~ m extra-uterino** extra-uterine chloasma; **~ m uterino** pregnancy chloasma, chloasma uterinum, dark patches on the face; **~ m hepático** *m* chloasma hepaticum
clomifeno *m* clomiphene
clon *m* clone; **~ m de cDNA** cDNA clone
clonación *f* cloning; **~ f al azar** shotgun cloning; **~ f de genes** gene cloning; **~ f en perdigonada** shotgun method of cloning; **~ f molecular** molecular cloning; **~ f posicional** positional cloning
clónico *adj* clonic
clonidina *f* clonidine
clono *m* clone
clonorchis *f* **sinensis** clonorchis sinensis, Chinese liver flukes, clonorchiasis
clonorquíasis *f* clonorchis sinensis, Chinese liver flukes, clonorchiasis
clopidogrel *m* clopidogrel
clorambucil *m* Chlorambucil
cloranfenicol *m* chloramphenicol
clorfeniramina *f* chlorpheniramine
clorhexidina *f* chlorhexidine
clorhidrato *m* hydrochloride
cloro *m* chlorine, bleach
clorodiazepóxido *m* chlordiazepoxide
clorofluorocarbono *m* chlorofluorocarbon, monohalogenocarbons
cloroformo *m* chloroform, trichloromethane
cloromielossarcomatosis *f* **de Sternberg** Sternberg chloromyelosarcomatosis
cloroplasto *m* chloroplast, chlorophyll body, chlorophyll granule
cloroquina *f* chloroquine
clorosis *f* chlorosis, green sickness
clorotrianiseno *m* chlorotrianisene, estrogen
clorpirifos *m* chlorpyrifos
clorpromazina *f* chlorpromazine
clortalidona *f* chlorthalidone, a diuretic
cloruro *m* chloride; **~ m cálcico** calcium chloride; **~ m de mercurio** $HgCl_2$, mercuric chloride, corrosive sublimate; **~ m de metiltioninio** methylene blue; **~ m de tridihexetil** tridihexethyl chloride, tridihexethyl iodide; **~ m mercúrico** $HgCl_2$, mercuric chloride, corrosive sublimate; **~ m mercurioso** calomel, mercurous chloride, dimercury dichloride
clorzoxazona *f* chlorzoxazone
clostridiopeptida *f* microbial collagenase
Clostridium *m* Clostridium; **~ m botulinum** Clostridium botulinum, Ermengen's bacillus; **~ m perfringens** Clostridium perfringens, Welch-Frankel's bacillus; **~ m septicum** Clostridium septicum, Ghon-Sachs bacillus, Sachs bacillus; **~ m tetani** Clostridium tetani, Nicolaier's bacillus
cloxacilina *f* cloxacillin
CMP *f* **ciclico** cCMP, cyclic nucleotide formed from cytidine triphosphate
coadaptación *f* coaptation
coagulación *f* coagulation, clotting; **~ f enzimática** enzymatic coagulation; **~ f extrinseca** extrinsic coagulation pathway; **~ f intravascular diseminada** disseminated

intravascular coagulation; ~ f **intrínseca** intrinsic coagulation

coagular v to coagulate

coagulasa f coagulase, staphylococcal clumping factor

coágulo m clot, coagulum; ~ m **de sangre** blood clot, coagulum, thrombus; ~ m **sanguíneo** blood clot, coagulum

coagulopatía f coagulopathy; ~ f **de consumo** coagulopathy, disseminated intravascular coagulation

coáltar m coal tar

coanas f pl posterior nares, choanae

coaptación f coaptation, coarctatio

coartación f coarctatio

cobalamina f cobalamin, vitamin B12, cyanocobalamin, anti-pernicious factor, animal protein factor, APF

cobertura f coverage

cobija f blanket

cobre m copper

coca f cocaïne plant, coca

cocaína f cocaine

cocainismo m **agudo** cocaine poisoning

coccidioidomicosis f coccidioidomycosis

coccidioidina f coccidioidin

coccidioidosis f coccidioidomycosis

coccidiosis f coccidiosis

coccigectomía f coccygectomy

cóccix m tailbone, coccyx

cociente m quotient; ~ m **inhibidor** inhibitory quotient

cóclea f cochlea

coclear adj cochlear

coco m coccus; ~ m **anaerobio** anaerobic coccus; ~ m **gramnegativo** gram-negative coccus; ~ m **grampositivo** gram-positive coccus

codeína f codeine

codificar v encode

código m code; ~ m **genético** genetic code; ~ m **postal** zip code, postal code

codo m elbow

codón m codon, triplet of nucleotides that specify a single amino acid; ~ m **ámbar** amber codon;

initiation codon; ~ m **de paro** stop codon; ~ m **de terminación** stop codon; ~ m **finalizador** stop codon; ~ m **traducible** sense codon

coeficiente m coefficient; ~ m **de absorción** absorption coefficient; ~ m **de absorción decimal lineal molar** molar linear decadic absorption coefficient; ~ m **de actividad** activity coefficient; ~ m **de actividad iónica** ionic activity coefficient; ~ m **de atenuación** attenuation coefficient; ~ m **de difusión** diffusion coefficient; ~ m **de distribución** distribution coefficient; ~ m **de fricción** frictional coefficient; ~ m **de sedimentación** sedimentation coefficient; ~ m **de variación** coefficient of variation; ~ m **osmótico** osmotic coefficient

coenzima f coenzyme

cofactor m cofactor

cognición f cognition, cognitive ability

cognitivo adj cognitive, understood

coherencia f coherence, consistency; ~ f **del pensamiento** coherent thought

cohorte f cohort

coiloniquia f koilonychia, thin, brittle fingernails

coincidente adj identical, analagous

coito m coitus, sexual intercourse, intercourse; ~ m **anal** anal sex, coitus per anum, anal intercourse; ~ m **interrumpido** coitus interruptus

cojear v limp, to, hobble, to; ~ f limping, lameness, claudication

cojín m **eléctrico** heating pad, warming pad

cola f tail; ~ f **del epidídimo** tail of the epididymis

colagenasa f collagenase; ~ f **intersticial** interstitial collagenase, matrix metalloproteinase; ~ f **microbiana** microbial collagenase, clostridiopeptidase, Clostridium histolyticum collagenase

colágeno m collagen; ~ m **pulmonar** lung collagen

colagenosis f collagen disease, connective-tissue disease

colagogo m cholagogue, promotes the flow of bile into the intestine

colangiografía f cholangiography, bile duct x-ray; ~ f **intravenosa** intravenous cholangiography; ~ f **percutanea transhepática** transhepatic percutaneous cholangiography

colangiopancreatografía f **retrógrada endoscópica** endoscopic retrograde cholangiopancreatography

colangitis f cholangitis, inflammation of the bile duct; ~ f **obliterante primaria** sclerosing cholangitis

colapsarse v buckle at the knees

colapso m fainting, swoon, collapse; ~ m **cardiovascular** cardiovascular collapse, cardiovascular failure

colchicina f colchicine, a poisonous alkaloid that inhibits mitosis

cold cream m cold cream

colecalciferol m vitamin D3

colecistectomía f cholecystectomy, removal of the gall bladder

colecistitis f cholecystitis, gall bladder inflammation; ~ f **enfisematosa** emphysematous cholecystitis; ~ f **gangrenosa** gangrenous cholecystitis; ~ f **glandular proliferativa** cholecystitis glandularis proliferans; ~ f **hidrópica** hydrops vesicae felleae; ~ f **supurada** suppurative cholecystitis

colecistografía f cholecystography, an imaging study for visualizing the gallbladder; ~ f **oral** cholecystogram, oral cholecystography

colectomía f colectomym, pancolectomy, extirpation of the entire colon

colelitiasis f cholelithiasis, gallstones, biliary calculus, biliary concretion

cólera m cholera; ~ m **infantil** cholera infantum

colerético m choleretic

colestasis f cholestasis, bile flow stoppage; ~ f **extrahepatico** extra-hepatic cholestasis

colesteremia f cholesterolemia, cholesteremia

colesterol m cholesterol, cholesterin; ~ m **de HDL** HDL colesterol; ~ m **de LDL** LDL cholesterol; ~ m **de VLDL** VLDL cholesterol; ~ ~ **oxidasa** f cholesterol oxidase

colesterolemia f cholesterolemia, cholesteremia

colesterosis f cholesterosis; ~ f **extracelular** extracellular cholesterosis

colgajo m **cutáneo** skin flap, flap of skin; ~ m **de corión** corium flap

colibacteria f coliform bacteria, coliform organism, bacterium coli

cólica f colic

cólico m colic, cramps; ~ m **flatulento** flatulent colic; ~ m **gaseoso** flatulent colic; ~ m **hepático** biliary colic, hepatic colic; ~ m **intestinal** colic of the large intestine, intestinal colic; ~ m **nefrítico** renal colic; ~ m **renal** renal colic; ~ m **uterino** uterine colic

colina f choline; ~ **-cinasa** f choline kinase; ~ **-oxidasa** f choline oxidase

colinérgico adj cholinergic

colinesterasa f choline esterase, CHEL, benzoylcholinesterase

colirio m eye drops, eyewash, collyrium

colistina f colistin

colita f tailbone, coccyx

colitis f colitis; ~ f **amebiana** amebic dysentery, amebic colitis; ~ f **asociada a antibióticos** antibiotic-associated colitis; ~ f **seudomembranosa** antibiotic-associated colitis; ~ f **ulcerosa** ulcerative colitis; ~ f **urémica** uremic colitis

collar m **de Venus** syphilitic leucoderma of the neck

collarín m **cervical** neck brace, cervical collar

coloboma f coloboma; ~ f **de Fuchs** Fuchs coloboma; ~ f **del iris** coloboma of the iris

colocar v to place, to put, to plant; ~ v **em cuarentena** to put in quarantine, to quarantine; ~ v **férula** to splint, to put in a cast or splint

colodión m collodion

coloidal adj colloidal

colon m colon; ~ m **ascendente** ascending colon; ~ m **descendente** descending colon; ~ m **inestable** spastic colon, irritable colon, irritable bowel syndrome; ~ m **irritable** spastic colon, irritable colon, irritable bowel syndrome; ~ m **sigmoideo** sigmoid colon; ~ m **transverso** transverse colon

colonia f colony

colonoscopía f colonoscopy

colopatía f colonopathy, colon disease

coloración f coloring, staining, pigmentation

colorrectal adj colorectal

colostomía f colostomy, an artificial anus

between colon and surface of the abdomen

colpitis f vaginitis, colpitis, inflammation of the vaginal mucosa; ~ **f granular de las vacas** granular vaginitis, nodular vaginitis, infectious vaginitis, granular venereal disease (of cows!); ~ **f micótica** colpitis mycotica, vaginal yeast infection

colposcopia f colposcopy (exam of cervix)

columna f column; ~ **f inmunoadsorbente** immunoadsorbent column; ~ **f preparada** packed column; ~ **f vertebral** spinal column, vertebral column

colutorio m gargle, mouthwash; ~ **m antibiótico** antibiotic mouthwash, antiseptic gargle; ~ **m antiséptico** antiseptic gargle, mouthwash

coma m coma; ~ **m acidótico** acidotic coma

comadrona f midwife, birth attendant

comatoso adj comatose

comba f bulge, protrusion

combinación f combination; ~ **f de impedimentos** combination of impairments

comedomastitis f comedomastitis

comedón m comedone, blackhead, pimple, (acne) pustule, furuncle

comensal m microorganism, microbe, commensal

comer v to ingest, to eat

comerse v **las uñas** to bite one's nails

comezón m itch, itching

comicidad f humor, merriment, laughter, mirth

comida f meal; ~ **f grasa** fatty food; ~ **f podrida** spoiled food

comisura f commissure; ~ **f del hipocampo** hippocampal commissure

como how, like

comorbilidad f comorbidity

comparación f comparison; ~ **f longitudinal** longitudinal comparision; ~ **f transversal** transversal comparison

compatible adj compatible

compensación f compensation

competitivo adj competitive; ~ m competitive

complejo m complex; ~ **m de inferioridad** inferiority complex, sense of inferiority; ~ **m hierro–dextrano** iron-dextran complex; ~ **m principal de histocompatibilidad** major

histocompatibility complex, MHC; ~ m **QRS** QRS complex, part of heart monitor readout

complementaridad f complementarity; ~ **f de las bases nucleicas** nucleic bases complementarity

complementario adj complementary, additional

complemento m complement

complianza f compliance; ~ **f pulmonar** pulmonary compliance

complicación f complication, sequela; ~ **f intraoperatoria** intraoperative complication

componente m component; ~ **m del complemento** complement component; ~ **m policlonal** polyclonal component

comportamiento m behavior; ~ **m autista** autistic behavior; ~ **m irracional** irrational behavior; ~ **m sexual** sexual behavior

compota f de manzanas apple sauce

comprensión f comprehension, understanding

compresa f compress, poultice; ~ **f higiénica** sanitary napkin

compresión f compression; ~ **f axial** axial compression; ~ **f cardíaca** cardiac compression; ~ **f del pecho** chest compression

comprimido m pill, tablet; ~ **m vaginal** vaginal tablet

compuesto m compound, body; ~ **m cetónico** ketone body; ~ **m orgánico** organic compound; ~ **m organoclorado** organic chlorine compound; ~ **m tricíclico** tricyclic antidepressant, tricyclic compound; ~ **m xenobiótico** xenobiotic compound

computadora f computer

computadorizado adj computerized

comunicación f communication; ~ **f interventricular** ventricular septal defect

con with; ~ **frecuencia** frequently; ~ **permiso** excuse me; ~ **pituita** slimy

concatémero m concatemer

concatenar v to concatenate

concentración adj joining; ~ **f** concentration, level; ~ **f absorbida** absorbed concentration; ~ **f ambiental prevista** predicted environmental concentration; ~ **f catalítica** catalytic concentration; ~ **f de actividad catalítica** catalytic activity concentration; ~ **f de células** cell count; ~ **f de leucocitos en**

sangre WBC count; ~ f de lípido en plasma
lipemia; ~ f de masa mass concentration;
~ f de número number concentration; ~ f de
proteína en líquido cefalorraquídeo CSF
protein content; ~ f de sustancia molarity,
substance concentration; ~ f eficaz effective
concentration; ~ f eficaz mediana median
effective concentration; ~ f inhibidora
inhibitory concentration; ~ f letal lethal
concentration; ~ f máxima peak, peak level,
spike; ~ f mínima trough level; ~ f molar
molar concentration; ~ f osmótica osmotic
concentration; ~ f plasmática plasma level;
~ f sérica serum level; ~ f subterapéutica
subtherapeutic level; ~ f terapéutica
therapeutic level; ~ f tisular concentration in
tissues; ~ f tóxica toxic level
concentrado m concentrate; ~ m enzimático
enzymatic concentrate
concepción f conception
conciencia f consciousness
conclusión f conclusion; ~ f por analogía
conclusion by analogy
concomitante adj accessory, concomitant
concoscopio m rhinoscope, conchoscope, nasal
speculum
concreción f concretion; ~ f pericárdica
pericardial concretion
concreto adj concrete
condensador m condenser
condición f condition, status
cóndilo m occipital condyle; ~ m del occipital
occipital condyle
condiloma m condyloma; ~ m acuminado
condyloma acuminatum, fig wart, genital
wart; ~ m plano condyloma latum
condón m condom
condritis f chondritis, inflammation of cartilage
condroblasto m chondroblast, an embryonic
cartilage-producing cell
condrocalcinosis f chondrocalcinosis,
pseudogout
condrocito m chondrocyte
condrodistrofia m chondrodystrophy
condrofibroma m chondrofibroma
condroitin f chondroitin, a mucopolysaccharide
constituent of chondrin
condroitina f chondroitin, a

mucopolysaccharide constituent of chondrin
condrolipoma m chondrolipoma
condroma m hialino hyalo-enchondroma
condromalacia f chondromalacia; ~ f de la
rótula chondromalacia patella, a progressive
erosion of cartilage in the knee joint
condromatosis f chondromatosis;
~ f osteogénica chondromatosis, skeletal
chondromatosis; ~ f sinovial synovial
chondromatosis
condromia m chondroma; ~ m bronquial
bronchial chondroma
condromyixfibroma m chondromyxofibroma,
chondromyxoid fibroma
condrosarcoma m chondrosarcoma, a
malignant neoplasm derived from cartilage
tissue (chondroblasts)
condrosdiaplasia f chondrodysplasia
condrosis f chondrosis
conducción f conduction, transfer; ~ f a los
desagües conduit of waste in enclosed piping
conductancia f conductance; ~ f eléctrica
electric conductance; ~ f específica specific
conductance
conductimetría f conductometry
conductividad f conductivity; ~ f eléctrica
electric conductivity; ~ f molar molar
conductivity
conducto m duct, passage; ~ m arterioso
artificial artificial ductus arteriosus Botalli;
~ m arterioso persistente patent ductus
Botalli, open ductus arteriosus Botalli;
~ m auditivo auditory canal, auditory meatus;
~ m biliar gall duct, ductus cholidocus; ~ m de
Alcock Alcock canal, pudendal canal;
~ m deferente vas deferens, sperm duct;
~ m excretor excretory duct; ~ m genital
genital canal; ~ m lagrimal lacrimal duct, tear
duct; ~ m medular espinal medullary canal;
~ m nasolagrimal nasolacrimal duct;
~ m onfalomesentérico omphalo-enteric
duct; ~ m óptico optic foramen, optic canal;
~ m pélvico birth canal; ~ m periodontal
periodontal cyst, dental root cyst;
~ m pudendo Alcock canal, pudendal canal;
~ m vaginal vaginal canal; ~ m vitelino
vitelline duct, umbilical duct
conectivitis f collagen disease, connective-

tissue disease
conferencia f lecture
confidencialidad f confidentiality
confiscación f confiscation
confluencia f confluence; ~ f **sinusal** confluence of the sinuses
confusión f confusion, confusional state, ideosynchysis; ~ f **alucinatoria** hallucinatory confusion; ~ f **arteriosclerótica** arteriosclerotic confusion
confuso adj confused
congelación f frostbite
congenital adj congenital; ~ **colectasia** f congenital colectasia, Hirschsprung disease
congénito adj congenital
congestión f congestion; ~ f **bronquial** bronchial congestion; ~ f **cerebral** cerebral congestion, cerebral engorgement; ~ f **nasal** nasal congestion; ~ f **pulmonar** pulmonary congestion; ~ f **sanguínea** blood congestion, passive hyperemia; ~ f **venosa** venous congestion
congoja f mental anguish, mental distress
congreso m conference
conidióforo m conidiophore
conjugación f conjugation, linkage
conjugado adj conjugated, joined
conjuntiva f conjunctiva
conjuntival adj conjunctival
conjuntivitis f conjunctivitis; ~ f **de la lepra** leprous conjunctivitis; ~ f **flictenular** herpes conjunctivae
conjunto m complex; ~ m **de síntomas** syndrome
conmigo with me
conmoción f concussion, commotion; ~ f **cerebral** brain concussion
connatural adj congenital
conocer v to know
conocimiento m consciousness
consanguinidad f blood relationship, family relationship
consejería f council, commission; ~ f **profesional** vocational counseling, career counseling
consejero m counselor, adviser; ~ m **matrimonial** marriage counselor, relationship therapist

consejo m counseling, advice; ~ m **genetico** genetic counseling; ~ m **médico** counseling
consentimiento m consent; ~ m **informado** informed consent; ~ m **informado previo** m prior informed consent
conservación f **del esperma** semen storage
conservador adj conservative; ~ m preservative
conservar v to conserve
constante f constant; ~ f **de afinidad** affinity constant; ~ f **de Avogadro** Avogadro's constant, Avogadro's number; ~ f **de desintegración** decay constant, disintegration constant; ~ f **de disociación** dissociation constant; ~ f **de distribución** distribution constant; ~ f **de equilibrio** equilibrium constant; ~ f **de Faraday** Faraday constant; ~ f **de masa atómica** atomic mass constant; ~ f **de Michaelis** Michaelis constant
constantemente adj permanent, constantly
constipación f obstipation, constipation
constitución f constitution; ~ f **genética** constitution, genetic makeup
constitucional adj constitutional
constituyente m ingredient, component, constituent
constricción f stricture, stenosis; ~ f **del esófago** esophageal stricture, esophageal stenosis, stricture of the esophagus
consulta f doctor's office, doctor's consulting room, doctor's practice; ~ f **del dentista** dental clinic
consultorio m **de medicina** medical practice, practising medicine, doctor's office; ~ m **médico** medical practice, practicing medicine, doctor's office, doctor's practice
consumidor m consumer; ~ m **de drogas** drug user
consumo m consumption; ~ m **de drogas** drug use, drug consumption, drug abuse; ~ m **de oxígeno** oxygen uptake, oxygen absorbtion, oxygen capacity
contacto m contact, touch; ~ m **de centelleo** scintillation counter; ~ m **de partículas** particle counter; ~ m **Geiger-Müller** Geiger-Müller counter
contagio m infection, contamination; ~ m **mutuo** cross infection, mutual infection
contagioso adj communicable, contagious

contaminación f carry-over, contamination; ~ f **alimentaria** radioactive contamination of the food chain; ~ f **bacteriana** bacterial pollution; ~ f **de la biosfera** pollution of the biosphere; ~ f **radioactiva** radioactive contamination

contaminar v to pollute, to contaminate

contaminado adj polluted, contaminated; ~ adj **por gérmenes** septic

contenido m content; ~ m **catalítico** catalytic content; ~ m **cervical** cervical pool; ~ m **de número** number content; ~ m **de sustancia** substance content; ~ m **duodenal** duodenal contents; ~ m **gástrico** gastric contents; ~ m **vaginal** vaginal contents

contestar v to respond

contexto m context, background; ~ m **genético** genetic background

continencia f continence; ~ f **periódica** periodic abstinence, rhythm method

contingencia f contingency

continuación f follow-up

continuado adj progressive

continuar v to continue

continuo adj continuous

contra against, versus

contracción f contraction; ~ f **de los bronquios** bronchoconstriction, constriction of air passages; ~ f **miocárdica** myocardial contraction, contractility of the heart, cardiac inotropism; ~ f **muscular** muscle contraction; ~ f **uterina** uterine contraction, myometrial contraction; ~ f **ventricular prematura** premature ventricular contraction, premature heartbeat

contracepción f contraception, birth control

contraceptivo m contraceptive; ~ m **oral** oral contraceptive

contracoloración f counterstain

contractilidad f contractility, ability to contract; ~ f **miocárdica** myocardial contractility

contractura f contracture, permanent tissue shortening; ~ f **de los dedos** finger contracture; ~ f **por aducción** adduction contracture; ~ f **por calor** heat cramps

contradictorio adj contradictory

contraer v to get, to catch, to make, to take on

contraindicación f contraindication, reason not to prescribe

contrainmunoelectroforesis f CIE; ~ f counterimmunoelectrophoresis

contrapresión f back pressure

contrariedad f setback, adversity

contrario adj adverse, harmful

contrarrestar v to counteract

contrastación f **del esperma** semen evaluation

contratranscrito m countertranscript

contraveneno m antidote

control m control; ~ m **de la calidad** quality control; ~ m **ambulatorio** ambulatory monitoring, ambulatory control; ~ m **externo de la calidad** external quality control; ~ m **interno de la calidad** internal quality control

controlar v to monitor

contundente adj contusive, blunt force, causing contusion

contusión f bruise, bruising, contusion; ~ f **cardíaca** contusion of the heart, traumatic injury of the heart; ~ f **cerebral** brain contusion; ~ f **medular** contusion of the spinal cord; ~ f **ocular** contusion of the eyeball

convalecencia f reconvalescence, convalescence

convencional adj conventional, normal

convergencia f ocular convergence; ~ f **ocular** convergence

conversión f conversion, hysteria

convertir v to convert, score

convulsión f convulsion, spasm

convulsiones f pl seizure, convulsions

conyugal adj conjugal, marital

cónyuge m spouse

coordinación f coordination, association; ~ f **neuromuscular** neuromuscular coordination

coordinador m chair, chairman, chairperson

coprocultivo m fecal culture, stool culture

coproporfirina f coproporphyrin

cópula carnal f intercourse

copular v to have intercourse, to have sex, to copulate, to make love

coqueluche f pertussis, whooping cough

coracoideo m coracoid process

corazón m heart; ~ m **artificial** artificial heart; ~ m **pulmonar** cor pulmonale

corcovado adj hunchback

corditis f chorditis; ~ f **tuberosa** tuberous chorditis

cordón m bundle, tract, sheaf of fibers; ~ m **amniótico** abdominal pedicle, pedicle of the allantois; ~ m **umbilical** umbilical cord

cordotomía f cordotomy, operation on the spinal cord

corea f chorea; ~ f **de Huntington** Huntington's chorea, Huntington's disease; ~ f **de la cabeza** spasmus nutans, nodding spasm; ~ f **gravidarum** chorea gravidarum

coriodemona f destructive placental mole, chorio-adenoma destruens, invasive hydatiform mole

coriogonadotropina f choriogonadotropin, CG

coriomamotropina f choriomammotropin, CS; ~ f chorionic somatomammotropin

corionitis f chorionitis

corioretinitis f chorioretinitis, choroidoretinitis; ~ f **macular** central choroidoretinitis; ~ f **por toxoplasma** toxoplasmatic chorioretinitis

coriza f catarrh, head cold, nasopharyngitis; ~ f **por yodo** iodic rhinorrhoea

córnea f cornea; ~ f **globosa** megalocornea, cornea globata; ~ f **guttata** endothelial corneal dystrophy, cornea guttata

cornete m nasal concha, turbinate bone; ~ m **dentario** dental infundibulum

coroiditis f choroiditis; ~ f **central** choroiditis; ~ f **difusa** choroiditis, disseminated choroiditis; ~ f **diseminada** choroiditis, disseminated choroiditis; ~ f **miópica** myopic choroiditis; ~ f **senil** senile guttate choroiditis, Hutchinson choroiditis

corona f crown (on teeth)

coronario adj coronary

coronariopatía f coronary artery disease

corpiño m bra, brassiere

corporal adj somatic, physical

corpúsculo m particle; ~ s m pl **de Malpighi** malpighian corpuscles, renal corpuscles

corrección f correction; ~ f **de entropión** entropion correction; ~ f **de galeradas** proof-reading

correctivo m correction

correlación f corelation

corresponder v to correspond

corriente f current, stream, draft; ~ f **eléctrica** electric current; ~ f **sanguínea** bloodstream, blood flow

corrosión f corrosion; ~ f **dérmica** dermal corrosion

corrosivo adj caustic, corrosive

corset m **lumbrosacro** back brace, back support

cortar v to cut, to chop, to slice

cortada f cut

cortadura f cut; ~ f **profunda** incised wound, stab wound, deep cut

corte m incision, cut; ~ m **en bisel** staggered cut

corteza f cortex; ~ f **adrenal** suprarenal cortex, adrenal cortex; ~ f **auditiva** auditory cortex, auditory projection area; ~ f **cerebelosa** cerebellar cortex; ~ f **motora** motor cortex; ~ f **prefrontal** prefrontal cortex; ~ f **suprarrenal** suprarenal cortex, adrenal cortex, the outer layer of the adrenal gland

cortical adj cortical

corticoid m corticoid, corticosteroid

corticoliberina f corticoliberin, CRF, corticotropin-releasing factor

corticosteroide m corticosteroid; ~ m **tópico** topical corticosteroid

corticoterapia f corticoid therapy

corticotrofina f [**fármaco**] corticotrophin

corticotropina f adrenocorticotropic hormone

cortisol m cortisol

cortisona f cortisone

corto adj short

cortocircuito m **cardiopulmonar** coronary artery bypass graft

corva f back of the knee, popliteal space, popliteal fossa

Corynebacterium m corynebacterium; ~ m **diphteriae** Klebs-Löffler's bacillus, Löffler's bacillus; ~ m **pseudodiphtericum** Hormann's bacillus; ~ m **pseudotuberculosis** Preisz-Nocard's bacillus

cosa f thing

cosintropina f cosyntropin, tetracosactrin

cosmético m cosmetic

cósmido m cosmid

cosquillear v to tickle

costilla f rib; ~ f **cervical** cervical rib; ~ f **falsa** false rib; ~ f **verdadera** true rib costra f scab on a wound, crust

cot cot value

coulomb f coulomb

coxa f vara adolescente adolescent coxa vara, knockknees of young people in rural areas

coxalgia f coxalgia

coxartrosis f coxarthrosis, disease of the hip joint

coyontura f joint

craneano adj cranial

cráneo m skull, cranium

craneofacial adj craniofacial

craniotomía f trepanation, craniotomy, trephination

cráter m crater

creatina f creatine; ~ -cinasa f CK, creatine kinase, CPK

creatinasa f creatinase

creatinemia f creatinemia

creatinina f creatinine; ~ -desaminasa f creatinine deaminase

creatininasa f creatininase

creatininio m creatininium

crecimiento m growth

crema f cream; ~ f de afeitar shaving cream; ~ f hidratante moisturizer

crepitación f crepitation; ~ f atelectásica atelectatic crepitation; ~ f cutánea crepitation of the skin; ~ f de retorno crepitus redux

crepitar v to pop

cresta f crest

criar v to bring up, raise; ~ v con pecho to breast feed a child, to nurse a baby

cribado m detection, research, screening; ~ m mamográfico mammography screening, breast cancer screening, mammogram

cricotirocotomía f crichothyrocotomy

crioanestesia f cryo-anesthesia, using cold as anesthetic

criocirugía f cryosurgery

criodesecación f lyophilization, freeze-drying

criógeno m cryogenic fluid

crioglobulina f cryoglobulin

criptococosis f cryptococcosis, torulosis

criptorquidea f undescended testicle, cryptorchism

criptosporidiosis f cryptosporidiosis

crisis f crisis, turning point in a disease; ~ f nerviosa nervous breakdown; ~ f sincopal vasovagal syncope

crisoterapia f chrysotherapy, aurotherapy

crisparse v to twitch, to jerk, to have a twitch

cristal m crystal

cristales m pl asmáticos de Charcot-Leyden Charcot-Leyden crystals, asthma crystals

cristalino adj vitreous, glassy; ~ m cataract

cristalización f crystallization

cristalizar v to crystallize

cristaluria f crystalluria, crystals in the urine

criterio m criterion, menstruation, periods

cromafin adj chromaffin, chromophil, pheochrome

cromátide f chromatid

cromatina f chromatin

cromatografía f chromatography; ~ f de adsorción adsorption chromatography; ~ f de afinidad affinity chromatography; ~ f de elución elution chromatography; ~ f de exclusión exclusion chromatography; ~ f de gases gas chromatography; ~ f en capa fina thin-layer chromatography; ~ f en columna column chromatography; ~ f en fase líquida liquid chromatography; ~ f planar planar chromatography

cromatógrafo m chromatograph

cromatograma m chromatogram

cromatólisis f karyolysis

cromóforo m chromophore

cromómero m chromomere

cromonema f cromonema

cromosoma m chromosome; ~ m Filadélfia Philadelphia chromosome

cromosómico adj chromosomal

cronaxia f chronaxy, chronaxie

crónico adj persistent, chronic

cronotropo adj chronotropic, affecting the time or rate

cruda f hangover

cruel adj inhuman, cruel

crujido m popping, clicking

cruor m sanguinis coagulated mass, cruor

crup m croup; ~ m diftérico diphtheritic croup; ~ m laríngeo m laryngotracheobronchitis, croup

cruposo adj croupous

cruzamiento *m* crossing; ~ *m* **múltiple** multiple crossing

cuadrado *adj* square

cuadril *m* hip, coxa

cuadro *m* square, picture; ~ *m* **clínico** clinical picture, complex of symptoms, clinical symptomatology, syndrome; ~ *m* **de agudeza visual** vision chart, eye chart; ~ *m* **de lectura** reading frame; ~ *m* **hemático** blood analysis, hemogram

cuajarones *m pl* **de sangre** blood clots

cualitativo *adj* qualitative

cualitología *f* qualitology

cualitometría *f* qualitometrics

cuando when

cuantía *f* magnitude

cuantitativo *adj* quantitative

cuánto how much

cuarenta *adj* fourty

cuarto *adj* fourth; ~ *adj* four

cuarto *m* room; ~ *m* **estéril** sterile room

cuaternario *adj* quaternary, fourth

cubeta *f* **para utensiles** kidney dish

cubital *adj* ulnar, cubital

cúbito *m* ulna

cubreobjetos *m* cover slip

cucharada *f* tablespoon

cucharadita *f* teaspoon

cuchillada *f* gash, knife wound, stab wound

cuchillo *m* knife; ~ *m* **de trinchar** carving knife

cuello *m* neck; ~ *m* **de matriz** cervix (uteri), neck of the uterus, womb neck; ~ *m* **del astrágalo** neck of talus; ~ *m* **del fémur** neck of femur; ~ *m* **lastimado** whiplash; ~ *m* **torcido** torticollis, twisting of head and neck; ~ *m* **uterino** cervix (uteri), neck of the uterus, womb neck

cuenca *f* bowl, basin, socket; ~ *f* **del ojo** eye socket

cuenta *f* bill, fee, invoice, count; ~ *f* **de Addis** Addis count

cuéntagotas *m* **medicinal** pipette, eyedropper, medicine dropper

cuerda *f* rope, cord

cuerdas *f pl* **vocales** vocal cords

cuerno *m* horn, antler

cuero *m* derma; ~ *m* **cabelludo** epicranium, scalp

cuerpo *m* body, cuerpo; ~ *m* **calloso** corpus callosum, connection between right & left cerebral hemispheres; ~ *m* **de Barr** chromatin body; ~ *m* **carotídeo** carotid body; ~ *m* **de inclusión** inclusion body; ~ *m* **extraño** strange object, foreign body; ~ *m* **lúteo** corpus luteum; ~ *m* **mamilar** mamillary body, mamillary plexus, corpora candicantia; ~ *m* **pituitario** cerebral hypophysis, pituitary gland, pituitary; ~ *m* **vítreo** vitreous humor

cuerpos *m pl* **aorticos** aortic bodies; ~ *m pl* **cetónicos** acetone bodies, ketone bodies; ~ *m pl* **de Nissl** Nissl's bodies, chromophil corpuscles

cuestionable *adj* questionable, implausible, debatable, not proven

cuestionario *m* questionnaire; ~ *m* **estadístico** statistical questionnaire; ~ *m* **médico** medical questionnaire, forms for patient to fill out

cuidado *m* care; ~ *m* **adoptivo** foster care, foster home care; ~ *m* **paliativo** palliative care; ~ *m* **pastoral** pastoral care

cuidadores *m pl* care givers, caregivers

cuidados *m pl* **del prematuro** care of premature infants; ~ *m pl* **dirigidos** managed care; ~ *m pl* **intensivos** acute care, intensive care; ~ *m pl* **posteriores** after care services, follow-up treatment; ~ *m pl* **postoperatorios** postoperative care, postoperative treatment

cuidadoso *adj* observant, attentive

cuidar *v* a to take care of

culdocentesis *f* culdocentesis

culdoscopia *f* culdoscopy

culebra *f* snake

culo *m* anal orifice, anus

columbimetría *f* coulometry

cultivo *m* culture; ~ *m* **celular** cell culture; ~ *m* **de la defecación** stool culture; ~ *m* **de la garganta** throat culture; ~ *m* **de la orina** urine culture; ~ *m* **discontinuo** batch culture; ~ *m* **inclinado** slant agar culture; ~ *m* **para anaerobios** anaerobic culture; ~ *m* **por picadura** stab culture; ~ *m* **portador** carrier-culture; ~ *m* **sanguíneo** blood culture

cumplimiento *m* compliance

cumulativo *adj* cumulative, increasing

cuñada *f* sister-in-law

cuñado *m* brother-in-law

cuneiforme adj cuneate, wedge-shaped
cura f cure, healing, recovery; ~ f **de hambre** hunger cure, fasting cure; ~ f **médicade urgencia** first aid
curación f recovery, getting well, cure, healing; ~ f **definitiva** definite recovery, persistent recovery; ~ f **holistica** holistic healing; ~ f **por creencia** faith healing; ~ f **por la fé** faith healing
curalotodo m panacea
curandería f quackery, fraudulence, charlatancy, deceit
curanderismo m charlatanism, quackery
curandero m healer, psychic healer, faith healer, spiritual healer, medicine man, witch doctor; ~ m **homologado** naturopathic healer
curar v to medicate, to treat with medicine, to heal, to cure
curarizar to curarize, to treat with curare, to paralyze using curare
curativo adj curative, curing, healing
curetaje m curettage, abrasion, D&C, scraping off; ~ m **del útero** uterine curettage, uterine abrasion
curita f adhesive plaster
curva f curve; ~ f **de calibración** calibration curve; ~ f **de dosis y respuesta** dose-effect curve; ~ f **de eficacia** operating characteristic curve; ~ f **de elución** elution curve; ~ f **de medida** measuring curve
custodia f custody; ~ f **de los hijo** custody of children
cutáneo adj cutaneous
cutis f cutis, complexion, skin; ~ f **anserina** cutis anserina, goose flesh; ~ **laxa** cutis laxa, dermatolysis, loose skin, dermatochalasis

D

daltónico adj color-blind
daltonismo m color blindness, discromatopsis, parachromatism
dañar v to injure, to harm, to abuse, to hurt
dañino adj harmful (to your health), noxious, detrimental, pernicious
daño m hurt, esion, injury, trauma, wound,

affected area; ~ m **fetal** fetal injury, fetal damage; ~ m **ocasionado a la fertilidad** impairment of fertility
dantroleno m dantrolene, a muscle relaxant
dapsona f dapsone, diaminodiphenylsulfone, a sulfone drug to treat leprosy
dar v to give; ~ v **el alta** to discharge (from a hospital); ~ v **el pecho** to breastfeed, to nurse, to lactate, to suckle; ~ v **la baja** to give a medical certificate; ~ v **la mamadera al néné** to give baby the bottle, to bottle-feed
darse v **en la cabeza** to bump one's head
DDT (dicloro-difenil-tricloroetano) m DDT, carcinogenic polychlorinated pesticide
de of, from, by; ~ **alto grado diferenciada** high-grade differentiated; ~ **bajo peso** underweight, skinny, too thin; ~ **corto plazo** short-term, temporary, transitory, brief; ~ **duración breve** short-term, temporary; ~ **gran potencia** highly potent; ~ **nuevo** again; ~ **primer paso** first pass; ~ **repente** adv suddenly
debajo de under
deber v may, shall
débil adj weak, flaccid, flabby, soft
debilidad f lassitude, weariness, fatigue, exhaustion, weakness; ~ f **corporal general** asthenia, weakness, loss of strength; ~ f **mental** impaired judgement, alteration in judgement, deficient judgement, dementia, loss of mental functions; ~ f **motora** motor debility, motor infantilism
debilitación f debilitation, weakness; ~ f **de la voluntad** ; ~ f **general** cachexia, wasting away
debilitado adj run-down, weakened, tired, dragging, worn out
debilitar v invalidate, to
debrisoquina f debrisoquine
decadencia f decline, decay, decadence; ~ **neural** shrinkage of neurons, degenerating neurons
decaído adj listless, wan, apathetic
decantación f elutriation, washing out; ~ f **de anticuerpos** elutriation of antibodies
decantar v to elutriate
decidua f decidua; ~ f **gravídica** decidua graviditatis; ~ f **menstrual** decidua menstrualis

decilitro *m* deciliter

décimo *adj* tenth

decir *v* to tell

declaración *f* declaration, statement; ~ *f de* **discapacidad** *f* impairment rating, degree of disablement; ~ *f* **de Helsinki** Helsinki Accord

decolorante *m* decolorizer

decoro *m* decorum, good taste

decorticación *f* decortication; ~ *f* **pleural** pleural decortication, pleurectomy

decrépito *adj* decrepit, to be worn out, feeble, infirm, sickly, doddering

decúbito *f* decubitus

decusación *f* decussation

dedo *m* finger; ~ *m* **anillo** ring finger; ~ *m* **anular** ring finger; ~ *m* **corazón** middle finger; ~ *m* **cordial** middle finger; ~ *m* **de zinc** zinc-finger; ~ *m* **del pie** toe; ~ *m* **en martillo** hammertoe; ~ *m* **gordo del pie** big toe, hallux; ~ *m* **índice** index finger; ~ *m* **meñique** little finger, pinky finger; ~ *m* **pequeño del pie** little toe

defecación *f* bowel movement, defecation, stool, feces; ~ *f* **sanguinolenta** blood in the stools, bloody stool, hematochezia

defecar *v* to move the bowels, to defecate

defecto *m* deficiency, lack, shortage; ~ *m* **congénito** congenital defect, birth defect; ~ *m* **cromosómico** chromosome defect, chromosome damage; ~ *m* **de dicción** speech disorder, speech defect; ~ *m* **de nacimiento** birth defect; ~ *m* **del cromosoma** chromosome defect, chromosome damage; ~ *m* **immunitario** immune dysfunction, immune deficiency

defensor *m* **del paciente** patient advocate

deficiencia *f* deficiency, impairment; ~ *f* **cardiaca** cardia deficiency; ~ *f* **cognitiva** cognitive handicap; ~ *f* **congénita** congenital deficiency; ~ *f* **enzimatica genetica** genetic enzymatic deficiency

deficiente *m* **mental** mentally deranged, psychotic, lunatic

déficit *m* deficit

deformación *f* deformation, warping; ~ *f* **del tórax** chest deflection

deformado *m* deformed

deforme *adj* distorted

deformidad *f* deformity, malformation; ~ *f* **de Madelung** carpus curvus, Madelung's deformity

degeneración *f* degeneration; ~ *f* **amiloidea** amyloid degeneration, amyloidosis; ~ *f* **axónica** axonal degeneration; ~ *f* **centrífuga** descending degeneration, centrifugal wallerian degeneration; ~ *f* **de las neuronas** shrinkage of neurons, degenerating neurons; ~ *f* **gris** degeneration, grey degeneration; ~ *f* **macular** macular degeneration, maculopathy; ~ *f* **mucoide** mucoid degeneration

degenerativo *adj* degenerative

deglución *f* deglutition, swallowing

deglutir *v* to swallow

degradación *f* degradation, break down; ~ *f* **abiótica** abiotic degradation; ~ *f* **anaerobia** anaerobic decay, anaerobic digestion, anaerobic degradation; ~ *f* **catabólica** catabolic degradation; ~ *f* **enzimatica** enzyme degradation

dehidratasa *f* **del ácido delta–aminolevulínico** delta-aminolevulinic acid dehydratase

dehidrocortisona *f* prednisolone, hydrometrocortine, metacortandralone

dehiscencia *f* dehiscence

dejar *v* to leave, to let, to lend

delantal *m* **de plomo** lead apron

delante *f* at the front

deleción *f* deletion; ~ *f* **génica** gene deletion

deletéreo *adj* deleterious, detrimental

delgado *adj* thin

delicado *adj* sickly, weak, frail, delicate

delineación *f* delineation; ~ *f* **cortical** cortical delineation

delirante *adj* light-headed, dizzy, woozy, lightheadedness

delirar *v* to be delirious

delirio *m* paranoia; ~ *m* **alcohólico** alcoholic delirium, delirium tremens; ~ *m* **de grandeza** megalomania, delusions of grandeur; ~ *m* **onírico** delirium, onirism, vesanic dementia, waking dream state

demanda *f* demand; ~ *f* **bioquímica** biochemical demand; ~ *f* **de oxígeno** oxygen demand

demencia f dementia, loss of mental functions; ~ f **senil** senile dementia; ~ f **senil alcohólica** alcoholic senile dementia

demora f delay, retard

demulcente adj demulcent, emollient, soothing, softening, sedative

dendrita f dendrite; ~ f **postsináptica** postsynaptic nerve fiber, postsynaptic dendrite

dendrítico adj dendritic, branching; ~ m dendritic, branching

denervación f denervation; ~ f **muscular** muscle denervation

dengue m dengue fever, breakbone fever

densidad f density; ~ f **de corriente eléctrica** electric current density; ~ f **relativa** relative density

densitometría f **de huesos** osteodensimetry, bone density test, bone densitometry

densitómetro m **de huesos** bone densitometer, osteometric densitometer

dentadura f teeth; ~ f **parcial fija** fixed paritial dental bridge, fixed bridgework; ~ f **postiza** full set of dentures, false teeth, denture

dentalgia f toothache, odontodynia, dentalgia

dentición f teething, dentition

dentista m dentist

dentro inside; ~ **de** in

dependencia f outhouse; ~ f **de drogas** addiction, drug addiction; ~ f **de heroina** heroin addiction; ~ f **de una droga** drug addiction, toxicomania

dependiente adj dependent

depilatorio m depilatory

depleción f depletion, exhaustion and dehydration; ~ f **grave** lymphocyte depletion

deporte m sports

deposición f bowel movement, defecation, stool, feces

depósito m reservoir

depósitos m pl **amiloides** amyloid plaques, senile plaques, amyloid deposits; ~ m pl **de calcio** calcium deposits

depresión f depression; ~ f **de involución** involutional depression, major depressive disorder

depresor m depressant; ~ m **de apetito** anorexiant, appetite suppressant, appetite depressant, anorectic agent

deprimido adj depressed

depuración f purification, clearance; ~ f **de creatininio** creatinine clearance; ~ f **de inulina** clearance of inuline; ~ f **de la sangre** blood purification; ~ f **hepática** hepatic clearance; ~ f **mucociliar** mucociliary clearance, mucociliary transport; ~ f **renal** renal clearance

derecho m right-handed; ~ m **de rehusar tratamiento** right to refuse medical treatment

deriva f drift; ~ f **antigénica** antigenic drift

derivación f derivation; ~ f **directa** direct lead; ~ f **yeyunoileal** jejunoileal bypass, anastomosis of the proximal part of the jejunum to the distal portion of the ileum

derivado m derivative; ~ m **de salicilato** salicylate derivative

dermabrasión f dermabrasion, surgical planing

dermatitis f dermatitis, skin inflammation; ~ f **alérgica** allergic dermatitis, allergic dermatosis; ~ f **alérgica de contacto** allergic contact dermatitis; ~ f **atópica** atopic dermatitis; ~ f **estásica** stasis dermatitis; ~ f **hiemalis** dermatitis hiemalis, winter itch, pruritus hiemalis; ~ f **hiperémica** hyperemic dermatitis; ~ f **lumínica** actinodermatitis, actinodermatosis; ~ f **melitocócica** Brucella dermatitis; ~ f **no alérgica de contacto** non-allergic contact dermatitis; ~ f **papilar maligna** Paget's disease, Paget carcinoma; ~ f **por ácaros** acarodermatitis, skin inflammation or eruption produced by mites; ~ f **pustulosa miliar estafilocócica** dermite pustuleuse miliaire staphylococcique; ~ f **radiográfica** radiodermatitis, X-ray dermatitis, dermatitis actinica; ~ f **seborreica** dysseborrheic dermatitis, seborrheic dermatitis

dermatofibroma m dermatofibroma; ~ m **lenticular** lenticular dermatofibroma

dermatofito m dermatophyte

dermatofitosis f dermatophytosis

dermatoglifia f **del ADN** genetic footprint, genetic imprint, DNA fingerprint

dermatolisis f cutis laxa, dermatolysis, loose skin, dermatochalasis

dermatología f dermatology

dermatológico adj dermatological, skin-related

dermatólogo m dermatologist

dermatomicosis f dermatomycosis, fungal skin infection

dermatopatía f dermatopathy, skin ailment

dermatopatología f dermatopathology, pathology of skin disease

dermatosclerosis f scleroderma, dermatosclerosis

dermatosis f dermatosis, skin desease; ~ f **degenerativa** degenerative eczema, sensitization dermatitis

dérmico adj dermal

dermis f dermis, derma; ~ f **reticular** dermis

dermografía f dermographia, using pressure or friction to write on skin

dermografismo m dermography

dermopatía f skin disease, dermatopathy

derrame m effusion; ~ m **pericárdico** pericardial effusion; ~ f **pleural** pleural effusion

desabrocharse v to unzip, to unbuckle

desacomodación f **horaria** jet lag

desahogo m relief, solace, balm, comfort

desajuste m misalignment

desalentado adj discouraged

desalentado m breathlessness, shortness of breath

desalineación f misalignment

desambientación f **fisiológica** jet lag

desangramiento m bleeding, blood loss, exsanguination; ~ m **en las narices** nosebleed, nasal hemorrhage

desanimado adj disheartened, demoralized, discouraged

desaparición f disappearance, extinction, disintegration or dissolution (of cells)

desarollo m development; ~ m **de los niños** child development, pedology; ~ m **psíquico** cognitive development

desasosiego m vague sensation of uneasiness

desayuno m breakfast

desbridamiento m débridement, removing infected or necrotic tissue

descalzo adj barefoot

descamación f desquamation, exfoliation, peeling

descansar v to rest

descanso m spare time, leisure time, time off

descarboxilación f decarboxylation; ~ f **oxidativa** decarboxylation

descendencia f offspring, progeny

descendentes m pl offspring, progeny

descenso m fall, drop, descent

descerebración f decerebration

descompensación f decompensation

descomposición f breakdown, decomposition, decompression; ~ f **abdominal** decompression; ~ f **oxidante** oxidative decomposition

descompuesto m **de estómago** stomach ache

descondicionamiento m **cardiovascular** cardiovascular deconditioning

descongestivo adj decongestant; ~ m **nasal** nasal decongestant, drug that shrinks the swollen membranes in the nose

descontaminación f decontamination

descontaminar v to decontaminate

descubrimiento m research, detection, screening

descubrir v to detect, to discover

descuento m discount

desdoblamiento m dissociation, separation

desecación f dryness, dessication

desecante adj siccative, desiccant

desecar v to dry out

desecho m waste, discharge; ~ m **vaginal** discharge (vaginal)

desechos m pl waste, discharge, trash; ~ m pl **infecciosos** infectious waste

desensibilización f desensitization; ~ f **terapia** desensitization therapy

deseo m wish, desire; ~ m **sexual** libido, sexual impulse; ~ m **vehemente** craving, state of addiction

desequilibrio m imbalance

desfavorable adj adverse, harmful, noxious, detrimental, pernicious, unfavorable

desfibrilación f defibrillation, restoring heart beat

desfibrilador m defibrillator; ~ m **implantable** implantable defibrillator; ~ m **llevadero** wearable defibrillator

desgarrar v to tear, to rip, to break; ~ **un músculo** to strain a muscle, to pull a muscle

desgarro m laceration, tear (wound), flesh

wound, avulsion; ~ *m* **de la vesícula biliar** rupture of gall bladder; ~ *m* **de un ligamento** straining of a ligament, rupture or tearing of a ligament; ~ *m* **ligamentoso** torn ligament

desgaste *m* abrasion, graze, curettage, decortication

desglose *m* breakdown, decomposition

deshidratación *f* dehydration, exsiccosis; ~ **f hipertónica** hypertonic dehydration; ~ **f isotónica** isotonic dehydration

deshidroepiandrosterona *f* dehydroepiandrosterone

deshumanización *f* dehumanizing, dehumanization

desinfección *f* disinfection; ~ **f de la vestimenta** disinfection of clothing; ~ **f de las manos** disinfection of hands; ~ **f de los instrumentos** disinfection of instruments

desinfectante *m* antiseptic, disinfectant

desinfectar *v* to disinfect, to sterilize

desinhibición *f* disinhibition

desintegración *f* disintegration; ~ **f de la inteligencia** loss of intelligence, disintegration of intelligence, mental deterioration

desinterés *m* disengagement, withdrawal

desintoxicador *adj* detoxifying

desintoxicar *v* to detoxify

desmayar *m* blackout, seeing black, fainting, losing consciousness

desmayar *v* to black out, to faint, to lose consciousness

desmayo *m* syncope, faint, fainting spell

desmectasia *f* pulled tendon, desmectasia, strained tendon

desmesurado *adj* excessive

desmielinación *f* demyelination, destruction or loss of the myelin sheath; ~ **f isquémica** ischemic demyelination

desmocráneo *m* desmocranium

desmoide *adj* desmoid, ligamentous

desmoralizado *adj* disheartened, demoralized, discouraged

desnaturalización *f* denaturation; ~ **f de proteínas** denaturation

desnaturalizar *v* to denature

desnudarse *v* to undress

desnudo *adj* nude, naked

desnutrición *f* inanition, starvation, malnutrition, hypothrepsia

desobstrucción *f* clearing

desodorante *m* deodorant

desogestrel *m* desogestrel

desorientación *f* disorientation; ~ **f espacial** spatial disorientation

desorientado *adj* disoriented

desosificación *f* deossification

desoxiadenosina *f* deoxyadenosine

desoxicitidina *f* deoxycytidine

desoxicorticosterona *f* deoxycorticosterone

desoxigenación *f* deoxygenation

desoxiguanosina *f* deoxyguanosine

desoxirribonucleasa *f* deoxyribonuclease, DNase

desoxirribonucleótido *m* deoxyribonucleotide

despacio *adj* slow

despegamiento *m* **cutáneo** degloving, skin detaching

desperdicio *m* waste

desperdicios *m pl* **inertes** inert waste

desperfecto *m* lesion, injury, trauma, wound, affected area

despersonalización *f* alienation, depersonalization, a dream-like feeling

despido *m* dismissal; ~ *m* **del hospital** discharge from the hospital

despigmentación *f* depigmentation

despistado *adj* maudlin, lackadaisical, apathetic

desplazado *adj* displaced

desplazamiento *m* luxation, dislocation, moving out of position, sprain, torsion; ~ *m* **de banda** band shift; ~ *m* **del umbral** threshold shift

despliegue *m* extension, moving apart

despolarización *f* depolarization; ~ **f postsináptica** postsynaptic depolarization; ~ **f ventricular** ventricular depolarization

despreciable *adj* negligible

desprendimiento *m* detachment, separation; ~ *m* **de retina** retinal detachment, detached retina

después de -; del nacimiento postnatal; ~ **del parto** postpartum, after childbirth

desrepresión *f* derepression

destellar *v* to blink one's eye, to wink, to nictitate

destete *m* weaning, end of breast feeding, ablaction

destilar to distill
detoxificación f detoxication, drug addiction treatment
destreza f skill; ~ f **cognitiva** cognitive skills; ~ f **manual** manual dexterity
destrozar v to wreak havoc
destrucción f destruction
desvaído adj decrepit, to be worn out, to be feeble, doddering
desvanecimiento m syncope, faint, fainting spell
desvestirse v to undress, to take off one's clothes
desviación f deviation; ~ f **de la norma** anomaly, abnormality, deviation; ~ f **lateral** lateral deviation; ~ f **sexual** perversion; ~ f **típica** standard deviation
desviado adj deviant
detección f detection, research, screening; ~ f **directa del antígeno fluorescente** direct fluorescent-antigen detection; ~ f **genética** genetic screening, presymptomatic genetic testing; ~ f **precoz** early detection, screening, preventive medical checkup; ~ f **prenatal** prenatal screening; ~ f **presintomática** pre-symptomatic screening; ~ f **selectiva** screening, detection; ~ f **sistemática del cáncer** routine screening for cancer; ~ f **serológica** serological screening
detectabilidad f detectability
detectar v to detect, to discover
detector m detector; ~ m **de centelleo** scintillation detector; ~ m **de partículas magnéticas** magnetic particle detector; ~ m **semiconductor** semiconductor detector
detergente m detergent
deterioro m deterioration; ~ m **del medio ambiente** environmental degradation; ~ m **físico** physical deterioration; ~ m **intelectual** mental deterioration
determinación f determination; ~ f **de los gases sanguíneos** arterial blood gas test, arterial blood gas level; ~ f **del sitio** localization, locating
determinante m determinant; ~ m **antigénico** antigenic determinant, antigenic site, epitope
detorsión f detorsion
detrás at the back

dexametasona f dexamethasone
dexfenfluramina f dexfenfluramine
dextrano m dextran
dextrina f dextrin
dextrocardia f dextrocardia
dextrosa f glucose, dextrose, grape sugar; ~ f **monohidratada** dextrose monohydrate
deyección f evacuation of the intestines, dejection, defecation
DHEA f **(dehidroisoandrosterona)** DHEA, dehydroisoandrosterone
día m day
diabetes f diabetes; ~ f **bronceada** hemochromatosis, diabetes-hemochromatosis syndrome; ~ f **de tipo I** insulin-dependent diabetes, type I diabetes, juvenile-onset diabetes; ~ f **de tipo II** type II diabetes; ~ f **insípida** diabetes insipidus; ~ f **insípida nefrogenica** nefrogenic diabetes insipidus, vasopressin-resistant diabetes; ~ f **latente** diabetes, asymptomatic diabetes; ~ f **mellitus** diabetes mellitus; ~ f **mellitus lipoatrofica** lipoatrophic diabetes; ~ f **mellitus dependiente de insulina** insulin-dependent diabetes
diabético adj diabetic
diacetato m diacetate
diacetilmorfina f heroin, diacetylmorphine
diacilglicerol m diacylglycerol
diacinesis f diakinesis
diáfisis f diaphysis
diaforesis f diaphoresis, sweating, perspiration
diafragma m diaphragm; ~ m **pesario** cervical cap, diaphragm, diaphragm pessary
diagnóstico m diagnosis; ~ m **constitucional** constitutional diagnosis; ~ m **de unidades** unit diagnostics; ~ m **diagnóstico o preventivo** screening, detection, preventive medical checkup; ~ m **diferencial** DD, differential diagnosis; ~ m **hematológico** blood diagnosis; ~ m **inmunológico** immunodiagnosis, immunodiagnostics; ~ m **por gammagrafía** gamma-indicator diagnosis; ~ m **por imágenes** diagnostic imaging; ~ m **por ultrasonido** ultrasound examination; ~ m **precoz** early diagnosis, early detection; ~ m **profundo** diagnostic workup; ~ m **provisorio** presumptive diagnosis,

tentative diagnosis; ~ m **radiológico**
diagnostic radiology; ~ m **sicológico**
psychological diagnosis

diagrama m diagram; ~ m **de bandas** banding
pattern

diálisis f dialysis; ~ f **de los riñones** kidney
dialysis; ~ f **peritoneal** peritoneal dialysis,
transperitoneal dialysis

diámetro m diameter; ~ m **transverso pélvico**
diameter of pelvic outlet

diana f target, dartboard

diapasón m tuning fork

diapédesis f diapedesis; ~ f **de leucocitos**
leucocyte diapedesis

diapositiva f slide

diarrea f diarrhea; ~ f **de heces ocres** diarrhea
with yellow-ochre feces; ~ f **entérica** enteral
diarrhea; ~ f **síquica** diarrhea, psychic diarrhea

diastematomelia f diastematomyelia

diástole f diastole

diastólico adj diastolic

diatermia f diathermy

diátesis f diathesis; ~ f **alérgica** allergic
diathesis; ~ f **angioespástico** angiospastic
diathesis; ~ f **de los tejidos conjuntivos**
diathesis of connective tissue;
~ f **fibrinolítica** fibrinolytic diathesis;
~ f **neuropática** neuropathic diathesis

diazinón m diazinon

diciembre m december

dicloxacilina f dicloxacillin

dicotomía f dichotomy

dictamen m report; ~ m **experto** expert opinion

dicumarol m dicumarol

didesoxicitidina f zalcitabine, dideoxycitidine

dídimo m didymus

didrogesterona f dydrogesterone,
isopregnenone

diecinueve adj nineteen

dieciocho adj eighteen

dieciséis adj sixteen

diecisiete adj seventeen

diencefálico adj diencephalic

diencéfalo m diencephalon

dienestrol m dienestrol

diente m tooth; ~ m **artificial** artificial tooth;
~ m **de leche** milk tooth, deciduous tooth,
baby tooth

diestro adj dextromanual; ~ m right-hander

dieta f diet; ~ f **baja en calorías** low-calorie
diet; ~ f **para diabéticos** diabetic diet;
~ f **pobre en colesterol** low-cholesterol diet;
~ f **rica en proteínas** high-protein diet; ~ f **sin
sal** salt-free diet

dietilcarbamazina f diethylcarbamazine

diez adj ten

difásico adj biphasic, two-phase

diferencia f difference; ~ f **de potencial**
potential difference

diferenciación f differentiation

dificultad f difficulty

difilobotríasis f diphyllobothriasis

difteria f diphtheria

difteroide adj diphtheroide

difundido adj widely distributed

difunto adj dead, deceased

difusión f spreading, diffusion

difuso adj diffuse

digerible adj digestible

digerir v to metabolize, to digest, to assimilate

digestible adj digestible

digestión f digestion

digestivo adj digestive

digitalización f digitalization

digitopuntura f acupressure, pressure point
massage

digitoxina f digitoxin

dignidad f dignity; ~ f **humana** human dignity

digoxina f digoxin

dihidroergotoxina f dihydroergotoxin

dihidrofolato–reductasa f dihydrofolate
reductase, tetrahydrofolate dehydrogenase

Dilantin Dilantin

dilatación f dilatation, stretching, expansion;
~ f **de los bronquios** bronchodilatation,
dilated state of a bronchus, widening of the
airways, broncholysis; ~ f **precordial**
precordial protrusion, protrusion of the
embryonic heart; ~ f **pupilar** pupillary dilation,
pupil dilation, wide eyes, mydriasis

dilatador m dilator; ~ m **uterino** uterine dilator

diltiazem m diltiazem, a teratogenic
benzothiazepine derivative with vasodilating
action

dilución f dilution; ~ f **homeopática**
homeopathic dilution

diluido *adj* watery, diluted
diluidor *m* diluter
diluyente *adj* diluent, excipient, inactive part of drug; ~ *m* diluent, excipient, inactive part of drug
dimensión *f* dimension; ~ *f* **de una magnitud** dimension of a quantity
dimetilcisteína *f* D-penicillamine
dinero *m* money
dinitrato *m* dinitrate; ~ *m* **de isosorbide** isosorbide dinitrate
dinitroclorobenceno *m* dinitrochlorobenzene
dinoprostona *f* dinoprostone
dinucleótido *m* dinucleotide
dióxido *m* dioxide; ~ *m* **de azufre** sulfur dioxide; ~ *m* **de carbono** carbon dioxide; ~ *m* **de titanio** titanium dioxide
dipiridamol *m* dipyridamole
dipirona *f* dipyrone
diplococo *m* diplococcus
diploide *adj* diploid
diploma *m* diploma
diplomelituria *f* diplomelituria
diplopagos *m pl* diplopagus
diplopía *f* diplopia, double vision
diplotena *f* diplotene
dirección *f* address
directivas *f pl* directives; ~ *f pl* **de adelanto** advance directives, medical power of attorney
directo *adj* direct
director *m* director, editor; ~ *m* **de una edición** editor
dirigir *v* to direct, to aim, to address
dirigido *adj* **hacia adelante** anterograde, moving forward
disartria *f* dysarthria, speech defect
discapacidad *f* disability; ~ *f* **cognitiva** cognitive impairment, cognitive dysfunction, cognitive defect; ~ *f* **del desarrollo** developmental disorder, developmental disturbance; ~ *f* **física** physical disability, physical handicap, physical incapacity; ~ *f* **laboral** work-related disability; ~ *f* **mental** mental impairment; ~ *f* **temporaria** temporary disability
discapacitado *adj* handicapped, disabled, impaired; ~ *m* **de la vista** visually impaired person; ~ *m* **del desarrollo** developmentally disabled person

discernir *v* to detect, to discover
discinesia *f* dyskinesia; ~ *f* **dolorosa** dyskinesia algera; ~ *f* **tardía** tardive dyskinesia
disco *m* disc; ~ *m* **herniado** herniated disc, slipped disc; ~ *m* **intervertebral** intervertebral disc; ~ *m* **lumbar herniado** lumbar herniated disc; ~ *m* **protruído** herniated disc, slipped disc
discoide *adj* discoid, disk-shaped
discrasia *f* dyscrasia
discrepancia *f* discrepancy
discromatopsia *f* color blindness, discromatopsis, parachromatism
discutible *adj* questionable, implausible, debatable, not proven
disdiemorrisis *f* dysdiemorrhysis
disemia *f* dysaemia, cynosis, blood toxemia
diseminación *f* dispersion, spreading, proliferation, propagation, dissemination, scatter
disentería *f* dysentery; ~ *f* **amebiana** amebic dysentery, amebic colitis
disertación *f* lecture
disestesia *f* cacaesthesia, dysesthesia
disfagia *f* dysphagia; ~ *f* **paradójica** paradoxical dysphagia
disfonía *f* dysphonia; ~ *f* **espástica** dysphonia spastica
disforia *f* dysphoria
disfunción *f* dysfunction, malfunction; ~ *f* **cognitiva** cognitive dysfunction, cognitive disorders; ~ *f* **orgánica** organ dysfunction; ~ *f* **sexual psicológica** psychological sexual dysfunction; ~ *f* **tiroidea** thyroid dysfunction
disfuncional *adj* dysfunctional
disgenesia *f* dysgenesis, malformation; ~ *f* **gonadal** gonadal dysgenesis
disgeusia *f* dysgeusia
disglobulinemia *f* dysglobulinemia, plasma cell dyscrasia
disgónico *adj* dysgonic
dishidrosis *f* dyshidrotic eczema, dyshidrosis, cheiropompholyx
disimilación *f* dissimilation, catabolism
dislalia *f* dyslalia
dislexia *f* dyslexia
dislocación *f* luxation, dislocation, moving out of position, sprain, torsion

dislocamiento *m* displacement

dismenorrea *f* dysmenorrhea; ~ **inflamatoria** inflammatory dysmenorrhea; ~ **sintomática** symptomatic dysmenorrhea

dismetría *f* dysmetria

disminución *f* decrease, reduction; ~ **de la audición** hypoacusis, slight deafness; ~ **de las pulsaciones** decrease in the pulse rate

disminuido *adj* handicapped, disabled, impaired to reduce, to bring down, to lessen

disminuir *v* to reduce, to bring down, to lessen

disnea *f* dyspnea; ~ **acidótica** acidotic dyspnea; ~ **espiratoria** expiratory dyspnea; ~ **por esfuerzo** dyspnea due to exertion, exertional dyspnea; ~ **urémica** uremic dyspnoea, uremic dyspnea

disociación *f* dissociation, separation; ~ **auriculoventricular** atrioventricular dissociation; ~ **bacteriana** bacterial dissociation; ~ **citoglobulínica** cytoglobulinic dissociation

disolución *f* dissolution, lysis; ~ **acuosa** aqueous solution; ~ **del núcleo celular** karyolysis

disolvente *m* solvent, dissolvent; ~ *m* **de pintura** paint thinner

disolventes *m pl* solvents

disonancia *f* dissonance; ~ **cognitiva** cognitive dissonance

disopiramida *f* disopyramide

dispareunia *f* dyspareunia, pain during coitus

disparo *m* gunshot

dispensador *m* dispenser

dispepsia *f* dyspepsia, indigestion, upset stomach; ~ **bílica** biliary dyspepsia; ~ **histérica** hysterical dyspepsia; ~ **parenteral** parenteral dyspepsia

dispersión *f* spreading

displasia *f* dysplasia; ~ **broncopulmonar** bronchopulmonary dysplasia; ~ **retiniana** retinal dysplasia

disponibilidad *f* availability; ~ **a pagar** willingness to pay

disposición *f* disposition, tendency

dispositivo *m* gadget, contrivance, apparatus, device; ~ *m* **de aspiracion de aire** air suction system

disrafia *f* spinal dysraphism; ~ **oculta** spina bifida occulta

disreflexia *f* dysreflexia

distal *adj* distal, peripheral

distención *f* distension, enlarging

distender *v* to distend, to swell

distensión *f* distension; ~ **muscular** ruptured muscle; ~ **vesical** vesical distension, swollen bladder

distinguir *v* to detect, to discover

distintivo *m* **de identificación** name tag, name badge, identity badge, nametag

distiquia *f* distichiasis, distichia

distiquiásis *f* distichiasis, distichia

distocia *f* dystocia; ~ **cervical** cervical dystocia; ~ **materna** maternal dystocia, difficult delivery

distonía *f* dystonia, lack of muscle tone; ~ **muscular deformante** torsion dystonia, dystonia musculorum deformans; ~ **neurovegetativa** neurovegetative dystonia; ~ **premenstrual** premenstrual dystonia, premenstrual syndrome, PMS

distopia *f* dystopia, congenitally abnormal position of an organ; ~ **ureteral** ureteral dystopia

distorsión *f* distortion, skewing; ~ **de la percepción** perception disorder, perceptual disturbance

distractibilidad *f* inability to concentrate, distractibility

distraído *adj* absent-minded, forgetful, distraught

distribución *f* distribution; ~ **al azar** randomization; ~ **de referencia** reference distribution

distrofia *f* dystrophy; ~ **de la córnea** corneal dystrophy; ~ **miotónica** myotonic dystrophia, Steinert's disease, Batten's disease, Batten-Steinert syndrome, autosomal dominant neuromuscular disorder; ~ **muscular** muscular dystrophy; ~ **muscular de Duchenne** Duchenne muscular dystrophy; ~ **muscular hiperplástica** hyperplastic muscular dystrophy

distrofina *f* dystrophin, a protein from skeletal muscle

disturbio *m* impairment, disturbance

disuria *f* dysuria, painful urination

D

disyunción f disjunction; ~ f **genética** genetic disjunction; ~ f **meiótica** meiotic disjunction

DIU m **(dispositivo intrauterino)** intra-uterine device, IUD, coil, loop; ~ m **que libera hormonas** hormone-releasing IUD

diuresis f urinary output, diuresis

diurético m diuretic

diurno adj daytime, diurnal

divergencia f divergence

diverticulitis f diverticulitis, inflammation of the colon

divertículo m diverticulum; ~ m **del colon** colonic diverticulosis; ~ m **de Meckel** Meckel's diverticulum; ~ m **esofágico** esophageal diverticulum; ~ m **uretral** ureteral diverticulum

divieso m boil, furuncle, bump, swelling, bruise

división f division; ~ f **de una célula** mitosis, cell division

divorciado adj divorced

DNA m DNA; ~ m **bicatenario** double-stranded DNA; ~ m **circular cerrado** closed circle DNA; ~ m **complementario** complementary DNA, copy DNA; ~ m **espaciador** spacer DNA; ~ m **expandido** extended DNA; ~ m **incompleto** gapped DNA; ~ **-ligasa** f DNA repair enzyme, DNA ligase; ~ m **monocatenario** simple strand DNA, simple strand DNA; ~ m **matador** killer DNA; ~ m **no repetido** non-repetitive DNA; ~ **-nucleotidilexotransferasa** f DNA nucleotidylexotransferase; ~ **-polimerasa** f DNA polymerase; ~ m **superhelicoidal** supercoiled DNA

doblarse v to flex, to bend inward, to lean forward, to bend over; ~ v **por atrás** to lean back, to bend backwards

doble adj double; ~ adj **hélice** double helix

doce adj twelve

doctor m doctor

documentar v to document

documento m document, form; ~ m **de identidad** identification

dolencia f pain

doler v to ache, to hurt

dolor m pain; ~ m **abdominal** abdominal pain, abdominalgia, pain in the belly; ~ m **agudo** acute pain; ~ m **anginoso** anginal pain, pain in the chest; ~ m **ardiente** burning pain, stinging pain, smarting sensation; ~ m **bajo de espalda** low back pain, low backache; ~ m **constante** ache, steady pain; ~ m **de cabeza** headache, cephalea; ~ m **de dientes** toothache, odontodynia, dentalgia; ~ m **de estómago** gastralgia, stomach ache, tummy ache; ~ m **de garganta** pharyngitis, sore throat, inflammation of throat, inflammation of the pharynx; ~ m **de muelas** tooth ache; ~ m **de oído** earache, otalgia; ~ m **de parto** labor pain; ~ m **de vientre** stomach ache, tummy ache, belly ache; ~ m **del costado** pain or stitch in the side, stitches in the side, flank pain; ~ m **en el talón** pain in the heel, calcaneodynia; ~ m **en la espalda** back pain, backache; ~ m **en un músculo** myalgia, muscle pain; ~ m **fantasma** phantom pain, phantom limb syndrome, phantom sensation; ~ **fuerte** severe pain, sharp pain; ~ m **inducido por presión** pressure pain, pain from being touched; ~ m **insoportable** unbearable pain; ~ m **insufrible** unbearable pain, insufferable pain; ~ m **intermenstrual** intermenstrual pain, mittelschmerz, intermenstrual bleeding and pain; ~ m **isquémica** ischemic pain; ~ m **leve** slight pain, mild pain; ~ m **ligero** slight pain, mild pain; ~ m **lumbar bajo** low back pain, low backache; ~ m **neuropático** neuropathic pain; ~ m **pélvico** abdominal pain, abdominalgia, pain in the belly; ~ m **persistente** persistent pain, chronic pain; ~ m **por compresión** pressure-induced pain; ~ m **posoperatorio** postoperative pain; ~ m **precordial** heartburn, pyrosis, cardialgia, pain in the heart area; ~ m **recio** severe pain, sharp pain; ~ m **torácico** chest pain

dolores m pl **del parto** labor pains; ~ m pl **menstruales** menstrual cramps; ~ m pl **articulares** joint ache

dolorido adj painful, aching, sore

doloroso adj painful, aching, sore

dominancia f dominance; ~ f **cerebral** cerebral dominance

domingo m Sunday

donación f donation; ~ f **alogénica** allograft, allogenic graft, allogenic transplant, homologous graft

donante m donor; ~ m **de espermas** sperm donor; ~ m **de órganos** donor; ~ m **de plasma** blood plasma donor; ~ m **de sangre** blood donor

donde where

dopamina f dopamine, a neurotransmitter

doparse v to take stimulants, to dope oneself

doping m doping

Doppler m doppler; ~ m **vascular** vascular doppler; ~ m **venoso** venous doppler

dormir v to be asleep, to sleep

dorsal adj dorsal

dorsalgia f back pain, backache, dorsalgia, notalgia

dorsiflexión f dorsiflexion

dorso m back; ~ m **de la mano** back of the hand, dorsum manus

dos adj two; ~ **veces** twice; ~ **veces al día** twice a day, bid (bis in die)

doscientos adj two hundred

dosificación f dosage

dosimetría f dosimetry; ~ f **biológica** biological dosimetry

dosis f dose; ~ f **absorbida** absorbed dose; ~ f **de ataque** loading dose; ~ f **de cebamiento** initial dose, loading dose; ~ f **de radiación absorbida** radiation absorbed dose, rad; ~ f **equivalente** dose equivalent; ~ f **excesiva** overdose, overdosing, overdosage; ~ f **homeopática** homeopathic dose; ~ f **inicial** initial dose, loading dose; ~ f **letal** lethal dose; ~ f **letal de radiación** lethal dose of radiation; ~ f **mediana efectiva** median effective dose; ~ f **normal** standard dose; ~ f **única** unit dose, a single dose

dotación f endowment, crew; ~ f **cromosómica** chromosome set; ~ f **médica** medical supplies, pharmaceutical supplies

doxapram m doxapram

doxepina f doxepin

doxiciclina f doxycycline

doxorrubicina f adriamycin, doxorubicin

D-penicilamina f D-penicillamine

dramamina f dramamine

drenaje m drainage, paracentesis, fluid removal; ~ m **linfático** lymphatic drainage, lymph drainage

drepanocitosis f sickle cell anemia, an inherited blood disorder characterized by chronic anemia and painful episodes

droga f drug; ~ f **adictiva** addictive drug, habit-forming drug, dependence-producing drug; ~ f **analgésica** pain killer, analgesic, pain reliever, painkiller; ~ f **antianginosa** antianginal, angina drug

drogadicción f drug addiction, toxicomania

drogadicto m addict, drug user, drug addict

drogas f pl drugs; ~ f pl **legales** legal drugs; ~ f pl **sintéticas** designer drugs, street drugs

droperidol m droperidol

ducha f shower

ductus m passage, duct

dudoso questionable, implausible, debatable, not proven

duelo m grief, grieving

dulce adj sweet

duodenectomía f duodenectomy

duodeno m duodenum

duodenoilostomía f duodeno-ileostomy

duodenopancreatectomía f Whipple's operation, duodeno-pancreatectomy

dúplex duplex

duplicación f replication, duplication

duplicidad f duplication; ~ f **verdadera** ureteral duplication, ureteral bifidy

duración f length, duration; ~ f **de la vida** longevity, length of life

duramadre f dura mater; ~ f **encefálica** dura mater of the brain; ~ f **espinal** spinal dura mater

durante during, while; ~ **la noche** overnight

durapatita f hydroxyapatite, durapatite

durazno m peach

duro adj hard; ~ adj **de oído** hard of hearing, hearing impaired

D-xilosa f D-xylose

E

eburnación f eburnation, osteoesclerosis

eccema f eczema; ~ f **postvacunal** postvaccinal eczema

eccémátide f eczematid; ~ f **pitiriasiforme** pityriasiform eczematid; ~ f **psoriasiforme** psoriasiform eczematid

ecchinococosis f echinococcosis; ~ f **hepática** echinococcosis of the liver

ECG, electrocardiograma m electrocardiogram

echinacea f echinacea, purple coneflower

echovirus m echovirus

eclampsia f eclampsia; ~ **del recién nacido** eclampsia neonatorum, eclampsia of a newborn child; ~ f **infantil** eclampsia neonatorum, eclampsia of a newborn child; ~ f **puerperal** puerperal sepsis, puerperal infection, puerperal eclampsia, puerperal abscess

ecocardiografía f echocardiography, ultrasonic recording of the size, motion, and composition of the heart

ecocardiograma m echocardiogram

ecografía f echography; ~ f **obstétrica** obstetrical ultrasound, fetal echography; ~ f **ocular** ocular ultrasonography; ~ f **prostática endorrectal** transrectal prostate ultrasonography; ~ f **renal** renal ultrasound, renal ultrasonography

ecopatia f echopraxia, echopathy, mimicking other peoples' movements

ectasia f ectasia, enlargement; ~ f **capilar** capillary dilation

ectodermo m ectoderm

ectólisis f ectolysis

ectoparásito m ectoparasite

ectopia f heterotopia, ectopy; ~ f **testicular** testicular ectopy; ~ f **ventricular** ventricular ectopia; ~ f **vesical** ectopia of urinary bladder, vesical ectopy

ectópico m ectopic

ectoplasma m ectoplasm

ecuación f equation; ~ f **de Henderson-Hasselbach** Henderson-Hasselbach equation; ~ f **de Nernst** Nernst equation

eczema m eczema, pruritic papulovesicular dermatitis; ~ m **alérgico** allergic eczema; ~ m **dishidrótico** dyshidrotic eczema, dyshidrosis, cheiropompholyx; ~ m **penfigoide** bullous pemphigoid, bullous eczema

edad f age; ~ f **de fallecimiento** age at death

edema m edema, swelling; ~ m **agudo pulmonar** acute pulmonary edema; ~ m **ambulante** calabar swelling; ~ m **angioneurótico** Quincke disease, angioneurotic edema; ~ m **cerebral de gran altura** high-altitude cerebral edema (HACE); ~ m **de hambre** hunger edema; ~ m **de la papila óptica** papilledema; ~ m **papilar** papilledema, papilloedema, swollen optical disk; ~ m **pulmonar** pulmonary edema, an accumulation of fluid in the lungs

edematoso adj edematous

editor m publisher

educación f education; ~ f **de la sensibilidad** sensitivity training

EEG (electroencefalograma) EEG (electroencephalography)

efectividad f efficacy, effectiveness

efectivo adj efficacious

efecto m effect; ~ m **biológico** biological effect; ~ m **citopático** cytopathic effect; ~ m **colateral** side effect, adverse reaction; ~ m **de eco** ghost image, echo image; ~ m **de la dosis** dosage effect; ~ m **Doppler** Doppler shift; ~ m **halo** halo effect; ~ m **positivo inotrópico** positive inotropic effect, affecting the force or energy of muscular contractions; ~ m **preclínico** preclinical effect; ~ m **teratógeno** teratogenic effect

efector m effector

efectuar v to make, to carry out; ~ v **medidas** to take measurements

efedrina f ephedrine

eficacia f efficiency; ~ f **biológica relativa, EBR** relative biological effectiveness, RBE; ~ f **de clonado** cloning efficiency

eficaz adj effective, efficient

eflectancia f eflectance

efluente m effluent

efusión f effusion

eje m **sagital** sagittal axis

ejecución f **en la horca** death by hanging

ejercicio m exercise; ~ m **físico** physical exercise, movement; ~ m **muscular** muscle building, strengthening, muscle training; ~ m **respiratorio** breathing exercise

ejes f **vasculares de grandes vasos** vascular axes of great blood vessels

él he

el *m*, la *f*, los *m pl*, las *fp* the

elaboración *f* de una serie de pruebas médicas workup, an intense diagnostic study

elaborar *v* to work up

elastasa *f* elastase; ~ *f* de leucocito lysosomal elastase, polymorphonuclear leukocyte elastase, PMN elastase; ~ *f* leucocitaria neutrophil elastase; ~ *f* pancreática pancreatic elastase, pancreatopeptidase

elasticidad *f* elasticity

elástico *adj* elastic, springy, supple, limber

elastina *f* elastin

elastosis *f* elastosis; ~ *f* distrófica elastosis dystrophica

electroendósmosis *f* electro-endosmosis

elección *f* election, selection

electivo *adj* elective, non-urgent (e.g. operation)

electricidad *f* electricity

electro-anestesia *f* electro-anesthesia

electrocardiografía *f* electrocardiography, heart monitor

electrocardiograma *m* electrocardiogram, ECG; ~ *m* de la pared torácica chest-wall ECG

electrocariotipo *m* electrokaryotipe

electrochoc *m* electric shock

electrocoagulación *f* surgical diathermy, electrocoagulation

electrocución *f* electrocution

electrodiálisis *f* electrodialysis

electrodo *m* electrode; ~ *m* de referencia reference electrode; ~ *m* enzimático enzyme electrode; ~ *m* indicador indicator electrode

electroencefalografía *f* electroencephalography

electroencefalograma *m* electroencephalogram

electroeyaculación *f* electro-ejaculation

electrofisiología *f* electrophysiology

electrofisiológico *m* electrophysiological, involving study of electrical phenomena in living bodies

electroforesis *f* electrophoresis; ~ *f* bidimensional en gel two-dimensional gel electrophoresis; ~ *f* cruzada crossover electrophoresis; ~ *f* de inversión de campo en gel field inversion gel electrophoresis; ~ *f* en

gel de agarosa agarose gel electrophoresis; ~ *f* en gel de poliacrilamida PAGE, polyacrylamide gel electrophoresis

electroftalmo *m* visual prosthesis, electrophthalm

electrogravimetría *f* electrogravimetry

electrólisis *f* electrolysis

electrólito *m* electrolyte, solution which conducts electricity

electromiografía *f* electromyography, EMG

electromiograma *m* electromyogram, EMG

electrónes *m pl* electrones

electrónica *f* biológica bionics

electronvolt *m* electronvolt

electropatología *f* electro-pathology

electroporación *f* electroporation

electropulsación *f* electropulsation

electroscopia *f* por resonancia magnética cerebral brain MRS, brain magnetic resonance spectroscopy

electroterapia *f* electrotherapeutics, electric stimulation therapy, electrotherapy

electrotransferencia *f* por adsorción electroblotting

elefantiasis *f* elephantiasis; ~ *f* filariensis filarial elephantiasis, true elephantiasis; ~ *f* piodérmica elephantiasis pyodermatica; ~ *f* sifilítica elephantiasis syphilitica; ~ *f* tuberosa elephantiasis tuberosa

elemento *m* element; ~ *m* catalytico catalytic element; ~ *m* transponible transposable element; ~ *m* traza oligoelement, trace element

elevado *adj* elevated

eliminación *f* elimination; ~ *f* de intrones intron splicing

eliminador *m* eliminator; ~ *m* de polvo dust eliminator, dust separator, dust collector, ventilator

elisa *f* ELISA, enzyme-linked immunosorbent assay

elixir *m* elixir; ~ *m* medicated elixir

ella she, her

ello it

ellos, ~as they

elongación *f* elongation

eluato *v* to eluate

elutriación *f* elutriation, washing out

elutriar v to elutriate

eluyente f eluent

emaciación f emaciation, extreme leanness

emagrecer v to lose weight

embajada f embassy

embarazada adj pregnant

embarazo m gestation, pregnancy, gravidity; ~ m **de alto riesgo** high-risk pregnancy; ~ m **dicigótico** dizygotic pregnancy; ~ m **ectópico** ectopic pregnancy; ~ m **en adolescencia** teenage pregnancy, adolescent pregnancy; ~ m **monocigótico** monozygotic pregnancy; ~ m **no deseado** unwanted pregnancy; ~ m **tuboabdominal** tubal pregnancy

embolectomía f embolectomy; ~ f **arterial** arterial embolectomy

embolia f embolism; ~ f **bacilar** bacterial embolism; ~ f **capilar** capillary embolism; ~ f **cerebral** cerebral infectious embolism; ~ f **gaseosa** air embolism, aerothrombosis, aeroembolism; ~ f **grasa** fat embolism; ~ f **parasitaria** parasitic embolism; ~ f **pulmonar** pulmonary embolism; ~ f **séptica** septic embolism

embolismo m embolism; ~ m **amniótico** amniotic embolism; ~ m **pulmonar** pulmonary embolism

embolización f embolization

émbolo m embolus; ~ m **tumoral** tumor cell embolus

embriaguez f drunkenness, inebriation

embrión m embryo; ~ m **viable** viable embryo

embrionario adj embryonic

embriopatía f embryopathy

embudo m funnel

emenagogos m pl emmenagogues

emergencia f emergency

emesis f vomiting

emético m emetic, substance to cause vomiting

emetropía f emmetropia, the normal refractive condition of the eye

emitancia f emittance

emoción f affect, emotion

emocional adj affective, emotional

emoliente adj soothing, relaxing, pacifying

emoliente f emollient, soothing lotion

empalme m **de proteína** protein splicing

empaquetamiento m packaging; ~ m **del DNA** DNA packaging

emparentado adj related by marriage

empaste m filling (in teeth)

empatía f empathy

empeine m pubic region, groin, instep; ~ m **abdominal** lower part of abdomen, pubic region, groin

empeoramiento m aggravation, exacerbation, worsening, disease progression

empezar v to start

empiema m empyema, pus in a body cavity; ~ m **articular** arthroempyesis; ~ m **pulmonar** purulent pleurisy, pleuropyesis, suppurative pleurisy, pyothorax

empírico adj empiric, based on experience

emplasto m plaster, medicated compress, poultice

empleado m employee

empoderamiento m empowerment

emprostótonos m emprosthotonos

empujar v to push

emulsión f emulsion, suspension of one liquid in another; ~ f **bacteriana** bacterial emulsion

emulsionar v to emulsify

en on, in, by; ~ **actividad** active; ~ **ayunas** fasting; ~ **casa** at home; ~ **dirección** in the direction of, towards; ~ **parto** in childbed; ~ **reposo** at rest, inactive; ~ **su lugar natural** in situ, in the normal place

enalapril m enalapril

enanismo m dwarfism, microsomia

enano m, **enana** f dwarf, midget

enantema f enanthem, enanthema, eruption on a mucous surface; ~ f **vesicular** vesicular enanthema

encapsidación f encapsidation

encarcerado adj ingrown, strangulated

encarnado m healing wound

encefálico adj encephalic

encefalina f enkephalin; ~ f **leucina** leucine enkephalin

encefalitis f encephalitis, brain inflammation

encéfalo m brain, cerebrum

encefalomielitis f encephalomyelitis; ~ f **diseminada** disseminated encephalomyelitis

encefalomiopatía f encephalomyopathy

encefalopatía f brain disease, encephalopathy;
~ f **alcohólica** alcoholic encephalopathy,
Wernicke's encephalopathy; ~ f **bilirrubínica**
bilirubin encephalopathy; ~ f **espongiforme**
spongiform encephalopathy (Creutzfeldt-
Jakob disease); ~ f **espongiforme bovina**
bovine spongiform encephalopathy, mad cow
disease; ~ f **espongiforme transmisible (EET)**
transmissible spongiform encephalopathy;
~ f **hipertensa** hypertensive encephalopathy;
~ f **saturnina** saturnine encephalopathy, lead
poisoning encephalopathy; ~ f **tóxica crónica**
chronic toxic encephalopathy

encendido adj on

enchinarse (la piel) to get goosebumps

encía f gum

encima de upon, on top

encogerse v to shrink

encondroma m enchondroma, true chondroma

encondromatosis f enchondromatosis

encontrar v to find

encopresis f encopresis, incontinence of feces,
usually psychological

endeble adj decrepit, to be worn out, feeble,
infirm, sickly, doddering

endémico adj endemic

enderezarse v to straighten up, to sit up

endocárdico adj endocardiac, endocardial

endocárdico m endocardium

endocarditis f endocarditis

endocrino adj endocrine

endocrinología f endocrinology

endocrinológico m endocrinologist

endodoncia f endodontics, endodontia

endodontista m endodontist

endoenzima f endoenzyme

endógeno adj endogenous, without obvious
external cause

endogenote endogenote

endolisina f endolysin

endometriosis f endometriosis; ~ f **de colón**
endometriosis of large intestine, colonic
endometriosis; ~ f **intratorácica** intrathoracic
endometriosis; ~ f **ovárica** ovarian
endometriosis, adenoma endometrioides
ovarii; ~ f **ureteral** ureteral endometriosis;
~ f **uterina** stromal adenomyosis,
adenomyoma of the uterus, uterine

endometriosis; ~ f **vesical** vesicular
endometriosis

endometritis f endometritis, inflammation of
the uterus

endonucleasa f endonuclease; ~ f **de
restricción** restriction endonuclease

endoparásito m internal parasite, endoparasite

endopeptidasa f endopeptidase

endoprótesis f bioprosthesis

endorfina f endorphin

endoscopia f endoscopy; ~ f **de las glándulas
salivales** endoscopic examination of the
salivary glands

endoscopio m endoscope; ~ m **de fibra óptica**
lexible fiberscope, optical-fiber endoscope,
laparoscope

endostosis f endostosis

endotelio m endothelium; ~ m **venoso alto**
endothelial venule, HEV

endotóxico adj endotoxic

endotraqueal adj endotracheal, intratracheal

endoxina f endoxin

endurecido m callous, hardened

endurecimiento m induration, hardening;
~ m **de las arterias** hardening of the arteries;
~ m, **callosidad** induration, hardening

enema m enema; ~ m **de bario** barium enema,
barium swallow, barium contrast study

energético adj energetic

energía f energy; ~ f **cinética** kinetic energy;
~ f **de excitación** excitation energy;
~ f **interna** internal energy; ~ f **libre** free
energy; ~ f **radiante** radiant energy

enero m January

enfadado adj angry

enfebrecido adj feverish

enfermedad f disease, illness; ~ f **cardiaca
isquémica** f ischemic heart disease, ischemic
myocardial disease; ~ f **catastrófica**
catastrophic illness; ~ f **celíaca** celiac disease;
~ f **cerebral** brain disease, encephalopathy;
~ f **cerebro-vascular** cerebrovascular disease;
~ f **contagiosa** communicable disease,
contagious disease; ~ f **contagiosa** infectious
disease; ~ f **crítica** critical illness;
~ f **cromosómica** chromosomal illness,

chromosomopathy; ~ f **crónica respiratoria** chronic respiratory disease; ~ f **curable** curable disease; ~ f **de Addison** Addison's disease; ~ f **de Albright** Albright-McCune-Sternberg syndrome; ~ f **de Alzheimer** Alzheimer's disease, Alzheimer dementia; ~ f **de Asperger** Asperger syndrome, Asperger's disease; ~ f **de autoinmunidad** autoimmune disease; ~ f **de Basedow** Parry's disease, Basedow's disease; ~ f **de Biett** lupus erythematosus, SLE, disseminated erythematosus lupus, erythematosus lupus, lupus, Biett disease; ~ f **de Bornholm** epidemic diaphragmatic pleurodynia, Bornholm disease, devil's grip; ~ f **de Bourneville** Bourneville syndrome, tuberous sclerosis; ~ f **de Bozzolo** multiple myeloma, plasmacytoma, myelomatosis, Kahler's disease, Huppert's disease, Bozzolo disease; ~ f **de Buerger** thromboangiitis obliterans; ~ f **de Corrigan** aortic insufficiency, Corrigan disease; ~ f **de Crohn** regional enteritis, regional ileitis, Crohn's disease; ~ f **de Dupuytren** Dupuytren's contracture; ~ f **de Gowers** Gowers disease, Gowers syndrome; ~ f **de Hageman** Hageman factor deficiency; ~ f **de Hanot** Hanot disease, Hanot cirrhosis; ~ f **de Hodgkin** Hodgkin's disease; ~ f **de Huntington** Huntington's chorea, Huntington's disease; ~ f **de Huppert el plasmacitoma** multiple myeloma, plasmacytoma, myelomatosis, Kahler's disease, Huppert's disease, Bozzolo disease; ~ f **de Kahler** multiple myeloma, plasmacytoma, myelomatosis, Kahler's disease, Huppert's disease, Bozzolo disease; ~ f **de Kerl-Urbach** extracellular cholesterilinosis; ~ f **de Kienböck** Kienböck's disease, osteonecrosis of the lunate bone; ~ f **de Köhler** Köhler's disease; ~ f **de la sangre** hemopathy, blood disease; ~ f **de la válvula cardiaca** heart valve disease; ~ f **de las vías urinarias** urinary tract disease; ~ f **de los maquinistas** cervicobrachial disorder, machinist's disease; ~ f **de Lou Gehrig** Lou Gehrig's disease, amyotrophic lateral sclerosis; ~ f **de Lyme** Lyme disease, ~ f **de Machado-Joseph** Machado-Joseph disease, spinocerebellar

ataxia type 3, autosomal dominant striatonigral degeneration; ~ f **de Mitchell** erythromelalgia, Mitchell disease; ~ f **de mohos** mycotic infection, mycosis; ~ f **de Niemann** Niemann-Pick disease; ~ f **de Paget** Paget's disease, Paget carcinoma; ~ f **de Parkinson** Parkinson's disease; ~ f **de priones** prion disease; ~ f **de Recklinghausen** neurofibromatosis, von Recklinghausen's disease, osteitis fibrosa cystica; ~ f **de Schaumann** benign lymphogranulomatosis, Boeck's sarcoid, lupus pernio, sarcoidosis, Besnier-Boeck disease; ~ f **de Scheuermann** Scheuermann's disease; ~ f **de Steinert** myotonic dystrophia, Steinert's disease; ~ f **de Tay-Sachs** Tay-Sachs disease; ~ f **de transmisión hídrica** water-borne disease; ~ f **de transmisión sexual** STD, sexual transmitted diseases, veneral disease; ~ f **de Weil** Weil's disease, a highly infectious disease caused by spirochetal bacteria; ~ f **de Whipple** intestinal lipodystrophy, Whipple's disease, ~ f **de Wilson** hepatolenticular degeneration, Wilson's disease; ~ f **debilitante** debilitating disease, debilitating disorder; ~ f **del arañazo de gato** cat scratch disease, cat scratch fever, benign lymphoreticulosis; ~ f **del colágeno** collagen disease, connective-tissue disease; ~ f **del corazón** heart disease; ~ f **del legionario** legionnaire's disease; ~ f **del pulmón** pneumopathy, lung disease; ~ f **del riñón** nephropathy, kidney disease, renal disease, nephritic disease; ~ f **del sueño** sleeping sickness; ~ f **endémica** endemic disease; ~ f **genética** genetic disease; ~ f **granulomatosa** granulomatous disease; ~ f **hemolítica** hemolytic disease; ~ f **hereditaria** hereditary disease; ~ f **infecciosa** infectious disease; ~ f **inflamatoria pélvica** PID, Pelvic Inflammatory Disease, adnexitis; ~ f **inflamatoriadel intestino** inflammatory bowel disease, IBD; ~ f **innata** inborn diseases; ~ f **intestinal** intestinal disease; ~ f **Letterer-Siwe** Letterer-Siwe disease, acute

form of Langerhans-cell histiocytosis;
~ f **metabólica** metabolic disease;
~ f **muscular** myopathy, muscle diease;
~ f **musculoesquelética** musculoskeletal
disorder / disease; ~ f **nerviosa** neuropathy,
nervous system disorder, neurological
disorder; ~ f **neurodegenerativa**
neurodegenerative disease; ~ f
neuromuscular neuromuscular diseases;
~ f **nutricional** nutritional disease;
~ f **periodóntica** periodontal disease,
periodontosis; ~ f **por reflujo gastroesofágico
(GERD)** gastroesophageal reflux disease;
~ f **psicosomática** psychosomatic illness;
~ f **pulmonar obstructiva crónica** COPD,
chronic obstructive pulmonary disease;
~ f **recesiva** recessive disease; ~ f **renal
crónica** chronic renal disease; ~ f **renal
poliquística** polycystic disease of the kidney,
polycystic renal disease; ~ f **transmisible**
communicable disease, contagious disease;
~ f **venérea** veneral diseases, STD;
~ f **yatrógena** iatrogenic disease
enfermera/o m/f nurse; ~ m/f **a cargo** nurse
case manager; ~ m/f **cargada del caso** nurse
case manager; ~ m/f **de cuidados intensivos**
intensive care nurse; ~ m/f **diplmada**
registered nurse; ~ m/f **instrumentista**
surgical orderly, operating-room orderly; ~ m/
f **militar** hospital orderly; ~ m/f **psiquiátrico**
psychiatric nurse; ~ m/f **supervisora** head
nurse, charge nurse
enfermería f infirmary, nursing
enfermeros m pl care givers, caregivers
enfermizo adj sickly
enfermo adj ill, sick, m sick; ~ m **mental**
mentally ill person, psychiatric patient
enfisema m emphysema; ~ m **bronquiolar**
bronchiolar emphysema; ~ m **mediastínico**
mediastinal emphysema; ~ m **pulmonar**
pulmonary emphysema
enflaquecimiento m weight loss, slimming
enfoque m **poliantigénico** antigenic approach
enfrentar v to cope with, to deal with
engordar v **de peso** to gain weight, to put on
weight
engorroso adj cumbersome

engrosamiento m thickening; ~ m **del tiroides**
struma, goiter, thyroid enlargement;
~ m **pleural** pleural thickening, pleuritic
callosity
enjuagar v to flush
enjuague m rinse; ~ m **bucal** mouthwash
enjugar v to dessicate, to dry out, to wipe
enlace m **iónico** ionic bond, adsorption
immobilization
enoftalmia f enophthalmos, recession of the
eyeball into the orbit
enoxacina f enoxacin
enrojecido adj reddish, reddened, erythroid
enrojecimiento m redness; ~ m **en la piel**
erythema, skin redness
ensanchamiento m dilatation, stretching,
expansion
ensangrentado adj bloody
ensayo m assay, analytical test; ~ m **biológico**
bioassay, biological testing; ~ m **clínico**
clinical trial, clinical experiment, clinical
assay; ~ m **clínico aleatorio** randomized
clinical trial; ~ m **de aptitud** proficiency
testing; ~ m **de toxicidad** toxicity test; ~ m **en
doble-ciego** double-blind comparative trial;
~ m **serológico** serological test
enseñar v to teach
entablazón f severe constipation
entablillar v to splint, to put in a cast or splint
entalpía f enthalpy
entender v to understand
enterocolitis f enterocolitis
enteritis f enteritis; ~ f **amebiana** amebic
enteritis; ~ f **regional** regional enteritis,
regional ileitis, Crohn's disease
entero, un a whole
enterobius m pinworm, intestinal nematode
worm
enterocolitis f enterocolitis
enterohepático adj enterohepatic
enteroinvasor m enteroinvasive
enteropatía f enteropathy; ~ f **exudativa**
exudative enteropathy, proteinlosing
enteropathy
enteropatógeno adj enteropathogenic
enteropeptidasa f enterokinase,
enteropeptidase
enterotoxigénico adj enterotoxigenic

enterotoxina f enterotoxin; ~ f **estafilocócica** staphylococcal enterotoxin

enterovirus m enterovirus

entidad f entity; ~ f **morbosa** morbid entity; ~ f **patológica** pathologic entity

entítico adj entitic

entorno m environment

entorpecer v to numb, to become numb, to stiffen

entramado m **fino de nylon** fine-mesh nylon gauze

entrar v to enter; ~ v **en calor** to limber up, to warm up

entrecruzamiento m crossing-over, crossover; ~ m **de fibrina** fibrin cross-linking

entrenamiento m training, workout, fitness training; ~ m **de la sensibilidad** sensitivity training; ~ m **en asertividad** assertiveness training

entrepiernas f pl crotch, groin

entresijo m genital region

entropía f entropy

entropión m entropion

entumecer v to numb, to become numb, to stiffen

entumecido m numbness, obnubilation

entumescimiento m numbness, obnubilation

enucleación f enucleation

enuresis f enuresis, bedwetting

envaramiento m rigidity, stiffness, numbness, obnubilation

envarar v to numb, to become numb, to stiffen

envasado m **aséptico** aseptic filling

envase m package, container; ~ m **de vidrio** cartridge, vial

envejecimiento m aging, getting older, senescence; ~ m **prematuro de la piel** accelerated skin aging, premature aging of the skin

envenenamiento m intoxication, poisoning; ~ m **por el xenón** xenon poisoning; ~ m **por nitroglicerina** nitroglycerine poisoning

envenenar v to poison

envoltura f bandage, surgical dressing; ~ f **abdominal** peritoneum; ~ f **proteica** protein coat

envolvente adj surrounding

enyesado m plaster cast (on a limb)

enyesadura f cast

enzima f enzyme; ~ f **alostérica** allosteric enzyme; ~ f **constitutivo** constitutive enzyme; ~ f **cortadora** cutting enzyme; ~ f **de conversión de la angiotensina** angiotensin converting enzyme, ACE; ~ f **de restricción** restriction enzyme; ~ f **llave** key enzyme

enzimas f pl **cardiacas** cardiac enzymes; ~ f pl **del hígado** liver enzymes

enzimoinmunoanálisis m EIA, enzyme immunoassay

eosina f eosine

eosinofilia f eosinophilia; ~ f **pulmonar** pulmonary eosinophilia

eosinofilocito m eosinophil, eosinophilocyte

epicanto m epicanthus, epicanthic fold

epicondilalgia f epicondylalgia

epicondilitis f epicondylitis, tennis elbow

epicóndilo m epicondyle

epidemia f epidemic disease

epidémico adj epidemic

epidemiología f epidemiology

epidemiólogo adj epidemiological, involving study of epidemics

epidemiólogo m involving study of epidemics

epidérmico adj epidermal, skin-related

epidermólisis f **ampollosa** epidermolysis bullosa

epididimitis f epididymitis

epidídimo m epididymis

epidural adj epidural, extradural

epifisario adj epiphyseal

epífisis f epiphysis, pineal body

epigastralgia f epigastralgia, upper abdomen pain

epigástrico adj epigastric

epigenético adj epigenetic

epiglotis f epiglottis

epilepsia f epilepsy; ~ f **cortical** cortical epilepsy, focal epilepsy, Jacksonian epilepsy, partial epilepsy; ~ f **generalizada** grand mal, generalized tonic-clonic seizure; ~ f **minor** petit mal, minor epilepsy; ~ f **mioclónica** idiopathic myoclonic epilepsy, symptomatic myoclonic epilepsy; ~ f **psicomotora** psychomotor epilepsy, temporal-lobe epilepsy

epiloia f Bourneville's disease

epinefrina f epinephrine, adrenalin

episiotomía f episiotomy, cut to vagina in

childbirth
episodio m episode
epistaxis f epistaxis, nosebleed, nasal hemorrhage
epitelio m epithelium; ~ **germinal** germinal epithelium; ~ **m germinativo** germinal epithelium
epitelioide adj epithelioid
epitelioma m skin cancer, malignant epithelioma, skin carcinoma; ~ **m glandular** adenomatous carcinoma, adenoepithelioma; ~ **m indiferenciado** undifferentiated epithelioma
epítope m antigenic determinant, antigenic site, epitope
EPOC COPD, chronic obstructive pulmonary disease
épulis f epulis, a benign tumor of the gums
equilibrio m balance; ~ **m acidobásico** acid-base balance; ~ **m muscular** muscle balance; ~ **m esquelético** skeletal balance, skeletal workup
equinococcia f **pulmonar** echinococcosis of the lung, alveolar echinococcosis
equinococosis f echinococcosis, hydatidosis
equipaje m luggage
equipo m **de reactivos** kit, reagents kit; ~ **m respiratorio adecuado** suitable respiratory equipment
equivalente m equivalent
ERA f **(audiometría electroencefalográfica)** ERA, evoked response audiometry
ercalciol ergocalciferol, vitamin D2
erección f penile erection; ~ f **del pelo** piloerection; ~ f **persistente** continuous erection
ergastoplasma m ergastoplasma, ergastoplasm, endoplasmic reticulum (rough surfaced)
ergonometría f ergonomics, ergonometry, human engineering
ergoterapeuta m occupational therapist
ergoterapia f occupational therapy, ergotherapy
ergotismo m ergotism, poisoning from ergot fungus
ergotoxina f ergotoxin
erisipela f erysipelas, St. Anthony's fire, onchocerciasis; ~ f **precoz** early erysipelas; ~ f **umbilical** umbilical erysipelas

erisipeloide m erysipeloid; ~ m **de Klauder** erysipeloid
eritema m erythema, redness of the skin; ~ **m cronico migrans** erythema chronicum migrans; ~ **m emotivo** emotional blush; ~ **m infeccioso** erythema infectiosumm; ~ **m multiforme** erythema multiforme, ~ **m nudoso** erythema nodoso; ~ **m solar** sunburn, solar dermatitis
eritrasma m eritrasma, erythrasma
eritroblastosis f **fetal** fetal erythroblastosis, erythroblastosis fetalis
eritrocianosis f erythrocyanosis
eritrocito m erythrocyte, red blood cell, red corpuscle, RBC
eritrocitos m pl red blood cells, erythrocytes; ~ **m pl homólogos centrifugados** packed red cells
eritrodermia f **ictiosiforme** erythrodermia ichthyosiforme congenitum; ~ f **maculopapulosa** macropapular erythrodermia
eritroenzimopatía f red cell enzymopathy, enzymatic deficiency of human erythrocytes
eritromelalgia f erythromelalgia, Mitchell disease
eritromicina f erythromycin
eritropoyesis f erythropoiesis
eritropoyetina f erythropoietin
eritrosedimentación f erythrocyte sedimentation rate, erythrosedimentation, ESR, sedimentation velocity
eritrosis f **facial** acne rosacea, facial erythrosis
ERM m **cerebral** brain MRS, brain magnetic resonance spectroscopy, magnetic resonance spectroscopy of the brain
erosión f erosion; ~ f **cromosómica** chromosome erosion; ~ f **dentaria** abrasion, graze, curettage, decortication, tooth erosion; ~ f **recidivante de la córnea** recurring erosion of the cornea
erradicación f eradication
erradicar v to eradicate, to eliminate
error m error; ~ m **absoluto** absolute error; ~ **m aleatorio** random error; ~ m **médico** medical malpractice; ~ m **relativo** relative error; ~ m **sistemático** bias, systematic error; ~ m **total** total error

eructar v to belch, to eructate

eructo m eructation, belching, burp, belch

erupción f eruption, break out, extrusion

escabiosis f scabies

escafoides m del carpo navicular bone, scaphoid bone; ~ m del tarso navicular bone, scaphoid bone

escala f scale; ~ f de adaptación accommodation range; ~ f de diferencias difference scale; ~ f del estado mental mental status questionnaire, mental status schedule; ~ f nominal nominal scale; ~ f ordinal ordinal scale; ~ f racional ratio scale

escaldado m en la boca soreness of the mouth

escaleras f stairs

escalofríos m pl chills, shivers, ague (perhaps due to malaria), shivering; ~ m pl incontrolables shivering attack, uncontrollable trembling

escamoso adj squamous, scaly

escáner m pelviano pelvic scan

escanografía f scan; ~ f cerebral brain scan, PET scan of brain

escápula f scapula, shoulder blade

escara f bedsore, decubitus ulcer, pressure sore

escariar v to scrape (the skin)

escasamente adv scantily, sparingly, scarcely, hardly; ~ diferenciada poorly differentiated

escayola f plaster of Paris

escherichia f coli escherichia coli, E. coli

escintigrafía f scintigraphy; ~ f al talio thallium scan; ~ f ósea skeletal scintigraphy

escintilograma m scintigram

escisión f excision, surgical removal, resection, cleavage

esclerodactilia f sclerodactyly, acroscleroderma

esclerodermia f scleroderma, dermatosclerosis; ~ f circunscrita circumscribed scleroderma

esclerosis f sclerosis, hardening by tissue cells; ~ f cerebral difusa cerebrosclerosis; ~ f cerebral tuberosa tuberous sclerosis, Bourneville's disease, hypertrophic tuberous cerebrosclerosis, epiloia; ~ f coroidiana choroid sclerosis, choroideremia; ~ f lateral amiotrófica amyotrophic lateral sclerosis, ALS, Lou Gehrig's disease; ~ f múltiple multiple sclerosis

escleroterapia f sclerotherapy

esclerótica f sclera, white of the eye; ~ f sclerotic, tumor-like hardening of the skin

escobillón m swab

escocimiento m burning pain, stinging pain, smarting sensation

escoliosis f scoliosis, abnormal lateral curvature of the spine; ~ f de la columna vertebral spinal scoliosis

escondido adj hidden, occult, concealed

escorbuto m scurvy

escoriación f dérmica degloving, skin detaching

escorpión m scorpion

escotadura f cerebelosa anterior semilunar notch (in the cerebellum

escotoma m scotoma, blind spot

escozor m burning pain, stinging pain, smarting sensation

escribir v to write

escritura f writing, handwriting; ~ f manual ilisível illegible handwriting

escroto m scrotum

escuchar v to listen

escudriñar v to research, to investigate, to examine

escuela f school

escupir v to spit, to expectorate

esfigmanómetro m no invasivo non-invasive sphygmomanometer

esfigmomanómetro m blood pressure meter, sphygmomanometer, hemadynamometer

esfincterotomía f sphincterotomy, excision of a sphincter

esfingomielina f sphingomyelin; ~ f fosfodiesterasa sphingomyelin phosphodiesterase

esfínter m sphincter; ~ m anal anal sphincter; ~ m de Hyrtl Hyrtl sphincter; ~ m del cardias cardial sphincter, diaphragm sphincter of the esophagus; ~ m hepatopancreatico Oddi's sphincter, the sphincter of the hepatopancreatic ampulla within the duodenal papilla; ~ m ileocólico ileocolic sphincter, ileocolic valve; ~ m pilorico pyloric sphincter, sphincter antri

esfirectomía f sphyrectomy

esfregar v to rub

esfuerzo m physical exertion, movement,

physical stress, exertion, strenuous activity;
~ *m pl* **físico** physical labor

esguince *m* ankle; ~ *m* **de tobillo** twisted ankle, sprained ankle

esguinzarse *v* **el tobillo** to sprain one's ankle

eso *m*, **esa** *f*, **eso, este, esta, -o, que** (comp) that (near)

esofagitis *f* esophagitis; ~ *f* **corrosiva** corrosive esophagitis

esófago *m* esophagus, gullet; ~ *m* **de Barrett** Barrett's esophagus

esofagocardiomiotomía *f* **extramucosa** Heller operation, Heller procedure

esofagogastrostrectomía *f* esophagogastrectomy

esofagostomía *f* esophagostomy

esos *m*, **-as** *f* those (near)

espacio *m* space; ~ *m* **hueco** cavity, hollow; ~ *m* **personal** privacy, confidentiality, private life, personal space; ~ *m* **subaracnoideo** subarachnoid space; ~ *m* **subdural** subdural space

espalda back

español *adj* Spanish

espanto *m* shock, fright

esparadrapo *m* adhesive plaster

esparganosis *f* sparganosis, Diphyllobothrium infection

espasmo *m* convulsion, spasm; ~ *m* **abdominal** abdominal cramp, gripe; ~ *m* **de la laringe** thymic asthma, Kopp's asthma, laryngismus, laryngeal spasm, spasm of the larynx, phrenoglottic spasm; ~ *m* **de los bronquios** asthma, bronchospasm, bronchial asthma; ~ *m* **esofagico difuso** diffuse esophageal spasm; ~ *m* **muscular** muscle cramp, muscle spasm

espasmódico *adj* spasmodic

espasmolítico *m* anti-spasm, spasmolytic

espasticidad *f* spasticity, muscle rigidity

espástico *adj* spastic

especialidad *f* speciality; ~ *f* **farmacéutic** proprietary medicine; ~ *f* **medicinal** specialty pharmaceutical product, proprietary medicinal product

especialista *f* specialist

especialización *f* **en la medicina** medical residency

especialmente especially, particularly

especie *f* species; ~ *f* **oportunista** opportunist species

especificación *f* specification

especificidad *f* specificity; ~ *f* **antigénica** antigenic specificity; ~ *f* **diagnóstica** diagnostic specificity; ~ *f* **metrológica** metrological specificity; ~ *f* **nosográfica** nosographic specificity; ~ *f* **nosológica** nosologic specificity

específico *adj* specific

especimen *m* specimen, sample

espectinomicina *f* spectinomycin

espectro *m* spectrum; ~ *m* **de absorción** absorption spectrum

espectrometría *f* photometry, spectrophotometry, spectrometry; ~ *f* **de absorción atómica** atomic absorption; ~ *f* **de absorción atómica de llama** flame atomic absorption spectrometry; ~ *f* **de absorción molecular** molecular absorption spectrometry; ~ *f* **de dispersión molecular** molecular dispersion spectrometry; ~ *f* **de emisión atómica de llama** flame atomic emission spectrometry, flame photometry; ~ *f* **de fluorescencia molecular** molecular fluorescence spectrometry; ~ *f* **de luminiscencia molecular** molecular luminiscence spectrometry; ~ *f* **de masas** mass spectrometry; ~ *f* **de reflectancia** reflectance spectrometry

espectrómetro *m* photometer, spectrophotometer, spectrometer; ~ *m* **de masas** mass spectrometer; ~ *m* **multinuclear** multinuclear nuclear magnetic resonance, NMR, spectrometer

espectroscopía *f* spectroscopy; ~ *f* **de emisión** emission spectroscopy; ~ *f* **de imágenes** imaging spectroscopy; ~ *f* **de interferencia** interference spectroscopy; ~ *f* **de masa** mass spectroscopy, mass spectrometry; ~ *f* **fotoelectrónica ultravioleta** ultraviolet photoelectron spectroscopy; ~ *f* **infraroja** infrared spectroscopy; ~ *f* **por resonancia magnética cerebral** magnetic resonance spectroscopy of the brain; ~ *f* **por resonancia magnética nuclear** nuclear magnetic resonance spectroscopy

espéculo *m* speculum; ~ *m* **bucal** mouth speculum; ~ *m* **laríngeo** laryngeal speculum; ~ *m* **nasal** rhinoscope, conchoscope, nasal speculum; ~ *m* **vaginal** vaginal speculum

espejuelos *m pl* glasses

esperanza *f* hope; ~ **de vida** life expectancy

esperma *m* semen; ~ *f* **fresco** fresh semen; ~ *f* **ultracongelado** frozen semen, frozen sperm

espermatocele *m* spermatocele

espermatocistitis *f* seminal vesiculitis, spermatocystitis

espermatogénesis *f* spermatogenesis, sperm-formation

espermatozoide *m* spermatozoid

espermicida *f* spermacide, sperm-killing contraceptive

espermidina *f* spermidine

espina *f* spina, spine; ~ **bifida** spina bifida, cleft spine; ~ *f* **dendrítica** dendritic spine; ~ *f* **dorsal** spine

espinaca *f* spinach

espinal *adj* spinal

espinilla *f* pimple, acne pustule, blackhead, pustule, furuncle, comedone, shin bone, tibia

espiración *f* expiration, breathing out; ~ *f* **prolongada** prolonged expiration

espiramicina *f* spiramycin

espirar *v* to breathe out

espirometría *f* spirometry, spirometric testing, measurement of volume of air inhaled or exhaled in the lung

espirómetro *m* spirometer

espiroqueta *f* spirochete, causes Lyme disease

esplenitis *f* spleen infection

esplenomegalia *f* spleen enlargement, splenomegaly

espliceosoma *f* spliceosome

esplínquer *m* sequencing primer linker, splinker

espolón *m* spur; ~ *m* **calcáneo** heel spur, calcanean spur; ~ *m* **traqueal** carina tracheae

espondilitis *f* spondylitis, vertebrae inflammation; ~ *f* **anquilosante** ankylosing spondylitis, Bechterew's disease; ~ *f* **deformante** ankylosing spondylitis deformans

espondilolistesis *m* isthmic spondylolisthesis

esponjoso *adj* cancellous, spongy, trabecular

espora *f* spore

esporádicamente *adj* irregularly

esporádico *adj* random, sporadic

esporicida *f* sporicide

esporotricosis *f* sporotrichosis, a chronic myotic infection

esporozoito *m* sporozoite

esposa *f* wife

esposo *m* husband

espuma *f* foam; ~ *f* **espermaticida** spermicidal foam

espundia *f* leishmaniasis, espundia

esputo *m* phlegm, viscid mucus, sputum, expectoration; ~ *m* **inducido** sputum induction

esquelético *adj* skeletal

esqueleto *m* skeleton

esquema *m* schema, outline, plan, pattern, schedule; ~ *f* **de administración del medicamento** dosage schedule; ~ *f* **de excreción de un medicamento** excretion pattern of a drug; ~ *m* **corporal** body scheme

esquiascopio *m* ophthalmoscope, retinoscope, skiascope

esquistosomiasis *f* schistosomiasis, bilharziasis; ~ *f* **intestinal** intestinal schistosomiasis; ~ *f* **urinaria** endemic hematuria, urinary schistosomiasis

esquizofrenia *f* schizophrenia

esquizofrenico *m* schizophrenic (person)

esta semana this week

estabilidad *f* stability; ~ *f* **biológica** biological stability

estabilización *f* stabilization

estación *f* **de cuarentena** quarantine center

estadiaje *m* staging; ~ *m* **del cáncer** cancer staging, the determination of the size and extent of cancer in the body

estadística *f* statistics

estadísticas *f pl* **vitales** vital statistics, demographic data, population statistics

estadístico *adj* statistic, statistical

estado *m* state, status; ~ *m* **actual** state of the art; ~ *m* **analgésico** analgesic state; ~ *m* **asistencial** welfare state; ~ *m* **asmático** status asthmaticus; ~ *m* **benefactor** welfare state; ~ *m* **civil** marital status, civil status; ~ **de ánimo** state of mind; ~ **de**

desconexión parcial shut-down state; ~ *m* **de equilibrio** steady state; ~ *m* **de reposo** stand-by state; ~ *m* **general** performance status, condition; ~ *m* **mental** state of mind; ~ *m* **precancerígeno** precancerous state

estafilococo *m* staphylococcus; ~ *m* **dorado** staphylococcus aureus

estafiloma *f* staphyloma

estándar *m* standard

estandarizar *v* to standardize

estar *v* to be; ~ *v* a **régimen** to be on diet; ~ *v* **amodorrado** to be drowsy; ~ *v* **boca abajo** lying prone, face down, prostrate; ~ *v* **borracho** to be drunk; ~ *v* **constipado** to have stuffy or runny nose, to have the sniffles; ~ *v* **de dieta** to be on diet; ~ *v* **destemplado** to feel queasy, to feel out of sorts, to feel shivery, to be unwell; ~ *v* **desvanecido** to feel faint, to be woozy; ~ *v* **en cuclillas** to squat; ~ *v* **enfermo** to feel ill, to be ill; ~ *v* **malo del corazón** to have a heart condition; ~ *v* **nauseabundo** feel nauseous, to, feel sick to one's stomach, to; ~ *v* **roto** to have a hernia; ~ *v* **sin aire** breathlessness, shortness of breath; ~ *v* **supino** lying supine, lying face up; ~ **dormido** *v* to be asleep, to sleep; ~ **envarado** *v* to feel bloated, to have gas; ~ **nauseado** *v* to be nauseated, to throw up, to vomit; ~ **postrado** lying prone, face down, prostrate; ~ **presente** to be present

estasis *f* stasis, keeping in check; ~ *f* **en la ventilación pulmonar** stasis of pulmonary ventilation

estatinas *f pl* statins, cholesterol-lowering drugs

este *m*, **esta** *f* this

esteatonecrosis *f* steatonecrosis, fat necrosis, adiponecrosis

esteatorrea *f* steatorrhea, excess fat in the motions

esteatosis *f* steatosis, fatty degeneration

estenosis *f* stenosis, duct narrowing; ~ *f* **arterial coronaria** coronary artery, coronary stenosis; ~ *f* **de la válvula pulmonar** pulmonic valve stenosis, stenosis of the pulmonary valve; ~ *f* **esofagica** esophageal stricture, esophageal stenosis, stricture of the esophagus; ~ *f* **mitral** mitral stenosis; ~ *f* **aórtica** aortic stenosis,

stenosis of aortic valve, narrowing of the aorta

estereopsis *f* stereoscopic vision, stereopsis

estereotaxia *f* stereotaxis

estereotipia *f* stereotypy

estéril *adj* sterile, clean

esterilidad *f* sterility; ~ *f* **irreversible** irreversible sterility; ~ *f* **irreversible comprobada** verified irreversible sterility

esterilización *f* sterilization; ~ *f* **eugénica** eugenic sterilization; ~ *f* **por calor** heat sterilization; ~ *f* **por óxido de etileno** ethylene oxide sterilization; ~ *f* **por vapor** steam sterilization

esterilizador *m* sterilizer; ~ *m* **por gas** gas sterilizer

esterilizar *v* to disinfect, to sterilize

esternón *m* breast bone, sternum

esteroide *m* steroid; ~ *f* **anabolica** anabolic steroid, androgenic steroid

esterol-O-aciltransferasa *f* cholesterol acyltransferase

estertor *m* stertorous respiration, stertor

estesioneuroblastoma *m* esthesioneuroblastoma

estética *f* **dental** cosmetic dentistry, dental aesthetics

estetoscopio *m* stethoscope; ~ *m* **esofágico** stethoscope

estiaje *m* drought (climate term, NOT a medical term)

estimulación *f* excitation, stimulation; ~ *f* **del cerebro profundo** deep brain stimulation; ~ *f* **eléctrica transcutánea de nervios** TENS transcutaneous electrical nerve stimulation; ~ *f* **exagerada** over-stimulation, hyperstimulation

estimulador *m* stimulator, pacemaker; ~ *m* **del cerebro profundo** brain stimulator, brain pacemaker, implantable pulse generator

estimulante *m* stimulant; ~ *m* **cardiaco** cardiac stimulant; ~ *m* **de crecimiento** growth stimulant; ~ *m* **del apetito** orexigenic, appetite-stimulating

estimular *v* to activate, to stimulate

estímulo *m* stimulus; ~ *m* **inadecuado** inadequate stimulus

estimulón *m* stimulon

estiramiento *m* distension, enlarging

estirar v to straighten up, to sit up

estirarse v to stretch (body part)

esto this

estoma m stoma, an artificial opening in the abdominal wall

estómago m stomach; ~ m **descompuesto** upset stomach; ~ m **revuelto** upset stomach, gastritis

estomas m pl stomata

estomatitis f stomatitis, mouth inflammation; ~ f **angular** angular cheilitis, angular cheilosis, angular stomatitis, exfoliative cheilitis; ~ f **herpética** herpetic stomatitis; ~ f **vesicular** vesicular stomatitis, an acute viral disease, especially of horses

estomatología f stomatology

estomatológico adj stomatological

estomio m stomion

estorbo m interference

estornudar v to sneeze

estornudo m sneeze

estos m, **–as** f these

estrabismo m strabismus, squint; ~ m **manifesto** heterotropy

estradiol m estradiol

estrangulación f strangulation; ~ f **de la hernia** hernial impaction

estrangulado adj ingrown, strangulated

estranguria f stranguria, characterized by slow, painful and sporadic passage of urine with associated tenesmus

estratificación f stratification

estrato m **de tejido** a layer of tissue

estrechez f stricture, narrowing

estregadura f scrape mark, scrub mark, scuff mark

estremecerse v to shiver, to tremble, to shake

estreñimiento m obstipation, constipation; ~ m **psicosomático** psychosomatic constipation; ~ m **severo** severe constipation

estreñir v to clog, to constipate

estreptococo m streptococcus; ~ m **betahemolítico** beta-hemolytic streptococcus; ~ m **fecal** fecal streptococcus; ~ m **hemolítico** hemolytic streptococcus; ~ m **piogénico** streptococcus pyogenes

estreptoquinasa f streptokinase, a thrombolytic agent

estrés m mental strain, stress; ~ m **del trabajo** job stress, overwork, tension; ~ m **psicológico** mental anguish, mental distress, psychic distress

estresante adj stressful, tiring

estría f vascular stria vascularis

estrías f pl linea albicante, stretch marks, striae atrophicae, striae cutis distensa

estribo m stirrup

estricto strict

estricturotomía f stricturotomy

estridor m stridor, respiratory sounds; ~ m **faríngeo** pharyngeal stridor

estrobilo m strobila

estrógeno m estrogen

estroma m stroma, the supporting tissue of an organ; ~ m **del iris** stroma of the iris; ~ m **linfoide** lymphoid stroma; ~ m **medular** medullary stroma

estrongiloidiasis f strongyloidiasis

estructural adj structural

estruma m struma, goiter, thyroid enlargement; ~ m **de Riedel** Riedel's thyroiditis, iron-hard tumor, a rare fibrous induration of the thyroid gland; ~ m **fibroso** fibrous struma, a goitre with fibrous hyperplasia

estudio m study; ~ m **clínico–farmacológico** clinical-pharmacological study; ~ m **comparativo** comparative study; ~ m **Doppler** doppler scanning; ~ m **genealógico** pedigree, genealogy

estudios m pl **de mutagenicidad** mutagenicity tests, genetic toxicity tests, mutagenicity testing

estufa f stove

estupidez f stupidity

estupor m stupor

estupro m rape (of a minor)

etanidazol m etanidazole, a nitroimidazole that sensitizes hypoxic tumor cells

etanol m ethanol

etanolamina f ethanolamine

etapa f stage, period; ~ f **de latencia** latency stage, window period, latency period; ~ f **de recuperación** convalescence, recovery phase

ética f ethics; ~ f **médica** medical ethics

étiología f etiology, study of disease cause,

causation, aetiology; ~ f multifactorial
multifactorial etiology; ~ f de asthme asthma
etiology

etnicidad f race, ethnicity

etoposida f etoposide

etosuximida f ethosuximide

ETS (enfermedad de transmisión sexual) STD,
sexual transmitted diseases, veneral diseases

eucariota adj eukaryotic

euforia f agitation, euphoria

eufrasia f common eyebright, euphrasy

eugenesia f eugenics

eugenésico adj eugenic

euglucemia f euglycemia

eugónico adj eugonic

eutanasia f euthanasia

evacuación f emptying, evacuation, emptying
the bowels, defecation; ~ f del estómago
evacuation of the stomach, emptying of the
stomach; ~ f intestinal evacuation of the
intestines, dejection, defecation

evaluación f assessment, evaluation;
~ f clínico-técnica clinical-technical
evaluation; ~ f de capacidad laboral
functional capacity evaluation; ~ f de la
calidad quality assessment; ~ f de la dosis/
respuesta dose/response evaluation;
~ f externa de la calidad external quality
assessment; ~ f médica independiente
independent medical examination, IME

evaporación f evaporation; ~ f requerida
required evaporation

evaporador m evaporator, vaporizer

eventración f eventration; ~ f raquítica rachitic
eventration

eversión f eversion; ~ f parcial del párpado
partial eversion of eyelids

evidencia f evidence

evidente adj manifest, visible, evident

evisceración f evisceration, gutting; ~ f de la
órbita evisceration of orbit, evisceration of the
eyeball

evocar v to evoke

evolución f evolution

exacerbación f aggravation, exacerbation,
worsening

exactitud f accuracy

exageración f exaggeration; ~ f de los reflejos
hyperreflexia, exaggerated reflexes

exagerar v to exaggerate, to overstate

examen m exam, examination;
~ m bacteriologico bacterial examination;
~ m con el microscopio micrography,
microscope examination; ~ m de la vista
vision test; ~ m médico medical test, lab test;
~ m respiratorio breathing test, breath test;
~ m sistemático routine examination;
~ m virológico virology workup, virological
examination

examinar v to check, to research, to investigate,
to examine

exantema m skin rash, hives, exanthema, rash;
~ m infeccioso infectious exanthema;
~ m quinino quinine exanthema

exartrosis f exarthrosis

excesivo adj excessive

exceso m excess; ~ adj de peso overweight, fat,
chubby, pudgy, portly, stout

excipiente m excipient, carrier (in the
pharmaceutical ndustry)base, basis, lower part,
vehicle

excisión f excision

excitación f excitation, stimulation

excitancia f radiante radiant excitance

exclusión f exclusion; ~ f postcigótica post-
zygotic exclusion; ~ f precigótica pre-zygotic
exclusion

exclusivo adj exclusive

excoriación f excoriation, abrasion

excrecencia f excrescence, outgrowth

excreción f discharge, secretion, excretion;
~ f de calcio en orina calciuria; ~ f de
glucosa en orina glucosuria; ~ f vaginal
vaginal discharge

excrementos m pl fecal matter, excrement,
feces

excretor m excretory

excusado m toilet, lavatory

exenteración f pélvica pelvic exenteration

exento adj free, exempt; ~ de virus virus free;
~ de olor free of odor

exéresis f exeresis, excision, abscision

exfoliación f exfoliation, desquamation

exhalar v to exhale, to breathe out

exicosis f exsiccosis, dehydration; ~ f por falta

de sal salt exsiccosis, dehydration due to salt deficiency

existencias f pl stock

exo-a-sialidasa f neuraminidase

exoceloma m exocelom, exocoelomic cavity

exocitosis f exocytosis

exocrino adj exocrine

exoenzima f exoenzyme

exoforia f exophoria

exoftalmía f exophthalmos; ~ **f de origen endocrino** endocrine exophthalmos; ~ **f paradójica** paradoxal exophthalmos

exógeno adj exogenous

exogenote exogenote

exón m exon

exónfalo m umbilical hernia, omphalocele

exonucleasa f exonuclease

exostosis f exostosis; ~ **f múltiple cartilaginosa** multiple hereditary exostoses; ~ **f múltiple hereditaria** multiple hereditary exostoses; ~ **f osteocartilaginosa** osteocartilaginous exostosis

exotoxina f exotoxin

exotropia f divergent strabismus, exotropia, divergent squint

expandarse v to radiate

expansión f expansion

expansor m expander; ~ **m plasmático** plasma expander, blood expander

expectorante m expectorant

expedientes m pl clinical records, medical records, patient records

experimentación f test; ~ **f con animales** test on animals

experimental experimental

experimentar v to test

expiración f breathing out, exhale

exploración f medical examination, examination, scanning; ~ **f ecográfica** ultrasound examination; ~ **f urodinámica** urodynamic examination

explorar v to scan

explotar v to burst, to break open

exposición f exhibition; ~ **f general** systemic exposure

expresión f expression; ~ **f del fenotipo recesivo** expression of the recessive phenotype; ~ **f tisular específica** tissue specific expression

expulsión f expulsion; ~ **f de la placenta** expulsion of the placenta

éxtasis m ecstasy pills

extendido adj widely distributed

extensión f moving apart, extension; ~ **f sanguínea** blood film

extensor m expander, upper body builder

extenuación f asthenia, weakness, loss of strength, debilitation

extenuante m **dolor crónico** debilitating chronic pain

exterior outside

externo adj external

extinción f extinction

extirpación f ablation, extirpation, removal of an organ by surgery, extraction, removal; ~ **f de los órganos sexuales** castration, neutering; ~ **f quirúrgica** extraction, removal

extirpar v to extirpate, to, excise, to

extracapsular extracapsular

extracción f removal, extraction; ~ **f de sangre** phlebotomy, bloodletting, blood-letting; ~ **f líquido–líquido** liquid-liquid extraction; ~ **f obstétrica por aspiración** obstetrical vacuum extraction

extracelular adj extracellular

extracorporal adj extracorporeal

extracto m extract; ~ **m de levadura** yeast extract; ~ **m medicinal** medicinal extract

extradural adj epidural, extradural

extraembrionario m extra-embryonic

extraer v to extract

extraño adj aberrant, irregular, abnormal

extrapiramidal adj extrapyramidal

extrarrenal extrarenal, outside the kidney

extrasístole f extrasystole; ~ **f ventricular** ventricular extrasystole

extrauterino adj extra-uterine

extravasación f extravasation, escape of blood or fluid into tissue

extravascular extravascular, outside a vessel

extremidad f **superior** upper extremity

extremidades f pl extremity

extremo adj extreme, m end; ~ **m cohesivo** sticky end, cohesive end; ~ **m romo** blunt end; ~ **m saliente** overhanging end

extrínseco extrinsic

exudación f exudation
exudado m exudate; ~ m **faríngeo** pharyngeal exudate; ~ m **fibrinoso** fibrinous exudate; ~ m **intersticial** interstitial exudate; ~ m **libre** free exudate; ~ m **ótico** otic exudate; ~ m **parenquimatoso** parenchymal exudate; ~ m **purulento** purulent exudate; ~ m **seroso** serous exudate; ~ m **uretral** urethral exudate
eyaculación f ejaculation; ~ f **precoz** premature ejaculation
eyaculado m to ejaculate
eyector m exhaust fan, exhauster, suction-pipe, ventilator

F

fabricación f production, manufacture
fabricante m manufacturer
faceta f **ósea** facet
facial adj facial
fácil adj easy
facilitación f facilitation; ~ f **presináptica** presynaptic facilitation; ~ f **social** social facilitation
facólisis f phacolysis
facticio adj artificial, factitous
factor m factor; ~ m **activador de macrófagos** MAF, Macrophage Activating Factor; ~ m **activador de plaquetas** PAF, platelet activating factor; ~ m **anti-hemofílico** antihemophilic globulin, antihemophilic factor A; ~ m **biótico** biotic factor; ~ m **causante** trigger, eliciting factor; ~ m **de absorción** absorption factor; ~ m **de coagulación** clotting factor, coagulation factor; ~ m **de crecimientoparecido a la insulina** insulin growth factor 1, IGF-1, insuline-like growth factor, somatomedin; ~ m **de crecimiento** growth factor, growth promotor; ~ m **de crecimiento derivado de plaqueta** PDGF, platelet-derived growth factor; ~ m **de crecimiento insulinoide** insulin-like growth factor; ~ m **de estrés** stressor; ~ m **de la coagulación** coagulation factor; ~ m **de necrosis tumoral** tumor necrosis factor; ~ m **de reflexión** reflection factor; ~ m **de**

riesgo risk factor; ~ m **de terminación** release factor; ~ m **de transcripción** transcription factor; ~ m **de transferencia** transfer factor; ~ m **de transmisión** transmission factor; ~ m **estimulador de colonias de granulocitos (G-CSF)** G-CSF, Granulocyte-Colony Stimulation Factor; ~ m **inhibidor de la migración de los macrófagos** macrophage migration inhibitory factor; ~ m **reumatoideo** rheumatoid factor; ~ m **VIII de coagulación** antihemophilic globulin, factor VIII, antihemophilic factor; ~ m **X de coagulación** Stuart factor
factores m pl **hematopoyéticos** blood growth factors, hematopoietic factors; ~ m pl **quimiotacticos de macrófagos** chemotactic factors
factura f bill, fee, invoice
facultativo adj facultative, optional, contingent
fago m phage, bacteriophage; ~ m **atenuado** temperate phage; ~ m **defectuoso** defective phage; ~ m **lambda** phage lambda; ~ m **tproductor** transducing phage
fagocitario adj phagocytic
fagocito m phagocyte, carrier cell, scavenger cell
fagocitosis f phagocytosis
faja f girdle, sash, strip; ~ f **de embarazada** pre-natal belt, pregnancy belt, maternity girdle; ~ f **de embarazo** pre-natal belt, pregnancy belt, maternity girdle; ~ f **médica** back brace, back support, medical belt; ~ f **para hernia** hernial truss, hernia bandage
falanges f pl phalanges
fálico adj phallic, penile
fallecido adj deceased
fallo m defect, flaw; ~ m **cardíaco** heart failure; ~ m **cardiovascular** cardiovascular collapse, cardiovascular failure
faloidina f phalloidine
falsa f **costilla** false rib; ~ f **memoria** false memory, mnemic delusion
falsear v buckle at the knees
falta f defect, flaw, deficiency, lack, shortage, deficit; ~ f **de alineación** misalignment; ~ f **de amor proprio** feelings of inadequacy; ~ f **de conocimiento** unconsciousness; ~ f **de contestar a la preguntas** failure to answer

questions; ~ f **de fuerza** asthenia, weakness, loss of strength; ~ f **de hálito** breathlessness, shortness of breath; ~ f **de ritmo regular** arrhythmia, irregular heartbeat; ~ f **de sangre** ferriprive, anemic, iron-deficient

familia f family; ~ f **de acogida** foster parents

familiar adj next of kin, blood relative

fangoterapia f medicinal mud, healing mudpack, fangotherapy, mud packs

fantasma m ghost image, echo image

farad m farad

faringe f pharynx

faringitis f pharyngitis, sore throat, inflammation of throat, inflammation of the pharynx; ~ f **crónica** chronic pharyngitis; ~ f **lateral** lateral pharyngitis, lateral angina

farmacéutico adj pharmaceutical adj

farmácia f druggist, pharmacist, chemist, pharmaceutics, pharmacy, drug store

fármaco m drug, pharmacon, medication, pharmaceutical; ~ m **a difusión regulada** sustained release drug, timed-release drug; ~ m **anorexígeno** anorexiant, appetite suppressant, appetite depressant, anorectic agent; ~ m **antiedema** edema agent, a drug to combat or prevent edema; ~ m **antiinflamatorio esteroideo** steroidal anti-inflammatory drug (SAID); ~ m pl **antiinflamatorio no esteroideo** non-steroidal anti-inflammatory drugs (NSAID); ~ m **de acción duradera** long-acting drug; ~ m **de liberación controlada** sustained release drug, timed-release drug; ~ m **hipolipidemiante** lipid-lowering medication, antihyperlipidemic agent, lipid lowering drug, hypolipidemic drug; ~ m **rebajador del nivel de colesterol** cholesterol-lowering agent, hypocholesterolemic agent; ~**inmunosupresor** m chemical immunosuppressive; ~ m **simpaticomimético** sympathomimetic drug

farmacocinética f pharmacokinetics

farmacodinamia f pharmacodynamics

farmacología f pharmacology; ~ f **clínica** clinical pharmacology; ~ f **homeopática** materia medica, homeopathic pharmacology; ~ f **bioquímica** biochemical pharmacology

farmacológico adj pharmacological

farsante m quack, charlatan, fraud

fascia f fascia; ~ f **de Buck** Buck fascia, fascia of the penis

fasciculación f fasciculation, twitch

fascículo m bundle, part, installment; ~ m **de His** atrioventricular bundle, fasciculus atrioventricularis, His' bundle, bundle of His

fasciitis f fasciitis; ~ f **necrotizante** necrotizing fasciitis, flesh-eating disease

fase f phase; ~ f **de eliminación** elimination phase; ~ f **de latencia** lag phase, latency, dormancy; ~ f **de recuperación** convalescence, recovery phase; ~ f **de secreción** luteal phase, progestational phase, secretory phase; ~ f **estacionaria** stationary phase; ~ f **móvil** mobile phase; ~ f **preclínica** preclinical phase, prodromal stage; ~ f **prodrómica** preclinical stage, prodromal stage; ~ f **terminal** final stage, end stage

fásmido m phasmid

fatal adj pernicious, malignant, fatal, harmful

fatiga f lassitude, weariness, fatigue, exhaustion; ~ f **auditiva** auditory fatigue; ~ f **mental** mental fatigue, psychological fatigue, stress; ~ f **sensorial** sensory fatigue; ~ f **síquica** mental fatigue, psychological fatigue

favismo m **por inhalación** airborne favism, inhalational favism

febrero m February

febrícula f low-grade fever

febril adj feverish, febrile

fecal adj fecal

fecha f date; ~ f **de caducidad** date of expiration, expiration date; ~ f **de la lesión** date of injury; ~ f **de la primera menstruación** menarche, first period, first menses; ~ f **de nacimiento** date of birth; ~ f **del accidente** date of injury; ~ f **del aniversario** anniversary date

fecundación f fertilisation; ~ f **extracorporal** in vitro fertilization; ~ f **in vitro** in vitro fertilization; ~ **del óvulo** impregnation, fertilization, making pregnant

feedback m feedback, constructive criticism, regulation

femenina adj female, feminine

femoral *adj* femoral

fémur *m* femur

fenacetina *f* phenacetin, aceto-phenetidin

fenciclidina *f* phencyclidine, PCP, angel dust

fenfluramina *f* fenfluramine, amphetamine derivative

fenilalanina *f* phenylalanine

fenilenodiamina *f* phenylenediamine

feniletilalamina *f* phenylethylamine

fenitoína *f* phenytoin, Dilantin, diphenylhydantoin

fenobarbital *m* phenobarbital, phenobarbitone

fenogreco *m* fenugreek, herb with medicinal properties

fenolftaleína *f* phenolphthalein

fenómeno *m* phenomenon; ~ *m* **de Raynaud** Raynaud's phenomenon, chilblains; ~ *m* **de rebote** rebound effect; ~ *m* **de recurrencia** flash-back phenomenon; ~ *m* **del umbral** threshold phenomenon; ~ *m* **físico** physical phenomenom

fenotiazina *f* phenothiazine

fenotípico *m* phenotypical

fenotipo *m* phenotype

fenoxibenzamina *f* phenoxybenzamine

fenoximetilpenicilina *f* penicillin V

feocromocitoma *m* pheochromocytoma

fermentación *f* fermentation; ~ *f* **láctica** lactic fermentation

fermento *m* **digestivo** digestive enzyme

feromona *f* pheromone

ferredoxina *f* ferredoxin

ferriprivo *adj* ferriprive, anemic, iron-deficien

ferritina *f* ferritin

ferroquelatasa *f* hæm synthetase, ferrochelatase, hem synthase

ferroxidasa *f* ceruloplasmin, ferroxidase

fértil *adj* fertile

fertilidad *f* fertility

férula *f* splint; ~ *f* **de abducción** abduction splint; ~ *f* **de cadera** hip splint; ~ *f* **de vendas enyesadas** plaster bandage splint, plaster splint; ~ *f* **de yeso** plaster splint; ~ *f* **del pie** foot splint; ~ *f* **digital** finger splint; ~ *f* **hinchable** inflatable splint; ~ *f* **oclusal** night guard, mouth guard, biteguard, occlusal splint, peridontal splint; ~ *f* **para la pierna** leg splint

fetal *adj* fetal

fetalismo *m* fetalism

fetidez *f* sickly smell, stink

feto *m* fetus

fetoplacentario *adj* fetoplacental

fetotóxico *adj* fetotoxic

fiabilidad *f* reliability; ~ *f* **de un instrumento** accuracy of a test

fibra *f* fiber; ~ *f* **fusiforme** spindle fiber (in mitosis); ~ *f* **del tejido conjuntivo** connective-tissue fiber; ~ *f* **muscular estriada** striated muscle fiber; ~ *f* **reticular** reticular fiber

fibrilación *f* fibrillation, twitch; ~ *f* **atrial** ventricular fibrillation; ~ *f* **ventricular** atrial fibrillation, atrial flutter

fibrina *f* fibrin, blood-clotting protein

fibrinógeno *m* fibrinogen, coagulation factor I; ~ *m* *pl* **anormal** abnormal fibringen

fibrinolisina *f* plasmin

fibrinolisis *f* fibrinolysis

fibrinolítico *adj* fibrinolytic

fibrinoplastina *f* fibrinoplastin, albuminous substance in the blood

fibroadenoma *m* adenofibroma, fibroadenoma

fibroblasto *m* fibroblast; ~ *m* **de la piel** skin fibroblast; ~ *m* **humano diploide** diploid fibroblast

fibroblastos *m* *pl* fibroblasts, connective-tissue cells

fibroelastosis *f* fibro-elastosis; ~ *f* **endocardico** endocardial fibro-elastosis

fibrocepiteloma *m* **premaligno** premalignant fibro-epithelial tumor

fibroma *f* fibroma (type of benign tumor); ~ *m* **bronquial** fibroma; ~ *m* **de celulas gigantes** giant cell fibroma; ~ *m* **nasofaringeo** nasopharyngeal fibroma; ~ *m* **uterino** uterine fibroma, uterine fibroid

fibromatosis *f* fibromatosis; ~ *f* **agresiva** aggressive fibromatosis

fibromiálgica *f* fibromyalgia, chronic fatigue syndrome, myalgic encephalomyelitis

fibronectina *f* fibronectin, a glycoprotein of high molecular weight

fibroscopio *m* **flexible** flexible fiberscope, optical-fiber endoscope, laparoscope

fibrosis *f* fibrosis; ~ *f* **con bridging** bridging fibrosis; ~ *f* **del miocardio** fibrosis of the myocardium; ~ f **endomiocardica** endomyocardial fibrosis; ~ f **intersticial pulmonar difusa** interstitial pulmonary fibrosis; ~ f **pulmonar** pulmonary fibrosis; ~ f **quística** cystic fibrosis

fibrositis f muscular rheumatism, fibrositis

ficaína f ficain

ficha f chip, token, card, sheet, record; ~ f **médica de evacuación** medical evacuation sheet

fichas f pl records; ~ f pl **clínicas** clinical records, case history, medical files; ~ f pl **médicas** clinical records, case history, medical files

fichero m **médico** clinical records, patient records

fiebre f pyrexia, fever; ~ f **a remitir** remittent fever; ~ f **adinámica** adynamic fever; ~ f **aftosa** foot and mouth disease, aphthous fever, hoof-and-mouth disease, epizootic aphtha; ~ f **amarilla** yellow fever; ~ f **de Ebola** Ebola virus hemorrhagic fever; ~ f **de Lassa** Lassa fever, an acute viral illness; ~ f **de montaña americana** Tick Bite Fever, American Mountain Fever; ~ f **de picadura de garrapata** fevers resulting from tick bites, Tick Bite Fever, Lyme disease; ~ f **del fundidor de cinc** zinc chills, zinc disease, zinc oxide chills, zinc fume fever, zinc shakes; ~ f **del heno** hay fever; ~ f **efímera** ephemeral fever; ~ f **escarlatina** scarlatina, scarlet fever; ~ f **estivootoñal** falciparum malaria, malignant malaria, malignant tertian malaria, subtertian malaria; ~ f **hemorrágica** hemorrhagic fever; ~ f **intermitente** intermittent fever; ~ f **postvacunal** postvaccinal fever; ~ f **reumática** rheumatic fever; ~ f **tifoidea** typhoid fever; ~ f **traumatica** traumatic fever, wound fever; ~ **amarilla** f yellow fever

fijación f fixation, obsession (psychology); ~ f **del complemento** complement fixation; ~ f **entrecruzada** crossover fixation

fijador m **externo** external fixation device

filiforme adj filamentous, filiform

filtración f filtration; ~ f **glomerular** glomerular filtration

filtrado m filtrate; ~ m **glomerular** glomerular filtrate

filtro m filtro; ~ m **interferencial** interference filter; ~ m **solar** sunscreen

fimbria f fimbria, (at the ends of the fallopian tubes and uterine tube), fingerlike structure

fimbrias f pl **bacteriales** bacterial fimbriae, short hairlike filaments on bacteria

final adj terminal

finalizador m **de cadena** chain terminator

finasterida f finasteride, Proscar (drug)

fingirse v enfermo to malinger, to feign illness, to shirk

fino adj thin, fine; ~ adj **destreza motora** fine motor skills; ~ adj **motricidad** fine motor skills

firma f signature

firme adj al tacto firm to the touch

fisiatra m physiatrist

fisiatría f physiatry

físico adj somatic, physical

fisicoquímico adj physicochemical

fisiología f physiology; ~ f **de la célula infectada** physiology of the host cell; ~ f **de la nutrición** physiology of nutrition; ~ f **de la reproducción** physiology of reproduction, reproductive physiology; ~ f **humana** human physiology

fisiológico adj normal, physiological

fisiologista m physiologist

fisiólogo f physiologist

fisión f fission, cleavage

fisiopatología f pathophysiology, physiopathology

fisioterapeuta m physical therapist

fisioterapia f physical therapy, physiatrics, physiotherapy

fisioterapista m physical therapist

fisonomía f physiognomy

fístula f fistula, abnormal passageway; ~ f **capilar** capillary fistula; ~ f **coledocoduodenal** choledochoduodenal fistula; ~ f **cólica** colonic fistula; ~ f **colónica** colonic fistula; ~ f **de las glandulas salivales** salivary fistula; ~ f **perineal** perineal fistula; ~ f **rectovaginal** rectovaginal fistula; ~ f **ureteral** ureteral fistula; ~ f **vesicouterina** vesico-uterine fistula; ~ f **vesicovaginal** vesicovaginal fistula

fisura f fissure, groove, sulcus, crack, split, line;
~ f **anal** anal fissure; ~ f **de la piel** rhagade,
lines; ~ f **primaria** primary sulcus of the brain,
primary fissue; ~ f **vertebral** cleft of vertebral
arches, fissure of vertebral arches

fitofármaco m phytopharmaceutical product,
herbal medicine

fitoterapia f phytotherapy, herbal treatment,
herbal medicine

flácido adj flaccid, flabby, soft

flatulencia f abdominal bloating, meteorism,
excessive gas, gas, flatulence, farting

flatulento adj flatulent

flavona f flavone

flavonoides m pl flavonoids, substances of plant
origin containing flavone

flebitis f phlebitis, vein inflammation

flebografía f phlebography, vein x-ray;
~ f **radiológica** venography, phlebography

flebosclerosis f phlebosclerosis

flebotomista f phlebotomist

flema f phlegm, viscid mucus, sputum

flemón m phlegmon; ~ m **de la barbilla**
phlegmon of the chin; ~ m **del mentón**
phlegmon of the chin

flexión f flexion; ~ f **de piernas** deep knee
bend; ~ f **del útero** uterine flexion

flexionarse v to flex, to bend inward

flictena f blister from burns, vesicle

flocoso adj floccose

flojo adj flaccid, flabby, soft, springy, supple,
limber

flora f flora; ~ f **dérmica** dermal flora;
~ f **intestinal** intestinal flora, bacterial content
of the intestine, colon bacteria, colonic flora;
~ f **indígena** indigenous flora

flu m flu, influenza

flucitosina f flucytosine

fluconazol f fluconazole

flufenazina f fluphenazine

fluido m **extracelular** extracellular fluid,
extracellular liquid

flujo m discharge, secretion, excretion, flux,
flow; ~ m **blanco** fluor albus, vaginal
discharge, nervous vaginal discharge;
~ m **continuo** continuous flow; ~ m **de
retorno** reflux, return flow; ~ m **discreto**
discrete flow; ~ m **espiratorio máximo** peak

expiratory flow rate, PEFR, peak flow rate;
~ m **laminar** laminar flow; ~ m **luminoso**
luminous flux; ~ m **maximal** peak flow, lung
power; ~ m **mucilaginoso** slime flux,
mucociliary clearance, mucociliary transport;
~ m **por presión** pressure flow; ~ m **radiante**
radiant flux; ~ m **sanguíneo** bloodstream, flow
of blood

flunitracepam m flunitrazepam

flúor m fluorine; ~ m **albus** fluor albus, vaginal
discharge, nervous vaginal discharge

fluoresceína f fluorescein

fluorimetría f fluorometry

fluorodeoxiglucosa f fluorodeoxyglucose

fluoroinmunoanálisis m fluorescence
immunoassay, FIA, fluoroimmunoanalysis;
~ m **de polarización** fluorescence polarization
immunoassay, FPIA; ~ m **de resolución tardía**
time resolved fluoroimmunoassay

fluoroscopia f fluoroscopy

fluoroscopio m fluoroscope, radioscopic
apparatus

fluorouracilo m fluorouracil

fluoruro m **de sodio** sodium fluoride

fluoxetina f fluoxetine (Prozac), an SSRI
antidepressant

flúter m flutter; ~ m **ventricular** ventricular
flutter

fluvastatina f fluvastatin, a cholesterol-
lowering drug

fluvoxamina f fluvoxamine (Luvox), an SSRI
antidepressant

fobia f phobia

foco m focus, focal spot, point, center;
~ m **clínico** clinical outbreak; ~ m **de
calcificación** calcium deposits; ~ m **primario**
primary outbreak

folacin m folic acid, pteroyl glutamic acid,
folacin, vitamin B9

folate m folic acid, pteroyl glutamic acid,
folacin, vitamin B9

folato m folate

foliberina f follicle-stimulating-hormone-
releasing factor; ~ f FSH-RF

foliculitis f folliculitis, follicle inflammation

folículo m follicle; ~ m **de Graaf** ovarian

follicle, graafian follicle; ~ *m* **linfoide** lymphoid follicle; ~ *m* **piloso** hair follicle; ~ *m* **ovárico** ovarian follicle, graafian follicle

folitropina *f* follicle-stimulating hormone, follitropin, FSH

fómite fomite

fonoaudiología *f* speech-language pathology

fontanela *f* fontanelle; ~ *f* **parietal** parietal fontanelle

foramen *m* foramen; ~ *m* **magnum** foramen magnum; ~ *m* **intervertebral** intervertebral foramen

fórceps *m* forceps

forma *f* form; ~ *f* **farmacéutica** pharmaceutical form; ~ **L f L** form

formaldehído *m* formaldehyde, formol

formiato *m* formate

formol *m* formaldehyde, formo

fórmula *f* formula; ~ *f* **adaptada** baby milk, infant milk, infant formula; ~ *f* **leucocitaria** differential white blood cell count, leukogram

formulación *f* formulation, presentation; ~ *f* **de preguntas** presentation of questions

formulario *m* document, formular, printed form

fórnix *m* fornix; ~ *f* **conjuntival** conjuntival fornix, fornix of conjunctiva; ~ *m* **de la faringe** pharyngeal fornix

forúnculo *m* boil, furuncle, bump, swelling, bruise

fosa *f* fossa; ~ *f* **acetabular** acetabular fossa; ~ *f* **epigástrica** epigastric fossa; ~ *f* **escafoidea** scaphoid fossa; ~ *f* **iliaca** iliac fossa; ~ *f* **peritoneal** peritoneal recessus; ~ *f* **romboidea** rhomboid fossa

fosfatasa *f* phosphatase; ~ *f* **ácida** acid phosphatase; ~ *f* **ácida prostática** prostatic acid phosphatase, PAP; ~ *f* **alcalina** alkaline phosphatase

fosfatidilcolina *f* phosphatidylcholine

fosfátidos *m pl* phospholipids, phosphatides

fosfato *m* phosphate; ~ **–acetiltransferasa** *f* phosphate acetyltransferase, phosphotransacetylase; ~ *m* **cálcico** calcium phosphate; ~ *m* **no esterificado** non-esterified phosphate

fosfolipasa *f* lipophosphodiesterase, phosphatidase, phospholipase

fosfolípido *m* phospholipid

fosfolípidos *m pl* phospholipids, phosphatides

fosfonato *m* phosphonate

fosfoproteínas *m pl* phosphoproteins

fosforilación *f* phosphorylation; ~ *f* **oxidante** oxidative phosphorylation

fosforilasa *f* phosphorylase; ~ **–cinasa** *f* phosphorylase kinase

fosforismo *m* phosphorus poisoning, phosphorism

fósforo *m* phosphorus

fosforotioato *m* phosphorothioate

fotalgia *f* photalgia

fotocélula *f* photocell

fotocoagulación *f* photocoagulation, photocautery

fotoferesis *f* extracorporeal photopheresis, extracorporeal photochemotherapy

fotofobia *f* photophobia, intolerance to light

fotólisis *f* photolysis; ~ *f* **del ADN** DNA photolysis

fotomultiplicador *m* photomultiplier

fotosensibilidad *f* photosensitivity

fotosensibilización *f* photosensitization

fototerapia *f* PDT, photodynamic therapy, phototherapy

fototransducción *f* phototransduction

fracaso *m* setback, adversity; ~ *m* **terapéutico** failure of treatment, lack of results from the therapy

fracción *f* fraction; ~ *f* **catalítica** catalytic fraction; ~ *f* **de eyección** ejection fraction; ~ *f* **de masa** mass fraction; ~ *f* **de número** number fraction; ~ *f* **de sustancia** substance fraction, mole fraction; ~ *f* **de volumen** volume fraction; ~ *f* **postmitocondrial** post-mitochondrial fraction; ~ *f* **saturante** saturation fraction

fraccionamiento *m* fractionation; ~ *m* **cellular** cell fractionation; ~ *m* **de plasma** fractionation of human blood plasma

fractil *adj* fractile

fractura *f* fracture; ~ *f* **cerrada** closed fracture; ~ *f* **compuesta** compound fracture; ~ *f* **de Colles** Colles fracture; ~ *f* **en abducción** abduction fracture; ~ *f* **por aducción** adduction fracture; ~ *f* **por arrancamiento** strain fracture; ~ *f* **por flexión forzada** bent fracture, hyperflexion fracture; ~ *f* **por**

torsión shearing fracture, spiral fracture; ~ f **simple** simple fracture; ~ f **subcapital** f infraarticular fracture; ~ f **subperióstica** subperiosteal fracture

fragmento m fragment; ~ m **de ADN repetitivo** DNA fragment

franjas f pl fringes

franjeado adj fimbriate, fringed

frasco m **medicinal** pill bottle, medicinal flask

fraude m **en la atención médica** medifraud, health care fraud, kickbacks

frecuencia f frequency; ~ f **de mutación** mutation rate; ~ f **de polimorfismo** polymorphism rate; ~ f **del pulso** pulse rate; ~ f **fenotípica** phenotypic frequency; ~ f **rotacional** rotational frequency; ~ **de inervación** f innervation frequency, the number of regular recurrent stimuli per second to a muscle fiber

fregar v to scrub, to wash, to clean

fregarse v **las manos antes de operar** to scrub up before surgery

frémito m fremitus; ~ m **en los bronquios** bronchial fremitus; ~ m **hidatádico** hydatid fremitus, hydatid thrill; ~ m **pleural** pleural fremitus

frenocardia f pulmonary dystonia

frenos m pl braces (dental)

frente f forehead, versus

fresa f strawberry

fricción f rubbing, friction

friccionar massage, to

frigidez f frigidity

frijoles m beans

frío adj catarrh, cold, nasopharyngitis

fríos m pl chills

frito adj fried

frotación f rub

frotamiento m rubbing, friction

frotar v to rub

frotarse v **los ojos** to rub one's eyes

frotis m smear; ~ f **cérvico-vaginal** cervical smear; ~ m **vaginal** cervical-vaginal swab

fructocinasa f fructokinase

fructosa f fructose; ~ **-bisfosfatasa** f fructose-bisphosphatase; ~ **-bisfosfato–aldolasa** f fructose 1-phosphate aldolase, fructaldolase B

fructosamina f fructosamine

frutas f pl fruit

fucsina f fuchsin, a red dye used as stain in histology and bacteriology

fuego m fire

fuente f para el lavado de emergencia de los ojos emergency eye wash fountain

fuera de outside, out

fuero adj strong

fuerte adj loud

fuerza f force; ~ f **analítica** analytical function; ~ f **centrífuga** centrifugal force; ~ f **de morbilidad** force of morbidity; ~ f **de sujeción** grip strength; ~ f **del campo eléctrico** electric field strength; ~ f **electromotriz** electromotive force; ~ f **electrostática** electrostatic force; ~ f **iónica** ionic strength; ~ f **vital** endurance, stamina

fumar v smoke, to

fumigar v fumigate

función f function; ~ f **analítica** analytical function; ~ f **cognitiva** cognitive function; ~ f **de calibración** calibration function; ~ f **de medida** measuring function; ~ f **mitocondrial** mitochondrial function; ~ **inadecuada** f inadequacy

funcionamiento m functioning; ~ m **de la tiroides** thyroid functioning; ~ m **performance**

funda f **de almohada** pillowcase

fundamental adj fundamental

fundamento m base, basis, lower part

fundoplicación f fundoplication

fungemia f fungemia

fungible adj fungible, interchangeable

fungicida m fungicide

fungistático adj fungistatic, fungus growth-preventing

fungus m fungus

furosemida f furosemide, frusemide

furúnculo m boil, furuncle, bump, swelling, bruise

furunculosis f boils, furunculosis

fusión f fusion; ~ f **de replicones** replicon fusion; ~ f **del DNA** DNA melting; ~ f **espinal** spondylosyndesis, spinal fusion

Fusobacterium m **fusiforme** Vincent's bacillus; ~ m **necrophorum** Schmorl's bacillus

futuro m future

G

gafas f pl glasses; ~ f pl **de lectura** reading glasses

galactocinasa f galactokinase

galactogénesis f lactogenesis, galactopoiesis

galactorrea f galactorrhea, excessive milk production

galactosa f galactose; ~ –**oxidasa** f galactose oxidase

galactosemia f galactosemia, udpglucose hexose-1-phosphate uridylyltransferase deficiency

galactosidasa f galactosidase, galactosyl hydrolase

galénico adj galenical, relating to Galen's methods

galerada f galley proof

galleta f biscuit, cookie

galvanocauterio m galvanocautery

gameto m gamete, sexual reproductive cell

gammaglobulina f gamma globulin

gammagrafía f radioisotope scanning, gammagraphy, ~ f **gástrica** gastrointestinal scan, gastrointestinal scintigraphy; ~ f **hepática** liver scan, hepatic scintigraphy; ~ f **pulmonar** pulmonary scintigraphy, scintigraphy of the lung, radioisotope scanning of the lung; ~ f **tiroidea** thyroid scan, thyroid scintigraphy

gamma-GTP f **(gamma glutamil transpeptidasa)** gamma glutamyl transpeptidase

ganas f pl **de vomitar** nausea, queasiness, feeling sick, feeling nauseated

gancho m **de huesos** bone hook

ganchos m pl **dentales** braces (dental)

ganciclovir m ganciclovir

ganglio m ganglion, knot; ~ m **espinal** spinal ganglion; ~ m **isquiático** ischiatic lymph node; ~ m **linfático** lymph node; ~ m **linfático de la áxila** axillary lymph node; ~ m **mediastínico** mediastinal lymph node, mediastinal lymph gland

ganglioma m ganglioneuroma, ganglionic neuroma

ganglioneuroblastoma m ganglioneuroblastoma

ganglioneuroma m ganglioneuroma, ganglionic neuroma

ganglios m pl ganglia, ganglions; ~ m pl **basales** basal ganglia; ~ m pl **linfáticos** lymph nodes, lymph glands

gangoso adj with a nasal twang, snuffling, nasal tone

gangrena f necrolysis, gangrene, necrosis; ~ f **cutánea diseminada** cutaneous gangrene; ~ f **gaseosa** gas gangrene

gap m **junctions sin alteración** junctional activity

garantía f guarantee, warranty, assurance; ~ f **de la calidad** quality assurance

gargajos m pl sputum, phlegm

garganta f throat

gargarismo m gargling

garrapata f tick

garras f pl claws (animal term)

garrotillo m acute laryngotracheobronchitis, croup, diphtheritic croup

gas m gas; ~ m **criogénico** cryogenic gas; ~ m **hilarante** nitrous oxide, laughing gas; ~ m **inerte** inert gas; ~ m **lacrimogeno** tear gas; ~ m **nervioso** nerve gas; ~ m **neurotóxico** neurotoxic gas; ~ m **tóxico** toxic gas, noxious gases

gasa f surgical gauze, gauze; ~ f **tubular** tubular gauze

gases m pl gases; ~ m pl **de la sangre** arterial arterial blood gases; ~ m pl **intestinales** intestinal gases

gasolina f gasoline

gasometría f **sanguínea** blood gas analysis, blood gas determination

gasteroscopio m gastroscope

gasto m **cardiaco** cardiac output, cardiac pressure output, cardiac minute ouput; ~ m **urinario** urinary output, diuresis

gastralgia f gastralgia, colic of the stomach

gastrectomía f **parcial** partial gastrectomy

gastricsina f gastricsine

gastrina f gastrin, peptide hormone secreted by the stomach

gastritis f upset stomach, gastritis; ~ **atrófica** atrophic gastritis, autoimmune gastritis; ~ **corrosiva** corrosive gastritis; ~ **hipertrófica gigante** giant hypertrophic gastritis, Menetrier disease; ~ **infecciosa** infective gastritis; ~ **química** corrosive gastritis; ~ **ulcerante** ulcerative gastritis

gastroduodenal adj gastroduodenal, stomach and gut-related

gastroenteritis f gastroenteritis, gastric flu

gastroenterocolitis f gastro-enterocolitis

gastroenterostomía f gastroenterostomy

gastroesofágico adj gastroesophageal, stomach and esophagus-related

gastrointestinal adj gastrointestinal

gastroscopía f gastroscopy

gastrostomía f gastrostomy; ~ **endoscópica percutánea** percutaneous endoscopic gastrostomy

gástrula f gastrula

gastrulación f gastrulation, a complex, coordinated series of cellular movements during embryonic development

gato m cat

gaznate m esophagus, gullet

gel m gel; ~ **de agar** agar gel; ~ **de sílice** silica gel; ~ **dérmico** skin gel; ~ **ocular** eye ointment

gelatina f jelly; ~ **vaginal** vaginal jelly, spermacidal jelly

gelatinoso adj gelatinous, glutinous

gemelos m pl twins; ~ **fraternos** dizygotic twins; ~ **pl identicos** monozygotic twins, 2 offspring developed from one fertilized ovum, identical twins; ~ **pl monocigótos** monozygotic twins, 2 offspring developed from one fertilized ovum, identical twins; ~ **pl unidos** conjoined twins

gemir v to moan, to groan

gen m gene; ~ **constitutivo** constitutive gene; ~ **discontinuo** split gene; ~ **de**

histocompatibilidad histocompatibility gene; ~ **m del complejo de histocompatibilidad** MHC genes; ~ **m indicador** reporter gene; ~ **m letal** lethal gene; ~ **m letal dominante** dominant lethal gene; ~ **m letal zigótico** zygotic lethal gene; ~ **m ligado** linked gene; ~ **m marcador** marker gene; ~ **m oncosupresor** tumor suppresor gene; ~ **m quimérico** chimeric gene; ~ **m recesivo** recessive gene; ~ **m regulador** regulator gene; ~ **m retrovírico** retroviral gene; ~ **m saltador** jumping gene; ~ **m suicida** suicide gene; ~ **m supresor de tumor** tumor suppressor gene; ~ **m trans-activador** transactivator gene; ~ **m variable** variable gene

genealogía f pedigree, genealogy

generador m generator; ~ **de oxígeno** oxygen generator

general common

genética f genetics; ~ **bioquímica** biochemical genetics, molecular genetics; ~ **médica** medical genetics; ~ **microbiana** microbial genetics; ~ **molecular** molecular genetics

genético adj genetic

genetista m geneticist

gengivitis f gingivitis; ~ **marginal** marginal gingivitis; ~ **neoplásica** neoplastic gingivitis

genital adj genital

genitales m pl private parts, genitalia, genitals, sex organs, reproductive organs

genitourinario adj genitourinary

genoma m genome; ~ **del hepatocito** hepatocyte genome, liver cell genome

genómica f genomics, genome study

genómico adj genomic

genoteca f gene library, gene bank; ~ **de cDNA** cDNA library; ~ **genómica** genomic library

genoterapia f genetic therapy

genotipo m genotype

gentamicina f gentamicin

geriatra m geriatrician, a specialist in geriatrics

geriatría f geriatrics, presbyatrics

geriátrico adj geriatric

germanio m germanium

gérmenes m pl germs, microbes

germicido adj germicidal

germinal adj germinal

germoplasma *m* germ plasm

gerontología *f* gerontology, the science of aging; ~ *f* **social** social gerontology

gerontológico *adj* gerontological

gestación *f* gestation, pregnancy, gravidity

gesticular *v* to gesticulate

gestión *f* management; ~ *f* **de la calidad** quality management

gesto *m* gesture; ~ *m* **expresivo** expressive gesture, expressive movement

gestodén *m* gestodene

g-glutamiltransferasa *f* gGT

GGT *f* **gamma glutamil transferasa** *f* GGT (gamma glutamyl transpeptidase)

giardiasis *f* giardiasis, Giardia lamblia infection

gimnasio *m* health club, fitness center

gimoteador *m* whiner, crybaby

ginecología *f* gynecology, gynaecology

ginecológico *adj* gynelogical; ~ *m* gynecologist, gynecological

ginecomastia *f* gynecomastia,, development of breasts in men

gingivitis *f* bleeding from the gums, gingivitis; ~ *f* **descamativa catamenial** desquamative intermenstrual gingivitis; ~ *f* **necrótica** necrotizing gingivitis

gingivopericementitis *f* periodontolysis, gingivopericementitis

ginkgo *m* **biloba** Ginkgo biloba, maidenhair tree, the source of extracts of medicinal interest

ginseng *m* ginseng

glabella *f* glabella

glándula *f* gland; ~ *f* **de Bartholin** Bartholin glands; ~ *f* **endocrina** endocrine gland; ~ *f* **mamaria** mammary gland; ~ *f* **parótida** paratid gland; ~ *f* **pineal** pineal gland, epiphysis; ~ *f* **pituitária** pituitary gland, pituitary; ~ *f* **prostática** prostate gland; ~ *f* **sebácea** sebaceous glands; ~ *f* **tiroidea** thyroid gland

glándulas *f pl* adrenales adrenal gland, suprarenal glands; ~ *f pl* **apocrinas** apocrine glands, sweat glands; ~ *f pl* **bucales** buccal glands; ~ *f pl* **cardiales** cardial glands; ~ *f pl* **de transpiración** sweat glands, perspiratory glands; ~ *f pl* **faríngeas** pharyngeal glands; ~ *f pl* **gastrica** gastric glands; ~ *f pl* **molares** molar glands; ~ *f pl* **palatinas** palatine glands; ~ *f pl* **salivales** salivary glands; ~ *f pl* **sudoríparas** sweat glands, perspiratory glands; ~ *f pl* **suprarrenales** adrenal glands, suprarenal glands

glaucoma *m* glaucoma; ~ *m* **capsular** capsular glaucoma, exfoliation syndrome

glenohumeral *adj* glenohumeral

glenosporosis *f* glenosporosis

gliadina *f* gliadin

glicemia *f* glycemia

glicerol *m* glycerol; ~ **–cinasa** *f* glycerol kinase

glicina *f* glycine

gliclazida *f* gliclazide, an oral sulfonylurea hypoglycemic agent which stimulates insulin secretion

glicoforina *f* glycophorin

glicohemoglobina *f* hæmoglobin A1, glycated hemoglobin, glycohemoglobin, glycosylated hemoglobin

glicopéptido *m* glycopeptide

glicoproteína *f* glycoprotein

glicosaminoglicano *m* glycosaminoglycan, mucopolysaccharide

glicósido *m* **hidrolasa** glycoside hydrolase

glimepirida *f* glimepiride

glioblastoma *m* **multiforme** glioblastoma multiforme, a type of brain tumor that derives from glial cells

glioma *m* glioma; ~ *m* **de Gibson** Gibson glioma; ~ *m* **del nervio óptico** glioma of the optic nerve; ~ *m* **nasal** nasal glioma; ~ *m* **periférico** peripheral glioma, neurinoma, neurilemmoma; ~ *m* **quístico** cystic glioma; ~ *m* **sólido** hard glioma; ~ *m* **telangiectásico** telangiectatic glioma

gliosis *f* gliosis

glipizida *f* glipizide

globina *f* globin

globo *m* balloon, globe; ~ *m* **del ojo** eyeball

globular *f* globular

globulina *f* globulin; ~ *f* **antilinfocitaria** antilymphocyte globulin

glóbulo *m* globule, blood cell, corpuscle; ~ *m* **blanco** white blood cell; ~ *m* **rojo** red blood cell, erythrocyte

glomeración *f* agglomeration

glomerular adj glomerular
glomérulo m renal cluster, glomerulus
glomerulonefritis f glomerulonephritis;
~ **f aguda** acute glomerulonephritis;
~ **f alérgica** allergic glomerulonephritis;
~ **f membranosa** membranous
glomerulonephritis
glomérulos m pl glomeruli
glomus m carotídeo carotid body, cluster of
chemoreceptive cells near the bifurcation of
the internal carotid artery
glonoinismo m nitroglycerine poisoning
glositis f glossitis, inflammation of the tongue
glosodinia f glossodynia, pain in the tongue
glosolalia f glossolalia
glossitis f glossitis, inflammation of the tongue
glotis f glottis, the vocal apparatus of the larynx
glucagón glucagon, hyperglycemic factor
glucano m glucan
glúcido m carbohydrate
glucocinasa f glucokinase
glucocorticoide m glucocorticoid
glucógeno m glycogen; ~ **-fosforilasa** f muscle
phosphorylase a and b, polyphosphorylase; ~ **-sintasa** f glycogen synthase
glucogenosis f glycogenosis, glycogen-storage
disease; ~ **f hereditaria** inherited glycogenosis
glucómetro m saccharimeter, mustmeter
gluconato m cálcico calcium gluconate
gluconocinasa f gluconate kinase,
gluconokinase
glucopirrolato m glycopyrrolate, a muscarinic
antagonist
glucoproteína f glycoprotein
glucosa f blood sugar, glucose, grape sugar,
dextrose; ~ **-1-deshidrogenasa** f glucose 1-
dehydrogenase; ~ **-6-fosfatasa** f glucose-6-
phosphatase; ~ **f isomerasa** glucose
isomerase; ~ **-oxidasa** f glucose oxidase
glucosamina f glucosamine
glucosidasa f amygdalase, glucosidase;
~ **f scindidora** trimming glycosidase
glucósido m carbohydrate, glycoside;
~ **m cardiotónico** cardiac glycoside
glucosilación f glycosylation, adding glycan
chains to proteins
glucosilceramidasa f glucocerebrosidase

glucosuria f glycosuria, sugar in the urine;
~ **f adrenal** adrenal glycosuria; ~ **f diabética**
diabetic glycosuria; ~ **f renal** renal glycosuria,
inability of the renal tubules to reabsorb
glucose completely
glucuronidasa f glucuronidase
glucuronosiltransferasa f UDP glucuronyl
transferase, glucuronosyltransferase
glucurrónido m de bilirrubina bilirubin
glucuronid
glutamato m glutamate
glutamiltransferasa f gamma GT, g-
glutamyltransferase
glutamina f glutamine
glutaminasa f glutaminase
glutatión f glutathione; ~ **-reductasa**
(NADPH) glutathione reductase (NADPH); ~ **-sintasa** f glutathione synthase
gluten m gluten, protein from wheat and other
cereals
glutetimida f glutethimide, a tranquilizer
GM-CSF GM-CSF, Granulocyte-Macrophage-
Colony Stimulation Factor
gnatología f gnathology
gollete m neck
golondrino m tumor in the armpit
golpe m impact, blow; ~ **m de calor** heatstroke,
siriasis; ~ **m de conejo** whiplash injury,
hyperextension of the neck
golpear v clapping, tapping, percussion, a
massage technique
goma f gum, rubber; ~ **f amoníaca** ammoniac
gum
gónada f gonad; ~ **f masculina** testis, testicle,
male gonad
gonadal adj gonadal, testicle-related or ovary-
related
gonadoliberina f gonadotropin-releasing
factor; ~ **f LH/FSH-RF**
gonadorelina f gonadorelin, FSH-releasing
hormone
gonadotropina f gonadotrophin,
gonadotropin; ~ **f coriónica humana** human
chorionic gonadotrophin; ~ **f hipofisarias**
pituitary gonadotrophin; ~ **f menopáusica
humana** f human menopausal gonadotrophin
gonadotropo adj gonadotrope, gonadotropic
gonfosis f gomphosis

gonioscopia *f* gonioscopy, eye examination

gonorrea *f* blennorrhagia, gonorrhea, clap, gonorrhoea

gonosomas *m pl* sex chromosomes

gordinflón *adj* overweight, fat, chubby, pudgy, portly, stout

gordo *adj* overweight, fat, chubby, pudgy, portly, stout

gordura *f* fat, fatness; ~ *f* **sobre el corazón** fatty heart

gorgoteo *m* **en el vientre** borborygmus, rumbling tummy, growling tummy

GOT *f* (**transaminasa glutamico–exaloacética**) Glutamic-Oxaloacetic Acid Transaminase, SGOT

gota *f* gout, drop; ~ *f* **metastásica** metastatic gout; ~ *f* **pendiente** hanging drop; ~ *f* **saturnina** lead poisoning, lead intoxication, plumbism; ~ *f* **visceral** abarticular gout, podagra

gotas *f pl* **óticas** ear drops, eardrops

goteo *m* dribbling; ~ *m* **de orina** urinary dribbling; ~ *m* **posnasal** postnasal drip

gotiera *f* night guard, mouth guard, biteguard, occlusal splint, peridontal splint, dental prosthesis

GPT *f* (**alanina transaminasa**) serum glutamate-pyruvate transaminase (SGPT), alanine transaminase

gracias thanks, thank you

gradiente *m* gradient; ~ *m* **de concentración** concentration gradient

grado *m* degree, grade; ~ *m* **Celsius** degrees Celsius; ~ **de disociación** degree of dissociation; ~ **de fuerza** intensity, strength; ~ **de tensión** intensity, strength

gradual *adj* gradual

gramnegativo *adj* gram negative

gramo *adj* gram

grampositivo *adj* gram positive

gran *f* large; ~ **extracción** *f* **podálica** complete podalic extraction; ~ **mal** *m* grand mal, generalized tonic-clonic seizure

grande *adj* massive, solid, large

granito *m* pimple, acne pustule, blackhead, furuncle

grano *m* pimple, acne pustule, blackhead, pustule, furuncle; ~ *m* **exuberante** granulation tissue, luxuriant caro

granulaciones *f pl* granulations; ~ *f pl* **aracnoideas** arachnoid granulations

granulado *m* granules, granulated

gránulo *m* granule; ~ *m* **de azufre** sulfur granule

granulocito *m* granulocyte; ~ *m* **acidófilo** neutrophil, white blood cell, eosinophil, acidocyte, acidophil, acidophilic cell; ~ *m* **eosinófilo** eosinophil granulocyte

granulocitopenia *f* granulocytopenia, lack of white blood cells

granuloma *m* granuloma; ~ *m* **anular** granuloma annulare; ~ *m* **apical** granuloma, dental granuloma; ~ *m* **de células gigantes** giant cell granuloma; ~ *m* **eosinófilo** eosinophilic granuloma; ~ *m* **piógeno** pyogenic granuloma

granulomatosis *f* **de Wegener** Wegener's granulomatosis

grapa *f* suture clip, staple; ~ *f* **de fijación** fixation plate; ~ *f* **para sutura** staple (surgical), suture clip, wound clip

grapadora *f* stapler, stapling gun; ~ *f* **desechable para sutura** disposable suture stapler; ~ *f* **lineal endoscópica** endoscopic linear stapler

grasa *f* fat; ~ *f* **dorsocervical** buffalo hump; ~ *f* **mineral** mineral oil

grasoso *adj* fatty, greasy

grave *adj* pernicious, malignant, fatal, harmful, severe, serious

gravedad *f* severity, criticality

gravemente *adv* seriously

gravidez *f* gestation, pregnancy, gravidity

gravimetría *f* gravimetry

gray *adj* gray

grieta *f* fissure, crack, split

gripe *f* flu, influenza

gris *adj* grey

griseofulvina *f* griseofulvin

grueso *adj* overweight, fat, chubby, pudgy, portly, stout, thick

gruñon *adj* irritable, cranky, touchy, short-tempered, in a bad mood

grupo *m* cluster, concentration, complex; ~ *m* **comparable** peer group; ~ *m* **de comparación** peer group; ~ *m* **de enlace** linkage group, liaison group; ~ *m* **de**

referencia control group; **~ m prostético** prostetic group; **~ m sanguíneo** blood type; **~ m testigo** control group

GTP phosphoenolpyruvate carboxylase, phosphopyruvate carboxylase

guanilato-cinasa f guanylate kinase

guanina f guanine

guanosina f guanosine; **~ 5'-monofosfato** f GMP, guanosine 5'-monophosphate; **~ ~ trifosfato** f guanosine triphosphate, GTP

guantes m pl gloves; **~ pl cirúrgicos** surgical gloves, surgeon's gloves; **~ m pl estériles** surgical gloves, surgeon's gloves

guardando m cama bed rest, confinement to bed

guardería f infantil day care center, nursery school

guata f cotton wad, cotton ball

guerra f war; **~ f biológica** germ warfare, biological warfare

guía f f guide; **~ f de incisión** f incision guide

gusano m worm; **~ m parásito** intestinal parasite, parasitic worm

gusto m sense of taste, ability to taste, gustation, taste

gutapercha f gutta percha

H

haber v to have

habitación f salubre healthful living environment

hábito m habit; **~ m malo** bad habit, addiction, craving

hábitos m pl de limpieza grooming

habituación f habituation; **~ f a las drogas** drug habit, drug addiction

habitual adj usual, periodic

habitus m habitus; **~ m tísico** habitus phthisicus

hablador adj talkative, loquacious, chatty

hablar v to speak

habones m pl hives, urticaria

hace v ago; **~ mucho tiempo** m long time ago; **~ poco** short time ago

hacer f to do; **~ v apósito en una herida** to dress a wound, to bandage a wound; **~ v del cuerpo** to defecate, to have a bowel movement; **~ v ejercicios** to work out, to exercise; **~ v frente a** to cope with, to deal with; **~ v gárgaras** to gargle; **~ v masajes** massage, to; **~ v pipí** to urinate, to piss, to pee

hacerse v cortar el pelo to get a haircut; **~ v el enfermo** to feign illness, to shirk, to

hachís m hashish

hacia towards; **~ a delante** forward; **~ atrás** backward

hados m pl puffiness around the eyes, bags / dark circles under the eyes

Haemophilus m ducreyi Ducrey's bacillus; **~ m influenzae** Weeks bacillus, Koch-Weeks bacillus, Pfeiffer's bacillus

hafefobia f haptophobia, fear of touching, haphephobi

halitosis f bad breath, halitosis

hallar v to find

hallazgos f pl) findings, results, observations

hallux m big toe, hallux; **~ m valgus** hallux valgus

halón m halogenated hydrocarbon, halon

haloperidol m haloperidol

halotano m halothane

hamamelis f hamamelis

hambre m hunger

hantavirus m hantavirus, Hantaan virus

haploide adj haploid

haplotipo m haplotype

hapteno m hapten

haptofobia f haptophobia, fear of touching, haphephobia

haptoglobina f haptoglobin

haptonomía f haptonomy, the science of affectivity

haragán m couch potato, stay-at-home, slug, lounger, lazybones, person who watches too much TV

hashish m cannabis, hashish

haz m cluster, concentration; **~ m de fibras** bundle, tract, channel, sheaf of fibers

HBsAg hepatitis B surface antigen, surface antigen of hepatitis B

HDL high-density lipoprotein, HDL

hebra f thread, fiber, strand; ~ f **codificadora** coding strand; ~ f **conductora** leading strand; ~ f **líder** leading strand

heces m pl stool, feces, excrement; ~ f pl **de ayuno** inanition feces, feces during fasting

héctico f frail consumptive, tuberculous person

heder v to stink, to smell bad

hediondez f sickly smell, stink

helarse v to be freezing cold

hélice f helix

Helicobacter m **pylori** helicobacter pylori, campylobacter pylori

helio m helium

helminto m helminth

hemaglutinación f hemagglutination

hemaglutinina f hemagglutinin

hemangioblastoma m hemangioblastoma

hemangioma m hemangioma, a benign tumor made up of blood vessels; ~ m **capilar** capillary hemangioma, capillaropathy; ~ m **cavernoso** cavernous hemangioma

hemangiosarcoma m hemangiosarcoma

hematemesis f hematemesis, vomiting blood

hematimetría f complete blood count, blood picture, hemogram, blood workup

hematocolpos m hematocolpos

hematocrito m hematocrit

hematófago adj hematophagous, blood-sucking

hematogonia f hematogone, hemocytoblast, blast cell

hematología f hematology, hæmatology; ~ f **clínica** biological hematology

hematológico adj hematological

hematólogo m hematologist

hematoma m hematoma; ~ m **cístico** hematmatous cyst; ~ m **periorbitario** peri-orbital hematoma; ~ m **pulsátil** throbbing hematoma, pulsatile hematoma; ~ m **subcapsular del hígado** subcapsular hematoma of the liver; ~ m **subdural** subdural hematoma; ~ m **subperióstico** subperiosteal hematoma

hematoplástico adj hematoplastic, hematopoietic

hematopoyesis f hematopoiesis, hemocytopoiesis

hematozequia f blood in the stools, bloody stool, hematochezia, tarry stool

hematuria f hematuria, blood in the urine; ~ f **angioneurótica** vasofunctional hematuria; ~ f **posoperatoria** postoperative hematuria; ~ f **vasofuncional** vasofunctional hematuria

hemeralopía f day blindness, hemeralopia

hemicrania f **oftalmopléjica** ophthalmoplegic hemicrania

hemimelia f hemimelia

hemiparesia f hemiparesis

hemipelvectomía f hemipelvectomy

hemiplejía f paralysis of one side, hemiplegia

hemipléjico adj hemiplegic

hemisferio m hemisphere; ~ m **cerebral** cerebral hemisphere; ~ m **dominante** dominant hemisphere

hemisomía f hemisomia

hemo m hem, hæm

hemoblasto m hematogone, hemocytoblast, blast cell

hemocitoblasto m hematogone, hemocytoblast, blast cell

hemocitómetro m counting chamber

hemocromatosis f hemochromatosis, diabetes-hemochromatosis syndrome

hemocultivo m blood culture

hemodiálisis f hemodialysis

hemofilia f hemophilia; ~ f **esporádica** sporadic hemophilia

hemofílico m hemophiliac, bleeder

hemoglobina f hæmoglobin; ~ f **fetal** fetal hemoglobin; ~ ~ **-monóxido** m **de carbono** carbon monoxide hemoglobin

hemoglobinómetro m hemoglobinometer

hemoglobinopatía f hemoglobinopathy

hemoglobinuria f hemoglobinuria, hemoglobin in the urine; ~ f **sintomática** symptomatic hemoglobinuria

hemograma f blood count, hemogram, complete blood count, CBC; ~ f **completo** full blood count, FBC, complete blood count

hemólisis f hemolysis, destruction of red blood cells; ~ f **beta** beta-hemolysis, ß-hémolyse

hemopatía f hemopathy, blood disease

hemoperfusión f hemoperfusion

hemopoyesis f blood cell production, hematopoiesis

hemopoyético *adj* hemopoietic, related to blood cell formation

hemoproteína *f* hemeprotein

hemoptisis *f* hemoptysis, coughing up blood

hemorragia *f* hemorrhage, bleeding, losing blood, exsanguination; ~ *f* **arterial** arterial bleeding; ~ *f* **capilar** capillary bleeding; ~ *f* **cerebral** cerebral hemorrhage; ~ *f* **crónica** chronic bleeding; ~ *f* **difusa** oozing hemorrhage; ~ *f* **gastrointestinal** gastro-intestinal bleeding; ~ *f* **histriónica** histrionic hemorrhage; ~ *f* **intermenstrual** metrorrhagia, breakthrough bleeding, intermenstrual bleeding; ~ *f* **intestinal** intestinal bleeding; ~ *f* **intracapsular** intracapsular hemorrhage; ~ *f* **intracraneal** intracranial hemorrhage, intracranial bleeding; ~ *f* **intradural** intradural bleeding; ~ *f* **nasal** nosebleed, bloody nose; ~ *f* **neuropática** neuropathic bleeding; ~ *f* **oculta** occult bleeding, occult blood; ~ *f* **por diapédesis** diapedetic bleeding; ~ *f* **premenstrual** premenstrual hemorrhage; ~ *f* **renal** renal hemorrhage, nephrorrhagia

hemorroidectomía *f* hemorrhoidectomy, excision of piles

hemorroides *f pl* hemorrhoids, piles

hemosiderina *f* hemosiderin

hemostasia *f* hemostasis, stagnation of blood flow

hemostasis *f* hemostasis, stagnation of blood flow

hemostático *adj* hemostatic, styptic, stopping bleeding

hemostático *m* hemostatic preparation

hemostáticos *m pl* styptics

hemoterapia *f* hemotherapy

hemoxímetro *m* hemoximeter, oximeter

hendidura *f* fissure, groove, sulcus

heno *m* **griego** fenugreek, herb with medicinal properties

henry henry

heparina *f* heparin

hepático *adj* hepatic

hepatitis *f* hepatitis; ~ *f* **amebiana** amebic hepatitis; ~ *f* **crónica** chronic hepatitis; ~ *f* **crónica activa** chronic active hepatitis; ~ *f* **infecciosa** infectious hepatitis, viral hepatitis; ~ *f* **mononuclear** mononuclear

hepatitis; ~ *f* **necrotizante** necrotic hepatitis; ~ *f* **recidivante** recurring hepatitis, recrudescent hepatitis; ~ *f* **tipo A / B / C / D** hepatitis A / B / C / D, inflammation of the liver; ~ *f* **tóxica** toxic hepatitis; ~ *f* **tóxica hepatocelular** *f* hepatocellular toxic hepatitis; ~ *f* **viral delta** delta hepatitis; ~ *f* **vírica** infectious hepatitis, viral hepatitis

hepatobiliar *adj* hepatobiliary, relating to liver and bile ducts

hepatocelular *adj* hepatocellular

hepatocito *m* hepatocyte, epithelial liver cell

hepatocolangiogastrostomía *f* hepatocholangiogastrostomy

hepatólogo *m* hepatologist - a physician who specializes in liver diseases

hepatoma *m* cancer of the liver, hepatoma

hepatomegalia *m* hepatomegaly

hepatonefritis *f* **tóxica** toxic hepatitis-nephritis

hepatopancreas *m* hepatopancreas

hepatosis *f* **colestática** cholestatic hepatosis

hepatotóxico *adj* hepatotoxic, poisonous to liver cells

herencia *adj* heredity, inheritance; ~ *f* **alternativa** crisscross inheritance; ~ *f* **citoplasmática** cytoplasmic inheritance, extra-nuclear inheritance, cytoplasmic heredity; ~ *f* **cromosómica** chromosomal inheritance; ~ *f* **gologínica** hologynic inheritance; ~ *f* **gonosómica** gonosomal heredity; ~ *f* **materna** maternal inheritance; ~ *f* **paterna** paternal inheritance; ~ *f* **poligénica** polygenic inheritance, multifactorial inheritance

herida *f* lesion, injury, trauma, wound, affected area; ~ *f* **causada por mordedura** bite wound, wound caused by a bite; ~ *f* **de arma blanca** stab wound, knife wound; ~ *f* **de arma de fuego** gunshot wound; ~ *f* **de bala** bullet wound; ~ *f* **desgarrada** laceration, tear (wound), flesh wound; ~ *f* **por arma de fuego** gunshot wound, bullet wound; ~ *f* **punzante** puncture wound

herido *adj* injured

herir *v* to wound, to injure

hermafrodita *m* hermaphroditic, both male and female

hermafroditismo *m* hermaphroditism

hermana f sister
hermano m brother
hermanos m pl siblings, brothers and sisters
hermético adj hermetic
hernia f hernia, rupture; ~ f **cerebral** cerebral herniation, cerebral hernia; ~ f **diafragmática** diaphragmatocele, diaphragmatic hernia; ~ f **discal** discopathy, disk herniation; ~ f **epigástrica** epigastric hernia; ~ f **escrotal** scrotal hernia; ~ f **estrangulada** strangulated hernia, incarcerated hernia; ~ f **femoral** femorocele, femoral hernia, crural hernia; ~ f **inguinal** inguinal hernia; ~ f **intermitente** intermittent hernia; ~ f **isquiática** ischiatic hernia, infrapiriforme hernia; ~ f **isquiorrectal** perineal hernia; ~ f **labial** labial hernia; ~ f **mediastina** mediastinal hernia; ~ f **obturadora** obturator hernia; ~ f **obturatriz** obturator hernia; ~ f **perineal** perineal hernia; ~ f **por deslizamiento** sliding hernia; ~ f **sinovial** synovial hernia; ~ f **suprapiramidal** suprapiriform hernia; ~ f **tentorial** tentorial hernia; ~ f **tonsilar** tonsillar herniation of the cerebellum; ~ f **trasvalvular** transvalvular hernia; ~ f **umbilical** umbilical hernia, omphalocele
herniación f herniation; ~ f **cerebral** cerebral herniation, cerebral hernia
heroína f heroin, diacetylmorphine
heroinomanía f heroin addiction
heroinómano m heroin addict
herpes m/f herpes; ~ m/f **conjuntival** herpes conjunctivae; ~ m/f **genital** genital herpes, herpes genitalis, herpes sexualis; ~ m/f **gutural** angina herpetica, vesicular pharyngitis; ~ m/f **neurálgico** neuralgic herpes; ~ m/f **simple** cold sore, herpes simplex, herpes labialis; ~ m/f **zoster** herpes zoster, shingles
herpesvirus m herpes virus
herramienta f tool; ~ f **de diagnóstico** diagnostic aid, diagnostic tool, diagnostic software
hertz m hertz
hervor m boiling; ~ m **de sangre** allergic reaction that results in a rash
hetacilina f hetacillin
heterocedasticidad f heteroscedaticity

heterocigoso adj heterozygous, heterozygotic
heterocigoto m heterozygote
heteroforia f heterophoria
heterógeno adj xenogenic, heterologous
heterogenote adj heterogenote
heteroimplante m heterograft, heteroplasty, xenograft, heterologous transplant, xenotransplant
heteropicnosis f heteropycnosis
heteroproteínas f pl heteroproteins
heteroquilia f heterochylia
heterotopia f heterotopia; ~ f **focal** focal heterotopia; ~ f **nodular** nodular heterotopia
heterótrofo adj heterotroph
hético m tuberculous person
hexacianoferrato (II) ferrocyanide
hexaclorofeno m hexaclorophene
hexocinasa f hexokinase, glucokinase
hexógeno adj hexogen
hialuronato-liasa f mucinase
hialuronoglucosaminidasa mucinase
hialuronoglucuronidasa mucinase
hibermetropía f hypermetropia, hyperopia
hibridación f hybridization; ~ f **de ácidos nucleicos** hybridization of nucleic acids; ~ f **de células somáticas** somatic cell hybridization; ~ f **in situ** in situ hybridization; ~ f **molecular** molecular hybridization; ~ f **por cruzamiento** cross-hybridization; ~ f **por superposición** overlap hybridisation
hibridoma m hybridoma
hidátide f hydatid
hidatidosis f hydatidosis (a parasitic disease)
hidramnios m hydramniose, hydramnion, an excessive amount of amniotic fluid
hidrargirismo m mercury poisoning, hydrargyrosis
hidrargirosis f mercury poisoning, hydrargyrosis
hidrartrosis f water on the knee, hydrarthrosis
hidratación f hydration
hidrato m hydrate; ~ m **de cloral** chloral hydrate
hidroalcohólico m hydroalcoholic, water and alcohol-related
hidroapéndice m hydro-appendix
hidrocarburo m pl hydrocarbon; ~ m **de fluoruro** chlorofluorocarbon,

monohalogenocarbon; ~ **m halogenado** halogenated hydrocarbon, halon

hidrocefalia f hydrocephalus; ~ **f concomitante** concomitant hydrocephalus

hidrocéfalo m hydrocephalus; ~ **m crónico** chronic hydrocephalus

hidrocele m hydrocele; ~ **m sintomático** symptomatic hydrocele

hidrocortisona f hydrocortisone

hidrocución f hydrocution, cold water shock, immersion syncope

hidrofílico adj hydrophilic

hidrofobia f hydrophobia

hidrófobo adj hydrophobic

hidrogenación f hydrogenation; ~ **f de grasas** hydrogenation of fats, hardening of fats

hidrógeno adj hydrogen

hidrogenocarbonato m sodium hydrogen carbonate, hydrogen carbonate, bicarbonate

hidrolasa f hydrolase; ~ **f peptídica** peptide hydrolase

hidrólisis f hydrolisis; ~ **f enzimática** enzyme hydrolysis, enzymatic hydrolysis

hidronefrosis f hydronephrosis; ~ **f congénita** congenital hydronephrosis; ~ **f dolorosa** painful hydronephrosis

hidropesía f hydrops; ~ **f fetal** fetal hydrops; ~ **f intermitente** intermittent hydrops

hidrosadenitis f hydrosadenitis; ~ **f supurativa** supurative hydrosadenitis, Verneuil's disease

hidrosalpinx m hydrosalpinx

hidrotermal adj hydrothermal

hidrotórax m pleurisy, pleuritis, hydrothorax

hidrotropía f hydrotropy, solubilization

hidrotrópico adj hydrotropic, causing hydrotropy

hidroxicloroquina f hydroxychloroquine

hidroxicobalamina f hydroxocobalamin, B12 vitamin

hidroxido m **de sodio** caustic soda, sodium hydroxide

hidroxilasa f hydroxylation

hidroxilo m hydroxyl

hidroxiprolina f hydroxyproline

hiedra f ivy; ~ **venenosa** poison ivy

hielo m ice

hierbas f pl herbs

hierbas f pl **medicinales** medicinal herbs, medicinal plants

hierro m iron

hierros m pl forceps, tweezers

hifa f hypha

hígado m liver; ~ **m amiloideo** amyloid liver; ~ **m nodular** hobnail liver

higiene f hygiene; ~ **f alimenticia** food sanitation, food hygiene; ~ **f de los alimentos** food sanitation, food hygiene; ~ **f oral** oral hygiene; ~ **f sexual** sexual hygiene, intimate care

higiénico adj hygienic

higroma m hygroma; ~ **m subdural** subdural hygroma

higromatosis f hygromatosis; ~ **f reumática** hygromatosis rheumatica

hija f daughter

hijo m son

hilaridad f humor, merriment, laughter, mirth

hilio m hilum; ~ **m pulmonar** pulmonary hilum, hilum of lung

hilo m **dental** dental floss

hilos m pl **orthopedicos** bone wires, steel wires

himen m hymen of vagina, claustrum virginale; ~ **m franjeado** fimbriate hymen; ~ **m imperforado** imperforate hymen; ~ **m lobular** lobate hymen; ~ **m perforado** perforated hymen

hinchado adj puffy, swollen, distended, bloated

hinchamiento m swelling, tumefaction, healing wound

hinchar v to swell, to bulge, to protrude

hinchazón f tumefaction, swelling; ~ **f de la papila óptica** papilledema, papilloedema, swollen optical disk; ~ **f del pie** swelling of the foot

hiosciamina f hyoscyamine

hiperactividad f hyperactivity

hiperacusia f hyperacousia, hyperacusis, loudness recruitment

hiperaldosteronismo m hyperaldosteronism; ~ **m primario** primary hyperaldosteronism, Conn's syndrome

hiperalgia f hyperalgesia

hiperbaro adj hyperbaric

hiperbilirrubinemia f hyperbilirubinemia; ~ **f intermitente** intermittent hyperbilirubinemia; ~ **f persistente** persistent hyperbilirubinemia

hipercalemia f hyperkalemia, excessive potassium in the blood

hipercapnia f hypercapnia

hipercinesia f hyperkinesia; ~ f **uterina** uterine hyperkinesia

hipercolesterolemia f hypercholesterolemia

hiperemesis f hyperemesis, excessive vomiting

hiperemia f hyperemia; ~ f **activa** active hyperemia, arterial hyperemia; ~ f **arterial** active hyperemia, arterial hyperemia; ~ f **pasiva** blood congestion, passive hyperemia; ~ f **venosa** venous hyperemia

hiperestesia f hyperesthesia; ~ f **dentaria** dental hyperesthesia

hiperestrogenismo m hyperoestrogenism; ~ m **femenino** feminine hyperoestrogenism; ~ m **viril masculino** masculine virile hyperoestrogenism

hiperextensión f hyperextension

hiperflexión f hyperflexion

hiperglicemia f hyperglycemia

hiperhidratación f hyperhydratation; ~ f **extracelular** extracellular hyperhydratation; ~ f **intracelular** intracellular hyperhydratation

hiperhidrosis f hyperhidrosis, excessive sweating; ~ f **facial** facial hyperhidrosis, sweaty face; ~ f **perineal** perineal hyperhidrosis

hipérico m St. John's wort

hiperinsulinemia f hyperinsulinemia

hiperinsulinismo m hyperinsulinism; ~ m **espontáneo** pernicious hyperinsulinism, Harris syndrome

hiperlipidemia f hyperlipidemia, increase in blood fat levels

hipernatrémia f hypernatremia

hipernutrición f overeating

hiperopia f hypermetropia, hyperopia

hiperortocitosis f hyperorthocytosis

hiperostosis f hyperostosis, abnormal bone thickening; ~ f **cortical deformante** Paget's disease, Paget carcinoma

hiperoxalemia f hyperoxalemia

hiperoxia f hyperoxia, excess of oxygen

hiperparatiroidismo m hyperparathyroidism; ~ m **óseo** hyperparathyroidism

hiperpatía f hyperpathia, excessive reaction to painful stimuli

hiperpigmentación f hyperpigmentation

hiperpirexia f hyperpyrexia, extreme fever

hiperpituitarismo m hyperpituitarism

hiperplasia f hyperplasia, increase in the number of normal cells in tissue; ~ f **adrenal congénita** congenital adrenal hyperplasia, CAH; ~ f **del endometrio** endometrial hyperplasia; ~ f **labial** labial hyperplasia; ~ f **prostática benigna** benign prostatic hyperplasia

hiperplástico adj hyperplastic

hiperprolactinemia f hyperprolactinemia

hiperprolinemia f iminoglycinuria, hyperprolinemia

hiperqueratosis f hyperkeratosis; ~ f **precancerosa** precancerous hyperkeratosis

hiperquinesia f hyperactivity, hyperkinesia

hiperreactividad f hyperreactivity; ~ f **bronquial** airway hyperresponsiveness, bronchial hyperreactivity

hipersecreción f hypersecretion

hipersensibilidad f hypersensitivity, over-sensitivity; ~ f **a los cacahuates** allergy to peanuts, peanut hypersensitivity; ~ f **al rebote** rebound tenderness; ~ f **de contacto** contact hypersensitivity; ~ f **retardada** delayed hypersensitivity; ~ f **tardia** delayed hypersensitivity

hipersexualismo m hypersexuality

hipersideremia f hypersideremia, iron overload

hipersomnia f hypersomnia

hipertelorismo m hypertelorism, abnormal increase in the interorbital distance

hipertensión f hypertension, high blood pressure, hypertonia; ~ f **arterial** arterial hypertension; ~ f **arterial pulmonar** pulmonary hypertension, pulmonary arterial hypertension; ~ f **climatérica** climacteric hypertension, menopause hypertension; ~ f **intracraneal** intracranial hypertension; ~ f **lábil** labile hypertension; ~ f **maligna** malignant hypertension; ~ f **pulmonar** pulmonary hypertension; ~ f **simpática** sympathetic hypertension

hipertermia f hyperthermia; ~ f **pasiva** passive hyperthermia

H

hipertiroidismo *m* hyperthyroidism, overactive thyroid

hipertónico *adj* hypertonic

hipertricosis *f* hypertrichosis, excess of hair growth

hipertrofia *f* hypertrophy, increase in the size of an organ; ~ *f* **de la pantorrilla** hypertrophic calf; ~ *f* **prostática benigna** benign prostatic hypertrophy, benign prostatic hyperplasia; ~ *f* **ventricular** ventricular hypertrophy

hipertrófico *adj* hypertrophic

hiperuricemia *f* hyperuricemia

hiperventilación *f* hyperventilation, excess of breathing

hipervitaminosis *f* hypervitaminosis, vitamin overdose

hipervolemia *f* hypervolemia, abnormal increase in blood volume

hipnosis *f* hypnosis; ~ *f* **terapéutica** therapeutic hypnosis

hipo *m* singultus, hiccup

hipoacusia *f* slight deafness, hypoacusis; ~ *f* **neurosensorial** labyrinthine hearing loss, inner-ear deafness, nerve deafness, sensorineural hearing loss

hipoaldosteronismo *m* hypoaldosteronism

hipoalgesia *f* hypoalgesia; ~ *f* **unilateral** hemihypalgesia, hemi-hypoalgesia

hipocaliemia *f* hypokalemia, low blood potassium

hipocampo *m* hippocampus, Ammon's horn; ~ *m* **menor** calcar avis

hipocapnia *f* hypocapnia

hipocondría *f* hypochondriasis

hipocratismo *m* hypocratism

hipocromático *adj* hypochrome

hipodenso *m* hypodense

hipodérmico *adj* hypodermic

hipofaringe *f* hypopharynx

hipofisario *adj* hypophyseal

hipofisectomia *f* hypophysectomy

hipófisis *f* hypophysis; ~ *f* **cerebral** cerebral hypophysis, pituitary gland

hipogástrico *adj* hypogastric

hipogastrio *m* hipogastrium, the lower part of the abdomen

hipoglicemia *f* hypoglycaemia, low blood sugar

hipoglotis *f* hypoglottis, underside of the tongue

hipoglucemia *f* hypoglycemia; ~ *f* **posprandial** postprandial hypoglycemia, poststimulative hypoglycemia

hipoglucemiante *adj* hypoglycemic, hypoglycaemic

hipogonadismo *m* hypogonadism, poorly developped genitals; ~ *m* **funcional prepuberal** functional prepuberal castration syndrome; ~ *m* **primario** primary hypogonadism, hypergonadotrophic hypogonadism; ~ *m* **secundario** secondary hypogonadism, hypogonadotrophic hypogonadism

hipomanía *f* hypomania, persistent slight hyperactivity

hipometabolismo *m* hypometabolism; ~ *m* **eutiroide** euthyroid hypometabolism

hipoplasia *f* hypoplasia, underdevelopment of tissues or organs

hipoproteinemia *f* hypoproteinemia; ~ *f* **idiopática** idiopathic hypoproteinemia

hipospadia *f* hypospadia

hipotalámico *adj* hypothalamic

hipotálamo *m* hypothalamus

hipotensión *f* hypotension, low blood pressure; ~ *f* **arterial** low blood pressure, hypotension, hypotonia; ~ *f* **controlada** controlled hypotension

hipotensivo *adj* hypotensive, with low blood pressure

hipotermia *f* hypothermia, low body temperature; ~ *f* **farmacológica** pharmacological hypothermia; ~ *f* **inducida** induced hypothermia, controlled hypothermia; ~ *f* **provocada** induced hypothermia, controlled hypothermia

hipótesis *f* hypothesis, theory

hipotiroidismo *m* hypothyroidism, underactive thyroid

hipotonía *f* hypotension, hypotonia, low blood pressure, loss of muscular tonicity; ~ *f* **ocular** intra-ocular hypotonia, intra-ocular hypotension

hipotrepsia *f* hypothrepsia, malnutrition

hipotrofia *f* hypotrophy

hipouricemia *f* hypouricemia, lack of uric acid in the blood

hipoventilación f hypoventilation, insufficient breathing
hipovitaminosis f hypovitaminosis, vitamin deficiency
hipovolemia f hypovolemia, low blood volume
hipoxantina f hypoxanthine
hipoxemia f hypoxemia, blood oxygen deficiency
hipoxia f hypoxia, tissue oxygen deficiency; ~ f **de altitud** high altitude hypoxia; ~ f **miocardica** myocardial hypoxia
hipromelosa f methylcellulose
Hirschsprung disease m congenital colectasia, Hirschsprung disease
hirsutismo m hirsutism, hairiness
hirudiniasis f hirudiniasis, a condition resulting from attack by leeches
hirudo m medicinal leech
hisopo m swab, Q-tip; ~ m **traqueal** tracheal swab
histamina f histamine
histaminoiontoforesis f histamine iontophoresis
histerectomía f hysterectomy, resection of the uterus
histeria f hysteria
histerosalpingografía f hysterosalpingography
histerosalpingooforectomía f hysterosalpingo-oophorectomy, adnexectomy
histeroscopia f hysteroscopy
histeroscopio m hysteroscope
histerotraquelectomía f hysterotrachelectomy
histidina f histidine; ~ f **descarboxilasa** decarboxylase
histiocito m histiocyte
histiocitosis f histiocytosis, the abnormal appearance of histiocyte cells in the blood; ~ f **de celulas de Langerhans** Langerhans cell histiocytosis, histiocytosis X; ~ f **maligna** malignant histiocytosis
histioquímica f histochemistry
histoautorradiografía f histoautoradiography
histocompatibilidad f histocompatibility, tissue compatibility
histología f histology
histológico adj histological
histona f histone
histopatología f histopathology

histoplasmosis f histoplasmosis; ~ f **diseminada** histoplasmosis
historia f history; ~ f **de caso familiar** family case history
historial m **médico** medical history
histótrofo adj histotrophic, histotropic
hocico m snout
hogar m **adoptivo** foster home
hojita f **de afeitar** razor blade
hola hello
holoprosencefalia f holoprosencephaly, arhinencephaly; ~ f **lobar** lobar holoprosencephaly
hombre m man
hombro m shoulder; ~ m **congelado** frozen shoulder, adhesive capsulitis
hombruna f virago, masculine woman
homeopatía f homeopathy
homeosecuencia f homeobox
homeostasis f homeostasis
homocedasticidad f homoscedasticity
homocigosis f homozygosis; ~ f **recesiva** recessive homozygosis
homocigoso adj homozygous, homozygotic
homocigoto m homozygote
homocistina f homocysteine - a non-essential amino acid
homodúplex homoduplex
homogéneo adj homogeneous, uniform
homogénesis f homogeny, homogenesis
homogenia f homogeny, homogenesis
homogenote adj homogenote
homoinjerto m allograft, allogenic graft, allogenic transplant, homologous graft
homología f homology
homólogo adj homologous
hondo adj deep
hongo m fungal, fungus; ~ m **dimórfico** dimorphic fungi
hongos m pl fungal infection
honorario m medical fee, honorarium, doctor's fee; ~ m pl **médico** medical fee, honorarium, doctor's fee
hora f hour, time; ~ f **de acostarse** bedtime
hormigueos m pl pins and needles, formication, tingling

hormona f hormone; ~ f **adrenocorticotropa**
ACTH, adrenocorticotropic hormone;
~ f **corticosuprarrenal** ACH, adrenal cortical
hormone; ~ f **del crecimiento** somatotrophin,
growth hormone; ~ f **del timo** thymic
hormone, thymus hormone; ~ f **estimulante**
stimulating hormone; ~ f **foliculoestimulante**
follicle-stimulating hormone, follitropin;
~ f **gastrointestinal** gastrointestinal hormone,
enteric hormone; ~ f **lactógena** lactogenic
hormone, lactation hormone, prolactin;
~ f **liberadora** releasing hormone; ~ f **luteinizante** luteinizing hormone,
interstitial cell-stimulating hormone, lutropin;
~ f **polipeptídica** polypeptide hormone;
~ f **tiroidea** thyroid hormone
hormonal adj hormonal
hormonas f pl hormones; ~ f pl **catabólicas**
catabolic hormones; ~ f pl **intestinales** enteral
hormones; ~ f pl **ováricas** ovarian hormones;
~ f pl **pituitarias** pituitary hormones;
~ f pl **sintéticas** synthetic hormones;
~ f pl **tiroideas** thyroid hormones
hormonoterapia f hormone therapy, hormonal
therapy
horquilla f hairpin; ~ f **de replicación**
replication fork
hospedero m host; ~ m **intermedio**
intermediate host
hospital m hospital, clinic; ~ m **de maternidad**
maternity clinic; ~ m **infantil** children's
hospital; ~ m **psiquiátrico** psychiatric hospital,
mental hospital
hospitalización f hospitalization, admission to
hospital
hostil adj hostile, antagonistic
hotel m hotel
hoy today
hoyito m **del chi** meatus of the urethra, urethral
meatus, hole through which urine passes
hueco m **poplíteo** back of the knee, popliteal
space, popliteal fossa
huella f trace, residue, impression, print; ~ f **de
escayola** impression of plaster cast;
~ f **digital** fingerprint; ~ f **genética** genetic
footprint, genetic imprint, DNA fingerprint;
~ f **genómica** genomic imprinting;
~ f **oligonucleotídica** oligonucleotide

fingerprint
huesecillo m ossicle, small bone
hueso m bone, bones; ~ m **biforme** sphenoid
bone; ~ m **coccígeo** coccyx, coccygeal bone,
tailbone; ~ m **de la rodilla** kneecap, patella;
~ m **del codo** olecranon, funnybone (in the
elbow); ~ m **del cuello** collarbone, clavicle;
~ m **del pecho** breast bone, sternum;
~ m **ganchoso** hamate bone, hooked bone;
~ m **ilíaco** ilium, hip bone; ~ m **lagrimal**
lacrimal bone; ~ m **malar** zygoma, jugal,
malar, cheek bone, zygomatic bone;
~ m **metacarpiano** metacarpal bone;
~ m **nasal** nasal bones; ~ m **occipital** occipital
bone; ~ m **púbico** pubic bone, pubis;
~ m **sacro** sacrum; ~ m **unciforme** hooked
bone
huesos m pl **del carpo** carpal bones, wrist
bones; ~ m pl **nasales** nasal bones;
~ m pl **parietales** cranial parietal bones
huesoso adj bony, osseous
huésped m host; ~ m **definitivo** definitive host
huesudo adj bony, osseous
huevo m egg; ~ m **pequeño** ovum, egg
humectabilidad f wettability
humedad f moisture; ~ f **libre** free moisture
humeral adj humeral
húmero m humerus
humeroscapular adj humeroscapular, shoulder-
related
humidificador m humidifier
humidofílico adj humidophilic
humo m smoke
humor m humor, merriment, laughter, mirth,
normal body fluid; ~ m **acuoso** aqueous
humor; ~ m **vítreo** vitreous humor
humoral adj humoral
huso m spindle; ~ m **acromático** mitotic
spindle; ~ m **de His** His spindle; ~ m **mitótico**
mitotic spindle, spindle fiber (in mitosis)
hypnotico adj hypnotic
hypocondríaco adj hypochondriac

I

ibuprofeno m ibuprofen

ictericia f jaundice, icterus; ~ f **colestática** cholestatic icterus; ~ f **fetal** fetal icterus, fetal jaundice

icterohemoglobinuria f icterohemoglobinuria

ictiosiforme adj ichthyosiform

ictiosis f ichthyosis, scaly skin; ~ **bulosa** f ichthyosis bullosa; ~ **congénita** f ichthyosis congenita

ictus m apoplexy, stroke, cerebrovascular accident

idea f idea; ~ f **delirante** delusional idea; ~ f **fija** obsession

ideación f ideation, capacity for forming ideas

ideas f pl **suicidas** suicidal ideation, contemplating suicide

idéntico identical, analogous

identificación f identification

ideomotor m ideokinetic, idiomotor

ideosínquisis f confusion, ideosynchysis

idiopático adj idiopathic, of unknown cause

idiosincrasia f idiosyncrasy, pecularity

idiotopo m idiotope, idiotypic determinant

igual adj homologous

ijar m, **ijada** f flank

ileítis f ileitis; ~ f **folicular** follicular ileitis; ~ f **regional** regional enteritis, regional ileitis, Crohn's disease

íleo m ileus, intestinal blockage; ~ m **biliar** gallstone ileus; ~ m **dinámico** dynamic ileus; ~ m **espástico** spastic ileus; ~ m **gástrico** gastric ileus; ~ m **paralítico** paralytic ileus; ~ m **por estrangulamiento** strangulation ileus; ~ m **por obstrucción** occlusive ileus; ~ m **posoperatorio** postoperative ileus; ~ m **séptico** septic ileus

ileocecostomía f ileocecostomy

íleon m ileum

ileostomía f ileostomy; ~ f **de descarga** divrting ileostomy

ileso adj unhurt

ilion m ilium, hip bone

iluminación f **de Köhler** Köhler illumination

iluminancia f illuminance

ilusión f illusion

ilusión f **mnésica** false memory, mnemic delusion; ~ f **óptica** optical illusion

imagen f image; ~ f **retiniana** retinal image; ~ f **por resonancia magnética** MRI, magnetic resonance imaging; ~ f **de compuerta** m gated imaging, image gating

imaginería f imaging; ~ f **cardiovascular** cardiovascular imaging; ~ f **diagnóstica** diagnostic imaging; ~ f **biomédica** biomedical imaging

IMAO MAOI, monoamine-oxidase inhibitor

imbecilidad f mental retardation, mental disorder, feeblemindedness, dementia, mental deficiency

imbibición f impregnation, fertilization, making pregnant

imersión f immersion, submersion

iminoglicinuria f iminoglycinuria, hyperprolinemia

imipramina f imipramine (Tofranil), a tricyclic antidepressant drug

impacto m impact; ~ m **ambiental** environmental impact; ~ m **ecológico** ecological impact; ~ m **único** single hit

impairment f impairment

impedancia f impedance

impedimento m handicap, delaying

impedir v to retard, to slow down, to delay

impenetrable adj hermetic, airtight

impétigo m impetigo; ~ m **variolosum** impetigo varicellosa; ~ m **folicular** impetigo folliculiris

implantación f implantation, implanting of a fertilized ovum, insertion, inserting; ~ f **del embrión maduro** nidation, fertilisation; ~ f **exitosa del injerto** engraftment

implante m implant; ~ m **biónico** bionic implant; ~ m **coclear** cochlear implant, cochlear prosthesis, cochlear apparatus; ~ m **de sustitución osteoarticular** joint replacement implant; ~ m **mamario de silicona** silicon breast implant; ~ m **osteoarticular de cadera** joint replacement

implicación f implication

importante adj relevant

impotencia f impotence; ~ f **masculina** male impotence, erectile dysfunction; ~ f **sintomática** symptomatic impotence

imprecisión f imprecision; ~ f **intraserial** within-run imprecision; ~ f **máxima tolerable** allowable maximum imprecision

impregnación f impregnation, fertilization,

making pregnant

impresión f impression; ~ f **aórtica** aortic impression; ~ f **de la dentadura** dental impression

impreso m printed form; ~ f **del pie** footprint; ~ f **genética** genetic footprint, genetic imprint, DNA fingerprint

impulso m impulse; ~ m **nervioso** nerve impulse; ~ m **propioceptivo** proprioceptive impulse

impurezas f pl impurities

imunocitoquímica f immunocytochemistry, technique for staining cells

imunohistoquímica f immunohistochemistry, technique for staining cells

in extremis in extremis, in articulo mortis, at the point of death

in situ in situ, at the original place, in the body

in vitro in vitro, in a test tube

in vivo in vivo, in the living body

inactividad f inertia

inactivo adj inactive

inadecuado adj inadequate, not apropriate, ill-suited

inaguantable adj unbearable, intolerable

inanición f inanition, starvation, malnutrition

inapetencia f loss of appetite, anorexia

incapacidad f impairment, handicap; ~ f **parcial** partial disability; ~ f **permanente** permanent disability; ~ f **profesional** work-related disability, occupational disability; ~ f **temporaria** temporary disability

incapacitado m disabled person, handicapped person

incarceración f incarceration, strangulated hernia

incautación f seizure, confiscation; ~ f **de heroína** seizure of narcotics, heroin seizure

incertidumbre f uncertainty

incesto m incest

incidencia f incidence, number of cases

incidental adj incidental, minor

incipiente adj incipient, beginning, in the early stages

incisión f incision, cut; ~ f **de Blalock** Blalock incision; ~ f **de Klapp** incision; ~ f **en huso** spindle-like incision

incisivo adj incisive, cutting

inciso m gash, knife wound, stab wound

incisura f notch

inclinación f addiction, preference; ~ f **sexual** sexual preference

inclinarse v to lean forward, to bend over; ~ v **en una ventana** to lean out of a window; ~ v **hacia adelante** to lean forward, to **inclusivo** adj inclusive

incoherente adj incoherent, unintelligible, disjointed

incólume adj unhurt

incomodidad f discomfort, uneasiness; ~ f **térmica** thermal stress, thermal discomfort, heat stress

incompatibilidad f incompatibility; ~ f **de medicamentos** drug incompatibility, drug antagonism

incompatible adj incompatible

incompetencia f incompetence, insufficiency; ~ f **del cuello uterino** incompetent cervix, insufficiency of the cervix

inconsciente adj unconscious

inconstante adj labile, unstable

incontinencia f incontinence, incompetence of the anal sphincter, anal sphincter incontinence, urinary incontinence; ~ f **por estrés** incontinence due to stress, stress urinary incontinence; ~ f **urinaria** urinary incontinence, incontinence of urine

inconveniente m drawback

incordio m inflamed lymph nodes, buboes (in the armpit)

incorporación f incorporation, inclusion

incubación f incubation

incubadora f incubator; ~ f **para prematuros** artificial incubator, incubator for newborn babies

incumplimiento m noncompliance

incurable adj incurable

indagar research, to, investigate, to, examine, to

indemnización f compensation; ~ f **de los accidentes de trabajo** workmen's compensation; ~ f **por accidente laboral** workers' compensation, workmen's compensation

independiente adj independent, autonomic; ~ m self-employed

indicación f indication, sign

indicaciones (pl f) instructions
indicador m indicator; ~ m **de contaminación fécal** indicator of fecal contamination
indicar v To indicate, to show
indicativo m indicative
índice m contents; ~ m **de Apgar** Apgar index, Apgar-score; ~ m **de embarazo** pregnancy rate; ~ m **de masa corporal** BMI, Quetelet's index, body mass index; ~ m **de Quetelet** BMI, Quetelet's index, body mass index; ~ m **de refracción** refractive index; ~ m **de supervivencia celular** survival rate; ~ m **del rendimiento cardíaco** cardiac output index; ~ m **mitótico** mitotic index; ~ m **terapéutico** therapeutic index
indiferente adj maudlin, lackadaisical, apathetic
indigestión f indigestion, a form of digestive symptoms
indirecto adj indirect
individual adj individual
individuo m individual; ~ m **de referencia** reference individual
indócil adj obstreperous, unruly, rambunctious
indolencia f indolence, absence of pain, painlessness, laziness
indolente adj indolent
indoloro adj painless
indometacina f indomethacin, non-steroidal anti-inflammatory agent (NSAID)
inducción f induction; ~ f **zigótica** f zygotic induction
inducido adj induced; ~ adj **por drogas** drug-induced, medication-induced
inductor m inducer; ~ m **gratuito** gratuitous inducer; ~ m **occipital** occipital inductor
induración f induration, hardening; ~ f **del pericardio** pericardial scar; ~ f **granular** granular induration, cirrhosis; ~ f **intersticial** f interstitial induration; ~ f **sifilítica** syphilitic induration, hard ulcer of primary syphilis
industria f industry; ~ f **farmaceutica** pharmaceutical industry
inercia f inertia
inerte adj inert
inervación f innervation, nerve distribution; ~ f **cardíaca** cardiac innervation
inespecífico adj nonspecific, non-specific
inestabilidad f instability

inestable adj labile, unstable
inexactitud f inaccuracy; ~ f **máxima tolerable** allowable maximum inaccuracy; ~ f **relativa** relative inaccuracy
infanticidio m infanticide, child murder
infantil adj infantile
infantilismo m infantilism
infarto m infarct, infarction, heart attack; ~ m **cerebral** cerebral infarction; ~ m **de miocardio** myocardial infarction, heart attack; ~ m **infectado** septic infarct
infausto adj unfortunate, unlucky
infección f infection; ~ f **cruzada** cross infection, mutual infection; ~ f **cutánea estafilocócica** staphylococcal skin infection; ~ f **de herida operatoria** postoperative wound infection; ~ f **de hongos** fungal infection; ~ f **de la herida** infected wound; ~ f **de las vías respiratorias** respiratory tract infection; ~ f **estreptocócica de la garganta** streptococcal throat infection; ~ f **herpérica** herpes infection; ~ f **hospitalaria** hospital acquired infection; ~ f **por borrelia** borreliosis, borrelia infection; ~ f **por gotitas** droplet infection; ~ f **respiratoria** respiratory infection; ~ f **urinaria** urinary infection, urinary tract infection
infecciosidad f infectivity, infectiousness
infeccioso adj infectious
infecundidad f infertility
infertilidad f infertility
infestación f infestation; ~ f **por insectos** insect infestation, insect outbreak
infibulación f **de la mujer** female infibulation
infiltración f infiltration; ~ f **cancerosa** cancerous infiltration; ~ f **en gotas** guttate infiltration; ~ f **paravertebral** paravertebral infiltration
infiltrado m infiltrate; ~ m **eosinófilo** eosinophilic infiltrate; ~ m **inflamatorio** inflammatory infiltrate; ~ m **linfocítico** lymphocytic infiltrate
inflamación f inflammation; ~ f **bacterial de la piel** impetigo, pyoderma; ~ f **de la glándula mamaria** mastitis, sore breasts; ~ f **de la laringe** laryngitis, sore throat, inflammation of throat; ~ f **de la mucosa oral** inflammation of the oral mucosa; ~ f **de la piel** dermatitis, skin

inflammation; ~ f **de la próstata** prostatitis, prostate inflammation, prostate infection; ~ f **de la vesícula biliar** cholecystitis, gall bladder inflammation; ~ f **de las glándulas** adenitis, gland inflammation; ~ f **de los vasos linfáticos** lymphangitis, lymphatic vessel inflammation; ~ f **de pelvis renal** pyelitis, inflammation of kidney; ~ f **de un músculo voluntario** muscle inflammation; ~ f **de un nervio** neuritis, nerve inflammation; ~ f **del cuello del útero** cervicitis, trachelitis; ~ f **del estómago** gastritis; ~ f **del iris** iridocyclitis, eye irritation; ~ f **del iris y del cuerpo ciliar** f iridocyclitis, eye inflammation; ~ f **del recto** proctitis, infection of rectum, sore bottom; ~ f **del riñón** nephritis, kidney inflammation; ~ f **infecciosa del tímpano** myringitis, inflammation of the eardrum; ~ f **pulmonar** bronchopneumonia, bronchial pneumonia

influenza f flu, influenza

información f information; ~ f **genética** genetic information

informática f **hospitalaria** medical LAN (local area network), hospital computer system

informatividad f informativity

informatizado adj computerized

informe m report; ~ m **del cirujano** surgeon's report; ~ m **del estado del hígado** liver profile, hepatic profile; ~ m **médico** medical report

infundíbulo m infundibulum

infundir v to infuse, to pour in, to suffuse

infusión f infusio, transfusion of liquids, intravenous drip

ingeniería f engineering; ~ f **bioquímica** biochemical engineering; ~ f **de proteínas** (genetic) protein engineering; ~ f **genética** genetic engineering, genetic manipulation

ingeniero m engineer; ~ m **biomédico** biomedical engineer

ingerir v ingest, to eat, to

ingestión f ingestion, swallowing

ingle f crotch, groin, inguinal region

inglés adj English

ingravidez f microgravity, weightlessness, zero gravity

ingrediente m ingredient, component

inguinal adj inguinal, pertaining to the groin, groin-related

inguinodinia f inguinodynia, pain in the groin

inhabitual adj unusual

inhalación f inhalation, breathing in

inhalador m inhaler, spray dispenser, moist vapor nebulizer, puff; ~ m **de aerosol** aerosol inhalation

inhalar v to inhale, to breathe in

inherente adj inherent, natural

inhibición f inhibition, stopping; ~ f **competitiva** competitive inhibition; ~ f **de la hemaglutinación** hemagglutination inhibition; ~ f **lateral** lateral inhibition; ~ f **no competitiva** non-competitive inhibition; ~ f **postsináptica** postsynaptic inhibition

inhibidor m inhibitor; ~ m **de agregacion plaquetaria** antiplatelet, platelet aggregation inhibitor; ~ m **de huso mitótico** spindle inhibitor; ~ m **de la monoaminooxidasa** MAOI, monoamine-oxidase inhibitor; ~ m **de la proteasa** protease inhibitor; ~ m **de la retrotranscriptasa** reverse-transcriptase blocker, reverse transcriptase inhibitor; ~ m **irreversible** irreversible inhibitor; ~ m **MAO** MAOI, monoamine-oxidase inhibitor; ~ m **reversible** reversible inhibitor; ~ m **selectivo de la reabsorción de serotonina** selective serotonin reuptake inhibitor

inhibina f inhibin

inhumano adj inhuman, cruel

inicial adj initial

injerto m graft; ~ m **de la piel** skin graft, epidermal graft; ~ m **heterólogo** heterogenous graft, xenograft, heterologous transplant, xenotransplant; ~ m **óseo** bone graft

inmadurez f immaturity

inmiscible immiscible, not mixable

inmovilización f immobilization, stopping movement, holding still, restraint, retention

inmortal adj immortal

inmovilización f immobilization; ~ f **por adsorción** ionic bond, adsorption immobilization

inmovilizar v to paralyze, to immobilize

inmune adj immune

inmunidad f immunity; ~ f a **fagos** phage

immunity; ~ f **celular** cell-mediated immunity, delayed hypersensitivity; ~ f **tisular** local immunity

inmunización f vaccination, immunization

inmunoadherencia f immune adherence

inmunoanálisis m immunoassay; ~ m **competitivo** competitive immunoassay; ~ m **heterogéneo** heterogeneous immunoassay; ~ m **homogéneo** homogeneous immunoassay; ~ m **no competitivo** non-competitive immunoassay; ~ m **secuencial** sequential immunoassay; ~ m **turbidimétrico** turbidimetric immunoassay

inmunocito m immunocyte, immune cell, immunocompetent cell

inmunocomplejo m immune complex; ~ m **circulante** circulating immune complex

inmunodeficiencia f immune deficiency, immunodeficiency

inmunodifusión f immunodiffusion; ~ f **indirecta** indirect immunodiffusion; ~ f **radial** radial immunodiffusion

inmunoelectrodifusión f immunoelectrodiffusion

inmunoelectroforesis f immunoelectrophoresis; ~ f **cruzada** crossed immunoelectrophoresis; ~ f **bidemensional** f two-dimensional immunoelectrophoresis

inmunoensayo m immunoassay

inmunoestimulante m immunostimulant

inmunofijación f immunofixation

inmunofluorescencia f immunofluorescence, fluorescence immunoassay, FIA

inmunogenicidad f antigenicity, immunogenicity

inmunógeno adj immunogenic, producing immunity

inmunoglobulina f immunoglobulin; ~ f **anti-D** anti-D immunoglobulin; ~ f **antitetánica** tetanus immunoglobulin; ~ f **homóloga** homologous immunoglobulin; ~ f **humana normal** human normal immunoglobulin

inmunohematología f immunohematology

inmunohemolisina f immunohemolysin

inmunología f immunology; ~ f **clínica** clinical immunology

inmunológico adj immunological, immunity study-related

inmunomodulación f immunomodulation

inmunoprecipitación f immunoprecipitation

inmunoquímica f immunochemistry

inmunorradiometría f immunoradiometry

inmunorrespuesta f immunoreaction, immune reaction

inmunosupresión f immunosuppression

inmunosupresor m immunosuppressant, drug to stop immune response

inmunoterapia f immunotherapy; ~ f **pasiva específica** specific passive immunotherapy

inmunotransferencia f immunoblot, immunoblotting

innato adj congenital, inherent, natural

inocuidad f harmlessness

inoculación f inoculation; ~ f **endodérmica** intradermal inoculation; ~ f **profiláctico** prophylactic inoculation

inocular v to inoculate, to vaccinate

inóculo m inoculum; ~ m **aclimatado** acclimatized inoculum

inocuo adj safe, harmless

inodoro m toilet, lavatory, water closet

inoperable adj inoperable

inorgánico adj inorganic, non-organic

inotrópico adj inotropic

inquietud f vague sensation of uneasiness

insalubre adj unsanitary, unhealthy, unclean

insecticida f insecticide

insecto m insect

inseguridad f lack of safety, insecurity; ~ f **al andar** unsteady gait, staggering gait

inseminación f insemination; ~ f **artificial** insemination by donor; ~ f **de prueba** test insemination

insensibilizar v to anesthetize, to numb up

inserción f insertion, inserting; ~ f **epitelial** epithelial attachment, junctional complex

insertar v to insert

inserto adj insert

insignificante adj negligible

insolación f sunstroke

insomne adj sleepless, insomniac

insomnio m insomnia, sleeplessness

insoportable adj unbearable, intolerable

inspección f examination

inspeccionar v to inspect

inspector m **médico** medical officer, examining

doctor, medical examiner, public officer
inspiración f inspiration, breathing in
instilación f trickling, instillation, to pour in by drops
instilar v to instill
instituciones f pl facilities; ~ f pl **de salud** health facilities
instrucción f instruction
instrumentación f instrumentation
instrumento m instrument; ~ m **analítico** analytical instrument; ~ m **de medida** measuring instrument
insuficiencia f insufficiency, inadequacy; ~ f **cardíaca** myocardial insufficiency, cardiac insufficiency; ~ f **cardíaca compensada** cardiac insufficiency, compensated heart failure; ~ f **cardíaca congénita** congenital heart heart failure; ~ f **cardíaca global** global cardiac insufficiency; ~ f **cervical** incompetent cervix, insufficiency of the cervix; ~ f **coronaria** coronary artery insufficiency; ~ f **de la válvula pulmonar** pulmonary regurgitation, pulmonary valve regurgitation, pulmonary valve insufficiency; ~ f **de multiples organos** multiple organ failure; ~ f **del cardias** cardial insufficiency, insufficiency of the cardial sphincter; ~ f **del tratamiento** failure of treatment, lack of results from the therapy; ~ f **del ventriculo** ventricular failure; ~ f **hepática aguda** acute liver failure; ~ f **hepatocelular** hepatocellular insufficiency; ~ f **orgánica** organic insufficiency, exertional insufficiency; ~ f **ovárica prematura** premature ovarian failure; ~ f **pancreática** pancreatic insufficiency; ~ f **placentaria** placental insufficiency; ~ f **renal** renal insufficiency; ~ f **renal aguda** chronic renal failure, kidney failure; ~ f **renal crónica** acute renal failure, kidney failure; ~ f **renal permanente** chronic kidney failure, anuresis, anuria; ~ f **respiratoria** respiratory failure, respiratory arrest; ~ f **suprarrenal** adrenal insufficiency; ~ f **testicular** testicular insufficiency; ~ f **velofaríngea** velopharyngeal insufficiency
insuficiente adj inadequate, insufficient

insuflación f inflation, blowing up; ~ f **intracraneal** intracranial insufflation
insuflador m insufflator; ~ m **de oxígeno** oxygen insufflator; ~ m **manual** manual insufflator
insufrible adj unbearable, intolerable
insulina f insulin, hormone that regulates blood sugar levels; ~ f **protamina de cinc** protamine zinc insulin
insulto m insult
intacto adj intact, whole
integrativo adj integrative
integridad f integrity, wholeness, preservation
integrina f integrin
integumentario adj of skin
integumentario f integumentary, of skin
integumento m integument; ~ m **común** common integument
inteligencia f intelligence
intensidad f intensity, strength
intensificación f enhancement
intensificador m enhancer
interacción f interaction
intercambiabilidad f interchangeability
intercambio m exchange; ~ m **de cromosomas** chromosome exchange
intercostal adj intercostal, between the ribs
interfase f interphase
interferencia f interference
interferón m interferon; ~ m **alfa** leucocyte interferon, lymphoblast interferon, alpha interferon; ~ m **del fibroblasto** fibroblast interferon, beta interferon; ~ m **gamma** gamma interferon, immune interferon; ~ m **inmune** gamma interferon, immune interferon; ~ m **leucocitario** leucocyte interferon, lymphoblast interferon, alpha interferon
interindividual adj interindividual, between individuals
intermediario adj intermediary
intermitente adj intermittent
internación f Admissions (in the hospital)
internado m internship, a medical training course in hospital
interneurona f interneuron, internuncial neuron, association neuron

interno *adj* internal, inner; ~ *m* **de hospital** intern (in a hospital)

interpersonal *adj* interpersonal, between individuals

interposición *f* interposition

interpretación *f* interpretation, explanation

intérprete *m* interpreter; ~ *m* **autónomo** freelance interpreter; ~ *m* **para sordos** interpreter for the deaf

interrupción *f* interruption, break; ~ *f* **del embarazo** abortion, miscarriage; ~ *f* **génica** gene disruption

intersticial *adj* interstitial, in gaps between tissue

intertrigo *m* intertrigo, chafing

intervalo *m* range, interval, space; ~ *m* **analítico** lineality range; ~ *m* **de medida** measurement range, measuring interval; ~ *m* **de referencia** reference range; ~ *m* **QT** QT interval; ~ *m* **terapéutico** therapeutic range

intervascular *adj* intervascular, between vessels

intervención *f* intervention; ~ *f* **en la crisis** crisis intervention; ~ *f* **quirúrgica** surgical intervention

intervenir mediate, to

intervertebral *adj* intervertebral, between two adjacent vertebrae

intesidad *f* intensity; ~ *f* **luminosa** luminous intensity; ~ *f* **radiante** radiant intensity

intestinal *adj* intestinal

intestino *m* intestine; ~ *m* **delgado** small intestine; ~ *m* **grueso** large intestine; ~ *m* **mayor** large intestine; ~ *m* **pequeño** small intestine

intestinos *m pl* bowels; ~ *m pl* intestines

íntima-pía *f* intima-pia

intimidar *v* to bully

intolerancia *f* intolerance; ~ *f* **medica** medical intolerance; ~ *f* **religiosa** religious intolerance

intoxicación *f* intoxication, poisoning; ~ *f* **accidental** accidental poisoning; ~ *f* **alcohólica** alcohol poisoning; ~ *f* **alimentaria** food poisoning; ~ *f* **de la sangre** bloodpoisoning, sepsis, toxemia

intraaracnoide *adj* intra-arachnoid

intracapsular *adj* intracapsular

intradermotuberculinización *f* intradermal tuberculin test

intraindividual *adj* intraindividual, within the individual

intramolecular *adj* intramolecular

intramuscular *adj* intramuscular, within the muscle

intraocular *adj* intraocular, within the eye

intraoperatorio *adj* intraoperative, operative, during the operation

intraperitonal *adj* intraperitoneal

intratable *adj* obstreperous, unruly, rambuncious

intratecal *adj* intrathecal, within the thecal sac surrounding the spinal cord

intratraqueal *adj* intratracheal

intrauterino *adj* intra-uterine

intravascular *adj* intravascular, within a blood vessel

intravenoso *adj* intravenous, within a vein

intrínseco *adj* intrinsic, internal, inner

intrón *m* intron

introversión *f* introversion; ~ *f* **autista** autistic introversion

intrusión *f* intrusion

intubación *f* intubation, inserting a tube; ~ *f* **ciega** blind intubation, endotracheal intubation; ~ *f* **endotraqueal** endotracheal intubation; ~ *f* **gástrica** gastric intubation, nasogastric intubation, esophageal intubation; ~ *f* **gastrointestinal** gastric intubation, nasogastric intubation, esophageal intubation

intususcepción *f* intussusception

inulina *m* inuline

invalidar *v* to invalidate

invasión *f* invasion

invasivo *adj* invasive, involving an operation

invención *f* invention, discovery

inversión *f* inversion; ~ *f* **genética** genetic inversion; ~ *f* **uterina parcial** inversion of uterus during birth

investigación *f* detection, research, screening; ~ *f* **médica** medical research; ~ *f* **médico-social** medico-social research

investigador *m* investigator

investigar to research, to investigate, to examine

invierno *m* winter

involución f involution; ~ f **cerebral orgánica** organic cerebral involution; ~ f **tumorosa** tumorous involution

involucro m sheathing, involucrum

inyección f injection, shot; ~ f **de refuerzo** f booster shot, hypervaccination, revaccination; ~ f **en flujo** flow injection; ~ f **endoneural** intraneural injection, endoneural injection; ~ f **epidural** epidural injection; ~ f **intracutánea** intracutaneous injection, intradermal injection; ~ f **intradérmica** intracutaneous injection, intradermal injection; ~ f **intravenosa** intravenous injection; ~ f **peridural** peridural injection; ~ f **rápida** bolus infusion; ~ f **secundaria** booster shot, hypervaccination, revaccination; ~ f **subcutánea** subcutaneous injection; ~ f **suboccipital** suboccipital injection

inyector m **a presión** jet injector, Dermo-Jet injector, needleless injector

ioduro-peroxidasa f iodide peroxidase, iodinase

ion m ion; ~ m **anfótero** zwitterion, amphoteric ion, zwitter ion, hybrid ion, dipolar ion; ~ m **fragmento** fragment ion; ~ m **híbrido** hybrid ion, zwitterion, amphoteric ion, zwitter ion, dipolar ion; ~ m **hidrógeno** hydrogenion

ionisación f ionization; ~ f **química** chemical ionization

ionoforesis f iontophoresis

ionograma ionogram

ipecacuana f ipecac, emetic

ir v to go

irascible adj irritable, cranky, touchy, short-tempered, in a bad mood

iridociclitis f iridocyclitis, eye inflammation

iritis f iritis; ~ f **séptica** septic iritis

IRM f MRI, magnetic resonance imaging; ~ f **cerebral** cerebral MRI, magnetic resonance imaging of the brain, MRI of the brain

irracionalidad f irrationality

irradiación f irradiation; ~ f **accidental** accidental irradiation

irradiancia f irradiance

irradiar v to irradiate

irregular adj irregular, unusual, atypical

irregularidad f anomaly, abnormality, deviation

irreversible adj irreversible

irrigación f irrigation, wash, washing; ~ f **colónica** rectal injection, colonic lavage, colonic irrigation; ~ f **de una herida** irrigating a wound

irritable adj irritable, cranky, touchy, short-tempered, in a bad mood

irritación f irritation; ~ f **cutánea** skin irritation

irritado adj distraught, upset

iscuria f urine retention; ~ f **espasmódica** ischuria spastica

islotes m pl **de Langerhans** islets of Langerhans

isoaglutinina f isoagglutinin

isoamilasa f isoamylase

isoanafilaxia f iso-anaphylaxis

isoelectroenfoque m isoelectrofocusing

isoenzima m/f isoenzyme, isozyme

isoesquizómero m isoschizomer

isofluorfato m DFP, isofluorphate, diisopropyl fluorophosphate

isoforma f isoform

isoinmunización f iso-immunoreaction; ~ f **feto-materna** isoimmunization

isoleucina f isoleucine

isoniacida f isoniazid, isonicotinylhydrazine

isopicnosis f isopycnose

isópteras f pl isopters

isosmótico adj isosmotic

isoterapia f isotherapy

isotónico adj isotonic

isótopo adj isotope

isótopo m isotope; ~ m **radiactivo** radioisotope

isquemia f ischemia, inadequate blood flow; ~ f **intestinal** intestinal ischemia, bowel ischemia, ischemia of the colon; ~ f **miocardica** mycardial ischemia

isquicapsular adj ischiocapsular

isquiocele f ischiatic hernia

isquión m ischial bone, ischium

ístmico adj isthmic

istmo m isthmus; ~ m **del útero** isthmus uteri

iteración f iteration

iterón m iteron

itiocifosis f ithyokyphosis

itrio m yttrium, a chemical element

J

jabón *m* soap; ~ *m* **de afeitar** shaving soap; ~ *m* **de tocador** toilet soap, a bar of soap
jabonoso *adj* soapy
jadeante *adj* out of breath, puffing & panting
jadear *v* to gasp, to have trouble breathing
jadeo *m* gasping for breath, panting
jalar *v* to pull
jalea *f* jelly; ~ *f* **espermaticida** spermacidal jelly, vaginal jelly; ~ *f* **real** royal jelly (from bees)
jaqueca *f* migraine; ~ *f* **clásica** classic migraine; ~ *f* **de la arteria basilar** basilar migraine, basilar artery migraine
jarabe *m* syrup; ~ *m* **de glucosa** glucose syrup, corn syrup; ~ *m* **de ipecacuana** syrup of ipecac; ~ *m* **para la tos** cough syrup
jardín *m* garden; ~ *m* **de infancia** kindergarden; ~ *m* **de infantes** day care center, nursery school
jaspeado *m* pressure marking, mottling
jefa *f* **de turno** head nurse, charge nurse
jeringa *f* syringe; ~ *f* **de Janet** wound and bladder syringe, Janet syringe; ~ *f* **hipodérmica** hypodermic syringe, hypodermic needle
jeringuilla *f* syringe, needle; ~ *f* **desechable** disposable syringe; ~ *f* **heparinizada** heparinized syringe; ~ *f* **para heridas** wound and bladder syringe; ~ *f* **para irrigación** irrigation syringe, vesicle syringe; ~ *f* **para punciones** puncture syringe; ~ *f* **uterina** uterine syringe
jiote *m* skin lesion with scaling
jocosidad *f* humor, merriment, laughter, mirth
joroba *f* hunchback, humpbacked; ~ *f* **de búfalo** buffalo hump
joule *f* joule
joven *adj* young, juvenile
joven *m/f* adolescent, juvenile, young, teenager
joyas *f* pl jewelry
juanete *m* bunion
jueves *m* Thursday
jugo *m* juice; ~ *m* **de manzana** apple juice; ~ *m* **gástrico** gastric juice
juicio *m* judgement; ~ *m* **clínico** clinical judgement

julio *m* July
junio *m* June
juntura *f* joint; ~ *f* **cartilaginosa** cartilaginous joint, amphiarthrosis
juramento *m* oath; ~ *m* **hipocrático** Hippocratic oath
juvenil *adj* adolescent, juvenile, young, teenager

K

kala-azar *m* tropical splenomegaly, kala-azar, visceral leishmaniasis
kanamicina *f* kanamycin
kelvin kelvin
keratitis *f* keratitis; ~ *f* **puntiforme superficial** superficial punctuate keratitis
ketamina *f* ketamine
ketoconazol *m* ketoconazole
kilo *m* kilogram
kinesiólogo *m* kinesiologist, physical therapist
Klebsiella *f* **pneumoniae** Klebsiella pneumoniae

L

la píldora the pill, oral contraceptive
lábil *adj* unstable, labile
labio *m* lip; ~ *m* **cucho** hare lip, cleft lip, cleft palate, uranoschisis, cheiloschisis; ~ *m* **fisurado** hare lip, cleft lip, cheiloschisis; ~ *m* **leporino** hare lip, cleft lip, cheiloschisis; ~ *m* **superior** upper lip
labios *m* pl lips, labia; ~ *m* pl **agrietados** chapped lips; ~ *m* pl **partidos** chapped lips
laboratorio *m* laboratory; ~ *m* **clínico** clinical laboratory; ~ *m* **de bacteriología** bacteriology laboratory; ~ *m* **de criminalística** crime lab; ~ *m* **de ensayo** testing laboratory; ~ *m* **de patología** pathological laboratory, pathology laboratory; ~ *m* **de referencia** reference laboratory; ~ *m* **de urgencias** emergency laboratory; ~ *m* **de virología** virology laboratory; ~ *m* **médico** medical laboratory; ~ *m* **microbiología** microbiology laboratory, microbiological laboratory
laceración *f* laceration, tear (wound), flesh

wound

lactación f lactation, milk production, breast feeding, nursing a baby

lactancia f lactation; ~ f **materna** breast feeding, nursing a baby

lactante m/f breast-fed infant, baby, suckling

lactar v to lactate, to nurse, to suckle, to breast feed a baby

lactato m lactate; ~ m **de calcio** calcium lactate; ~ m **de magnesio** magnesium lactate; ~ m **de sodio** sodium lactate; ~ m **deshidrogenasa** LDH, lactate dehydrogenase; ~ m **sódico** sodium lactate

lactoalbúmina f milk protein

Lactobacillus m **acidophilus** Lactobacillus acidophilus, Döderlein's bacillus; ~ m **plantarum** Lactobacillus plantarum

lactoferrina f lactoferrin

lactogénesis f lactogenesis, galactopoiesis

lactogenio m lactogen; ~ m **placentario** placental lactogen, chorionic somatomammotropin

lactosa f lactose, milk sugar

ladilla f phthirus pubis

lágrima f tear (eye)

lagrimal adj lacrimal, tear-related, pertaining to tears

lágrimas f pl **artificiales** artificial tears, ophthalmic solution, eye drops

lambliasis f giardiasis, Giardia lamblia infection

lamentarse v to moan, to groan

lamer v lick, to

laminectomía f laminectomy

lamparones m pl skin lesions

lanceta f blood lancet; ~ f **para vacunar** lancet for vaccination; ~ f **ultrasónica** lancet

lanolina f lanolin, wool wax, wool grease

lansoprazol m lansoprazole

lanugo m lanugo, the downy hair covering a fetus

laparoscopia f laparoscopy, keyhole surgery

laparoscopio m lexible fiberscope, optical-fiber endoscope, laparoscope

laparotomía f laparotomy

larga adj long; ~ f **suboccipital** suboccipital injection; ~ f **vida** longevity, long life, length of life

largura f length

laringe f larynx, voicebox; ~ f **artificial** artificial larynx, artificial voicebox

laringectomía f laryngectomy

laringismo m laryngismus, laryngeal spasm

laringitis f laryngitis, sore throat, inflammation of throat

laringoscopio m laryngoscope; ~ m **fiberoptico** fiber optic laryngoscope; ~ m **rígido** rigid laryngoscope

laringospasmo m laryngeal spasm, spasm of the larynx

laringotraqueítis f acute laryngotracheobronchitis, croup, diphtheritic croup; ~ f **infecciosa** infectious laryngotracheitis

larva m **migrans** cutaneous larva migrans, creeping eruption

lascas f pl bone chips, bone fragments

láser m laser; ~ m **de electrones libres** free-electron laser; ~ m **de excímero** excimer laser

lasitud f lassitude, weariness, fatigue, exhaustion

lastimadura f lesion, injury, trauma, wound, affected area

lastimar v to injure, to harm, to abuse, to hurt, to wound

latencia f latency, dormancy, a period in which the infection is present in the host without producing overt symptoms

lateral adj lateral, sideway, towards the side

latido m beat, beating, throb, throbbing; ~ m **cardiaco** heart beat; ~ m **del corazón** pulsation, heartbeat; ~ m **rítmico** pulsation

latir v to throb

laurilsulfato m **de amonio** ammonium lauryl sulfate

lavado m lavage; ~ m **bronquial** bronchial lavage; ~ m **del estómago** gastric lavage; ~ m **del útero** uterine lavage, embryo flushing; ~ m **gástrico** gastric lavage; ~ m **tubárico** hydrotubation

lavativa f enema

laxante adj laxative, remedy for constipation, vacuant

laxitud f burnout, exhaustion, inability to cope, weariness

laxo adj flaccid, flabby, soft; ~ m sling (for arm)

lazo *m* knot, bow, lasso; ~ *m* **de inversión** inversion loop

L-dopa *f* L-dopa, levodopa, natural form of dopa & immediate precursor of dopamine

le her, him

leche *f* milk; ~ *f* **de vaca** cow's milk; ~ *f* **irradiada** irradiated milk; ~ *f* **materna** mother's milk, breast milk, milk from a woman's breast; ~ *f* **para lactantes** baby milk, infant milk, infant formula

lecho *m* **de muerte** deathbed

lecitina *f* phosphatidylcholine

lectura *f* reading; ~ *f* **mínima** readability

leer *v* to read

legrado *m* curettage, D&C, abrasion, scraping off; ~ *m* **uterino** uterine curettage, uterine abrasion

leiomioma *m* leiomyoma; ~ *m* **uterino** uterine leiomyoma

leiomiosarcoma *m* leiomyosarcoma

leishmaniasis *f* leishmaniasis, Leishmania infection; ~ *f* **cutaneomucosa americana** espundia, mucocutaneous leishmaniasis americana, pian-bois; ~ *f* **cutánea** cutaneous leishmaniasis; ~ *f* **visceral** tropical splenomegaly, kala-azar, visceral leishmaniasis

lejía *f* lye, caustic soda, bleach; ~ *f* **de sosa** lye, caustic soda, sodium hydroxide; ~ *f* **sódica** sodium lye, soda lye

lejías *f pl* **residuales al sulfito** sulphite waste liquor, sulfite waste liquor (a byproduct of the paper industry)

lencería *f* underwear

lengua *f* tongue; ~ *f* **geográfica** geographic tongue, benign migratory glossitis, exfoliatio areata linguae; ~ *f* **materna** mother tongue

lenguaje *m* language; ~ *m* **corporal** mime, body language, facial expression; ~ *m* **hablado** spoken language; ~ *m* **infantil** infantile language, baby talk

lente *f* lens; ~ *f* **de contacto** contact lens

lentes *f pl* glasses; ~ *f pl* **binoculares** binocular magnifying glass, binocular loupe; ~ *f pl* **gas-permeables** gas-permeable lenses

lenticular *adj* lenticular, related to a lens, lentil shaped

lentificador *m* silencer

léntigo *m* pigmentary mole, naevus pigmentosus, lentigo; ~ *m* **de vejez** senile lentigo, liver spots

lepra *f* leprosy, Hansen's disease

leptospira *m* **de Noguchi** Noguchi leptospira

leptospirosis *f* leptospirosis, Weil's disease, infectious jaundice

leptotena *f* leptotene

lesbiana *f* lesbian

lesión *f* injury, lesion; ~ *f* **a la cabeza** head injury; ~ *f* **cardíaca** cardiac defect; ~ *f* **cerebral** brain damage brain dysfunction, intracranial disorder; ~ *f* **de ligamentos** torn ligamnet; ~ *f* **de los nervios periféricos** peripheral nerve injury; ~ *f* **del latigazo** whiplash; ~ *f* **del menisco** tear of the meniscus, meniscus rupture; ~ *f* **fetal** fetal injury, fetal damage; ~ *f* **glomerular** glomerular lesion; ~ *f* **interna por golpe** bruise, bruising, contusion; ~ *f* **laboral** occupational injury, industrial injury, accident at work; ~ *f* **mortal** fatal injury, fatality, fatal accident; ~ *f* **neoplásica** neoplastic lesion; ~ *f* **obstétrica** birth injury, birth trauma; ~ *f* **ocular** eye injury, ocular injury; ~ *f* **reumática temprana** early rheumatic lesion

letal *adj* lethal

letargo *m* latency, dormancy, lethargy

leucemia *f* leukemia; ~ *f* **aguda** acute leukemia; ~ *f* **aguda linfoide** acute lymphocytic leukemia, acute B-cell leukemia; ~ *f* **aguda mieloide** acute myeloid leukemia, AML; ~ *f* **granulocítica crónica** chronic leucemia aguda mieloide, chronic granulocytic leukemia; ~ *f* **indiferenciada** undifferentiated leukemia; ~ *f* **linfática** lymphoblast leukemia (ALL), lymphogenous leukaemia, lymphoid leukemia; ~ *f* **linfocítica** lymphoblast leukemia (ALL), lymphogenous leukaemia, lymphoid leukemia; ~ *f* **linfógena** lymphoblast leukemia (ALL), lymphogenous leukaemia, lymphoid leukemia; ~ *f* **linfoide** lymphoblast leukemia (ALL), lymphogenous leukaemia, lymphoid leukemia; ~ *f* **linfoide crónica** chronic lymphocytic leukemia, chronic B-cell leukemia; ~ *f* **mieloblástica** acute myeloblast leukemia, myelocytic leukemia; ~ *f* **mieloblástica crónica** chronic myelogenous leukemia; ~ f **mielocítica** myeloid leukemia, myelocytosis, myelocitic leukemia; ~ f **mielógena** myeloid leukemia, myelocytosis, myelogenous leukemia; ~ f **mieloide** myeloid leukemia; ~ f **mielomonocítica** myelomonocytic leukemia; ~ f **monoblástica** AMOL, monoblast leukemia; ~ f **neutrofílica crónica** chronic neutrophilic leukemia

leucil-aminopeptidasa f leucine aminopeptidase, leucyl aminopeptidase, leucyl peptidase

leucina f leucine

leucocítico adj leukocytic, white blood cell-related

leucocito m leucocyte, white blood cell, leukocyte, WBC; ~ m **neutrofilo** neutrophil, white blood cell; ~ m **polimorfonuclear** polymorphonuclear leukocyte

leucocitosis f leukocytosis, increased white blood cell count; ~ f **reactiva** reactive leucocytosis

leucodermia f leukoderma, achromia, localized depigmentation

leucoencefalopatía f leukoencephalopathy; ~ f **multifocal progresiva** progressive multifocal leukoencephalopathy

leucopenia f leukopenia, reduced white blood cell count

leucoplaquia f leukoplakia, leukoplasia, white patch on a mucous membrane, leukokeratosis

leucoplasia f leukoplasia, white patch on a mucous membrane, leukokeratosis; ~ f **del fumador** smokers' leukoplakia, smoker's tongue precancerous condition

leucoqueratosis f leukoplakia, leukoplasia, white patch on a mucous membrane, leukokeratosis

leucorrea f leukorrhea, vaginal discharge, fluor albus

levantamiento m lifting; ~ m **de pesos** weight lifting

levantar v to get up, to stand up

levodopa m L-dopa, levodopa, natural form of dopa & immediate precursor of dopamine

levonorgestrel m levonorgestrel

liasa f lyase

liberación f release, liberation; ~ f **del**

compuesto activo release of the active component

líbido f libido, sexual impulse; ~ f **disminuida** reduced libido, decreased sex drive

libre adj free

licofelone m licofelone, antiinflammatory osteoarthritis treatment

licopeno m lycopene, red pigment & antioxidant found in tomatoes, isomeric with carotene

licor m liquid, liquor, fluid, solution

lidocaína f lidocaine

L-iduronidasa f L-iduronidase

ligación f ligation

ligador m linker

ligadura f ligation, ligature; ~ f **tubarica** tubal ligation, tubal ligature, having her tubes tied

ligamento m ligament; ~ m **cruciforme** cruciate ligament; ~ m **peroneoastragalino** tibiofibular ligament

ligamentoso adj desmoid, ligamentous

ligamiento m linkage

ligando m ligand; ~ m **biológico** biological ligand

ligatura f ligation, ligature; ~ f **de las trompas** tubal ligation, tubal ligature, having her tubes tied

ligero adj light, mild

límbico adj limbic, edge-related, border

limfoedema m lymphoedema, lymphedema, limitación f limitation, limit

límite m limitation, limit; ~ m **de detección** detection limit, limit of detection, sensitivity; ~ m **de referencia** reference limit

limón m lemon

limpiador m cleaner; ~ m **de tuberia** drain cleaner; ~ m **de baños** toilet cleaner

limpiar v to clean

limpiarse los dientes to brush one's teeth

limpieza f cleaning

lincomicina f lincomycin

línea f line; ~ f **celular** cell line; ~ f **celular leucémica** leukemia cell line; ~ f **de base** baseline; ~ f **de precipitación** precipitin line

linealidad f linearity

linear adj linear

líneas f pl stretch marks, striae; ~ f pl **glabellares** glabellar lines

lineico adj lineic

linfa f lymph, plasma, normal body fluid
linfadenectomía f lymphadenectomy, adenotomy
linfadenitis f lymphadenitis
linfadenopatía f lymphadenopathy, lymph node disease, swollen lymph glands
linfangioleiomiomatosis f lymphangioleiomyomatosis
linfangitis f lymphangitis, lymphatic vessel inflammation
linfoblasto m lymphoblast
linfocina f lymphokine
linfocítico adj lymphocytic, white blood cell-related
linfocito m lymphocyte, lymphoid cell, lymphoid leucocyte; ~ m B B cell, B lymphocyte; ~ m **coadyuvante** helper lymphocyte; ~ m **colaborador** helper lymphocyte, helper cell, T4 cell; ~ m **de sangre periférica** peripheral blood lymphocyte; ~ m **folicular** follicle lymphocyte; ~ m **maduro** mature lymphocyte; ~ m T T lymphocyte, T-cell; ~ m T **citotóxico** killer T cell, cytotoxic T lymphocyte, cytotoxic T cell; ~ m T **supresor** suppressor T cell; ~ m T4 helper lymphocyte, helper cell, T4 cell
linfocitoma m lymphocytic lymphoma, lymphocytoma
linfocitosis f lymphocytosis; ~ f **del hambre** hunger lymphocytosis
linfogranuloma m lymphogranuloma; ~ m **venéreo** venereal lymphogranuloma, lymphogranuloma venereum
linfoide adj lymphoid
linfokina f lymphokine
linfoma m lymphoma, cancer of the lymph system; ~ m **asintomático de bajo grado** asymptomatic low-grade lymphoma; ~ m **cerebral** cerebral lymphoma, brain lymphoma; ~ m **de Burkitt** Burkitt's lymphoma, non-Hodgkin's lymphoma caused by the Epstein-Barr virus; ~ m **de célula T cutáneo** cutaneous T-cell lymphoma; ~ m **difuso** diffuse lymphoma, lymphosarcoma; ~ m **linfocítico** lymphocytic lymphoma; ~ m **maligna** malignant lymphoma; ~ m **no Hodgkiniano** non-Hodgkin's lymphoma

linfonódulos m pl lymphnoduli, lymph nodules, lymph glands
linfopatía f **venérea** lymphogranuloma venereum
linfosarcoma m diffuse lymphoma, lymphosarcoma
linfotoxina f lymphotoxin, substance released by lymphocytes that is cytotoxic to other cells
linterna f **de bolsillo** penlight
liofilización f lyophilization, freeze-drying
lipasa f lipase; ~ f **pancreática** pancreatic lipase
lípido adj fat; ~ m lipid
lipodistrofia f lipodystrophy, fat metabolism disturbance
lipofibroma m fibrolipoma, lipofibroma
lipófilo adj lipophilic, with an affinity for fat
lipolisis f lipolysis, breakdown of fat
lipoma m lipoma, a benign fatty tumor
lipomatosis f lipomatosis
lipomatoso adj lipomatous, characterized by the presence of a lipoma
lipoproteína f lipoprotein, complex of fat and protein; ~ f **de baja densidad** LDL, low-density lipoprotein; ~ **–lipasa** f clearing factor lipase
liposoluble adj lipo-soluble, fat-soluble, soluble in fat
liposoma m liposome, fatty or oily globule
liposucción f liposuction
lipotropina f lipotropic hormone
liquenificación f lichenification, skin hardening and thickening
líquido adj liquid, fluid, solution
líquido m fluid; ~ m **amniótico** amniotic fluid; ~ m **ascítico** ascitic fluid; ~ m **biológico** biological fluid, body fluid; ~ m **cefalorraquídeo** cerebrospinal fluid; ~ m **cerebroespinal** cerebrospinal fluid; ~ m **espinal** spinal fluid; ~ m **extracelular** extracellular fluid, extracellular liquid; ~ m **intracelular** intracelular fluid; ~ m **pericárdico** pericardial fluid; ~ m **peritoneal** peritoneal fluid; ~ m **pleural** pleural fluid; ~ m **prostático** prostatic fluid; ~ m **sinovial** joint fluid, synovial fluid; ~ m **tisular** tissue fluid
lisina f lysine
lisis f lysis, process of disintegration or dissolution (of cells); ~ f **ósea** bone lysis

liso *adj* smooth

lisogenia *f* lysogeny, lysogenicity, relationship between a temperate bacteriophage & a bacterium

lisogénico *adj* lysogenic

lisosoma *m* lysosome, cellular organelle that contains various hydrolytic enzymes, present in almost all cells

lisozima *f* lysozyme, in saliva, important antibacterial defence,

lista *f* list; ~ **f de comprobaciones** check list; ~ **f de espera** waiting list

listeria *f* listeria

listeriosis *f* listeriosis, Listeria monocytogenes infection

litiasis *f* nasal rhinolith, nasal calculus; ~ **f salival** salivary calculi, salivary calculus

lítico *adj* lytic, pertaining to cell destruction

lítico *m* lithium

litotripsia *f* lithotripsy; ~ **f extracorporal con onda de choque** extracorporeal shock-wave lithotripsy; ~ **f percutánea ultrasónica** percutaneous ultrasonic lithotripsy

litro *m* liter

livedo *m* livedo, mottling; ~ **f reticularis** cutis marmorata

lividez *f* lividity

lívido *adj* livid, grayish blue, black & blue

livor *m* mortis livor mortis, postmortem lividity

L-lactato-deshidrogenasa *f* lactic acid dehydrogenase

llaga *f* sore

llenado *m* filling; ~ **m vesical** fullness of the bladder

llenar *v* to fill, to run

lleno *adj* full

llorar *v* to cry

llorón *m* whiner, crybaby

llorona *f* whiner, crybaby

lluvia *f* rain

lo mismo same

lobectomía *f* lobectomy; ~ **f cerebral** cerebral lobectomy; ~ **f temporal bilateral** bilateral temporal lobectomy

lóbulo *m* lobe; ~ **m de la oreja** earlobe; ~ **m frontal** frontal lobe; ~ **m hepático** hepatic lobe; ~ **m inferior** lower lobe; ~ **m temporal** temporal lobe

local *adj* local, topical, regional, applied to the surface; ~ **m en cuarentena** quarantine station, isolation place

localidad *f* town

localización *f* localization, locating

localizar *v* to detect, to discover

loción *f* lotion; ~ **f para los ojos** eye drops, eyewash, collyrium

loco *m* maniac, lunatic, disturbed person

locomotor *m* locomotor, pertaining to movement, movement-related

locorregional *adj* locoregional

locura *f* **de desdoblamiento** schizophrenia

locus *m* locus; ~ **m complejo** complex locus

logit logit

logopedia *f* speech pathology, language pathology

logoterapeuta *m* **médico** speech therapist

logoterapia *f* speech therapy, speech training

lombriz *f* worm; ~ **f intestinal** intestinal parasite, parasitic worm

lomefloxacina *f* lomefloxacin

lomo *m* loin, upper part of back (usually an animal term)

longevidad *f* longevity, long life, length of life

longitud *f* length; ~ **f de onda** wavelength

loquaz *adj* talkative, loquacious, chatty

loquios *m* pl lochia, post-birth vaginal discharge

loracepam *m* lorazepam, anxiolytic benzodiazepine, ativan

loratidina *f* loratidine

los dos both

lovastatina *f* lovastatin

lúbrico *adj* slippery, oily, greasy

luciferasa *f* luciferase

luético *adj* luetic, syphilitis-related, pertaining to syphilitis

lugar *m* place; ~ **m de nacimiento** place of birth

luliberina *f* LH-RFL, luteinizing hormone-releasing factor, luliberin

lumbago *m* lumbago

lumbalgia *f* back pain, backache

lumbar *adj* lumbar

lumen *m* lumen, inside of a tube

luminiscencia *f* luminiscence

luminoinmunoanálisis *m* luminiscence immunoassay, luminoimmunoassay

luminómetro *m* luminometer

lunes *m* Monday

lupa *f* magnifying glass; ~ *f* binocular binocular loupe, binocular magnifying glass

lupia *f* encysted tumor

lupino *m* lupus, systemic lupus erythematosus

lupus *m* lupus; ~ *m* eritematoso discoide discoid lupus erythematosus; ~ *m* eritematoso diseminado disseminated lupus erythematosus; ~ *m* eritematoso sistémico systemic lupus erythematosus, SLE

luto *m* grief, grieving

lutropina *f* instertitial cell-stimulating hormone, luteinizing hormone, lutropin, LH

luxación *f* luxation, dislocation, moving out of position, sprain, torsion; ~ *f* de la clavícula luxation of the clavicle; ~ *f* de la muñeca wrist luxation, radiocarpal joint luxation; ~ *f* de la rótula luxation of the patella, dislocation of the kneecap; ~ *f* espontánea por distensión spontaneous distension luxation; ~ *f* por distensión distension luxation; ~ *f* radiocarpiana wrist luxation, radiocarpal joint luxation; ~ *f* temporomaxilar luxation of the temporomandibular joint

M

maceración *f* maceration, soaking, softening of tissues

machismo *m* machismo, sexism, male chauvinism

macindol *f* mazindol

macizo *adj* massive, solid

macrobiótico *m* macrobiotic

macrocefalia *f* macrocephaly, megalencephaly

macrocitemia *f* macrocythemia, macrocytosis, megalocytosis

macrocitosis *f* macrocythemia, macrocytosis, megalocytosis

macroconidia *f* macroconidia

macrófago *m* macrophage; ~ *m* para cuerpos extraños foreign body macrophage; ~ *m* alveolar alveolar macrophage, alveolar phagocyte, dust cell

macrofitas *f* pl macrophytes

macroglobulina *f* macroglobulin

macroglobulinemia *f* macroglobulinemia

macrólido *m* macrolide

macromolécula *f* macromolecule; ~ *f* biológica biological macromolecule

macrón *m* macron, macroscopic particle

macroscópico *adj* macroscopic

mácula *f* macule, small, flat spot; ~ *f* lútea macula lutea, yellow spot on retina

macular *v* to stain, to color

maculopapular *adj* maculopapular

madre *f* mother; ~ *f* lactante nursing mother, breastfeeding mother; ~ *f* portadora surrogate mother; ~ *f* subrogada surrogate mother

maduración *f* ripening; ~ *f* del folículo follicle ripening; ~ *f* del RNA RNA processing

madurez *f* maturity

magnesio *m* magnesium

magnitud *f* quantity; ~ *f* adimensional dimensionless quantity; ~ *f* biológica biological quantity; ~ *f* bioquímica biochemical quantity; ~ *f* de base base quantity; ~ *f* derivada derived quantity; ~ *f* influyente influence quantity; ~ *f* relativa relative quantity; ~ **particular** particular quantity

magro *adj* underweight, skinny, too thin

magulladura *f* bruise, bruising, contusion

mal, malo *adj* bad, evil

mal *adv* badly, wrongly, *m* malady, illness, disease; ~ *m* aliento bad breath, halitosis; ~ *m* articulado slurred speech, slurred articulation; ~ *m* de altura altitude sickness; ~ *m* de descompresión decompression sickness; ~ *m* de hiel gall bladder disease; ~ *m* de ijar pain in the side, stitches in the side, flank pain; ~ *m* de montaña mountain sickness; ~ *m* del apendice appendicitis; ~ *m* parto miscarriage, spontaneous abortion

mala *f* cama miscarriage, spontaneous abortion; ~ *f* nutrición malnutrition, inanition; ~ *f* respuesta inmunitaria dysfunction of the immune response

malabsorción *f* malabsorption, poor digestion; ~ *f* de glucosa y galactosa glucose-galactose malabsorption malapareamiento m mismatch

malaria f malaria

maldivisión f misdivision

maléolo m ankle joint

malestar m malaise, vague illness, discomfort, uneasiness; ~ m postural postural discomfort

maletín m de urgencia first aid kit, first aid chest

malformación f malformation; ~ f estructural structural anomaly

malignidad f malignancy, potential of a tumor to metastasize, cancerous tumor

maligno adj pernicious, malignant, fatal, harmful

malla f metálica stent wire mesh stent; ~ f para cirugía surgical mesh, a woven synthetic fabric of open texture used in surgery for repair, reconstruction or substitution of tissue

malmandado adj obstreperous, unruly, rambunctious

malnutrición f malnutrition; ~ f proteico-calórica protein-calorie malnutrition, protein-caloric malnutrition; ~ f secundaria secondary malnutrition

malo adj bad

malsano adj morbid, unhealthy

maltodextrina f maltodextrin, dextri-maltose

mama f breast

mamadera f baby bottle, nursing bottle, infants' feeding bottle

mamario adj mammary, breast-related, pertaining to the breasts

mamelón m nipple f

mamila f nipple m

mamilar adj nipple-related, mammillar

mamografía f mammography

mamograma m mammography screening, breast cancer screening, mammogram

mamoplastía f breast surgery mammaplasty

mañana f morning, tomorrow

mancha f macule, small spot, staining; ~ f amarilla macula lutea, yellow spot on retina; ~ f roja de nacimiento red birthmark, port-wine stain, naevus

manchar v to stain, to color

manchas f pl spots; ~ f pl de café con leche café au lait spots

mandíbula f jaw, mandible, lower jawbone

manejo m management; ~ m de casos case management, patient management

manguito m cuff, bandlike fibrous tissue surrounding joint; ~ m de presión cuff; ~ m del rotador rotator cuff

maní m peanut

manía f mania

maníaco adj manic

maníaco m maniac, lunatic, disturbed person

maniático adj fastidious, fussy

manifestación f phenomenon

manifiesto adj manifest, visible, evident

maniobra f maneuver, skilled manual procedure; ~ f de Heimlich Heimlich maneuver; ~ f de Valsalva Valsalva's maneuver

manipulación f manipulation; ~ f genética genetic engineering, genetic manipulation; ~ f génica gene manipulation

manipular v to manipulate, to handle

mano f hand

manometría f manometry; ~ f del intestino delgado manometry of the small intestine; ~ f esofágica esophageal manometry

manopla f washcloth, bath mitt

manosa f mannose

manotear v to gesticulate

manteca f lard

mantequilla f butter

manual adj manual

manual m manual; ~ m de procedimientos procedures manual

manubrio m manubrium

manzana f apple

mapa m map; ~ m peptídico peptide map; ~ m cromosómico genetic map, chromosome map; ~ m genético genetic map, chromosome map

mapeo m cerebral brain mapping

maquillarse v to put on make-up, to do one's face; ~ f machine, apparatus

marasmo m marasmus, cachexia; ~ m nutricional nutritional marasmus

marca f mark; ~ f de nacimiento birthmark, nevus, naevus

marcado adj labelling; ~ m génico gene tagging

marcador *m* marker; ~ *m* **genético** genetic marker; ~ *m* **indirecto** surrogate marker; ~ *m* **linfocitario** lymphocyte marker; ~ *m* **tumoral** tumor marker

marcaje *m* **terminal** end-labeling

marcapaso *m* pacemaker

marcapasos *m* **cardíaco** cardiac pacemaker

marcas *f pl* **de presión** pressure marking, mottling

marcha *f* gait; ~ *f* **atáxica** ataxic gait; ~ *f* **cerebelosa** cerebellar gait, staggering; ~ *f* **de funámbulo** heel to toe; ~ *f* **hemiplégica** hemiplegic gait; ~ *f* **inestable** unsteady gait, staggering gait; ~ *f* **sobre los talones** walking on one's heels, pes calcaneus

marco *m* **de lectura** reading frame; ~ *m* **de lectura cerrado** closed reading frame

mareado *adj* light-headed, dizzy, woozy, lightheadedness

mareos *m* dizziness, vertigo

marihuana *f* marijuana

marrón *adj* brown

martes *m* Tuesday

marzo *m* March

más *adv* more; ~ **que** *adv* more than; ~ **o menos** so so; ~ **pequeño** minimal; ~ **tarde** later

masa *f* mass, concentration; ~ *f* **anexial** adnexal tumor, adnexal mass; ~ *f* **atómica** atomic mass; ~ *f* **atómica relativa** relative atomic mass; ~ *f* **coagulada** coagulated mass, cruor; ~ *f* **corporal** body weight; ~ *f* **de tejidos blandos** mass of soft tissue; ~ *f* **molar** molar mass; ~ *f* **molecular** molecular mass; ~ *f* **molecular relativa** relative molecular mass; ~ *f* **ósea** bone density, bone mass; ~ *f* **pelviana** pelvic mass; ~ *f* **sanguínea** vascular mole, blood mole; ~ *f* **volúmica** volumic mass

masaje *m* massage; ~ *m* **cardíaco** cardiac massage, heart massage; ~ *m* **cardíaco externo** external cardiac compression, heart massage, closed chest cardiac massage; ~ *m* **de la espalda** back massage, backrub; ~ *m* **del dorso** back massage, backrub; ~ *m* **facial** facial massage

masajista *f* massage therapist

máscara *f* mask; ~ *f* **de protección respiratoria** respiratory mask, protective breathing gear, breathing apparatus; ~ *f* **para reanimación** resuscitation mask; ~ *f* **protectora** surgical mask

mascarilla *f* **respiratoria** respiratory mask, protective breathing gear, breathing apparatus

masculinidad *f* virilism, masculinity

masculinización *f* virilization, masculinization

masculino *adj* virile, manly, masculine, male

másico *adj* massic

masivo *adj* massive, solid

mastectomía *f* mastectomy; ~ *f* **segmenta** lumpectomy, tylectomy

masticable *adj* chewable

masticación *f* mastication, chewing; ~ *f* **de la hoja de coca** chewing coca leaves

masticar *v* to chew

masticatorio *m* masticatory, chewing-related

mastitis *f* mastitis, sore breasts

mastocito *m* mast cell, mastocyte; ~ *m* **tisular** connective tissue mastocyte

mastodinia *f* breast pain, mazodynia, mastodynia

mastoiditis *f* mastoiditis, inner ear infection

mastopatía *f* **fibroquística** fibrocystic mastitis, disease of the breast

masturbación *f* masturbation

masturbarse *v* to masturbate

mata *f* **de pelo** tuft of hair

matarse *v* to commit suicide

matasanos *m* quack, charlatan, fraud

materia *f* materia; ~ *f* **gris del cerebro** gray matter in the brain; ~ *f* **médica** materia medica, homeopathic pharmacology

material *m* material; ~ *m* **de calibración** calibration material; ~ *m* **de control** control material; ~ *m* **de referencia** reference material

matón *m* bully

matraz *m* flask; ~ *m* **aforado** calibrated flask, volumetric flask; ~ *m* **de Erlenmeyer** conical flask, Erlenmeyer flask; ~ *m* **de filtración** filter flask

matriz *f* matrix, basic material, cast; ~ *f* **del pelo** dermal papilla, hair bulb, hair matrix; ~ *f* **extracelular** extracellular matrix

matrona *f* midwife, birth attendant

maxilar *adj* maxillary, pertaining to the upper jaw; ~ *m* **inferior** lower jawbone, mandible; ~ *m* **superior** upper jaw, jawbone

máxima *f* **mejoría médica** maximum medical improvement

máximo *adj* maximal; ~ *m* maximum; ~ *m* **mejoramiento médico** MMI, Maximum Medical Improvement; ~ **error** *m* **tolerable** maximal allowable error

mayo *m* May

mayor *f* **parte (de)** most

me me

mecánica *f* mechanics; ~ *f* **pulmonar** pulmonary mechanics, lung mechanics, respiratory mechanics; ~ *f* **respiratoria** pulmonary mechanics, lung mechanics, respiratory mechanics

mecanismo *m* mechanism; ~ *m* **de casete** cassette mechanism; ~ *m* **de defensa** defense mechanism

mecanización *f* mechanization

mecanorreceptor *m* mechanoreceptor

mecisteína *f* methyl-cisteine

meconio *m* meconium, first fetal excretion of a newborn

media *f* **(aritmética)** mean

mediador *m* mediator

medial *adj* median, average

mediana *adj* average, median

mediante by

mediar *v* to mediate

mediastino *m* mediastinum, inter-pleural cavity, mediastinal cavity

medicación *f* medication, medicament, medicine

medicado *adj* medicated, medicinal

medicamentar *v* to medicate, to treat with medicine

medicamento *m* pharmacon, drug, medicament, medicine; ~ *m* **a base de** medication based on; ~ *m* **activo** active medicament; ~ *m* **confeccionado** preparation; ~ *m* **de alta tecnología** technology medicinal product; ~ *m* **de largo período de utilización** medicine

for long-term use; ~ *m* **de uso humano** medicine for human use; ~ *m* **genérico** generic medication, generic medicine; ~ *m* **homeopático** homeopathic remedy; ~ *m* **OTC** OTC, over-the-counter drug, non-prescription medication

medicar *v* to medicate, to treat with medicine

medicina *f* medication, medicament, medicine; ~ *f* **alternativa** alternative medicine, non-conventional medicine; ~ *f* **de grupo** collective medical practice, group practice; ~ *f* **del trabajo** industrial medicine, occupational medicine; ~ *f* **espacial** space medicine, aerospace medicine; ~ *f* **deportiva** sports medicine; ~ *f* **hiperbárica** hyperbaric medicine; ~ *f* **hospitalaria** hospital-based medicine; ~ *f* **intensiva** acute care, intensive care; ~ *f* **interna** internal medicine; ~ *f* **laboral** industrial medicine, occupational medicine; ~ *f* **legal** forensic medicine, legal medicine, medical jurisprudence; ~ *f* **nuclear** nuclear medicine; ~ *f* **paralela** alternative medicine, non-conventional medicine; ~ *f* **preventiva** predictive medicine; ~ *f* **social** social medicine; ~ *f* **veterinaria** veterinary medicine

medicinal *adj* medicated, medicinal

medicinar *v* to medicate, to treat with medicine

medición *f* measurement; ~ *f* **de la tensión arterial** blood pressure measuring

médico *adj* medical; ~ *m* doctor, physician; ~ *m* **adscrito** attending physician, treating physician; ~ *m* **asesor** medical officer, examining doctor, medical examiner; ~ *m* **asistente** physician's assistant, PA; ~ *m* **autorizado** panel doctor, approved medical practitioner; ~ *m* **consultante** consulting physician; ~ *m* **curante** attending physician, treating physician; ~ *m* **de atención primaria** primary care physician; ~ *m* **de aviación** flight surgeon; ~ *m* **de cabecera** general practitioner; ~ *m* **de consulta** consulting physician; ~ *m* **de familia** family

doctor; ~ *m* **de la empresa** company doctor;
~ *m* **de urgencia** emergency physician;
~ *m* **especialista** medical specialist;
~ *m* **generalista** general practitioner;
~ *m* **intensivista** critical care physician;
~ *m* **principal** primary care physician;
~ *m* **solicitante** requesting doctor;
~ *m* **tratante** attending physician, treating physician

medida *f* measurement, measure

medidas *f pl* **de precaución** precautionary measures

medio, –a *adj* half

medio *m* medium, means, substance, middle;
~ *m* **conservante** preservation medium;
~ *m* **de aislamiento** isolation medium; ~ *m* **de contraste** contrast medium (barium or iodine); ~ *m* **de cultivo** culture medium;
~ *m* **de diferenciación** differentation medium; ~ *m* **de enriquecimiento** enrichment medium; ~ *m* **de reanimación** resuscitation medium; ~ *m* **de transporte** transport medium; ~ *m* **para motilidad** motility medium; ~ *m* **preparado** ready-to-use medium; ~ *m* **seco** dry medium

medir *v* to measure

medula *f* marrow, medulla; ~ *f* **dorsal** spinal cord; ~ *f* **espinal** spinal cord; ~ *f* **oblongata** myelencephalon, medulla oblongata; ~ *f* **ósea** bone marrow; ~ *f* **roja** red bone marrow

medular *adj* medullary, marrow-related

meduloblastoma *m* medulloblastoma

megacarioblasto *m* megakaryoblast

megacariocito *m* megakaryocyte

megacolon *m* megacolon, colon enlargement;
~ *m* **congénito** congenital colectasia, Hirschsprung disease

megaencefalia *f* macrocephaly, megalencephaly

megaloblástico *adj* megaloblastic, large abnormal red blood cell

megalocitosis *f* macrocythemia, macrocytosis, megalocytosis

megalomanía *f* megalomania, delusions of grandeur

megalouréter *m* megaloureter, congenital megaureter

megauréter *m* megaureter, congenital megaureter

meiosis *f* meiosis

mejilla *f* cheek

mejor *adj* better

melamina *f* **formaldehído** melamine formaldehyde

melanina *f* melanin, pigment produced in a melanocyte

melanoblasto *m* melanoblast, precursor of a melanocyte or melanophore

melanocarcinoma *m* malignant melanoma, naevo-carcinoma, melanoblastoma

melanocítica *adj* melanocytic

melanocito *m* melanocyte, epidermal cell that produces melanin

melanodermia *f* melanoderma; ~ *f* **del arsénico** arsenic melanosis

melanófagos *m pl* melanophages, histiocytes that have phagocytosed melanin

melanoliberina *f* melanotropin-releasing factor, MFR

melanoma *m* melanoma, skin melanoma;
~ *m* **maligno** malignant melanoma

melanosis *f* melanosis, abnormal pigmentation

melanostatina *f* melanotropin release-inhibiting factor

melanotropina *f* MSH, melanocyte-stimulating hormone

melanuria *f* melanuria, the presence of melanins in the urine

melatonina *f* melatonin, a hormone secreted by the pineal gland

melena *f* melaena, blood-stained stools

melfalan *m* melphalan, melphalanum, sarcolysine

mella *f* nick

melocotón *m* peach

membrana *f* membrane; ~ *f* **alantoidea** allantoic membrane; ~ *f* **basilar** basilar membrane; ~ *f* **celular** cell membrane, cell surface; ~ *f* **flácida** flaccid part of tympanic membrane; ~ *f* **lipídica** lipid membrane; ~ *f* **mucosa** mucous membrane; ~ *f* **obturatriz** obturator membrane; ~ *f* **plasmática** plasma membrane, plasma lemma, outer membrane; ~ *f* **presináptica** presynaptic membrane; ~ *f* **sinovial** synovium, joint-lubricating membrane, synovial membrane

memoria f memory; ~ f **declarativa** explicit memory, declarative memory; ~ f **explícita** explicit memory, declarative memory; ~ **implícita** implicit memory, procedural memory; ~ f **inmunológica** immunological memory; ~ f **visual** visual memory

menarca f menarche, first period, first menses

menarquía f menarche, first period, first menses

meninges f pl meninges

meningioma m meningiome, meningioma

meningitis f meningitis; ~ f **aséptica** aseptic meningitis, viral meningitis; ~ f **basal** basilar meningitis; ~ f **cerebroespinal** cerebrospinal meningitis; ~ f **cerebroespinal epidémica** meningococcal cerebrospinal meningitis, meningococcal meningitis; ~ f **concomitante** concomitant meningitis; ~ f **espinal** spinal meningitis, perimyelitis; ~ f **viral** aseptic meningitis, viral meningitis

meningocele m meningocele, meningeal herniation

meningo–encefalitis f amoebic meningoencephalitis

meniscectomía f diskectomy, surgical removal of an intervertebral disk

menisco m meniscus (plural, menisci)

menopausia f climacterium, menopause; ~ f **precoz** early menopause, climacterium praecox

menopáusico adj menopausal

menores m pl **de edad** minors, not yet of age

menorragia f menorrhagia, heavy periods

menos less

menotropina f menotropin

mensajero m messenger; ~ m **proteinico** protein messenger

menstruación f menstruation, periods; ~ f woman's period, menstrual flow, menstration, periods

mental adj mental, physic

mentón m chin

meperidina f meperidine, isonipecaine, pethidine

mercadotecnia f marketing

mercurio m Hg, mercury, quicksilver; ~ m **colloidal** colloidal mercury

mericismo m rumiación

merienda f supper, tea

merolico m medicine man, witch doctor

mes m month

mesa f table; ~ f **basculante** tilt table; ~ f **de reconocimiento** examination table

mesénquima f embryonal connective tissue, mesenchyme

mesentérico adj mesenteric, involving the skin attaching various organs to the body

mesilato m **de doxazosin** doxazosin mesylate

mesométrio m parametrium

mesotelioma m mesothelioma; ~ m **peritoneal** peritoneal mesothelioma

mesquino m common wart, verruca vulgaris

mesurando m mesurand

meta f objective; ~ **–análisis** m meta-analysis

metabolismo m metabolism, permutation; ~ m **de ayuno** fasting metabolism, basal metabolic rate, basal metabolism; ~ m **de la purina–pirimidina** purine-pirimidine metabolism; ~ m **del calcio** calcium metabolism; ~ m **del hierro** iron metabolism; ~ m **energético** energy metabolism, bioenergetics; ~ m **férrico** iron metabolism; ~ m **máximo** peak metabolism

metabolito m metabolite, intermediate catabolic product; ~ m **biodisponible** bioavailable metabolite

metabolización f metabolization, processing

metabolizar v to metabolize

metacarpos m pl metacarpals

metadona f methadone

metafase f metaphase; ~ f **de la médula ósea** bone marrow metaphase; ~ f **mitótica** mitotic metaphase

metáfisis f metaphysis, transitional zone at which the diaphysis and epiphysis of a long bone come together

metahemoglobina f methemoglobin ferrihemoglobin, a blood pigment

metahemoglobinemia f methemoglobinemia, presence of methemoglobin in the blood, resulting in cyanosis

metales m pl metals; ~ m pl **pesados** heavy metals

metamielocito m metamyelocyte

metamioglobina f metmyoglobin

metanefrina f metanephrine

metanfetamina f methamphetamine,

methedrine, methylamphetamine, central nervous system stimulant and sympathomimetic

metanol *m* methanol, methyl alcohol; ~ *m* **acidificado** acidified methanol

metaplasia *f* metaplasia, abnormal tissue change

metas *f pl* goals, aims; ~ *f pl* **del tratamiento** goals of treatment, aims of treatment

metástasis *f* metastasis, disease site transfer; ~ *f* **ósea** bone metastasis

metastatizar *v* to metastasize, to spread by metastasis

metatarso *adj* metatarsal

metatarsos *m pl* metatarsals

meteorismo *m* bloating, meteorism, excessive gas; ~ *m* **abdominal** abdominal bloating, meteorism of large intestine

meter *v* to put

meterse *v* **el dedo en la nariz** to pick one's nose

metformina *f* metformin

meticilina *f* meticillin

metilanfetamina *f* methamphetamine, methedrine, methylamphetamine

metilcetona *f* methylketone

metildopa *f* methyldopa

metilergometrina *f* methylergonovine

metilfenidato *m* ritalin, methylphenidate, a drug used to treat hyperactive children

metilfenobarbital *m* mephobarbital

metilglioxalasa *f* methylglyoxalase, lactoylglutathione lyase

metilmorfina *f* codeine, methylmorphine

metilprednisolona *f* Medrol, methylprednisolone

metilsalicilato *m* methyl salicylate

metiona *m* methione

metionina *f* methionine; ~ – **adenosiltransferasa** *f* methionine adenosyltransferase

metirapona *f* metyrapone

metoclopramid *m* metoclopramide

método *m* method; ~ *m* **analítico** analytical method; ~ *m* **continuo** continuous method; ~ *m* **de medición** method of measurement; ~ *m* **de Ogino** periodic abstinence, rhythm method; ~ *m* **de referencia** reference

method; ~ *m* **de tratamiento** method of treatment; ~ *m* **definitivo** definitive method

metotrexato *m* methotrexate

metoxiadrenalina *f* methoxyadrenalin

metoxinoradrenalina *f* methoxynoradrenalin

metro *m* meter

metrología *f* metrology

metronidazol *m* metronidazole

metrorragia *f* metrorrhagia, breakthrough bleeding, intermenstrual bleeding; ~ *f* **perterapéutica** endometrial breakthrough bleeding

mezcla *f* mixture, blend; ~ *f* **de cloroformo y aire** chloroform-air mixture; ~ *f* **de glucosa y fructosa** invert sugar; ~ *f* **vorticial** vortex mix

mezclas *f pl* **medicinales** medicamentous mixtures

mezlocilina *f* mezlocillin

mi my

mialgia *f* myalgia, muscle pain

miasis *f* myiasis, fly maggot disease; ~ *f* **furunculoide** warble tumor; ~ *f* **vaginal** colpomyiasis

miastenia *f* myasthenia, muscle weakness; ~ *f* **gravis** myasthenia gravis

micción *f* urination, micturition, pissing

micela *f* micelle

micetoma *f* mycetoma

micobacteria *f* mycobacterium

micobacteriosis *f* mycobacteriosis

micolisina *f* mycolysin, pronase

micología *f* mycology

micológico *adj* mycological, fungus study-related

miconazol *m* miconazole

micosis *f* mycosis, fungal disease; ~ *f* **fungoide** mycosis fungoides, chronic malignant T-cell lymphoma of the skin; ~ *f* **profunda** systemic mycosis, systemic fungal infection; ~ *f* **vaginal** vaginomycosis, vaginal yeast infection

micótico *adj* mycotic

microbiano *adj* microbial, microbic

microbio *m* microorganism, microbe, germ

microbiología *f* microbiology; ~ *f* **clínica** clinical microbiology

microbiológico *adj* microbiological

microbiólogo *m* microbiologist

micróbios m pl germs, microbes
microcalcificación f microcalcification
microcauterio m micro cautery
microcefalia f microcephaly, microcephalia
microcirculación f microcirculation, blood flow in fine vessels
microcirugía f microsurgery; ~ f **subcelular** subcellular microsurgery
microencapsulación f microencapsulation
micrófalo m microphallus
microfilamentos m pl microfilaments, actin filaments
microfilaria f acanthocheilonema, microfilaria
microflora f microbial flora, microflora
microglia f neuroglial cells, microglia, astroglia, astrocytes
micrografía f micrography, microscope examination
microgramo m microgram, millionth of a gram
micrómetro m micrometer; ~ m **ocular** ocular micrometer
micronizar v to grind, to micronize, to reduce to a fine powder
microorganismo m germ, microbe, microorganism; ~ m **comensal** commensal microorganism
micropipeta f micropipette
microplaquita f microchip
microquímica f microchemistry
microscopía f microscopy; ~ f **de campo claro** brightfield microscopy; ~ f **de campo oscuro** dark-field microscopy; ~ f **de contraste de fases** phase-contrast microscopy; ~ f **infrarroja** infrared microscopy; ~ f **óptica** light microscopy
microscópico adj microscopic
microscopio m microscope; ~ m **binocular** binocular microscope; ~ m **de polarización** polarizing microscope; ~ m **electrónico** electron microscope; ~ m **operatorio** operating microscope, corneal microscope, surgical microscope; ~ m **óptico** light microscope; ~ m **protónico** proton microscope; ~ m **quirúrgico** operating microscope, surgical microscope
microsecuenciación f microsequencing
microsomal adj microsomal
microsomía f microsomia, dwarfism

microsporum m microsporum, a type of parasitic fungus
microtoxicosis f mycosis fungoides, chronic malignant T-cell lymphoma of the skin
microtúbulo m microtubule
microvellosidad f microvillus, protrusion from a cell
midriasis f pupil dilation
midriático adj mydriatic, pupil-dilating medication
miedo m anxiety, fear; ~ m **al abandono** separation anxiety, fear of abandonment; ~ m **mórbido** morbid fear, situation anxiety
mielina f myelin
mieloblasto m myeloblast
mielocito m myelocyte
mielocitosis f myeloid leukemia, myelocytosis, myelocitic leukemia
mielodisplasia f myelodysplasia
mielograma m myelogram, bone marrow examination
mieloma m myeloma, bone marrow cancer; ~ m **de célula plasmática** plasma cell myeloma; ~ m **múltiple** multiple myeloma, plasmacytoma, Kahler's disease
mielomatosis f myelomatosis, myeloma, bone marrow cancer
mielomeningocele m myelomeningocele
mielopatía f myelopathy, any disease affecting the spinal cord
mieloplaxa f multinucleated giant cell
mielosupresión f myelosuppression, arrest of bone marrow activity
mielotóxico adj myelotoxic, destructive to bone marrow
miembro m member, male sex organ, penis; ~ m **artificial** prosthesis, artificial limb
miércoles m Wednesday
migraña f migraine; ~ f **basilar** basilar migraine, basilar artery migraine; ~ f **en racimos de Horton** cluster headache, Horton's headache; ~ f **hemipléjica** hemiplegic migraine, classic migraine
miiasis f **rampante** creeping myiasis
mil adj thousand
miligramo m milligram
milímetro m millimeter
millón m million

mimado *adj* fastidious, fussy
mimetismo *m* mimicry; ~ *m* **molecular** molecular mimicry
mímica *f* facial expression
mina *f* mine; ~ *f* **terrestre** land mine
mineralización *f* mineralization
mineralocorticoide *m* mineralocorticoid, hormones
minerva *f* cervical collar, neck brace
mingitorio *m* urinal (in men's room)
minicromosoma *f* minute chromosome, double-minute
minimizar to minimize
mínimo *adj* minimal
mínimo *m* minimum
minociclina *f* minocycline, antibiotic
minusvalía *f* physical disability, physical handicap, physical incapacity
minusvalidez *f* disability
minusválido *m* handicapped, disabled, impaired; ~ *m* disabled person, handicapped person
minuto *m* minute
miocardio *m* myocardium
miocardiopatía *f* myocardial disease; ~ *f* **alcohólica** alcoholic myocardiopathy; ~ *f* **gravídica** gestational myocardiopathy; ~ *f* **hipertrófica** hypertrophic myocardiopathy, hypertrophic cardiomyopathy
miocardiosclerosis *f* myocardial sclerosis
miocarditis *f* myocarditis, heart muscle inflammation
mioclonia *f* myoclonus, involuntary muscle contractions; ~ *f* **del pequeño mal** myoclonic seizure, myoclonic absence
mioglobina *f* myoglobin
mioma *m* myoma, fibroid tumor; ~ *m* **uterino** uterine fibroids
miomectomía *f* myomectomy; ~ *f* **Czerny** Czerny myomectomy, Czerny enucleation
miometrio *m* myometrium, tunica muscularis uteri
miopatía *f* myopathy, muscle diease
miope *adj* nearsighted, myopic
miopía *f* myopia, near-sightedness, short-sighted; ~ *f* **de altura** high-altitude myopia
miorrelajante *m* muscle relaxant, neuromusclar depolarizing agent

miosina *f* myosin, myosin protein; ~ *f* **de músculo esquelético** skeletal muscle myosin
miosis *f* miosis, constriction of the pupil
miositis *f* myositis, muscle inflammation
miótico *adj* miotic; ~ *m* miotic, anti-glaucoma treatment
miotonía *f* myotonia; ~ *f* **atrófica** myotonic dystrophy; ~ *f* **congénita** congenital myotonia, hereditary myotonia
mirar *v* to look
miringotomía *f* tympanotomy, myringotomy, tympanocentesis; ~ *f* **de aspiración** aspiratory myringotomy
mis (pl) my
miscible *adj* miscible, mixable
mismo like
misoprostol *m* misoprostol
mitocondria *f* mitochondria, mitochondrion, chondriosome, plastosome
mitosis *f* mitosis, cell division; ~ *f* **anastral** bone marrow mitosis; ~ *f* **de médula osea** anastral mitosis
mixoblastoma *m* myxoma, colloid tumor
mixoma *m* myxoma, colloid tumor; ~ *m* **quístico** cystic myxoma
mocarditis *f* myocarditis
moco *m* mucus, phlegm, snot; ~ *m* **endocervical** endocervical mucus
modelo *m* model; ~ *m* **clínico** clinical model; ~ *m* **de rotura y reunión** break and reunion model
moderado *adj* moderate
modificación *f* modification, change, alteration
modificador *m* modifier
modificar *v* modify, to
modo *m* way, manner; ~ *m* **de andar** gait
modorra *f* somnolence, sleepiness
modulador *m* modulator; ~ *m* **de la respuesta inmunitaria** immune response modulator
moho *m* negro black mold, stachybotrys
mojabilidad *f* wettability
mojado *adj* wet
mola *f* mole; ~ *f* **hidatídica** hydatid mole; ~ *f* **hidatidiforme** hydatid mole; ~ *f* **hidatiforma** hydatiform mole; ~ *f* **maligna** malignant mole; ~ *f* **metastásica** metastasizing mole
molal molal

M

molalidad f molality

molar adj to grind, to micronize, to reduce to a fine powder

molde f template

molécula f molecule; ~ f **CD4** CD4 molecule; ~ f **protéica** protein molecule; ~ f **ubiquita** ubiquitous molecule

molecular adj molecular

molestar v to fase, to disturb

molestia f discomfort, uneasiness; ~ f **al orinar** urinary discomfort

mollera f soft spon on baby's head, fontanelle

molturar adj to grind, to micronize, to reduce to a fine powder

molusco m contagioso molluscum contagiosum

momento m moment; ~ m **de inercia** moment of inertia

moneda f coin

moniliasis f urogenital candidiasis, urogenital candidosis

monitorización f monitoring, keeping close tabs on a patient; ~ f **farmacoterapéutica** TDM, therapeutic drug monitoring; ~ f **Holter** Holter monitoring, 24 hour wearable ECG monitor (cardiology)

monitorizar v to monitor

monoanima f **oxidasa** MOA, monoamine oxidase

monoblasto m monoblast

monocito m monocyte; ~ m **circulante** circulating monocyte

monocromador m monocromator

monogamia f monogamy

monógamo adj monogamous

monoinsaturados m pl monounsaturates, mono-unsaturated fatty acids

mononeuritis f mononeuritis

mononitrato m **de tiamina** thiamin mononitrate

mononucleosis f mononucleosis; ~ f **infecciosa** infectious mononucleosis, glandular fever, monocytic angina, monocuclear leukocytosis, Epstein-Barr disease

mononucleótido m **de flavina** flavin mononucleotide; ~ m **de nicotinamida** nicotinamide mononucleotide

monoterapia f monotherapy, single-drug-treatment, one drug therapy

monóxido m **de carbon** carbon monoxide

monstruo m monster

montar v to ride, to assemble, to put together; ~ v **a horcajadas** to straddle, to have one leg on each side

moquera f snot, nasal mucus

Moraxella f **lacunata** Morax-Axenfeld's bacillus

morbididad f morbidity, diseased state, incidence of disease, rate of sickness

mórbido adj morbid, unhealthy

morboso adj pathological

mordedura f bite wound, wound caused by a bite; ~ f **de perro** dog bite; ~ f **de serpiente** snake bite

morder v to bite one's nails

morderse v **las uñas** to bite one's nails

mordisco m bite

moretón m bruise, bruising, contusion

morfina f morphine

morfinomanía f morphine addiction

morfinomimético m morphinomimetic, simulating effects of morphine

morfología f morphology; ~ f **celular** cell morphology; ~ f **sanguínea** blood morphology

Morganella f **morganii** Morgan's bacillus

morir v **desangrado** v to bleed to death, to bleed profusely

morir v to die, to pass away; ~ v **de hambre** to starve to death

mortal adj lethal

mortalidad f mortality rate, mortality

mosca f **tsétsé** tsetse fly

mosquitero m mosquito netting, fly screen, insect screening, bednet

mosquito m mosquito; ~ m **anofeles** anopheline mosquito, anopheles

mostaza f mustard; ~ f **nitrogenada** nitrogen mustard

motilidad f motility, ability to move spontaneously

motivo m motif; ~ m **de ADN** DNA motif

motor adj motor, mobile; ~ m motor, mobile

mover v to move

movilidad f mobility; ~ f **eléctrica** electric mobility; ~ f **electroforética** electrophoretic mobility

movilización f mobilization, loosening

movimiento m exercise, movement; ~ m **del**

mediastino mediastinal shift
movimientos m pl **estereotipados** stereotypy of movements
MRI MRI, magnetic resonance imaging
mucho adj a lot, lots (of)
muchos adj many, much
mucilaginoso adj mucociliary, mucous membrane and hair-related
mucina f mucin
muco m mucus; ~ m **anal** anal mucus; ~ m **cervical** cervical mucus; ~ m **nasal** nasal mucus
mucociliar adj mucociliary, mucous membrane and hair-related
mucocutáneo adj mucocutaneous
mucolítico adj mocolytic
mucolítico m mucolytic, drug liquidating phlegm
mucopolisacarida f glycosaminoglycan, mucopolysaccharide
mucopurulento adj mucopurulent, containing mucus and pus
mucosa f mucosa, mucous membrane; ~ f **gástrica** gastric mucosa, stomach lining; ~ f **intestinal** f intestinal mucosa; ~ f **secretoria** secretory mucosa
mucosidad f **del utero** endometrium (in the uterus), tunica mucosa uteri
mucoso adj gelatinous, glutinous
mucus m mucus, phlegm
mudo adj mute
muela f molar; ~ f **del juicio** wisdom tooth, dens serotinus
muerte f death; ~ f **cardíaca** cardiac death; ~ f **cardíaca repentina** cardiac death; ~ f **cerebral** brain death; ~ f **de la célula** cell reproductive death; ~ f **fetal** stillbirth, fetal death; ~ f **súbita del lactante** death syndrome (SIDS), crib death; ~ f **violenta** violent death
muerto adj dead, deceased
muerto m death
muestra f specimen, sample; ~ f **comercial** trade sample; ~ f **de biopsia** biopsy sample; ~ f **de exudado cervical** cervical smear; ~ f **de referencia** reference sample; ~ f **de tejido** tissue specimen; ~ f **primaria** primary sample; ~ f **testigo** known sample
muestreador m sampler

muestreo m sampling
muguet m oral candidiasis, oral thrush
mujer f woman; ~ f **embarazada** pregnant woman, expectant mother; ~ f **maltratada** battered wife, victim of domestic violence; ~ f **nulipara** nulliparous woman
muleta f crutch
multianalizador m multiparametric analyzer
multidosis f multidose
multineuritis f disseminated neuritis
multípara adj multiparous, woman who has had 2 or more babies
múltiple multiple
multiplexado adj multiplexing
multiplicación f proliferation, multiplication
multivalente m multivalent; ~ m **de translocación** translocation multivalent
muñeca f wrist; ~ f **compliante** compliant wrist, flexible wrist
muñón m (exarticulation) stump
mupirocina f mupirocin
muramidasa f muramidase
murino m **monoclonal** monoclonal murine
murmullo m murmur; ~ m **distólico** diastolic murmur
musculación f muscle building, strengthening, muscle training
muscular adj well-muscled, muscular
musculatura f musculature, muscles; ~ f **pélvica** pelvic muscles
músculo m muscle; ~ m **auxiliar** auxiliary muscle; ~ m **bíceps** musculus biceps brachii, biceps; ~ m **ciliar** ciliary muscle; ~ m **de cierre** sphincter; ~ m **de contracción involuntaria** smooth muscle, non-striated muscle, organic muscle; ~ m **de contracción voluntaria** striated muscle, voluntary muscle; ~ m **estriado** striated muscle, voluntary muscle; ~ m **jalado** pulled muscle; ~ m **liso** smooth muscle, non-striated muscle, organic muscle; ~ m **pectoral** pectoral muscle
musculos m pl muscles; ~ m pl **esqueléticos** skeletal muscles, red striated muscles; ~ m pl **faciales** facial muscles, mimetic muscles; ~ m pl **perineales** musculature of pelvic floor
muslo m thigh
mutación f mutation; ~ f **aceleradora** up

M

mutation; ~ *f* **ámbar** amber mutation;
~ *f* **completa** null mutation; ~ *f* **constitutiva**
constitutive mutation; ~ *f* **de genomio**
genome mutation; ~ *f* **del marco de lectura**
frame-shift mutation; ~ *f* **deletérea**
deleterious mutation; ~ *f* **directa** forward
mutation; ~ *f* **en un punto específico** site-
specific mutation; ~ *f* **génica** genome
mutation; ~ *f* **imperceptible** silent mutation;
~ *f* **lentificadora** down-promoter mutation,
down mutation; ~ *f* **multicéntrica** multisite
mutation; ~ *f* **ocre** ochre mutation; ~ *f* **ópalo**
opale mutation; ~ *f* **parcial** leaky mutation;
~ *f* **por inserción** insertion mutation;
~ *f* **puntual** point mutation, single site
mutation; ~ *f* **restauradora** back mutation;
~ *f* **sin sentido** nonsense mutation;
~ *f* **superrepresiva** surrepressive mutation;
~ *f* **sustitutiva** missense mutation;
~ *f* **termosensible** thermosensitive mutation;
~ *f* **transicional** transition mutation;
~ *f* **voluminosa** gross mutation
mutagénesis *f* mutagenesis; ~ *f* **dirigida**
directed mutagenesis, site-specific
mutagenesis; ~ *f* **específica puntual** site-
directed mutagenesis; ~ *f* **insercional**
insertional mutagenesis; ~ *f* **inversa** surrogate
genetics; ~ *f* **sitio dirigida** site-directed
mutagenesis, site-specific mutagenesis
mutágeno *adj* mutagenic; ~ *m* mutagen,
mutagenic agent
mutante *f* mutant
mutismo *m* mutism, dumbness, congenital alalia
mutón *m* muton
muy very; ~ **bien** very well; ~ **potente** highly
potent
muzolimina *f* muzolimine, a pyrazole diuretic
Mycobacterium bovis mycobacterium bovis;
~ *m* **leprae** mycobacterium leprae;
~ *m* **paratuberculosis** mycobacterium
paratuberculosis; ~ *m* **tuberculosis**
mycobacterium tuberculosis

N

nacido *adj* born, newborn; ~ *m* **muerto** fetal

death
nacimiento *m* birth, childbirth, delivery
nada nothing; ~ **por boca** n.p.o. (nihil per os)
NADH-peroxidasa *f* NADH peroxidase
nadir *m* nadir, low point
**NADP (metilenotetrahidrofolato-
deshidrogenasa)** NADP,
methylenetetrahydrofolate dehydrogenase
nafcilina *f* nafcillin
nalgas *f pl* cheeks, buttocks
nanodispositivo *m* medical nanodevice, medical
nanorobot
nanomedicina *f* bionanotechnolgy,
nanomedicine, medical nanotechnology
nanómetro *m* nanometer, nanon
nanon *m* nanometer, nanon
nanorrobot *m* medical nanodevice, medical
nanorobot
nanotecnologia *f* molecular nanotechnology
nanotube *m* nanotube
naproxeno *m* naproxen
naranja *adj* orange
narcolepsia *f* narcolepsy, sleep epilepsy
narcomanía *f* drug addiction
narcosis *f* narcosis; ~ *f* **por éter** ether narcosis,
etherization
narcótico *adj* narcotic, morphine-like drug
narices *f pl* nostril, nostrils
nariz *f* nose
nasal *adj* nasal, pertaining to the nose
nasalizado *adj* with a nasal twang, snuffling,
nasal tone
násico *adj* with a nasal twang, snuffling, nasal
tone
nasofaringe *f* nasopharynx, nasopharyngeal
cavity
nasolacrimal *adj* nasolacrimal
natremia *f* natremia
natriuresis *f* natriuresis, excretion of sodium by
kidneys
natriuria *f* natriuria
naturaleza *f* nature
naturista *f* naturopath, a practitioner of
naturopathy
naturópata *m* naturopath, a practitioner of
naturopathy
naturopatía *f* naturopathy, natural medicine
náusea *f* nausea, queasiness, feeling sick, feeling

nauseated

nebulización f **por inhalación** inhalation mist, inhalant

nebulizador m inhaler, spray dispenser, moist vapor nebulizer, puff, atomizer, evaporator, vaporizer

necesidad f need, necessity, emergency; ~ f **de oxígeno** oxygen demand

necesitar v to need

necrólisis f necrolysis, gangrene, necrosis; ~ f **epidérmica tóxica** necrotizing fasciitis, flesh-eating disease

necropsia f necropsy, autopsy, post mortem, postmortem examination

necrosis f necrosis, necrolysis; ~ f **fosfórica** phosphonecrosis; ~ f **grasa** steatonecrosis, fat necrosis, adiponecrosis; ~ f **hematopoyética infecciosa** infectious hematopoietic necrosis, IHN; ~ f **por coagulación** ischemic necrosis, caseation necrosis, coagulation necrosis; ~ f **tubular** tubular necrosis

nefelometría f turbidimetry, nephelometry

nefelómetro m nephelometer

nefrectomía f nephrectomy, extirpation of a kidney

nefritis f nephritis, kidney inflammation; ~ f **lipomatosa** lipomatous nephritis

nefrocalcinosis f nephrocalcinosis

nefrogénico adj nefrogenic

nefrógeno adj nephrogenous

nefrolito m nephrolith, kidney stone

nefrolitos m pl nephroliths, kidney stones

nefrología f nephrology

nefrólogo m nephrologist, kidney specialist

nefrón m nephron

nefropatía f nephropathy, kidney disease, renal disease; ~ f **poliquística** polycystic disease of the kidney, polycystic renal disease; ~ f **saturnina** nephropathy secondary to lead exposure; ~ f **tubular** tubular necrosis; ~ f **tubulointersticial** acute tubulo-interstitial nephropathy

nefrorrafia f renal suture

nefrorragia f renal hemorrhage, nephrorrhagia

nefrosclerosis f nephrosclerosis of kidney; ~ f **posinfarto** cirrhosis of infarcted kidney

nefrosis f nephrosis; ~ f **amiloidea** amyloid nephrosis; ~ f **de Epstein** Epstein nephrosis,

Epstein's syndrome; ~ f **gravídica** gestation nephrosis

nefrótico adj nephrotic

nefrotomía f renal incision, nephrotomy

nefrotoxicidad f nephrotoxicity

nefrotóxico adj nephrotoxic, destructive to the kidneys

negativo adj negative; ~ adj **falso** false negative; ~ adj **verdadero** true negative

negro adj black

Neisseria f **gonorrhoeae** gonococcus

neófito m neophyte, new user, beginner, novice

neoformación f growths

neogénesis f neogenesis, tissue regeneration

neomicina f neomycin, aminoglycoside antibioticcomplex produced by Streptomyces fradiae

neonatal adj neonatal, pertaining to newborns, newborn

neoplasia f neoplasia, neoplasm, tumor; ~ f **del colon y recto** colorectal cancer; ~ f **epitelial** epithelial neoplasm, skin cancer

neoplásico adj neoplastic

neoplasma m neoplasia, neoplasm, tumor; ~ m **del esófago** esophageal neoplasm, tumor of the esophagus; ~ m **maligno** malignant neoplasm, malignant tumor, malignancy

neovascularización f neovascularization; ~ f **de la córnea** corneal neovascularization; ~ f **retiniana** retinal neovascularization

nervio m nerve; ~ m **auditivo** auditory nerve, cochlear nerve, acoustic nerve; ~ m **ciático** sciatic nerve; ~ m **crural** femoral nerve, crural nerve; ~ m **eferente** efferent nerve; ~ m **femoral** femoral nerve, crural nerve; ~ m **frénico** phrenic nerve, motor nerve of the diaphragm; ~ m **glosofaríngeo** glossopharyngeal nerve; ~ m **lagrimal** lacrimal nerve; ~ m **obturador** obturator nerve; ~ m **olfatorio** olfactory nerve; ~ m **óptico** optic nerve, visual nerve; ~ m **periférico** peripheral nerve; ~ m **raquídeo** spinal nerves; ~ m **sensorial** sensory nerves; ~ m **trigémino** trigeminal nerve, trifacial nerve; ~ m **vago** vagus nerve, pneumogastric nerve, tenth cranial nerve; ~ m **vesticular** vestibular nerve

nerviosismo m nervousness

netilmicina f netilmicin

neumococemia f bronchopneumonia, bronchial pneumonia

neumoconiosis f pneumoconiosis, silicosis; ~ f **masiva progresiva** massive progressive pneumoconiosis

neumología f respiratory medicine

neumomediastino m pneumomediastinum

neumonía f pneumonia; ~ f **bacteriana** bacterial pneumonia; ~ f **estafilocócica** staphylococcus pneumonia; ~ f **por aspiración** aspiration pneumonia; ~ f **por pneumocystis carinii** pneumocystis carinii pneumonia; ~ f **química** chemical pneumonitis, chemical worker's lung, chemical pneumonia; ~ f **viral** viral pneumonia

neumonitis f pneumonitis; ~ f **por radiación** radiation pneumonitis; ~ f **química** chemical pneumonitis, chemical worker's lung, chemical pneumonia

neumopatía f pneumopathy, lung disease; ~ f **bacteriana** bacterial pneumonia; ~ f **por hipersensibilidad** extrinsic allergic alveolitis, allergic interstitial pneumonitis, hypersensitivity pneumonitis

neumotórax m pneumothorax; ~ m **de tensión** tension pneumothorax; ~ m **valvular** valvular pneumothorax

neural adj neural

neuralgia f neuralgia; ~ f **cervicobraquial** cervicobrachial neuralgia; ~ f **crural** crural neuralgia; ~ f **del nervio trigémino** trigeminal neuralgia, tic douloureux, prosopalgia; ~ f **facial** facial neuralgia, opalgia, pain in the eye

neurálgico adj neuralgic

neuraminidasa f neuraminidase

neurastenia f neurasthenia, nervous exhaustion; ~ f **espinal** spinal neurasthenia

neurectomía f neurectomy, excision of part of a nerve

neurilema f Schwann's sheath, neurolemma, neurilemma

neurinoma f peripheral glioma, neurinoma, neurilemmoma

neuritis f neuritis, nerve inflammation; ~ f **gravídica** pregnancy neuritis; ~ f **óptica** optic neuritis, neuritis of the optic nerve; ~ f **óptica retrobulbar** retrobulbar neuritis; ~ f **vestibular** vestibular neuritis

neurobiología f neurobiology

neuroblasto m neuroblast

neuroblastoma m neuroblastoma; ~ m **olfatorio** esthesioneuroblastoma

neurociencia f neuroscience; ~ f **cognitiva** cognitive neuroscience

neurocirugía f neurosurgery

neurocisticercosis f neurocysticercosis

neurocitoma f peripheral glioma, neurinoma, neurilemmoma

neurodepresor m CNS depressant, central nervous system depressant

neurodermatitis f neurodermatitis

neurofibromatosis f neurofibromatosis, von Recklinghausen's disease, osteitis fibrosa cystica

neurofílico adj neurotropic

neurofisiología f neuro-physiology

neurohormona f neurohormone

neurolema f Schwann's sheath, neurolemma, neurilemma

neuroléptico m neuroleptic, major tranquilizer, antipsychotic

neuroleptoanalgesia f neuroleptanalgesia

neurología f neuroscience

neurológico adj neurological

neurolúes m paretic neurosyphilis

neuroma m neuroma; ~ m **acústico** acoustic neuroma, tumor of the acoustic nerve; ~ **falso** m false neuroma

neuromuscular adj neuromuscular

neurona f neuron, nerve cell; ~ f **artificial** artificial neuron; ~ f **cortical** central motor neuron, upper motor neuron; ~ f **eferente** efferent neuron; ~ f **motora** motor neuron; ~ f **presináptica** presynaptic neuron; ~ m **sensorial** sensory neuron; ~ f **superior** central motor neuron, upper motor neuron

neuronal adj neuronal

neuropatía f neuropathy, nervous system disorder; ~ f **diabética** diabetic neuropathy; ~ f **periférica** peripheral neuropathy

neuropatología f neuropathology

neurópilo *m* neuropil, neuropilem
neuropsicología *f* neuropsychology
neuroquirurgo *m* neurosurgeon
neurosifilis *f* paretic neurosyphilis
neurosis *f* neurosis; ~ **f de ansiedad** anxiety neurosis, anxiety reaction, free-floating anxiety; ~ **f infantil** childhood neurosis; ~ **f traumática** traumatic neurosis, post-catastrophe syndrome
neurótico *adj* neurotic
neurotomía *f* neurotomy, excision of a nerve; ~ **f del nérvio periférico** neurotomy of the peripheral nerve
neurotóxico *adj* neurotoxic
neurotransmisor *m* neurotransmitter
neurotrópico *adj* neurotropic
neurotropo *adj* neurotropic
neurovegetativo *adj* neurovegetative
neutralización *f* neutralization
neutrófilo *adj* neutrophil
neutrófilo *m* neutrophilocyte
neutrofilocito *adj* neutrophil
neutrofilocito *m* neutrophilocyte; ~ *m* **segmentado** segmented neutrophil
neutropenia *f* neutropenia, low white blood cell count
nevirapina *f* nevirapine, Viramune
nevo *m* naevus, nevus; ~ *m* **flameo** capillary hemangioma, capillaropathy
nevus *m* naevus, nevus; ~ *m* **despigmentado** amelanotic nevus, nevus depigmentosus; ~ *m* **varicoso ósteo-odontohipertrófico** osteo-odontohypertrophic-varicose nevus syndrome
newton *m* newton
niacina *f* niacin, nicotinique acid, B vitamin
niacinamida *f* niacinamid, nicotinamide
nicotina *f* nicotine
nicotinamida *f* niacinamid, nicotinamide
nicturia *f* nocturia, nycturia
nidación *f* nidation
nieve *f* snow
nigua *f* chigger
niña *f* girl, child; ~ **f del ojo** pupil
niño *m* boy, child; ~ *m* **autisto** autistic child; ~ *m* **delicado** delicate child; ~ *m* **enfermizo** sickly child; ~ *m* **indadaptado** maladjusted child

nistagmo *m* ocular nystagmus, wonky eyes, nystagmu; ~ *m* **ocular** ocular nystagmus, wonky eyes, nystagmus
nitrato *m* nitrate; ~ *m* **de peroxibenzoílo** peroxybenzoyl nitrate, peroxy benzoyl nitrate; ~ *m* **potásico** saltpeter, potassium nitrate
nitrofurantoína *f* nitrofurantoin
nitrógeno *m* nitrogen; ~ *m* **y úrea** *f* **sanguínea** blood urea nitrogen, BUN
nitroimidazol *m* nitroimidazole
nitrosamina *f* nitrosamine
nitrosourea *f* nitrosourea
nivel *m* level; ~ *m* **de creatinina** creatinine level; ~ *m* **de glucemia** blood sugar level; ~ *m* **de glucosa en sangre** blood glucose level; ~ *m* **plasmático crítico de fibrinógeno** critical plasma fibrinogen level
no no; no; ~ **activo** *adj* passive, not active; ~ **característico** *adj* nonspecific, non-specific; ~ **cooperativo** *adj* uncooperative; ~ **cornezuelo** *m* non-ergot; ~ **embriagado** *adj* sober, not drunk; ~ **específico** *adj* nonspecific, non-specific; ~ **general** *adj* local, topical, regional; ~ **nocivo** *adj* atoxic, nontoxic, not poisonous; ~ **palpable** *adj* non-palpable, impalpable; ~ **positivo** *adj* negative; ~ **unido** *adj* unbound; ~ **venenoso** *adj* atoxic, non-poisonous
noche *f* evening, night
nociceptor *m* nociceptor
nocivo *adj* harmful (to your health), noxious, detrimental, pernicious
nocturnal *adj* nocturnal, nightly
nocturno *adj* nocturnal, nightly
nodriza *f* wet nurse, nurse hired to breast feed a baby
nodular *adj* nodose, nodular, with nodes, knotty
nódulo *m* nodule, node, nodus; ~ *m* **del ordenador** milker's nodule, pseudocowpox; ~ *m* **linfático** lymphatic nodule; ~ *m* **reumático** rheumatic nodule; ~ *m* **tumoral** tumor nodule
nombre *m* first name; ~ *m* **farmacéutico internacional** international non-proprietary name, common name, chemical generic name
noradrenalina *f* noradrenaline
norepinefrina *f* norepinephrine
noretisterona *f* norethisterone

N

norfloxacina f norfloxacin

norleucina f norleucine

norma f rule, regulation, standard, norm; **~ f de funcionamiento** performance standard

normal adj normal, physiological

normalización f normalization

normalmente normally

normotenso adj normotensive, with normal blood pressure

nortriptilina f nortriptyline

nos us

nosocomial adj nosocomial, disease contracted in hospital

nosología f nosology

nosotros m pl, **–as** fp we

notalgia f dorsalgia, notalgia, back pain, dorsodynia

notar v to notice

noveno adj ninth

noventa adj ninety

noviembre m November

novobiocina f novobiocin

novocaína f novocain

nube f cloud; **~ f del ojo** punctate cataract

nuca f nape of the neck

nucleasa f nuclease; **~ f de Aspergillus** endonuclease (Aspergillus)

nucléido f nuclide

núcleo m core, nucleus; **~ m gracilis** gracile nucleus, nucleus gracilis; **~ m interfásico** interphase nucleus; **~ m no divisional** interphase nucleus

nucleófilo adj nucleophile

nucleohistona m nucleohistone

nucleolo m nucleolus

nucleoplasma m nucleoplasm, nucleoplasma

nucleósido m nucleoside; **~ m difosfato** nucleoside diphosphate; **~ –fosfato–cinasa** nucleoside-phosphate kinase

nucleosoma m nucleosome

nucleótido m nucleotide; **~ m celular** cellular nucleotide

nucleótidos m pl nucleotides

nucleotomía f discectomy; **~ f lumbar percutánea automatizada** automated percutaneous lumbar discectomy; **~ f percutánea automatizada** automated percutaneous

lumbar discectomy, automated percutaneous discectomy

nudillo m back of the hand, dorsum manus, knuckle

nudo m nodule, node, nodus, knot; **~ m de Aschoff-Tawara** atrioventricular node, Aschoff-Tawara node; **~ m sinoauricular** sinoatrial node, sinus node

nuestro adj our

nueve adj nine

nuevo adj new

nuez m de adán Adam's apple, laryngeal prominence

nulípara adj nulliparous, never having given birth

nulípara f nulliparous, never having given birth

nulo adj nil

número m number; **~ m atómico** atomic number; **~ m de Avogadro** Avogadro's constant, Avogadro's number; **~ m de carga** charge number; **~ m de entidades** number of entities; **~ m de masa** mass number; **~ m de onda** wavenumber; **~ m de teléfono** telephone number; **~ m de transporte** transport number; **~ m de vueltas helicoidales** twisting number; **~ m único** unique number

numular adj nummular, coin-like

nutación f nutation

nutrición f nutrition; **~ f enteral** enteral nutrition; **~ f parenteral** parenteral nutrition, parenteral feeding

nutricionista f nutritionist

nutriente m nutrient, nutrition

nutrimento m nutrient, nutrition

nutritivo adj trophic, nutrition-related

O

o or

obesidad f obesity, being overweight

obeso adj obese

objetivo m objective; **~ m de inmersión** immersion objective, immersion lens

objeto m thing

obnubilación f numbness, obnubilation, mental

numbness, stupor, grogginess
observación f observation
observaciones f pl observations
observador adj observant, attentive
observancia f compliance
observar observe, to
obsesión f obsession
obstetra–ginecólogo m obstetrician &
gynecologist, ob-gyn doctor
obstetricia f obstetrics; ~ **y ginecología** f
obstetrics & gynecology
obstétrico adj obstetrical
obstrucción f blockage, block, blocking,
obstruction, barrier; ~ f **aérea** airway
obstruction; ~ f **biliar** biliary obstruction,
obturation of bile ducts; ~ f **esofágica** blocked
esophagus; ~ f **tubaria** tubal obstruction;
~ f **tubular** tubular obstruction; **intestinal** f
ileus, intestinal blockage
obtención f **de la impronta** footprinting; ~ f **de
las huellas digitales** fingerprinting
obtener v to get
obturador m obturator
ocasional adj occasional
occipucio m occiput
ochenta adj eighty
ocho adj eight
oclusión f occlusion, momentary closure, bite,
the act of closing; ~ f **intestinal** intestinal
obstruction, occlusion of the bowel;
~ f **permanente de la arteria coronaria** fixed
coronary artery occlusive disease;
~ f **tubárica** tubal occlusion; ~ f **venosa**
venous occlusion
octacosanol m octacosanol
octavo adj eighth
octubre m October
ocular adj ocular
oculista m ophthalmologist
oculógiro adj oculogyric
oculógiro m involving circular eye movements
oculomucocutáneo adj oculomucocutaneous
oculto adj hidden, occult, concealed
odontalgia f toothache, odontodynia,
dentalgia
odontoide adj odontoid
odontología f dentistry
odontoplastía f orthodontics, orthodonture,

orthodontic work, orthodontology
ofloxacina f ofloxacin
oftálmico adj ophthalmic
oftalmología f ophthalmology
oftalmológico adj ophthalmological
oftalmoplejia f ophthalmoplegia, paralysis of
the muscles of the eye
oftalmorrea f ophthalmorrhea
oftalmoscopia m manual hand ophtalmoscope
oftalmoscopio m ophthalmoscope, retinoscope,
skiascope; ~ m **eléctrico** electric
ophthalmoscope
ohm m ohm
oído m ears, hearing; ~ m **interno** inner ear
ojo m eye; ~ m **a la funerala** black eye;
~ m **artificial** ocularprosthesis, artificial eye,
prosthetic eye; ~ m **morado** black eye
ojos m pl eyes; ~ m pl **de soldador** welder's
eyes; ~ m pl **inc** puffiness around the eyes,
bags / dark circles under the eyes
oleandomicina f oleandomycin
olécranon m funny bone, olecranon, funnybone
(in the elbow)
oler v to smell
olfacción f olfaction, sens of smell, olfactory
organ
olfato m olfaction, sens of smell, olfactory
organ, olfactory, smell
oligodendroglía f oligodendrocytes,
oligodendroglia
oligoelemento m oligoelement, trace element,
essential trace element
oligofrenia f mental retardation, mental disorder,
feeblemindedness, dementia, mental
deficiency
oligomenorrea f oligomenorrhea, infrequent
periods
oligonucleótido m oligonucleotide;
~ m **antisentido** antisense oligonucleotide
oligosonda f oligoprobe
oliguria f oliguria, kidney depression
olor m odor, smell, aroma, fragrance, odour,
offensive odor, stench, bad smell, stink;
~ m **corporal** body odor, smell of sweat;
~ m **empalagoso** sickly smell, a stink
olvidadizo adj absent-minded, forgetful
ombligo m navel, umbilicus
ombudsman m ombudsman

omeprazol *m* omeprazole

omfalotomía *f* omphalotomy

omóplato *f* scapula, shoulder blade

OMS *f* **(Organización Mundial de la Salud)** World Health Organization, WHO

once *adj* eleven

onceavo *adj* eleventh

oncocercosis *f* onchocerciasis, river blindness, onchocercosis, blinding filariasis

oncogén *m* oncogene; **~** *m* **vírico** viral oncogene

oncogénico *adj* oncogenic, carcinogenic, tumorigenic

oncolítico *adj* oncolytic

oncología *f* oncology; **~** *f* **clínica** clinical oncology; **~** *f* **genética** genetic oncology; **~** *f* **molecular** molecular oncologyc; **~** *f* **pediátrica** pediatric oncology

oncólogo *m* oncologist, cancer specialist

oncótico *adj* oncotic

oncovirus *m* oncogenic virus, tumor virus, oncovirus

onda *f* wave; **~** *m pl* **cerebrais** brain waves

onfalocito *m* omphalosite

onicatrofia *f* atrophy of the nails

onicoclasia *f* onychoclasis

onicoclasis *f* onychoclasis

onicofagia *f* onychophagia

onicólisis *f* onychlysis

onido *m* **asmático** rhonchus, wheezing, whistling

oniquia *f* onychia; **~** *f* **maligna** onychia maligna; **~** *f* **piógena** pyogenic onychia

onirismo *m* delirium, onirism, vesanic dementia, waking dream state

ooforectomía *f* ovariectomy, oophorectomy, excision of an ovary, spaying

ooforitis *f* oophoritis, inflammation of the ovaries

opalescente *adj* opalescent, opal-like

opalgia *f* opalgia, pain in the eye

operación *f* operation, intervention; **~** *f* **aséptica** aseptic operation; **~** *f* **cesárea** C-section, caesarean, caesarean section; **~** *f* **contínua** continuous operation; **~** *f* **de Blalock-Taussig** Blalock-Taussig operation, Blalock-Taussig procedure; **~** *f* **de Dandy** suboccipital trigeminal rhizotomy, Dandy's operation; **~** *f* **de descompresión** decompressive operation; **~** *f* **de Heller** Heller operation, Heller procedure; **~** *f* **de Herzberg** Herzberg operation; **~** *f* **de Jansen** Jansen operation; **~** *f* **de urgencia** emergency surgery, emergency operation; **~** *f* **por grupos** batch operation

operador *m* operator

operar *v* to operate

opérculo *m* operculum; **~** *m* **frontoparietal** frontoparietal operculum; **~** *m* **rolándico** frontoparietal operculum; **~** *m* **temporal** temporal operculum

operón *m* operon

ophthalmoplegic *adj* ophthalmoplegic

opiáceo opiate, opioid

opiata *f* opiate, opioid

opio *m* opium, papaveretum

opioide *m* opiate, opioid

opistótonos *m* opisthotonos, backward spasm

opoponaco *m* valerian

oportunista *f* opportunistic

opresión *f* oppression, difficulty in breathing; **~** *f* **en el pecho** difficulty in breathing, tightness of the chest

opsina *f* opsin

opsonización *f* opsonization

óptico *adj* optic; **~** *m* optician

opticociliotomía *f* opticociliotomy

óptimo *adj* optimal

optometrista *m* optometrist, optician

oral oral, mouth-

orbital *adj* orbital

ordenador *m* computer; **~** *m* **central** host computer

oreja *f* ear, outer ear

orfón *m* orphon

organismo *m* organism; **~** *m* **modificado genéticamente** genetically modified organism; **~** *m* **transgénico** transgenic organism, a genetically modified organism

organito *m* subcellular organelle

organización *f* organization; **~** *f* **de atención médica** HMO Health Maintenance Organization; **~** *f* **del seguro de salud** Plan Physician Only, Preferred Provider Organization, PPO

órgano *m* organ; **~** *m* **análogo** analogous

organ; ~ **m de los sentidos** sensory organ, sense organ; ~ **m olfativo** olfactory organ, sense of smell; ~ **m olfatorio** sense of smell, olfactory; ~ **m vital** vital organ
organoclorado *m pl* chlorinated hydrocarbon
organogénesis *f* organogenesis
organoléptico *adj* organoleptic
organoplastía *f* organogenesis
orgánulo *m* organelle; ~ **m subcelular** subcellular organelle
orgasmo *m* orgasm
orientación *f* orientation; ~ **f espacial** spatial orientation; ~ **f profesional** vocational counseling, career counseling
orificio *m* orifice; ~ **m ciego de la dentadura** foramen caecum of tooth; ~ **m de salida de un proyectil** exit of gunshot wound; ~ **m esofágico del estómago** cardial sphincter
originario *adj* primary, first, main
orina *f* urine; ~ **f azul** cyanuria, blue urine, indicanuria; ~ **f del chorro medio** midstream urine, MSU; ~ **f sanguinolenta** hematuria, blood in the urine, bloody urine; ~ **f turbia** cloudy urine
orinal *m* urine bottle, urinal
orinar *v* to urinate
ORL *f* otorhinolaryngology, ENT, ear nose & throat medicine
ornitina *f* ornithine
oro *m* gold
orofacial *adj* orofacial, mouth & face-related
orofaringe *f* oral part of pharynx, oropharynx
orquialgia *f* testicular pain
orquidectomía *f* orchidectomy, orchiectomy, oscheotomy, testectomy
orquitis *f* orchitis, inflammation of the testicle
ortesis *f* orthosis
ortodoncia *f* orthodontics, orthodonture, orthodontic work, orthodontology
ortofonista *f* speech therapist
ortopédico *adj* orthopedic, correcting deformity
ortopedista *f* orthopedist, chiropodist
ortostático *adj* orthostatic
orzuelo *m* stye, sty; ~ **m del ojo** hordeolum, sty on eyelid
oscuro *adj* dark
osículo *m* ossicle, small bone
osificación *f* ossification, bone formation

osificante *adj* ossifying
osmolalidad *f* osmolality
osmometría *f* osmometry
ósmosis *f* osmosis; ~ **f inversa** reverse osmosis
osmótico *adj* osmotic
osteítis *f* osteitis; ~ **f deformante** Paget's disease, Paget carcinoma; ~ **f fibroquística** neurofibromatosis, von Recklinghausen's disease, osteitis fibrosa cystica; ~ **f fibroquística** osteitis fibrosa cystica, Recklinghausen disease; ~ **f paratiroidea** osteitis fibrosa cystica, Recklinghausen disease
ostensible *adj* manifest, visible, evident
osteoarthritis *f* osteoarthritis, arthritis, arthrosis; ~ **f degenerativa** degenerative osteoarthritis
osteoartrosis *f* osteoarthrosis; ~ **f cervical** cervical osteoarthritis, osteoarthritis in the neck vertebrae
osteoblasto *m* osteoblast, osteocyte
osteocalcina *f* osteocalcin
osteocito *m* osteocyte
osteoclastic *adj* osteoclastic
osteoclasto *m* osteoclast
osteocondrodisplasia *f* osteochondrodysplasia
osteocondrofibroma *m* fibrosing osteochondroma, osteochondrofibroma
osteocondroma *m* osteochondroma; ~ **m fibroso** fibrosing osteochondroma, osteochondrofibroma
osteocráneo *m* osteocranium, the bony part of the skull
osteodistrofia *f* osteodystrophy, defective bone formation; ~ **f renal** renal osteodystrophy
osteoesclerosis *f* eburnation, osteoesclerosis
osteofibroma *m* fibroma, fibroma ossificans
osteófito *m* osteophyte
osteofitosis *f* osteophytosis; ~ **f vertebral** spinal osteophytosis
osteogénesis *f* osteogénesis; ~ **f por distracción** distraction osteogénesis; ~ **f por estimulación eléctrica** electrically stimulated osteogenesis
osteogénico *adj* osteogenic
osteógeno *adj* osteogenic
osteohalistéresis *f* halisteresis, osteohalisteresis
osteólisis *f* osteolysis; bone dissolving
osteoma *m* osteoma; ~ **m cutáneo** osteosis

0

cutis; ~ *m* **osteoide** osteoid osteoma;
~ *m* **sinusal** sinusal osteoma
osteomalacia *f* osteomalacia
osteomielitis *f* osteomyelitis; ~ **esclerosante**
sclerosing osteomyelitis; ~ *f* **hematógena**
aguda hematogenous osteomyelitis;
~ *f* **piógena** pyogenic osteomyelitis;
~ *f* **serosa** serous osteomyelitis
osteonecrosis *f* osteonecrosis; ~ *f* **aséptica**
aseptic epiphyseonecrosis, aseptic
osteonecrosis
osteopatía *f* osteopathy
osteopetrosis *f* osteopetrosis, osteopoikilosis
osteopoiquilía *f* osteopoikilosis
osteopoiquilosis *f* osteopoikilosis
osteoporosis *f* osteoporosis
osteoradionecrosis *f* radionecrosis of the bone
osteosarcoma *m* osteogenic sarcoma,
osteosarcoma
osteosíntesis *f* osteosynthesis
osteotomía *f* osteotomy
ostitis *f* osteitis
otalgia *f* earache, otalgia
otitis *f* otitis, ear inflammation; ~ *f* **crónica**
chronic otitis; ~ *f* **media** otitis media,
~ *f* **media aguda** acute otitis media
otoño *m* autumn
otoplastia *f* otoplasty
otorrea *f* otorrhea, otorrhoea, weeping ear,
secretory otitis media, serous otitis media
otorrhea *f* otorrhoea, otorrhoea, weeping ear,
secretory otitis media, serous otitis media
otorrinolaringología *f* otorhinolaryngology,
ENT, ear nose & throat medicine
otosclerosis *f* otosclerosis, progressive deafness
otoscopio *m* otoscope
ototóxico *adj* ototoxic
otra vez again
otro *adj* other
óvalo *adj* oval
ovárico *adj* ovarian
ovariectomía *f* ovariectomy, oophorectomy,
excision of an ovary, spaying
ovario *m* ovary; ~ *m* **poliquístico** polycystic
ovary
ovariotomía *f* ovariectomy, oophorectomy,
excision of an ovary
ovaritis *f* oophoritis

ovulación *f* ovulation
óvulo *m* ovum, egg, ovule; ~ *m* **fecundado**
spermatovum, fertilized ovum; ~ *m* **vaginal**
vaginal insert, vaginal suppository, ovule
oxacepán *m* oxazepam
oxacilina *f* oxacillin
oxalato *m* oxalate
oxandrolona *m* oxandrolone
oxazolidinona *f* oxazolidinone
oxibutinina *f* oxybutynin; ~ *m* **hidrocloruro**
oxybutynin hydrochloride
oxicarbonemia *f* carbon monoxide poisoning,
carboxyhemoglobinemia
oxicodona *f* oxycodone
oxidación *f* oxidation, adding oxygen;
~ *f* **biológica** bio-oxidation, biological
oxidation; ~ *f* **del medicamento** drug
oxidation; ~ **-reducción** *f* redox, oxidation-
reduction
óxido *m* oxide; ~ *m* **de cinc** zinc oxide;
~ *m* **nitroso** nitrous oxide, laughing gas;
~ *m* **potásico** potash, potassium oxide;
~ *m* **pulga** lead dioxide, plumbic anhydride;
~ **cúprico** *m* cupric oxide, copper oxide
oxidorreducción *f* redox, oxidation-reduction
oxidorreductasa *f* oxidoreductase
oxifenciclimina *f* oxyphencycline
oxigenación *f* oxygenation; ~ *f* **de la**
membrana extracorpórea extracorporeal
membrane oxygenation; ~ *f* **hiperbárica**
hyperbaric oxygenation; ~ *f* **de la sangre**
arterial arterial oxygen saturation, oxygen
saturation of hemoglobin
oxígeno *m* oxygen
oxihemoglobina *f* oxyhaemoglobin
oximetazolina *f* oxymetazoline
oximetolona *f* oxymetholone
oximetría *m* oximetry; ~ *m* **del pulso** pulse
oximetry
oxímetro *m* oximeter
oximioglobina *f* oxymyoglobin
oximorfona *f* oxymorphone
oxitetraciclina *f* oxytetracycline
oxitócico *adj* oxytocic, hastening labor
oxitocina *f* oxytocin
oxiuro *m* pinworm, intestinal nematode worm
ozono *m* ozone
ozonosfera *f* ozone layer, ozonesphere

ozonoterapia *f* ozone therapy
ozostomía *f* bad breath, halitosis, foul breath

P

paciente *m/f* patient; ~ *m/f* **ambulatorio** outpatient, ambulatory patient; ~ *m/f* **comprometido** compromised host; ~ *m/f* **en riesgo** risk patient; ~ *m/f* **externo** outpatient, ambulatory patient; ~ *m/f* **hospitalizado** inpatient; ~ *m/f* **mental** mentally ill person, psychiatric patient
padecer (de) *v* to suffer (from); ~ **de estrés** to be stressed out; ~ **del corazón** have heart trouble
padrastro *m* hangnail
padre *m* father
padres *m pl* parents; ~ *m pl* **adoptivos** foster parents, foster family
pagofagia *f* pagophagia
país *m* country
pájaro *m* bird
paladar *m* palate; ~ *m* **blando** soft palate; ~ *m* **duro** hard palate, roof of the mouth; ~ *m* **hendido** cleft palate, uranoschisis; ~ *m* **suave** soft palate
palatino *adj* palatine, palatal
paleta *f* scapula, shoulder blade
paliativo *m* palliative therapy, palliative treatment, palliative care
pálido *adj* pale
palindrómico *adj* palindromic, recrudescent, recurring
palíndromo *m* palindrome
palma *f* palm; ~ *f* **de la mano** palm of the hand
palmar *adj* palmar, volar
palmitato *m* palmitate
palmoplantar *adj* palmoplantar; **keratosis** *f* **difusa** palmoplantar diffuse keratosis
palo *m* stick
palpable *adj* palpable, tangible
palpación *f* palpation; ~ *f* **del abdomen** abdominal palpation
palpar *v* palpate, to touch, to
palpebral *adj* palpebral

palpitación *f* palpitation, heart beat; ~ *f* **cardíaca** heart palpitation, cardiac anxiety, palpitation of the heart, heart throb
palpitaciones *f pl* throbbing pain, palpitations, increased heart rate
paludismo *m* malaria
pan *m* bread
panacea *f* panacea
panadizo *m* panaritium, inflammation around the fingernail, whitlow, felon; ~ *m* **interdigital** foot rot, interdigital panaritium
pañales *m pl* diapers
panax *m* ginseng
pancolectomía *f* colectomy, pancolectomy, extirpation of the entire colon
páncreas *m* pancreas
pancreatectomía *f* pancreatectomy
pancreatitis *f* pancreatitis, inflammation of the pancreas; ~ *f* **hemorrágica aguda** pancreatic apoplexy, hemorrhagic apoplexy of the pancreas
pancreatogastrostomía *f* pancreaticogastrostomy
pancr(e)ozimina *f* cholecystokinin, pancreozymin
pandemia *f* pandemic, holo-endemic, widespread epidemic
pandémico *adj* pandemic, holo-endemic
paniculitis *f* panniculitis, inflammation of fat under the skin; ~ *f* **mesentérica** mesenteric panniculitis
panmielopatía *f* panmyelopathy, panmyelophthisis; ~ *f* **alérgica** allergic panmyelopathy; ~ *f* **lupoide** lupoid panmyelopathy
panmieloptisis *f* panmyelopathy, panmyelophthisis
paño *m* cloth, duster; ~ *m* **para lavarse** washcloth, bath mitt
pantalla *f* screen, shade; ~ *f* **de la computadora** computer screen; ~ *f* **luminiscente** luminescent screen; ~ *f* **radioscópica** fluoroscopic screen
pantimediás *f pl* women's panties, women's underwear
pantoprazole *m* pantoprazole
pantorilla *f* calf

panza f belly, stomach, paunch, tummy
papaína f papain, thiol protease made from Carica papaya (pawpaws)
papas f pl potatoes
papel m paper; ~ m **de excusado** toilet paper; ~ m **higiénico** toilet paper
paperas f pl parotiditis, mumps, parotitis, swollen glands
papila f papilla; ~ **del gusto** taste bud; ~ f **dental** dental papilla; ~ f **dérmica** cutaneous papilla; ~ f **de Santorini** minor duodenal papilla; ~ f **óptica** papilla of the optic nerve; ~ f **filiforme** filiform papilla; ~ f **pilosa** hair papilla, papilla pili
papilar adj papillary
papiledema m papiledema, papilloedema, swollen optical disk
papilitis f papillitis, inflammation of the optic disk
papillocarcinoma m papillocarcinoma
papilomatosis f peritoneal papillomatosis
papilomavirus m papillomavirus
pápula f papule, mole
papulosis f papulosis; ~ f **atrófica** atrophic papulosis; ~ f **atrófica maligna** papulosis atrophica maligna, Degos-Delort-Tricot syndrome
paquete m package, parcel; ~ m **linfático** lymphatic bundle
paquipleuritis f pachipleuritis
paquitena f pachytene
par m pair, couple; ~ m **cromosómico** pair of chromosomes; ~ m **iónico** ion pair
para to, for
paraanestesia f paraanesthesia
paraaórtico adj para-aortic
paracentesis f paracentesis, fluid removal, abdominal tap; ~ f **de la córnea** corneal puncture
paracetamol m acetaminophen, paracetamol
parada f stop, arrest; ~ f **cardíaca** cardiac arrest
paradójico adj paradoxical
paradontólisis f periodontolysis, periodontoclasia, pyorrhoea alveolaris parodontitis, gingivopericementitis, dysparodontia
parafrenia f paraphrenia, dementia precoz
parafrenitis f paraphrenitis

paraganglios m pl paraganglions; ~ m pl **cromafines** chromaffin paraganglions, near the sympathetic ganglia; ~ m pl **no cromafines** parasympathetic paraganglia, nonchromafin paraganglia, glomus typmpanicum; ~ m pl **parasimpáticos** parasympathetic paraganglia, nonchromafin paraganglia, glomus typmpanicum
paragonimiasis f paragonimiasis, oriental lung fluke disease, infection with paragonimus trematodes
paralelaje m **ocular** ocular parallax
paralelismo m parallelism
paralelo adj parallel
paralgesia f paraesthesia, paresthesia
parálisis f palsy, paralysis; ~ f **agitante** Parkinson's disease; ~ f **capsular** capsular hemiplegia, capsular paralysis; ~ f **cerebral** cerebral palsy, athetosis; ~ f **de Bell** facial paralysis, Bell's palsy; ~ f **de Duchenne Erb** Duchenne-Erb paralysis; ~ f **del nervio motor ocular externo** abducens paralysis; ~ f **facial** facial paralysis, Bell's palsy; ~ f **laríngea saturnina** lead-induced laryngeal paralysis; ~ f **por plomo** lead palsy, lead paralysis; ~ f **saturnina** lead palsy, lead paralysis
paralizar v to paralyze, to immobilize
paramédico m paramedic, emergency medical technician, ambulance attendant
parametría f parametritis, pelvic pelvic
parametritis f parametritis, pelvic pelvic
parámetro m parameter, criterion
paramorfina f dimethylmorphine, thebaine, paramorphine
paranoia f paranoia; ~ f **de persecución** persecution paranoia
paranoico m **sensitivo** sensitive paranoiac, reference delusion
paranoide adj paranoiac; ~ adj paranoiac
paraoxón m paraoxon
paraplejía f paralysis, palsy, paraplegia
parapléjico adj paraplegic, m paraplegic
pararreflexia f paraflexia, dysreflexia; ~ f **vestibular cruzada** crossed vestibular dysreflexia, crossed vestibular nystagmus
parasimpático adj parasympathetic
parasimpaticolítico adj parasympatholytic

parasimpaticomimético *adj* parasympathomimetic

parasimpatolítico *adj* parasympatholytic

parasitario *adj* parasitic

parásito *m* parasite; ~ *m* **de heridas** facultative parasite; ~ **estricto** obligate parasite; ~ *m* **facultativo** facuitative parasite, wound parasite; ~ *m* **intestinal** intestinal parasite, parasitic worm

parasitología *f* parasitology

parasomnia *f* parasomnia

paratifoideo *adj* paratyphoid

parathion *m* parathion

paratirina *f* parathormone, parathyrin, parathyroid hormone, PTH

paratiroideo *adj* parathyroid

paraureteral *adj* paruretera1

paraurétrico *adj* paruretera1

paraureteritis *f* para-urethritis

paravenoso *adj* paravenous

paraventricular paraventricular

paravesical *adj* paravesical

parche *m* patch; ~ *m* **de nicotina** nicotine patch, transdermal patch; ~ *m* **de ojo** eye patch; ~ *m* **transdérmico** transdermal patch

pared *f* wall; ~ *f* **del estomago** wall of the stomach, gastric wall; ~ *f* **intestinal** wall of the intestine; ~ *f* **uterina** uterine lining, uterine wall

paregórico *m* paregoric

pareja *f* partner (sex), pair, couple

parénquima *m* parenchyma, functional tissue of an organ, storage tissue

parenteral *m* parenteral, not by mouth

parentesco *m* blood relationship, family relationship

paresia *f* paresis, partial paralysis; ~ *f* **edematosa** hydroparesis

parestesia *f* paraesthesia, paresthesia

pariente *adj* relative, blood relative

parientes *m pl* relatives

parietal *adj* parietal

parihuelas *f pl* gurney, stretcher cart, wheeled stretcher

parihuelas *f pl* stretcher, litter

parkinsonismo *m* parkinsonism

parlanchín *adj* talkative, loquacious, chatty

paro *m* arrest, stoppage, shutdown, breakdown; ~ *m* **cardíaco** cardiac arrest; ~ *m* **cardíaco inducido** induced cardiac arrest, stopping the heart during surgery; ~ *m* **respiratorio** respiratory failure, respiratory arrest, respiratory impairment

parodontología *f* periodontics, periodontology

parodontosis *f* periodontal disease, periodontosis

paroniquia *f* paronychia, inflammation of the nail skin

parótida *f* parotid, situated near the ear

parótidas *f pl* mumps

parotitis *f* parotitis, mumps, swollen glands

paroxístico *adj* paroxysmal

parpadear *v* to blink one's eye, to wink, to nictitate

párpado *m* eyelid

parte *f* part, portion; ~ **del cuerpo** region, body part; ~ *f* **elemental** particle

partera *f* midwife, birth attendant

partes *f pl* **blandas** soft tissues; ~ *f pl* **nobles** genitals, sex organs, reproductive organs; ~ *f pl* **ocultas** genitals, sex organs, reproductive organs; ~ *f pl* **privadas** genitals, sex organs, reproductive organs

participante *m* participant

partícula *f* particle; ~ *f* **formadora de colonia** CFU; ~ *f* **submicrónica** sub-micron particle

particularmente especially, particularly

partículas *f pl* foreign matter

parto *m* labor, delivery, parturition, birth, childbirth, birthing; ~ *m* **prematuro** premature birth, premature delivery

parvovirus *m* parvovirus

pasado over; ~ *adj* **de peso** overweight, fat, chubby, pudgy, portly, stout; ~ *m* **mañana** day after tomorrow

pasajero *adj* fleeting, passing, short-term, temporary, transitory, brief

pasaporte *m* passport

pasas *f pl* raisins

pascal *m* pascal

pasivo *adj* passive

paso *m* passage, transit; ~ *m* **de luz** pathlenght

pasta *f* **de Buckley** Buckley paste; ~ *f* **de impresión** impression paste, mould putty, stent's mass, Luralite paste; ~ *f* **de Viena** Vienna paste; ~ *f* **dentífrica** toothpaste

pastel m pie, cake
pasteurella f **pestis** Pasteurella pestis, Yersinia pestis, bacteria that causes bubonic plague;
~ f **tularensis** Francisella tularensis, Pasteurella tularensis
pasteurelosis f pasteurellosis
pastilla f pill, tablet, lozenge; ~ f **revestida** coated tablet
pastillas f pl **masticables** chewable tablets;
~ f pl **para dolor de cabeza** headache tablets
pata f paw, foot (animal term)
patacón m welt
pataleta f to have a fit, to throw a fit
patatús m fainting, swoon, collapse
patchuli m patchouli oil
patela f kneecap, patella
pato m bedpan
patógeno adj pathogen
patología f pathology; ~ f **dentaria** dental pathology; ~ f **experimental** experimental pathology; ~ f **molecular** molecular pathology; ~ f **perinatal** birth defect
patológico adj pathological
patólogo m clinical pathologist, pathologist
patrón m/F boss, employer, owner, m pattern, standard; ~ m **arbitrario** arbitrary standard;
~ m **de calibración** calibration standard;
~ m **primario** primary standard;
~ m **secundario** secondary standard
patulina f patulin, clavacin, claviformin
pavulon m pavulon
peachimetría f pH-metry
peachímetro m pH-meter
peca f freckle
pecho m chest, thorax, breast
pecoso adj freckled, freckly
pectasa f pectin esterase, pectin acetyl esterase, pectase
pectina f pectin
pectinato adj pectinate
pedar v to fart, to pass wind, to cut one, to break wind
pedialyte Pedialyte
pediatra m pediatrician
pediatría f pediatrics, paediatrics
pediátrico adj paediatric, pediatric
pedículo m petiole, peduncle; ~ m **ilíaco** iliac pedicle; ~ m **mesoabdominal** abdominal

pedicle, pedicle of the allantois;
~ m **vertebral** collum arcus vertebrarum, pedicle of vertebral arch
pediculosis f louse (singular), lice (plural), pediculosis; ~ f **pubis** pediculosis pubis
pedo m fart, wind, expelled gas, flatus
pedodoncia f pedodontics
pedología f child development, pedology
pedúnculo m petiole, peduncle; ~ m **cerebral** crus of cerebrum; ~ m **cerebeloso** peduncle of cerebellum
pefloxacina f pefloxacine
pegajoso adj communicable, contagious, sticky
pelagra f pellagra
película f film, movie; ~ f **liquida** liquifilm, thin liquid layer of coating
peligro m risk, danger, hazard; ~ m **en el lugar de trabajo** workplace hazard
peligroso adj risky, dangerous, pernicious, malignant, fatal, harmful
pellizcar v to pinch
pelo m hair; ~ m **de animales** animal hair;
~ m **radical** hair root, hair follicle
pelos m pl body hair; ~ m pl **púbicos** pubic hair, pubic hairs
peludo adj hairy, pilous
pélvico adj pelvic
pelvimetría f pelvimetry; ~ f **clínica** clinical pelvimetry; ~ f **radiográfica** X-ray pelvimetry
pelvis f pelvis, hip, coxa; ~ f **ginecoide** gynecoid pelvis; ~ f **masculina** masculine pelvis, pelvis of a man
pene m penis
penetración f penetration; ~ f **cutánea** cutaneous penetration
penetrancia f penetrancy
penetrante adj incisive, cutting
pénfigo m serious skin disease, pemphigus;
~ m **brasileño** Brazilian pemphigus, pemphigus brasiliensis; ~ m **brómico** bromine pemphigus;
~ m **eritematoso** pemphigus erythematosus, Senear-Usher disease; ~ m **foliáceo** pemphigus foliaceus
penfigoide adj pemphigoid
penfigoid f **bulloso** bullous pemphigoid, bullous eczema
penicilina f penicillin
penicilinasa f penicillinase

pensamiento *m* thought; ~ *m* **abstracto** abstract thinking; ~ *m* **autista** autistic thinking; ~ *m* **incoherente** incoherent thinking, confusion, incoherent ideation; ~ *m* **paradójico** paradoxical thinking thinking
pensar *v* to think
pentagastrina *f* pentagastrin
pentosa *f* pentose
pentoxifilina *f* pentoxifylline
peor worse
pepino *m* cucumber
pepsina *f* pepsin
péptico *adj* peptic
peptidil-dipeptidasa A *f* ECA
péptido *m* peptide; ~ *m* **antibacteriano** antibacterial peptide; ~ *m* **antigénico** antigenic peptide; ~ **C** *m* C peptide
pequeño *adv* little, small
pera *f* pear
percepción *f* sensation, perception; ~ *f* **auditiva** auditory perception; ~ *f* **de la profundidad** depth perception
percolación *f* percolation
percusión *f* clapping, tapping, percussion, a massage technique
percutáneo *adj* percutaneous, through the skin
perder *v* to lose, to leak, to miss; ~ *v* **el conocimiento** to lose consciousness, to faint
pérdida *f* loss, waste; ~ *f* **de inteligencia** loss of intelligence, disintegration of intelligence, mental deterioration; ~ *f* **de la consciencia** expansion of consciousness; ~ *f* **de la voz** aphonia, loss of voice; ~ *f* **de memoria** memory loss, loss of memory, amnesia; ~ *f* **de peso** weight loss, slimming, loss of weight; ~ *f* **de sangre** loss of blood
pérdidas *f pl* **blancas** fluor albus, vaginal discharge, nervous vaginal discharge; ~ *f pl* **vaginales tras el parto** lochia, post-birth vaginal discharge
perenne *adj* perennial, all the time, persistent
pereza *f* indolence, laziness
perezoso *adj* maudlin, lackadaisical, apathetic
perfenacina *f* perphenazine
perfil *m* biochemical profile; ~ *m* **bioquímico** biochemical profile; ~ *m* **de imprecisión** *m* imprecision profile; ~ *m* **plasmático** plasma profile

perfluorocarbono *m* perfluorocarbon
perforación *f* perforation; ~ *f* **del tabique nasal** perforation of the nasal septum
perfusión *f* perfusion, through passage of fluid, infusion, drip-feeding; ~ *f* **de cloruro de sodio** saline infusion
perianal *adj* perianal
periapendicitis *f* perithyphlitis, periappendicitis
periarteritis *f* arteritis; ~ *f* **herpética** herpetic arteritis
periartritis *f* periarthritis, joint inflammation; ~ *f* **de cadera** periarthritis of the hip
pericardiocentesis *f* pericardiocentesis, puncture of the pericardium, pericardial tap, pericardicentesis
pericardio *m* pericardium
pericardiocentesis *f* pericardiocentesis, puncture of the pericardium, pericardial tap, pericardicentesis
pericardiostomía *f* pericardiostomy, pericardial window technique
pericarditis *f* pericarditis, inflammation of the pericardium; ~ *f* **adhesiva** adherent pericardium; ~ *f* **ameboide** amoebic pericarditis; ~ *f* **constrictiva** adherent pericardium; ~ *f* **postinfarto de miocardio** pericarditis due to myocardial infarction; ~ *f* **reumática** rheumatic pericarditis
pericondrio *m* perichondrium
peridural *adj* peridural
periférico *adj* peripheral
perilla *f* **(del ojo)** hordeolum, sty (on eyelid)
perimielitis *f* spinal meningitis, perimyelitis
perinatal *adj* shortly after birth, perinatal
perinatología *f* perinatology, perinatal medicine
perineal *adj* perineal
perineo *m* pelvic floor, floor of the pelvis
perineoplastía *f* perineoplasty, plastic surgery of pelvic floor
perineotomía *f* episiotomy, cut to vagina in childbirth
periódico *adj* cyclic, periodic, regular
período *m* period; ~ *m* **de arranque** start-up time; ~ *m* **de permanencia** residence time; ~ *m* **de recuperación** recovery time, recovery period; ~ *m* **de remisión** disease-free interval,

P

remission, remittence, period of remission;
~ *m* **fértil de la mujer** child bearing period;
~ *m* **improductivo** down time; ~ *m* **latente**
latent period, latent time, inactive period;
~ *m* **refractario** refractory period;
~ *m* **ventana** latency stage, window period,
latency stage

periodontitis *f* periodontitis, alveolitis,
inflammation of the periodontal membrane,
periodontitis simplex

periodontoclasia *f* periodontolysis,
periodontoclasia, pyorrhoea alveolaris
parodontitis, gingivopericementitis,
dysparodontia

periodontosis periodontal disease, periodontosis

perioperativo *adj* perioperative

perioral *adj* perioral

periorbitario *adj* periorbital

periosteofito *m* periostitis ossificans

periostio *m* periosteum

periostoma *m* periostitis ossificans

peristalsis *f* peristalsis

peristáltico *adj* peristaltic

peritiflitis *f* perithyphlitis, periappendicitis

peritoneo *m* peritoneum

peritoneocentesis *f* peritoneal puncture

peritoneoscopia *f* peritoneoscope,
peritoneoscopy

peritonitis *f* peritonitis, inflammation of the
peritoneum

periumbilical *adj* periumbilical

periuretritis *f* para-urethritis

perivascular *adj* perivascular

perixoma *m* peroxisome

perjudicial *adj* to be detrimental

perla *f* nodule, node, nodus (in the hypodermis),
pearl

perlático *m* paralysis, palsy

perlesía *f* paralysis, palsy

permanente permanent, constantly

permeabilidad *f* permeability; ~ **capilar**
capillary permeability

permeable *adj* permeable, pervious, porous

permiso *m* permission

pernicioso *adj* harmful (to your health),
noxious, detrimental, pernicious, malignant

pernio *m* chillblains, pernio

pero *m* but

peroné *m* fibula

peroneo *adj* peronial

peroperatorio *adj* intraoperative, operative,
during the operation

peroral *adj* peroral, by mouth, orally

peroxidación *f* peroxidation; ~ **f lipídica** lipid
peroxidation

peroxidasa *f* peroxidase; ~ *f* **catalítica** catalytic
peroxidase

peróxido *m* peroxide; ~ **de benzoilo** benzoyl
peroxide, benzoic peroxyde

peroxisoma *m* peroxisome

perpetuo perennial, all the time, persistent

perro *m* dog

perseverante *adj* persistent, chronic

persistente *adj* persistent, chronic, recalcitrant,
all the time, perennial

persona *f* person; ~ *f* **accidentada** injured
person, casualty; ~ *f* **con desventaja**
handicapped person, disabled person; ~ *f* **con**
discapacidad mental mentally disabled
person, mentally handicapped person; ~ *f* **con**
impedimento disabled person, handicapped
person; ~ *f* **seropositiva** HIV-positive person

personal *m* staff; ~ *m* **sanitario** health
professional, health worker, medical
practitioner

personalidad *f* personality; ~ *f* **ciclotímica**
cyclothymic personality

perspiración *f* perspiration; ~ *f* **insensible**
insensible perspiration, breathing of the skin

perturbar *v* to fase, to disturb

pertussis *f* pertussis, whooping cough

perversión *f* perversion

pesadilla *f* nightmare

pesado *adj* heavy

pesario *m* check pessary, a birth control device,
pessary

pescado *m* fish

pescuezo *m* neck; ~ *m* **de un animal** neck of an
animal

peso *m* weight; ~ *m* **al nacer** birth weight;
~ *m* **atómico** atomic weight; ~ *m* **molecular**
molecular weight

pesquisar *v* to research, to investigate, to
examine

pestañas *f pl* eyelashes

pestañear *v* to blink one's eye, to wink, to

nictitate

peste f plague; ~ f **bubónica** bubonic plague, an acute febrile, infectious fatal disease caused by the bacillus Yersinia pestis; ~ f **porcina** swine fever, hog cholera

petacón adj overweight, fat, chubby, pudgy, portly, stout

petequia f petechia, purplish red spot

petidina f meperidine

petiolus m petiole, peduncle

petit mal petit mal, minor epilepsy

petrolatum crude petroleum jelly, petrolatum

pezón m nipple

pH m pH; ~ m **de equilibrio** pH balance, pH equilibrium; ~ m **del cuerpo** pH of the body, acid–base balance of the organism

phanryngitis phanryngitis

phosphatemia f phosphatemia

phosphaturia f phosphaturia

phtirius m **pubis** phthirus pubis

piamadre f pia mater

picadura f sting; ~ f **de abeja** bee sting; ~ f **de insecto** insect bite, insect sting; ~ f **de mosquito** mosquito bite; ~ f **de piojo** flea bite; ~ f **de pulga** flea bite; ~ f **de medusa** f jellyfish sting

picante (adj) itchy, itching, spicy

picazón m itch, itching, pruritus, tingling

picnosis f pyknosis

pico m beak, peak, peak level, spike, pick

picor m itch, pruritus

picornavirus m picornavirus, pico-RNA-virus

pie m foot; ~ m **de atleta** athlete´s foot; ~ m **de inmersión** immersion foot, trench foot, paddy foot, trenchfoot; ~ m **de trinchera** immersion foot, trench foot, paddy foot, trenchfoot; ~ m **espinoso** spinous foot, an affliction of horses & cattle; ~ m **pendular** foot drop, dropped foot, paralysis of the dorsal extensor muscles of the foot and toes; ~ m **valgo** pes valgus, duck feet; ~ m **varo** varus foot

piedra f calculus, stone; ~ f **del riñón** nephrolith, kidney stone

piel f skin; ~ f **artificial** artificial skin; ~ f **seca** dry skin

pielitis f pyelitis, inflammation of kidney

pielografía f excretion pyelography,

pielography, ureteropyelography; ~ f **intravenosa** infusion urography

pielonefritis f pyelonephritis

pierna adj left-handed, flower limb, leg, lower extremity; ~ f **artificial** leg prosthesis, artificial leg

piernas f pl **inquietas** restless legs

pigeonnau m tanner's disease, chrome ulceration, chrome ulcer

pigmentación f pigmentation, skin coloring, skin color

pigmento m pigment; ~ m **biliar** bile pigment

píldora f pill, tablet; ~ f **anticonceptiva** the pill, oral contraceptive, birth control pill; ~ f **de dieta** diet pill; ~ f **de dormir** sleeping pill, hypnotic, soporific; ~ f **para sacar el agua** water pills

pilocarpina f pilocarpine

piloerección f piloerection

píloro m pylorus, narrow outlet of stomach

pilorospasmo m pylorospasm

piloso adj hairy, pilous

pimiento m pepper

pinchar v to prick, to stick, to puncture

pinchazo m pinprick, pricking

pinchazos m pl pins and needles, formication, tingling

pinocitosis f pinocytosis, cell drinking

pintura f pl paint

pinzas f pl forceps, tweezers; ~ f pl **arteriales** arterial tweezers; ~ f pl **para depilar** depilating tweezers; ~ f pl **para manejar el algodon** cotton ball holder, dressing forceps

piocina f pyocin

piocinotipia f pyocin typing

piodermia f pyoderma, piodermia

piodermitis f pyoderma, piodermia

piógeno adj purulent, pusy, pyogenic

piojo m louse (singular, plural: lice); ~ m **ladilla** crab louse, pubic louse

piotórax m purulent pleurisy, pleuropyesis, suppurative pleurisy, pyothorax

piperacilina f piperacillin

piperonal m piperonal, heliotropin

pipeta f pipette, eyedropper, medicine dropper; ~ f **aforada** calibrated pipet, volumetric pipet; ~ f **de inhalación** f carry-over inhaler

piramidal adj wedge-shaped

P

pirámide *m* age-sex pyramid; ~ *m* **de población** age-sex pyramid

pirexia *f* pyrexia, fever

piridoxal *adj* pyridoxal

piridoxina *f* pyridoxine

pirizinamida *f* pyrazinamide

pirógeno *adj* pyrogenic, fever inducing

piroplasmosis *f* piroplasmosis, tick fever, babesiosis, Babesia infection

pirosis *f* heartburn, pyrosis, cardialgia, pain in the heart area

piruvato *m* pyruvate; ~ ~ **-carboxilasa** *f* pyruvate carboxylase; ~ **-cinasa** *f* pyruvate kinase; ~ **-descarboxilasa** *f* pyruvate decarboxylase; ~ ~ **-deshidrogenasa** *f* pyruvate dehydrogenase; ~ **-oxidasa** *f* pyruvate oxidase

pisar *v* to walk on; ~ **v en falso** to take a misstep; ~ **v mal** take a misstep, to

piso *m* floor, storey; ~ *m* **pélvico** pelvic floor, floor of the pelvis

pitiriasis *f* pityriasis, scaling of the skin

pituita *f* phlegm, viscid mucus

pivampicilina *f* pivampicillin

placa *f* sheet, plate; ~ *f* **de coadaptación** coaptation plate; ~ *f* **de microtitulación** microtiter plate; ~ *f* **dental, sarro** dental plaque, tartar; ~ *f* **de osteosíntesis** bone plate; ~ *f* **ecuatorial** equatorial plate; ~ *f* **metafásica** metaphase plate; ~ *f* **ósea** osteotomy plate, bone plate; ~ *f* **pleural** pleural plaque

placas *f pl* plaques; ~ *f pl* **seniles** amyloid plaques, senile plaques, amyloid deposits; ~ *f pl* **de Peyer** *f pl* lymphatic nodules of the vermiform appendix

placebo *m* placebo

placenta *f* afterbirth, placenta

plan *m* plan; ~ *m* **radioterapéutico** radiology treatment plan; ~ *m* **terapéutico** treatment plan

plana *f* page; ~ *f* **mayor** staff; ~ *f* **relajación** night guard, mouth guard, biteguard, occlusal splint, peridontal splint, dental prosthesis

planeamiento *m* planning

planificación *f* planning; ~ *f* **familiar** family planning, reproductive health care, planning for birth control

plano *adj* flat; ~ *m* plane, plan, map; ~ *m* **sagital** sagittal plane, vertical plane which is in parallel with the median plane of the body

planta *f* floor, ground, plant; ~ *f* **del pie** sole of the foot, plantar surface

plantar *adj* plantar

plantas *f pl* **medicinales** medicinal herbs, medicinal plants

plantilla *f* staff; ~ *f* **ortopédica** orthopedic insert, insole; ~ *f* **para el calzado** insole

plaqueta *f* blood platelet, thrombocyte

plasma *m* plasma; ~ *m* **estable** quiescent plasma; ~ *m* **granuloso** granular plasma, endoplasma; ~ *m* **hemático** blood plasma, human plasma; ~ *m* **sanguíneo** blood plasma, human plasma; ~ *m* **seminal** seminal plasma

plasmacito *m* plasmacyte, plasmocyte

plasmaféresis *f* plasmapheresis, plasma exchange

plasmalema *f* plasma membrane, plasma lemma, outer membrane

plasmalógeno-sintasa *f* plasmalogen synthase

plasmaproteína *f* plasma protein, blood protein

plásmide *m* plasmid

plásmido *m* plasmid; ~ *m* **autorreplicable** runaway plasmid; ~ *m* **de resistencia** resistance transfer factor; ~ *m* **desarmado** inactive plasmid; ~ *m* **multicopia** multicopy plasmid; ~ *m* **primero** prime plasmid; ~ *m* **vector** plasmid vector

plasmina *f* fibrinolysin, fibrinase

plasminógeno *m* profibrinogen, profibrinolysin

plasmoblasto *m* plasmablast

plasmocito *m* plasmacyte, plasmocyte, plasma cell

plasmocitoma *m* multiple myeloma, plasmacytoma, Kahler's disease, Huppert's disease, Bozzolo disease; ~ *m* **solitário** solitary plasmacytoma

plasmodium *m* malariae Plasmodium malariae

plastía *f* **del labio** cheiloplasty, lip surgery

plasticidad *f* plasticity; ~ *f* **fisiológica** physiological plasticity; ~ *f* **genética** genetic plasticity

plastosoma *m* mitochondria, mitochondrion, chondriosome, plastosome

plata *f* silver

plátano *m* banana
platispondilia *f* platyspondylia, platispondilia
pleomórfico *adj* pleomorphic
pletismografía *f* plethysmography
pleura *f* pleura; ~ *f* **parietal** parietal pleura; ~ *f* **visceral** visceral pleura, pulmonary pleura
pleurectomía *f* pleural decortication, pleurectomy
pleuresía *f* pleurisy, pleuritis, hydrothorax; ~ *f* **eosinófila** eosinophil pleurisy; ~ *f* **exudativa** exudative pleurisy; ~ *f* **hemorrágica** hemorrhagic pleurisy; ~ *f* **parietal** parietal pleurisy
pleuritis *f* pleurisy, pleuritis, hydrothorax
pleurodesis *f* pleurodesis
plexo *m* plexus, network; ~ *m* **hemorroidal** prostatic venous plexus; ~ *m* **hipogástrico** hypogastric plexus; ~ *m* **mamilar** mamillary body, mamillary plexus, corpora candicantia; ~ *m* **solar** solar plexus, celiac plexus; ~ *m* **vaginal** vaginal plexus; ~ *m* **venoso** venous plexus
plica *f* plica, fold of skin or tissue, plication, plicature
pliegue *m* plica, fold of skin or tissue, plication, plicature; ~ *m* **de Hasner** lacrimal fold, plica lacrimalis, Hasner's fold, Cruveilhier's valve; ~ *m* **sinovial** synovial fold
plomo *m* lead
plumbismo *m* lead poisoning, lead intoxication, plumbism
plurinucleado *adj* multinuclear
pneumonía *f* pneumonia; ~ *f* **cruposa** croupo-influenzal pneumonia
pneumonitis *f* **intersticial linfoide** interstitial lymphocytic pneumonia
población *f* population; ~ *f* **de referencia** reference population
pocillo *m* mug, bowl, dish; ~ *m* **de microvaloración** microtiter well
poco *adj* a little, *adv* little, small; ~ **a poco** gradual
pocos *adj* few
podálico *adj* pedal, foot related
poder *m* potency, sexual ability; ~ *m* **sexual** potency, sexual ability
poder *v* can (to be able to), may
podólogo *m* podiatrist, chiropodist

polarografía *f* polarography
polen *m* pollen
poliadenoma *m* multiple adenoma; ~ *m* **velloso** multiple villous adenoma
poliaminas *f pl* polyamines; ~ *f pl* **biógenas** biogenic polyamines; ~ *f pl* **biogénicas** biogenic polyamines
poliartritis *f* polyarthritis, severe arthritis
policía *f* police
policitemia *f* polycytemia, policitemia; ~ *f* **saturnina** saturnine polyglobulism
policondritis *f* polychondritis; ~ *f* **recidivante** atrophic polychondritis, chronic polychondritis
polidactilia *f* polydactyly, polydactylism
polidipsia *f* chronic thirst polydipsia, chronic thirst
polifarmacia *f* polypharmacy,
poligamia *f* polygamy, the practice of having several wives
poligénes *m pl* polygenes, multiple factor
poliglobulia *f* polycytemia, policitemia; ~ *f* **saturnina** saturnine polyglobulism
poliinsaturados *m pl* polyunsaturates, polyunsaturated fatty acids
poliligador polylinker
polimerización *f* polymerization; ~ *f* **iónica** ionic polymerization
polimixina *f* polymyxin
polimórfico *adj* polymorphic
polimorfismo *m* polymorphism; ~ *m* **genético** genetic polymorphism
polineuritis *f* polyneuritis; ~ *f* **alcohólica** alcoholic polyneuritis, potatorum polyneuritis; ~ *f* **amiloida familiar** familial amyloid polyneuropathy
poliomielitis *f* polio, poliomyelitis, infantile paralysis
poliosis *f* **medicamentosa** medicated canities
polipéptido *m* polypeptide, amino acid polymer; ~ *m* **inhibidor gastrico** gastric inhibitory peptide
pólipo *m* polyp; ~ *m* **adenomatoso** adenomatous polyp; ~ *m* **anal** anal polyp; ~ *m* **benigno** benign polyp; ~ *m* **coanal** choanal polyp, nasal polypus; ~ *m* **del cólon** intestinal polyp, polyp in the colon; ~ *m* **nasal** nasal polyp; ~ *m* **uretral** urethral polyp
poliquimioterapia *f* combination chemotherapy

P

poliquistosis f renal polycystic kidney disease

politerapia f polytherapy

política f policy; ~ f **de la calidad** quality policy

politoxicomanía f multiple addiction, multiple drug abuse, polytoxicomania

poliuria f polyuria

polivalente adj polyvalent

póliza f policy; ~ f **de seguro** insurance policy; ~ f **estimada** benefit policy

pollo m chicken

polvo m dust; ~ m **de amianto** asbestos dust; ~ m **de talco** talcum powder

polvos m pl **lácteos** milk powder; ~ m pl **lácteos** powdered milk; ~ m pl **para bebés** baby powder

polyomavirus m polyomavirus

pomada f ointment, paste, pomade, salve; ~ f **analgésica** analgesic ointment; ~ f **antiinflamatoria** anti-inflammatory ointment; ~ f **oftálmica** eye ointment; ~ f **para quemadura** burn ointment

pómulo m cheek bone, zygomatic bone

poner v to put, to set; ~ **-se** v **tenso** to tense up, to stiffen

poplíteal f popliteal; ~ f **fossa** back of the knee, popliteal space, popliteal fossa

por for; ~ **boca** peroral, by mouth; ~ **eso (conj)** so; ~ **favor** please; ~ **la mañana** in the morning; ~ **la noche** at night, in the night; ~ **la tarde** in the afternoon; ~ **qué** why; ~ **vía bucal** orally; ~ **vía oral** orally

porcentaje m rate, percentage; ~ m **de embarazos** pregnancy rate

porción f portion, share, piece

porfiria f prophyria; ~ f **cutánea tardía** porphyria cutanea tarda

porfirina f porphyrin

poros m pl pores

porosidad f porousness, porosity; ~ f **capilar** capillary porosity

poroso permeable, pervious, porous

porotos m beans

porque because

portacama f **rodante** gurney, stretcher cart, wheeled stretcher

portador m carrier, vehicle of infection

transmission, excipient; ~ m **asintomático** asymptomatic carrier, symptom-free carrier; ~ m **crónico del virus** chronic carrier of the virus; ~ m **de gérmenes** germ vector, germ carrier; ~ m **de la infección** germ vector

portaobjetos m slide

posición f position

positivo adj positive; ~ adj **falso** false positive; ~ m **verdadero** true positive

posmenopáusico adj postmenopausal

posnatal adj postnatal

posología f statement of dose, posology, dosage regimen, overall dosage, dosage schedule

posparto postpartum, after childbirth

posprandial adj postprandial, after dinner

postefecto m aftereffect

postemilla f abscess in the mouth

postergar v to procrastinate

posterior posterior

postilla f scab on a wound, crust

postoperatorio adj postoperative, postsurgical

postponer todo procrastinate, to

postquirúrgico adj postoperative, postsurgical

postrado m prone position, face-down position; ~ adj **en cama** bedridden, confined to bed

postraumático adj posttraumatic, post-traumatic

postrero adj terminal

post-traumático adj post-traumatic, posttraumatic

póstumo adj posthumous

postura f position; ~ f **antálgica** relieving posture; ~ f **en el trabajo** work posture; ~ f **incómoda** postural discomfort; ~ f **mala** improper posture, false posture, bad posture

postural adj postural, posture-related

potasio m potassium

potencia f potency, sexual ability, power; ~ f **radiante** radiant power

potenciación f potentiation, potentialization

potencial adj potential adj

potencial m potential; ~ m **de electrodo** electrode potencial; ~ m **eléctrico** tension, tone; ~ m **electrocinético** electrokinetic potential; ~ m **evocado** potential; ~ m **postsináptico** postsynaptic potential; ~ m **químico** chemical potential

potenciales *m pl* **evocados auditivos** brainstem evoked responses; ~ *m pl* **evocados auditivos del tronco cerebral** auditory brainstem evoked potentials; ~ *m pl* **evocados visuales** visually evoked potentials

potenciación *f* potentialization, potentiation

potenciometría *f* potentiometry

práctica *f* practice; ~ *f* **médica** medical practice, practising medicine

practicabilidad *f* practicability

practicar *v* to practice, to practise; ~ **el coito** *v* have intercourse, to, to have sex, to, to copulate, to, make love, to

precalentarse *v* to limber up, to warm up

precalicreína *f* prekallikrein, Fletcher factor

precarga *f* preload, heart muscle tension

precipitación *f* precipitation; ~ *f* **de proteínas** precipitation of proteins; ~ *f* **inmunoelectroforética** immunoelectrophoretic precipitation

precipitina *f* precipitin

precisión *f* precision; ~ *f* **de movimiento** *f* accuracy of movement

preclínico *adj* preclinical

precordial *adj* precordial, heart and chest-related

precordialgias *f pl* heart trouble, heart complaint

precursor *m* precursor, forerunner

predeterminación *f* **del sexo** gender selection

predicción *f* prediction; ~ *f* **de la enfermedad** disease prediction

predictor *m* predictor

predisposición *f* predisposition, tendency; ~ **genética** *f* genetic predisposition

prednisolona *f* prednisolone, hydroretrocortine, metacortandralone

prednisona *f* prednisone, dehydrocortisone, retrocortine, metacortandracin, deltacortisone

preeclampsia *f* preeclampsia

preferencia *f* preference; ~ **codónica** codon bias

pregunta *f* question

preliminar *adj* preliminary

prematuro *adj* premature, *m* premature infant, premature baby

premedicación *f* premed, premedication

premenstrual *adj* premenstrual

prenatal *adj* prenatal, prebirth, before birth

preocupación *f* concern, apprehension, worry

preoperatorio *adj* preoperative, before an operation

preparación *f* preparation; ~ *f* **para cirugía** surgical preparation, pre-operative treatment; ~ *f* **permanente** permanent preparation; ~ *f* **preoperatorio** preoperative preparation; ~ *f* **sanguínea** blood preparation

preparado *m* preparation; ~ *m* **alimenticio** readymade food; ~ *m* **homeopático** homeopathic preparation

prepucio *m* foreskin, prepuce

prerigor *m* livor mortis, postmortem lividity

presbicia *f* presbyopia, far-sightedness

presbiopía *f* presbyopia, far-sightedness

présbite farsighted, far-sighted

prescribir prescribe, to

prescripción *f* medication, medicament, medicine, prescription, medical prescription; ~ *f* **de drogas** prescription for drugs

presentación *f* presentation, angle (of the fetus); ~ *f* **de nalgas** breech birth, breech delivery, breech presentation; ~ *f* **de pie** footling presentation; ~ *f* **pélvica** breech birth, breech delivery, pelvic presentation, breech presentation, ~ *f* **podálica** footling presentation

presente present

preservativo *m* condom

presidente *m* chair, chairman, chairperson, president

presináptico *adj* presynaptic, before a nerve joint

presión *f* pressure, tension, tone; ~ *f* **alta** high blood pressure; ~ *f* **arterial** blood pressure; ~ *f* **atmosférica** atmospheric pressure; ~ *f* **baja** low back pain, low blood pressure; ~ *f* **capila** capillary blood pressure; ~ *f* **coloidosmótica** colloid osmotic pressure; ~ *f* **de invalidez** disability benefit; ~ *f* **de retorno** back pressure; ~ *f* **diastólica** diastolic pressure, afterload (of blood pressure); ~ *f* **elevada** hypertension, high blood pressure, hypertonia; ~ *f* **hepática en cuña** hepatic venous pressure; ~ *f* **intracraneal** intracranial pressure; ~ *f* **intraocular** intraocular pressure,

ophthalmotonus; ~ f **intratorácica**
intrathoracic pressure; ~ f **osmótica** osmotic
pressure; ~ f **osmótica coloidal** colloidal
osmotic pressure; ~ f **parcial** partial pressure;
~ f **positiva continua de las vías
respiratorias** continuous positive airway
pressure; ~ f **sanguínea** blood pressure;
~ f **transtorácica** transthoracic pressure;
~ f **ventricular** ventricular pressure

prestación f benefit, performance

prestaciones f pl **sanitarias** health care, medical
care, healthcare services

presunto adj presumptive

prevalencia f prevalence

prevención f prophylaxis, disease prevention,
prevention; ~ f **del embarazo** birth control;
~ f **médica** preventive medicine, preventive
care

preventivo adj prophylactic

previos previous

priapismo m continuous erection, priapism

prick m test skin-prick test

prima f premium, bonus; ~ f **de seguro**
premium

primario first

primavera f spring

primero adj primary, first, main; ~ f **dentición** f
milk teeth, deciduous teeth, baby teeth

primeros m pl **auxilios** primary care, primary
health care, first aid

primidona f primidone

primo, -a m/f cousin

primosoma f primosome

primovacunación f primary vaccination, first
vaccination

principal adj first, primary

principiante m neophyte, new user, beginner,
novice

principio m first; ~ m **activo** active principle,
active ingredient; ~ m **de medición** principle
of measurement

prión m prion, proteinaceous infectious particle

privacidad f privacy, confidentiality, private life,
personal space

privación f deprivation, loss or lack; ~ f **de
oxígeno** oxygen deprivation; ~ f **psíquica y**

social psychosocial deprivation; ~ f **sensorial**
sensory deprivation; ~ f **voluntaria**
abstinence, going without, refraining

privada f bathroom, toilet

privado adj private

proangiotensina f proangiotensin

probeta f test tube; ~ f **macrográfica** specimen
for macroscopic examination

probit probit

problema m problem; ~ m **de visión** vision
problem; ~ m **nutricional** nutritional
disturbance, dietary deficiency, nutritional
disorder; ~ m **respiratorio** difficulty in
breathing

procaína f procaine

procariota f prokaryotic cell, prokaryote, cytode

procedimiento m procedure; ~ m **analítico**
laboratory test, analytical procedure;
~ m **cruento** invasive procedure; ~ m **de
diagnóstico no invasivo** invasive diagnostic
procedure, non-invasive method of diagnosis;
~ m **de diagnóstico** diagnostic procedure;
~ m **de medida** measurement procedure,
laboratory test; ~ m **de referencia** reference
procedure; ~ m **microbiológico**
microbiological process; ~ m **terapéutico**
method of treatment

proceso m process; ~ m **analítico** analytical
process; ~ m **de identificación** identification
process

procrastinar procrastinate, to

procreación f procreation, child bearing

proctitis f proctitis, infection of rectum, sore
bottom; ~ f **hemorroidal** hemorrhoidal
proctitis

proctología f proctology

proctólogo m proctologist

proctoscopio m proctoscope

prodrómico adj prodromal

producción f production, manufacture

productivo adj productive

producto m product; ~ m **de degradación**
degradation product, product of catabolic
degradation; ~ m **de solubilidad** solubility
product; ~ m **fitofarmacéutico**
phytopharmaceutical product, herbal
medicine; ~ m **liofilizado** lyophilisate, freeze-
dried, lyophilizate; ~ m **para la higiene**

femenina feminine hygiene product;
~ *m* **precursor** drug precursor, precursor
product; ~ *m* **sanitario** medical device
proenzima *m/f* proenzyme, zymogen, zymogenic
bacteria
profago *m* prophage, probacteriophage
profármaco *adj* prodrug
profesión *f* profession, occupation; ~ *f* **de
comadrona** midwifery, the practice of
assisting women in childbirth
profesional *adj/m* professional; ~ *m* **sanitario**
health professional, health worker, medical
practitioner, health care provider
profesor *m* instructor, teacher
profibrinolisina *f* profibrinogen, profibrinolysin
profiláctico *adj* prophylactic
profilaxis *f* prophylaxis; ~ *f* **dental** caries
prophylaxis; ~ *f* **por gamaglobulina** gamma
globulin prophylaxis
profobilinógeno *m* porphobilinogen
profundidad *f* depth; ~ *f* **espiratoria** expiratory
depth
progenie *f* offspring, progeny
progenitura *f* offspring, progeny
progeria *f* progeria, premature aging, senile
nanism, Hutchinson-Gilford disease
progesterona *f* progesterone, female hormone
progestina *f* progestin
progestógeno *m* progestogen, female hormone
prognosis *f* prognosis, outlook, the future
programa *m* program
progranulocito *m* progranulocyte
progresión *f* progression; ~ *f* **de enfermedad**
disease progression
progresivo *adj* progressive
proinsulina *f* proinsulin
prolactina *f* prolactin, lactotropic hormone,
lactotropin, mammatropic hormone,
mammatropin, PRL
prolactinoma *f* prolactinoma, lactotropin
prolactoliberina *f* prolactin-releasing factor,
PRF
prolactostatina *f* prolactin release-inhibiting
factor
prolapso *m* prolapse; ~ *m* **de la uretra** prolapse
of urethra; ~ *m* **de la válvula aortica** aortic
valveprolapse; ~ *m* **hemorroidal** hemorrhoidal
prolapse; ~ *m* **mitral** mitral valve prolapse

proliferación *f* proliferation, multiplication
proliferativo *adj* proliferative
prolifero *adj* proliferative
prolina *f* proline, amino acid, pyrrolidine-2-
carboxylate
prolinfocito *m* prolymphocyte
prolongación *f* prolongation, extension, tailing;
~ *f* **del apareamiento** branch migration;
~ *f* **del cebador** primer extension
prolongado *adj* continuous
promedio *m* mean, average; ~ *m* **de vida** life
expectancy
promegacariocito *m* promegakaryocyte
promegaloblasto *m* promegaloblast
prominente *adj* prominent, protruding
promiscuidad *f* promiscuity; ~ *f* **sexual** sexual
promiscuity, having multiple sexual partners
promiscuo *adj* promiscuous
promonocito *m* promonocyte
promotor *m* promoter; ~ *m* **del crecimiento**
growth factor, growth promotor;
~ *m* **divergente** divergent promoter
pronación *f* pronation
prono lying prone, face down, prostrate
pronormoblasto *m* pronormoblast
pronosticado *adj* prognostic
pronóstico *adj* prognostic, *m* prognosis, outlook,
the future; ~ *m* **del tiempo** weather forecast;
~ *m* **grave** poor prognosis
pronto soon
propagación *f* spreading, diffusion;
~ *f* **bacteriana** bacterial dissemination,
propagation of bacteria
propanolol *m* propanolol
propensión *f* addiction
propenso *m* **a accidentes** accident-prone
properdina *f* properdin, complement factor P
propiedad *f* property; ~ *f* **patógena** pathogenic,
capable of causing disease
propio *adj* adequate
propionato *m* propionate; ~ *m* **de
testosterona** testosterone propionate
propionibacterium *m* propionibacterium
proplasmocito *m* proplasmacyte
proporción *f* proportion, ratio, rate; ~ *f* **de
reincidentes** relapse rate
proporcional *adj* proportional
propranolol *m* propranolol

propriocepción f proprioception, proprioceptive awareness

proptosis f exophthalmos, proptosis, protruding eyes

propulsar adj propulsive, driving

prosopalgia f trigeminal neuralgia, tic douloureux, prosopalgia

prosoplejía f facial paralysis, Bell's palsy

prostaglandina f prostaglandin, fatty acid

próstata f prostate

prostatectomía f prostatectomy; ~ f **total** prostatic extirpation, removal of the prostate gland, total prostatectomy

prostatismo m prostatism, prostate trouble

prostatitis f prostatitis, prostate inflammation, prostate infection; ~ f **congestiva** congestive prostatitis

proteasa f proteolytic enzyme, protease, protein-cleaving enzyme

protección f segregation, prevention, protection

protector m protective, protector; ~ m **citológico** cytoprotective agent

proteína f protein; ~ f **activadora del catabolismo** catabolite activator protein; ~ f **amiloide** amyloid peptide, amyloid protein; ~ f **C reactiva** C reactive protein, CRP; ~ f **celadora** molecular chaperone, chaperone protein; ~ f **crioprecipitable** cryoprecipitable protein; ~ f **de Bence Jones** Bence Jones protein; ~ f **de fase aguda** acute-phase protein; ~ f **de la leche** milk protein; ~ f **de la membrana celular** membrane protein; ~ f **del plasma** plasma protein, blood protein; ~ f **del virión** viral protein, virion protein; ~ f **desenrolladora** unwinding protein; ~ f **desestabilizadora** destabilizing protein; ~ f **gravídica** gestational protein; ~ f **HMGA** HMG-AT-hook protein, HMGA protein; ~ f **membranal** membrane protein; ~ f **no histórica** non-histone protein NHP; ~ f **quinasa** protein kinase; ~ f **recombinante** recombinant protein; ~ f **receptora de AMP cíclico** cyclic AMP receptor protein; ~ f **transportadora** carrier protein, transport protein

proteináceo adj proteinaceous

proteinemia f proteinemia

proteinosis f proteinosis; ~ f **alveolar**
pulmonar pulmonary alveolar proteinosis

proteinuria f proteinuria

proteólisis f proteolysis

proteolítico adj proteolytic, proteincleaving

proteómica f proteomics

prótesis f prosthesis, artificial limb; ~ f **arterial** arterial prosthesis, vascular prosthesis, synthetic artery; ~ f **auditiva** auditory apparatus; ~ f **cosmética** cosmetic prosthesis; ~ f **de cadera** hip joint prosthesis, hip joint arthroplasty, hip replacement; ~ f **de la extremidad inferior** leg prosthesis, artificial leg; ~ f **de Norszewski** visual prosthesis, electrophthalm; ~ f **de Starr-Edwards** Starr-Edwards valve, Starr-Edwards ball valve prosthesis; ~ f **neuromuscular** neuromuscular prosthesis; ~ f **valvular cardíaca** artificial heart valve, heart valve replacement; ~ f **vascular** arterial prosthesis, vascular prosthesis, synthetic artery

Proteus m **vulgaris** proteus vulgaris

protirelina f protirelin

protocolo m protocol; ~ m **terapéutico** therapeutic protocol; ~ m **toxicofarmacológico** pharmaco-toxicological protocol

protodiastólico adj protodiastolic, prediastolic

protooncogén m proto-oncogene, cellular oncogen

protoporfirina f protoporphyrin; ~ f **de cinc** zinc protoporphyrin

prototrofo adj prototroph

protozoos m pl protozoon

protrombina f prothrombin, blood factor II, coagulation factor II

protrombinasa f thrombokinase, factor xa, thromboplastin, prothrombinase

protrusión f bulge, protrusion; ~ f **precordial** precordial protrusion, protrusion of the embryonic heart

protuberancia f bulge, protrusion

provirus m integrated retroviral DNA, provirus

provocación f provocation; ~ f **con pilocarpina** pilocarpine provocation

proximal adj proximal, nearest

próximo/a adj next; ~ f **semana** next week

proyección f projection, casting, throwing;
~ f de imágenes por resonancia magnética
MRI (magnetic resonance imaging)
proyectivo adj projective
proyecto m planning
prueba f test; ~ f aleatoria en doble–ciego
randomized double-blind trial; ~ f analítica
laboratory test; ~ f calórica caloric test;
~ f con azul de metileno methylene blue
test; ~ f confirmatoria confirmatory test;
~ f de ADN DNA test; ~ f de alcoholemia
alcohol test, determination of blood alcohol
level; ~ f de antígeno leucocitario humano
Human Leukocyte Antigen Test; ~ f de
asimilación assimilation test; ~ f de Coombs
Coombs' test, Coombs reaction; ~ f de
degranulación degranulation test; ~ f de
degustación sensory evaluation; ~ f de
detección VIH HIV screening test; ~ f de
difusión en agar agar diffusion test; ~ f de
ejercicio stress test; ~ f de embarazo
pregnancy test; ~ f de emulsificación
emulsification test; ~ f de epicutánea skin
testing, epicutaneous test, patch test; ~ f de
fijación del complemento CF test; ~ f de
heces stool sample; ~ f de hemaglutinación
hemagglutination test; ~ f de
histocompatibilidad histocompatibility test;
~ f histocompatibilidad cruzada cross
match; ~ f de inmunodifusión
immunodiffusion test; ~ f de la actividad
bactericida bactericidal activity test; ~ f de la
aglutinación directa direct agglutination
test; ~ f de la asimilación de glúcidos
carbohydrate assimilation test; ~ f de la
catalasa catalase test; ~ f de la
coaglutinación coagglutination test; ~ f de la
inhibición de la hemaglutinación
hemagglutination inhibition test; ~ f de la ji
al cuadrado chi square test; ~ f de la
microaglutinación microagglutination test;
~ f de la neutralización neutralization test;
~ f de la penetración capilar hair penetration
test; ~ f de la perfusión salina sodium
chloride perfusion test; ~ f de la
precipitación precipitation test; ~ f de la

sinergia synergy test; ~ f de mutagenicidad
mutagenicity test; ~ f de orina urine sample;
~ f de pap pap smear; ~ f de Papanicolau pap
smear; ~ f de paternidad paternity test, proof
of paternity; ~ f de provocación challenge
testing, provocation test; ~ f de
radioalergosorbencia RAST; ~ f de
radioinmunosorbencia radioimmunosorbent
test, RIST; ~ f de sensibilidad sensitivity test;
~ f de Sereny Sereny test; ~ f de Widal Widal
test; ~ f del anticuerpo fluorescente
fluorescent–antibody test; ~ f del antígeno
específico de la próstata prostate-specific
antigen testing, PSA testing; ~ f del cultivo
linfocítico mixto MLC test; ~ f del hidrógeno
espirado hydrogen breath test; ~ f directa de
inmunofluorescencia direct
immunofluorescence test; ~ f directa del
anticuerpo fluorescente direct fluorescent-
antibody test; ~ f doble ciego double blind
study; ~ f funcional functional test;
~ f indirecta de la aglutinación indirect
agglutination test; ~ f indirecta de la
hemaglutinación indirect hemagglutination
test; ~ f intradérmica intracutaneous test,
intradermal test, IDT; ~ f psicométrica
psychometric test; ~ m de
radioalergosorbencia radioallergosorbent test
pruebas f pl medical tests, lab tests;
~ f pl cruzadas cross matching, cross-
agglutination test; ~ f pl cruzadas
sanguíneas blood crossmatching
prurítico adj itchy, itching, pruritic
pruritis f invernal dermatitis hiemalis, winter
itch, pruritus hiemalis
prurito m pruritus, itching, itch; ~ m anal anal
pruritus, anal itching; ~ m genital genital
pruritis
psamoma m psammoma
pselismo m stuttering, stammering
pseudoclaudicación f spurious claudication
pseudocolinesterase f pseudocholinesterase
pseudoefedrina f pseudoephedrine
pseudolinfoma m Burkitt's lymphoma, non-
Hodgkin's lymphoma caused by the Epstein-
Barr virus
Pseudomonas m **pseudomallei** Whitmore's
bacillus

pseudoqueloide *m* **postvacunal** vaccination keloid, postvaccinal pseudokeloid

pseudoquiste *m* pseudocyst; ~ **m pancreático** pancreatic pseudocyst, pseudocyst of the pancreas

pseudotumor *m* phantom tumor, pseudotumor, false tumor

psico-analítico *adj* psychoanalytical

psicodiagnóstico *m* **de Rorschach** Rorschach test

psicodrama *f* **espontánea** spontaneous role-playing, group therapy where people act out emotional situations

psicofármaco *m* psychoactive drugs, psychotropic drug

psicofísica *f* psychophysics

psicofisiología *f* psychophysiology

psicógeno *adj* psychogenic

psicoléptico *m* psycholeptic

psicología *f* psychology; ~ **f clínica** clinical psychology, medical psychology; ~ **f evolutiva** developmental psychology; ~ **f industrial** industrial psychology; ~ **f médica** medical psychology; ~ **f social** social psychology

psicológico *adj* psychological

psicólogo *m* psychologist; ~ **m clínico** clinical psychologist, medical psychologist; ~ **m diplomado** state-certified psychologist

psicomotor *m* psychomotor

psicomotricidad *f* psychic & motor functions, psychomotoricity, psychomotor activities

psicopático *adj* psychotic, insane

psicopatología *f* mental pathology, pathopsychology

psicopedagogía *f* educational psychology

psicosis *f* psychosis, mental illness; ~ **f afectiva** affective psychosis; ~ **f ansiosa** anxiety psychosis; ~ **f esquizofrenica** schizophrenic psychosis; ~ **f funcional** functional psychosis

psicosocial *adj* psychosocial

psicosomático *adj* psychosomatic

psicotecnia *f* psychotechnics, psychotechnology

psicotécnica *f* psychotechnics, psychotechnology

psicoterapéutica *f* psychotherapeutic

psicoterapia *f* psychotherapy, psychological counseling; ~ **f de grupo** group therapy, group psychotherapy

psicótico *adj* psychotic, insane, lunatic

psicotrópico *adj* psychotropic, mood-altering

psiquiatra *m/f* psychiatrist

psiquiátrico *adj* psychiatric

psíquico *adj* psychic

psoraleno *m* psoralen

psoriasis *f* psoriasis

pterigión *m* pterygium

ptialismo *m* excessive salivation, ptyalism, sialorrhoea

ptomaina *f* ptomaine

ptosis *f* ptosis, droopy upper eyelid; ~ **f del páncreas** pancreatoptosis

pubertad *f* puberty; ~ **f tardía** delayed puberty

pubescente *adj* pubescent

pubis *m* pubic bone, pubis

pudenda *f* vulva

puente *m* bridge; ~ **m cromosómico** chromosomal bridge; ~ **m de Chayes** Chayes fixed-movable bridge, Chayes saddle bridge, Chayes attachment; ~ **m dental m fixed** parietal dental bridge, fixed bridgework; ~ **m fijo desarmable de Chayes** Chayes fixed-movable bridge, Chayes saddle bridge, Chayes attachment

puerco *m* pork

puerperio *m* puerperium, confinement

pues *(conj)* still

puesto *m* stand

pulgar *m* thumb

pulmón *m* lung; ~ **m de acero** electrophrenic respirator, iron lung; ~ **m de harina de pescado** fishmeal worker's lung; ~ **m de los criadores de aves** pigeon breeder's lung; ~ **m del granjero** farmer's lung, farmer's lung disease, moldy-hay disease

pulmonar *adj* pulmonary, pulmonic

pulmonía *f* pneumonia

pulpa *f* pulp; ~ **f dentaria** dental pulp, pulp of a tooth

pulsación *f* pulsation, heartbeat

pulsar *v* to throb

pulso *m* pulse; ~ **m arterial** arterial pulse; ~ **m capilar** capillary pulse, nail pulse; ~ **m carótido** carotid pulse; ~ **m irregular** irregular pulse

pulverizador *m* spray; ~ **m de parihuelas** stretcher-mounted sprayer

punción f puncture; ~ f **arterial** arterial puncture; ~ f **biopsia** needle biopsy, aspiration biopsy; ~ f **biopsia pleural** pleural needle biopsy; ~ f **biopsia sinovial** synovial needle biopsy; ~ f **de la carina** carina puncture; ~ f **de la vejiga** puncture of the bladder; ~ f **exploradora guiada por ecografía** echo-guided fine-needle biopsy; ~ f **lumbar** spinal tap, lumbar puncture, Quincke's puncture; ~ f **medular** lumbar splenic puncture, sternal puncture; ~ f **pleural** pleural aspiration; ~ f **vesical** puncture of the bladder, capillary puncture

puño m fist

puntear v to stipple to fleck, to pluck, to head, to lead

punteado m **compuesto unilateralmente** unilateral compound pitting

punto m stitch, dot; ~ m **caliente** hot spot; ~ m **del pie** ball of the foot; ~ m **isoeléctrico** isoelectrical point; ~ m **más bajo** nadir, low point

puntos m pl **de sutura** stitches, sutures

punzada f severe pain, sharp pain

punzadas f pl stabbing pain

pupila f pupil

pureza f purity; ~ f **de la especie** purity of species

purga f gastric lavage

purgante adj laxative, remedy for constipation, vacuant

purgativo adj purgative, strong laxative

purina f purine

púrpura f purpura, blood spots; ~ f **trombocitopénica idiopática** idiopathic thrombocytopenic purpura

purulento adj purulent, pusy, pyogenic

pus f pus, thick yellowish fluid

pústula f pustule; ~ f **de acné** pimple, acne pustule, blackhead, furuncle; ~ f **maligna** malignant carbuncle, contagious carbuncle

pustuloso adj pustular, pimply, boil-like

Q

qi m qi, chí, life breath, vital energy

quadrillo m hip bone

que than

qué what; ~ **which**

quedar v to be, to stay; ~ v **caliente** to become hot; ~ v **sin aliento** to gasp, to have trouble breathing

queilitis f angular cheilitis, angular cheilosis, angular cheilitis, exfoliative cheilitis; ~ f **glandular** glandular cheilitis; ~ f **impetiginosa** impetiginous cheilitis; ~ f **solar** solar cheilitis

queja f complaint

quelación f chelation; ~ f **del hierro** iron chelation

quelante m chelating agent; ~ m **como la penicilamina** chelating agent (such as penicillamine); ~ m **del hierro** iron chelator

queloide m keloid, cheloid, cheloma, raised scar

quemado adj run-down, weakened, tired, dragging, worn out

quemadura f burns, burn wounds, brand; ~ f **de tercer grado** third degree burn wounds; ~ f **del sol** sunburn, solar dermatitis; ~ f **ocular** ocular burn; ~ f **química** chemical burn

quemante adj caustic, corrosive

quemosis f chemosis of conjunctiva

queratectomia f keratectomy

querático adj keratinous

queratina f keratin

queratinizado m enteric coating, a coating on tablets

queratinocito m keratinocyte

queratitis f keratitis; ~ f **dendrítica** follicular staphylococcus queratosis, dendritic keratitis; ~ f **leprosa** leprotic keratitis; ~ f **xerótica** xerotic keratitis

queratoconjuntivitis f keratoconjunctivitis

queratoidociclitis f kerato-iridocyclitis

queratolítico m keratolytic, product to produce skin shedding

queratoplastia f cornea transplant, corneal transplant

queratosis f keratosis; ~ f **actínica** actinic keratosis, solar keratosis, keratoma senilis, senile keratosis; ~ f **folicular** keratosis follicularis, follicular keratosis; ~ f **folicular estafilocócica** follicular staphylococcus queratosis, dendritic keratitis; ~ f **hereditaria** hereditary keratosis; ~ f **labial** keratosis labialis; ~ f **pigmentada** keratosis pigmentosa; ~ f **seborreica** seborrheic keratosis; ~ f **senil** actinic keratosis, keratoma senilis, senile keratosis; ~ f **solar** solar keratosis

queratotomía f keratotomy; ~ f **radial** radial keratotomy

queromanía f **expansiva** expansive querulous paranoia

queso m cheese

quequina queuine

quién who

quieto inactive

quieto adj quiescent, inactive, at rest

quigong m Qi-Gong, Qigong, Chinese energy control therapy

quijada f upper jaw, jawbone

quilomicrón m chylomicron

quiluria f chyluria

quimera f chimera

química f chemistry; ~ f **analítica** analytical chemistry; ~ f **clínica** clinical chemistry; ~ f **en fase sólida** dry chemistry; ~ f **médico-legal** chemistry

químico adj chemical

químico m chemical

quimiluminiscencia f chemoluminescence, chemi-luminescence

quimiocina f chemokine

quimioluminiscencia f chemiluminescence

quimiometría f chemometrics

quimioprofilaxia f chemoprevention, the use of natural or laboratory-made substances to prevent cancer, chemoprophylaxis

quimiorreceptor m chemoreceptor

quimiotáctico adj chemoattractant

quimiotaxis f chemotaxis

quimioterapia f chemotherapy; ~ **adyuvante** adjuvant chemotherapy; ~ f **de mantenimiento** maintenance chemotherapy; ~ f **de sostén** maintenance chemotherapy

quimioterápico f chemotherapeutic

quimo m chyme

quimotripsina f chymotrypsin

quinasa f kinase

quince adj fifteen

quinidina f quinidine

quinientos adj five hundred

quinina f kinin

quinolón m quinolone

quinolona f quinolone

quinto/a adj fifth; ~ f **de la tos ferina** attack of whooping cough; ~ f **enfermedad** erythema infectiosumm, fifth disease

quirófano m operating room, automated operating room, O.R.

quiropodalgia f acrodynia, pink disease, Raw beef hands and feet, Feer's disease

quiroponfólix f dyshidrotic eczema, dyshidrosis, cheiropompholyx

quiropráctica f chiropractic, chiropraxis, therapeutic treatment of the spinal column

quiropráctico m chiropractor

quirúrgico adj surgical

quisquilloso adj irritable, cranky, touchy, short-tempered, in a bad mood

quiste m cyst; ~ m **aracnoideo** arachnoid cyst, leptomeningeal cyst; ~ m **de páncreas** pancreatic cyst; ~ m **dermoide** dermoid cyst; ~ m **hidatádico** hydatid cyst; ~ m **ovario** ovarian cyst; ~ m **pancreático** pancreatic cyst; ~ m **pericárdico** pericardial cyst; ~ m **renal** renal cyst; ~ m **subchondral** subchondral cyst, solitary bone cyst; ~ m **testicular** testicular cyst

quitar v to remove, to take off/away

R

rabadilla f tailbone, coccyx

rabdomiolisis f rhabdomyolysis, necrosis or disintegration of skeletal muscle

rabdomiosarcoma m rhabdomyosarcoma

rabia f rabies

racimo m cluster, concentration

rad f radiation absorbed dose, rad

radiación f radiation; ~ f **concomitante** concomitant radiation; ~ f **corpuscular** particle radiation; ~ f **ionizante** ionizing radiation; ~ f **no ionizante** non-ionizing radiation; ~ f **solar ultravioleta** solar ultraviolet radiation; ~ f **ultravioleta** ultraviolet radiation; ~ f radiotherapy, radiation therapy

radical m radical; ~ m **de los ácidos grasos** fatty acid radical; ~ m **hidroxilo** free hydroxyl radical; ~ m **libre** free radical; ~ m **libre de oxígeno** oxygen-free radical

radiculitis f radiculitis

radiculopatía f radiculopathy, nerve root avulsion

radio m radius; ~ m **centrífugo** centrifugal radius; ~ m **occipital** occipital radius

radioactividad f radioactivity

radiodermitis f radiodermatitis, X-ray dermatitis, dermatitis actinica

radiofármaco m radiopharmaceutical

radiografía f radiography, X-ray; ~ f **de tórax** chest X-ray; ~ f **del aparato urinario** urinary tract X-ray

radioinmunoanálisis m radioimmunoassay, RIA

radiología f radiology

radiológico adj radiological

radiólogo m radiologist

radioluminescencia f radioluminescence

radiomarcado m radioactive tagging

radionucleido m radionuclide

radiooncólogo m radiation oncologist

radio-oncólogo m radiation oncologist

radioterapia f radiation therapy, radiotherapy

radiotransparente adj radiolucent, radiotransparent

radisótopo m radioisotope

radón m radon

rágade f rhagade, line

raíces m pl **de los cuerpos cavernosos del clítoris** crus of clitoris

raigón m dental broken-off tooth, remaining root structure

raíz m root; ~ f **lateral** lateral root; ~ f **medial** medial root; ~ f **sensitiva** sensitive nerve root; ~ f **nerviosa** nerve root

rama f ramus, branch

ramificado adj dendritic, branching

ranchero m farmer

ranitidina f ranitidine

ranura f groove, slot

rañura f fissure, crack, split

rápido adj fast

raquianaestesia f spinal anesthesia, subarachnoid anaesthesia; ~ f **epidural** epidural anaesthesia, peridural anaesthesia, caudal anesthesia; ~ f **epidural** epidural epidural anesthesia; ~ f **peridural** peridural anesthesia

raquitismo m rickets (illness); ~ m **fetal** fetal rickets, fetal rachitis

rasgo m character trait, characteristic; ~ m **pedológico** pedological trait

rasguño m scratch

rash m skin rash, hives, exanthema

raspado m abrasion, graze, curettage, decortication, curettage; ~ m **bronquial** bronchial brushing

raspador m xyster, raspatory, rugina

raspar v to scrub, to wash, to clean

rastreador m tomographic scanner; ~ m **del cuerpo entero** whole body scanner

rastreo m dredging, dragging, tracking; ~ m **genómico de malapareamiento** genomic mismatch scanning

ratón m **transgénico** transgenic mouse

rayas f pl stretch marks, striae; ~ f pl **de sangre** streaks of blood

rayo m ray, beam; ~ m **láser** laser beam; ~ m **g** g-ray

rayos m pl rays, beams; ~ m pl **gamma** gamma rays, gamma radiation; ~ m pl **x** radiography, X-ray; ~ m pl **x del tórax** chest x-ray

raza f race, ethnicity

razón f ratio; ~ f **de verosimilitud** likelihood ratio

reabsorción f reuptake, reabsorption

reacción f reaction; ~ f **adversa** adverse reaction; ~ f **anafilactóide** anaphylactoid reaction; ~ f **cruzada** cross reaction; ~ f **de autoinmunidad** autoimmune reaction, autoimmune response; ~ f **de conversión** conversion reaction; ~ f **de Coombs** Coombs reaction; ~ f **de fijación del complemento** complement fixation reaction; ~ f **de hipersensibilidad** hypersensitivity reaction; ~ f **de polimerización en cadena** polymerase chain reaction; ~ f **de relleno** fill-in reaction; ~ f **en cadena** chain reaction; ~ f **en cadena de la polimerasa** polymerase chain reaction; ~ f **en cadena por la ligasa** ligase chain reaction; ~ f **enzimática** enzymatic reaction; ~ f **histérica** hysterical reaction

reactante *adj* reactant

reactivación *f* reactivation

reactivar *v* to reactivate, to stimulate

reactividad *f* reactivity

reactivo *m* reagent

reagina *f* reagin

real *adj* actual

reanimación *f* rebreathing; ~ **cardíaca** cardiac rescussitation; ~ **f cardiopulmonar** cardiopulmonary resuscitation, CPR; ~ **f de urgencia** emergency life support, resuscitation

reanimar *v* to resuscitate, to revive

rebasar *v* overflow, to

rebelde *adj* recalcitrant, persistent, refractory

reborde *m* ledge, flange, rim; ~ **de tejido** plica, fold of skin or tissue, plication, plicature

recaída *f* relapse, reoccurrence

recambio *m* turnover, renewal

receptor *m* receptor, recipient, receiver; ~ **adrenérgico** adrenoreceptor, adrenergic receptor; ~ **m alfaadrenérgico** alphaadrenergic receptor; ~ **m alfa** alpha receptor; ~ **m antigénico** antigenic receptor; ~ **m dendrítico** dendriceptor; ~ **m H2 de histamina** histamine H2 receptor; ~ **m hormonal** hormone receptor; ~ **m opiáceo** opioid receptor, opiate receptor; ~ **m purinérgico** purinergic receptor; ~ **m sensorial** sensory receptor

receta *f* prescription; ~ **f médica** medical prescription

recetar *v* to prescribe

rechazo *m* rebound effect; ~ **de un injerto** graft rejection, rejection of a transplant; ~ **m lateral** lateral separation

recibir *v* to get

recidiva *f* case of relapse, recurrence

recidivante *adj* palindromic, recrudescent, recurring

recidivista *m* recidivist

recién *adv* newly, just; ~ **nacido** *m* newborn baby

reclamación *f* claim, complaint; ~ **f de pago** claim for payment; ~ **f fraudulenta** fraudulent claim

recogida *f* collection; ~ **f de saliva** saliva trap

recombinación *f* recombination; ~ **f conservativa** conservative recombination; ~ **f cruzada** crossing-over, crossover

recombinador *m* recombinator

recombinante *adj* recombinant

reconocer *v* to recognize

reconocimiento *m* inspection, examination, recognition, search; ~ **m clínico** clinical examination; ~ **m de gametos** gamete recognition; ~ **m de la función pulmonar** pulmonary function test; ~ **m de la próstata** prostate examination; ~ **m del recto** rectal examination; ~ **m físico** physical examination, medical examination; ~ **m génico** gene targeting; ~ **m médico** general physical examination, check-up, medical examination

reconstitución *f* reconstitution, regeneration, rehydrating of plasma

recordatorio *m* follow-up

récord *m* record; ~ **m médico** clinical record, medical record, patient record

recreación *f* pastimes, leisure activities, hobbies, recreational activities

recrudescimiento *m* recrudescence

rectal *adj* rectal

rectilinealidad *f* rectilinearity, linearity

recto *m* rectum

rectoscopio *m* proctoscope

rectosigmoidoscopia *f* rectosigmoidoscopy

rectovesical *adj* rectovesical

recuento *m* count; ~ **m de células** cell count; ~ **m de cromosomas** chromosome count, number of chromosomes; ~ **m de eritrocitos** erythrocyte count, red blood cell count; ~ **m de los glóbulos blancos de la sangre** white blood cell count; ~ **m de los glóbulos rojos de la sangre** red blood cell count; ~ **m de plaquetas** platelet count; ~ **m de quistes** cyst count; ~ **m diferencial leucocitario** differential blood count, white blood cell count, WBC; ~ **m leucocitario** leucocyte count; ~ **m sanguíneo completo** complete blood count

recuperación *f* recovery, getting well, recuperation; ~ **f espontanea** spontaneous recovery

recuperar *v* **la sobriedad** to sober up

recuperarse to recover, to recuperate, to get

well

recurrente *adj* recurrent

recurso *m* resource; ~ *m* **de origen genómico** genomic resource

red *f* net, network, plexus; ~ *f* **capilar alveolar** alveolar capillary plexus; ~ *f* **de difracción** diffraction grating; ~ *f* **de fibras reticulares** reticular network; ~ *f* **de información hospitalaria** hospital information network, medical LAN; ~ *f* **médica local** medical LAN (local area network), hospital computer system

redaños *m pl* guts

redondo *adj* round

reducción *f* reduction

reducir *v* to attenuate, to reduce, to weaken; ~ *v* **a polvo fino** to grind, to micronize, to reduce to a fine powder

reductasa *f* reductase

redundancia *f* redundancy

reeducación *f* re-education; ~ *f* **física** rehabilitation, re-education, rehabilitative medicine; ~ *f* **funcional** functional rehabilitation, professional rehabilitation

reevaluación *f* revaluation

referencia *f* reference

referencias *f pl* **médicas atribuibles** opposable medical references, OMR

referir *v* to tell, recount; ~ *v* **un paciente** refer a patient

reflejo *m* reflex; ~ *m* **anal** anal reflex; ~ *m* **axónico** axon reflex; ~ *m* **clónico** clonic reflex; ~ *m* **costopectoral** pectoral reflex; ~ *m* **cutáneo** skin reflex; ~ *m* **cutáneo abdominal** abdominal skin reflex; ~ *m* **cutáneo deltoideo** external reflex of the deltoid; ~ *m* **de deglutir** swallowing reflex; ~ *m* **de los aductores** adductor reflex; ~ *m* **de prensión palmar** grasping reflex; ~ *m* **de vómitar** vomiting reflex; ~ *m* **del seno carotídeo** carotid sinus reflex; ~ *m* **exteroceptivo** exteroceptive reflex; ~ *m* **palmomental** palm-chin reflex, palmomental reflex; ~ *m* **palmomentomano** palm-chin reflex, palmomental reflex; ~ *m* **patelar** patellar reflex, knee jerk reflex; ~ *m* **pilomotor** pilomotor reflex, pilomotor reaction; ~ *m* **propioceptivo** proprioceptive reflex; ~ *m* **psicogalvanico** electrodermal

response, psychogalvanic response, EDR; ~ *m* **pupilar** pupillary reflex; ~ *m* **senocarotídeo** carotid sinus reflex; ~ *m* **vegetativo** vegetative reflex

reflETor *m* reflective

refletoro *adj* reflective

reflexología *f* reflexology

reflexoterapia *f* spinal reflexotherapy

reflujo *m* reflux, return flow; ~ *m* **al esófago** esophageal reflux, esophageal regurgitation; ~ *m* **hepatoyugular** hepatojugular reflux; ~ *m* **mitral** mitral regurgitation, mitral reflux

reforzado *adj* enhanced

refractario *adj* refractory, *m* refractory

refractometría *f* refractometry

refregar *m* to rub

refrescamiento *m* **de sangre** introduction of fresh blood, blood replacement

refrescos *m pl* sodas, soft drinks

regalo present

regeneración *f* neogenesis, tissue regeneration; ~ *f* **lesionada** reconstitution, regeneration; ~ *f* **ósea** bone regeneration, fracture healing

régimen *m* régime, diet; ~ *m* **de eliminación** elimination diet

región *f* region, body part; ~ *f* **cromosómica** region of chromosomes, chromosomal region; ~ *f* **occipital** occipital zone, occipital region; ~ *f* **umbilical** umbilical region

regional *adj* local, topical, regional

registro *m* register, list, record; ~ *m* **de las operaciones** surgical journal; ~ *m* **Holter** Holter monitoring, 24 hour wearable ECG monitor (cardiology)

registros *m pl* clinical records, medical records, patient records; ~ *m pl* **médicos** clinical records, medical records, patient records

regla *f* rule, woman's period, menstrual flow, criterion, menstruation, periods

reglamento *m* regulation; ~ *m* **sanitario internacional** international health regulation

regoldar *v* to belch, to eructate

regresar *v* to come back

regresión *f* regression

regüeldo *m* belch, eructation, burp

regulación *f* feedback, constructive criticism, regulation; ~ *f* **del catabolismo** catabolic repression, catabolite repression

R

regular adj cyclic, periodic, regular
regularmente adj regularly
regulón m regulon
regurgitación f regurgitation, bringing back up; ~ f **del esófago** esophageal reflux, esophageal regurgitation
rehabilitación f rehabilitation, re-education, rehabilitative medicine; ~ f **de toxicómanos** rehabilitation of drug addicts; ~ f **funcional** functional rehabilitation; ~ f **profesional** professional rehabilitation; ~ f **vocacional** vocational rehabilitation
rehidratación f rehydration
reincidencia f relapse, reoccurrence, case of relapse
reinfección f reinfection
reinserción f **en la sociedad** social rehabilitation, assimilation into society
rejuvenecer v to rejuvenate
relación f connection, relation; ~ f **afectiva** emotional bonding, affective rapport, affective bond; ~ f **reflexiva** reflexive relation
relaciones f pl **espaciales** spatial relations; ~ f pl **humanas** social interaction, interpersonal relations; ~ f pl **interpersonales** interpersonal relations
relajación f relaxation
relajante adj relaxing
relajante m relaxant; ~ m **de acción muscular** muscle relaxant, neuromusclar depolarizing agent; ~ m **muscular** muscle relaxant, neuromuscular depolarizing agent
relajarse v to relax
relativamente adj comparatively
relato m report, tale, story; ~ m **médico** medical report; ~ m **operatorio** surgeon's report
relevante adj relevant
relieve m relief; ~ m **acústico** hearing relief; ~ m **endocárdico** endocardial cushion
relleno m filling stuffing; ~ m **de la columna** column packing
reloj m clock, watch; ~ m **biológico** biological clock
remate m cap
remedio m relief, solace, balm, comfort; ~ m **homeomiasmático** homoeomiasmatic remedy

remisión f remission; ~ f **espontánea** spontaneous remission
remodelación f reorganization, remodeling; ~ f **axónica** axonal reorganization, axonal remodeling; ~ f **ventricular** ventricular remodeling
renal adj renal
renaturalización f renaturation
rendimiento m output rate; ~ m **cardíaco** cardiac output, cardiac pressure output, cardiac minute ouput; ~ m **de la transpiración** transpiration efficiency
renina f renin
renovascular adj renovascular
renquear v limp, to hobble, to
reógrafo m impedance plethysmograph, rheograph
Reovirus m reovirus, Respiratory Enteritic Orphan virus, REO virus
reparación f repair, reparation; ~ f **de un malapareamiento** mismatch repair; ~ f **del DNA** DNA repair; ~ f **mutágena** mutagenic repair; ~ f **por escisión** patch repair; ~ f **por recombinación** recombination repair
repentino adj sudden, abrupt
reperfusión f reperfusion; ~ f **miocardica** myocardial reperfusion
repetibilidad f repeatability
repetición f repeat; ~ f **de la quinta tos ferinosa** double pertussis attack; ~ f **directa** direct repeat; ~ f **dispersa** dispersed repeat; ~ f **en tándem** tandem repeat
repetido adj cyclic, periodic, regular
repetidor m repetitive
repleción f repletion
replicación f replication, duplication; ~ f **del ADN** DNA replication; ~ f **semiconservativa del ADN** semi-conservative DNA replication
replicador m replicator
replicón m replicon
repollo m cabbage
reposo m rest, repose; ~ m **en cama** bed rest, confinement to bed
represar v to repress, to restrain, to suppress
representación f representation, delegation; ~ f **cromosómica** chromosome paint
represión f repression; ~ f **catabólica** catabolic repression, catabolite repression

reprimir v to repress, to restrain, to suppress
reproducción f procreation, reproduction
reproducibilidad f reproducibility
reptante v crawling, creeping, moving on hands and knees
repugnante adj sickening, disgusting, repugnant
repulsivo adj sickening, disgusting, repulsive
resaca f hangover
resbaladizo adj slippery, oily, greasy
resbaloso adj slippery, oily, greasy
resecar v to dry out
resección f excision; ~ f articular articular resection; ~ f colorrectal transanal colorectal dragging resection; ~ f del cardias cardiectomy, resection of the cardia; ~ f del intestino delgado resection of small intestine, bowel resection; ~ f ileocecal ileocecal resection; ~ f troncular simpática resection of the sympathetic trunk; ~ f ureteral ureteral resection
reserva f stock
reservorio m reservoir
resfriado m catarrh, cold, nasopharyngitis
resfriarse v to catch a cold
resfrío m cold, nasopharyngitis
residencia f house, residence; ~ f de transición halfway house; ~ f médica medical residency
residente m resident, medical resident, physician in residency training
residual adj residual, trace
residuo m residue, remainder; ~ m extraíble extractable residue; ~ m peligroso hazardous waste, toxic waste
residuos m pl residue, traces; ~ m pl de hospitales hospital waste, infectious waste; ~ m pl inertes inert waste
resistencia f resistance, endurance, stamina, hardening; ~ f a antibióticos antibiotic resistance; ~ f a la meticilina methicillin resistance; ~ f cruzada cross resistance; ~ f eléctrica electric resistance
resistente adj resistant; ~ adj a la meticilina methicillin resistant
resistividad f resistivity; ~ f eléctrica electric resistivity
resollar v to wheeze, to gasp, to have trouble breathing

resolución f resolution; ~ f temporal temporal resolution, resolution time
resonancia f resonance; ~ f magnética metabólica nuclear magnetic resonance tomography, NMR
resorción f resorption; ~ f de glucosa glucose resorption
respigón f hangnail
respiración f respiration; ~ f acidótica acidotic respiration; ~ f anhelosa stertorous respiration, stertor; ~ f artificial artificial respiration; ~ f artificial por boca mouth-to-mouth resuscitation method; ~ f asistida artificial respiration; ~ f diafragmática diaphragmatic breathing, deep breathing, abdominal breathing; ~ f laboriosa labored breathing, difficulty in breathing; ~ f lenta bradypnea, slow breathing; ~ f paradójica paradoxical respiration; ~ f sibilante wheezing, whistling
respirador m ventilator, artificial respirator, breathing appliance; ~ m de altitud high-altitude respirator; ~ m electrofrénico electrophrenic respirator, iron lung, cuirass respirator, Drinker respirator
respirar v to breathe; ~ v con dificultad to wheeze; ~ v hondo to take a deep breath; ~ v profundo to take a deep breath
respiratorio adj respiratory
responder v to respond
respuesta f reply, response; ~ f alérgica allergic reaction, allergic response; ~ f de autoinmunidad autoimmune reaction, autoimmune response; ~ f de Babinski Babinski's sign, paradoxical extensor reflex; ~ f de protección inmunitaria protective immune response; ~ f inmunitaria mediada por células cell-mediated immune response; ~ f supresora immune suppressor response
restablecerse v to recover, to recuperate, to get well
restablecimiento m recovery, getting well, recuperation
restañar v la sangre to stanch, to stop the flow of blood; ~ v las heridas to heal the wounds
restitución f recovery, getting well, recuperation

restituir v to return, to restore; ~ v **la salud** to heal, to cure

restricción f restriction; ~ f **del CMH** histocompatibility complex restriction, MHC restriction; ~ f **del DNA** DNA restriction; ~ f **física** restraint, retention, immobilization

restringido adj local, topical, regional, applied to the surface

resucitación f resuscitation, emergency life support; ~ f **cardiopulmonar** cardiopulmonary resuscitation, CPR

resucitar v to resuscitate, to revive

resuello adj to be short of breath, puffing; ~ m breath, audible respiration

resultado m result, effect, finding, observation; ~ m **clínico** clinical outcome, health outcome

resumen m abstract

retachar v to throb

retardación f **mental** mental retardation, dementia, mental deficiency

retardado adj mentally retarded

retardo m retardation, delaying

retención f restraint, retention, immobilization, uptake, absorbing, retention; ~ f **de orina** urine retention; ~ f **hídrica** water retention, fluid retention

retículo m **endoplasmatico granular** ergoplasma, ergastoplasm, endoplasmic reticulum (rough surfaced); ~ m **endoplásmico** endoplasmic reticulum; ~ m **glial** glial reticulum

reticulocito m reticulocyte

retina f retina

retinal adj retinal

retinal f vitamin A aldehyde

retinitis f retinitis; ~ f **pigmentaria** pigmentary retinopathy; ~ f **por citomegalovirus** cytomegalovirus retinitis

retinoblastoma m retinal glioma, retinoblastoma

retinol f retinol, vitamin A

retinopatía f retinopathy; ~ f **diabética** diabetic retinopathy; ~ f **pigmentaria** pigmentary retinopathy

retirar v **la reclamación** to withdraw the claim

retorno m return; ~ m **venoso** venous return, the return of blood to the heart

retortijón m abdominal cramp, gripe; ~ **de tripas** stomach cramps

retortijones m pl menstrual cramps

retracción f retraction

retractor m retractor; ~ m **de mandibulas** jaw retractor

retrasar v to retard, to slow down, to delay

retraso m delay, retard, delaying; ~ m **mental** mental retardation, mental disorder, mental deficiency

retrete m outhouse

retroacción f feedback, constructive criticism

retroactivo adj retroactive

retroalimentación f feedback, constructive criticism; ~ f **bioquímica** biochemical feedback; ~ f **psicológica** positive feedback, constructive criticism

retrobulbar adj retrobulbar

retrógrado adj backwards, retrograde

retroperitoneal adj retroperitoneal

retrosternal adj retrosternal, behind the breastbone

retrotranscriptasa f reverse transcriptase, RNA-dependent DNA polymerase

retrotransposón m retroposon

retrovirus m retrovirus; ~ m **exógeno** exogenous retrovirus

reumatismo m rheumatism; ~ m **muscular** muscular rheumatism, fibrositis

reumatoide adj rheumatic, rheumatoid

reumatología f rheumatology

reunión f conference

revacunación f booster shot, hypervaccination, revaccination

revalorización f revaluation

revascularización f revascularization; ~ f **cerebral** cerebral revascularization; ~ f **miocardica** myocardial revascularization

reventarse v to burst, to break open

reversible adj reversible

reversión f reversion; ~ f **antigénica** antigenic reversion

revés m setback, adversity

revestido m **con una tapa de pelicula** film-coated (pill, tablet)

revestimiento m **del estómago** gastric mucosa, stomach lining; ~ m **proteico** protein coat

revestir v to cover, to sheathe

revisión m review, revision; ~ m **por expertos** peer review

revulsivo adj revulsive, causing revulsion

rhinosporidium m rhinosporidium

ribavirin m ribavirin

ribete m border, addition; ~ m **de Burton** Burton's line

ribetes m pl **falopianos/uterinos** fimbriae, at the ends of the fallopian tubes & uterine tube

riboflavina f riboflavin

ribonucleasa f ribonuclease; ~ f **pancreática** pancreatic ribonuclease, pancreatic RNase

ribonucleoproteína f ribonucleoprotein

ribosa f ribose; ~ **-fosfato-pirofosfocinasa** f PRPP synthetase

ribosoma m ribosome

ribosonda f riboprobe

ribozima f ribozyme

ricina f ricin, a protein phytotoxin from the seeds the castor oil plant

rickettsia f rickets

riesgo m risk; ~ m **de cáncer gastrointestinal** risk of gastrointestinal cancer; ~ m **de exposición al amianto** risk of exposure to asbestos; ~ m **de irradiación** radiation hazard

rifampicina f rifampicin

rigidez f stiffness, rigidity; ~ f **cataléptica** rigid cataplexy, cataleptic rigidity; ~ f **del hombro** stiffness of the shoulder; ~ f **lumbar** lumbar rigidity; ~ f **pulmonar** pulmonary rigidity; ~ f **rigidez matutina** morning stiffness

rigor m stringency; ~ m **mortis** rigor mortis, cadaveric rigidity

rigoroso adj strict

riña f fight

rinconera f quack midwife, unskilled midwife

rinitis f rhinitis; ~ f **alérgica** allergic rhinitis, hay fever, allergic coryza, rhinitis in an allergic person, sniffles; ~ f **atrófica** atrophic rhinitis; ~ f **vasomotora** vasomotor rhinitis

rinoescleroma m rhinoscleroma

rinofaringitis f rhinopharyngitis, inflammation of the space behind the nose

riñón m kidney; ~ m **poliquístico** polycystic kidney, polycystic renal disease

rinoplastia f cosmetic surgery of the nose, rhinoplasty

rinorrea f rhinorrhea, runny nose

rinoscopio m rhinoscope, conchoscope, nasal speculum

rinosporidiosis f rhinosporidiosis

rinovirus m rhinovirus, picornaviridae that largely infect the upper respiratory tract

ritidectomía f rhytidoplasty, face lift, rhytidectomy

ritidoplastia f rhytidoplasty, face lift, rhytidectomy

ritmo m rhythm; ~ m **circadiano** circadian rhythm; ~ m **idioventricular** ventricular rhythm, idioventricular rhythm

rizotomía f rhizotomy

RMN f **(resonancia magnética nuclear)** nuclear magnetic resonance, NMR; ~ f **cerebral** cerebral MRI, magnetic resonance imaging of the brain, MRI of the brain

RNA m RNA; ~ m **antisentido** antisense RNA; ~ m **de transferencia** transfer RNA; ~ m **espaciador** spacer RNA; ~ m **mensajero** messenger RNA; ~ **-polimerasa dirigida por DNA** DNA-directed RNA polymerase; ~ m **ribosómico** ribosomal RNA

robot m robot; ~ m **médico** medical robot, surgical robot

robótica f robotic; ~ f **médica** surgical robotics, medical robotics; ~ f **quirúrgica** surgical robotics, medical robotics

robustez f robustness

roce m rub, rubbing, friction; ~ m **pericárdico** pericardial rustling sound, pericardial murmur

rodilla f knee

rodilleras f pl knee pads

rodopsina f rhodopsin, an integral membrane protein found in the discs of retinal rods & cones, visual purple

rojizo adj reddish, reddened, erythroid

rojo adj red

romadizo m head cold

romper v to burst, to break open

roncar v to snore, snoring

roncha f rash, exanthema, blister, bulla, bleb, pomphus, welt (on the skin), weal

ronco adj hoarse, husky, scratchy (voice)

roncus m rhonchus, wheezing, whistling

ronquera f hoarseness, scratchy throat, raucousness

ronquido m to snore, snoring; ~ m **por**

R

obstrucción obstruction snoring

ropa f clothing, clothes; **~ f interior** underwear

ropas f pl **de hospital** hospital scrubs, hospital clothing; **~ f pl esterilizadas** sterile clothing; **~ f pl manchadas o salpicadas** contaminated clothing

rosácea f acne rosacea, facial erythrosis

rostro m face

rotador m **del hombro** rotator cuff

rótula f kneecap, patella

rotura f rupture; **~ f cardíaca** cardiorrhexis, rupture of the heart; **~ f celular** cell disruption, cell breakage; **~ f de un tendón** rupture of a tendon; **~ f del tímpano** eardrum rupture, burst eardrum; **~ f muscular** muscle rupture; **~ f uterina** uterine rupture, metrorrhexis

rozadura f intertrigo, chafing

rubéola f German measles, rubella

rubor m blushing, turning red-faced, emotional blush, erythema pudicitiae, flush

ruborícese m blushing, turning red-faced, emotional blush, erythema pudicitiae

rudimentario adj vestigial, greatly reduced from the original ancestral form and no longer functional

ruido m noise; **~ m de aleteo** buzzing, ringing in the ears, tinnitus; **~ m de bazuqueo** gurgling sound; **~ m de molino** gurgling sound; **~ m raspante** rasping murmur

rumiación f rumination, merycism

ruptura f rupture

ruta f route, road

rutinariamente routinely, usually

S

sábado m Saturday

sábana f sheet, bedsheet

sabandijas f pl louse (singular), lice (plural)

sabañón m chillblains, pernio

saber v to know

sabio adj sensible, wise

sabor m taste, flavor; **~ m malo en la boca** a bad taste in the mouth

saburra f sordes

sacar v to take out, to get out; **~ v la lengua** to stick one's tongue out; **~ v muestra de sangre** drawing blood, blood letting, phlebotomy; **~ v sangre** drawing blood, blood letting, phlebotomy

sacarina f saccharin; **~ f sódica** sodium saccharine

saco m sac; **~ m amniótico** amniotic sac; **~ m pericardio** pericardial sac, parietal pericardium

sacoradiculografía f saccoradiculography

sacrolumbar adj sacrolumbar

sacudida f impact, blow; **~ f violenta** commotion, concussion

sacudir v to jar, to jolt, to bump, to jostle

sáculo m saccule, sacculus

safranina f safranin

sal f salt; **~ f común** sodium chloride, table salt; **~ f de litio** lithium salts; **~ f de magnesio** magnesium sulphate; **~ f de sodio** sodium chloride, table salt; **~ f inglesa** smelling salts; **~ f revulsiva** smelling salts

sala f hall, room, lounge, doctor's waiting room; **~ f de autopsias** autopsy room, coroner's inquest suite; **~ f de emergencia** emergency room, emergency unit, emergency service, emergency medical services; **~ f de enfermos infecciosos** infectious diseases; **~ f de operaciones** operating room, automated operating room, O.R. **~ f de recuperación** recovery room, recovery station

salado adj saline, salty

salazopirina f sulfasalazine, Salozapyrin, Azulfidine

salbutamol m salbutamol

salchicha f sausage

salicilato m salicylate

salicismo m salicylism, salicylic acid poisoning (chronic

saliente adj prominent, protruding

salino m saline, salty

saliva f saliva

salivación f salivation

salival adj salivary

salmonela f salmonella

Salmonella f enteriditis Gartner's bacillus; **~ f typhi** Eberth's bacillus; **~ f typhimurium** Nocard's bacillus

salmonelosis f salmonellosis
salpingitis f salpingitis, inflammation of the fallopian tubes
salpingólisis f salpingolysis, breaking down of adhesions in the uterus
salpingo–ooforitis f salpingo-oophoritis
salpingo–ovaritis f salpingo-oophoritis
salpullido m rash, hives, exanthema
saltarín adj springy, supple, limber
salubre adj healthful, healthy
salubridad f health, wellness
salud f health, wellness; ~ f física physical health; ~ f holística holistic medicine, holistic health; ~ f mental mental health; ~ f reproductiva reproductive health
saludable adj able-bodied, healthy, physically fit, having a sound, strong body
salurético adj saluric, encouraging sodium and chlorine in urine
sanador m, **-a** f quacksalver healer, psychic healer, faith healer, spiritual healer
sanar v to heal, to cure
sanarse v to recover, to recuperate, to get well
sanativo adj healthful, healthy
sanatorio m sanatorium
sangrado m bleeding, losing blood, exsanguination
sangrar v to bleed; ~ v por la nariz epistaxis, nosebleed
sangre f blood, total blood; ~ f arterial arterial blood; ~ f cortocircuitada shunt blood, bypass blood; ~ f desoxigenada deoxygenated blood; ~ f hemolisada lacked blood, hemolyzed blood; ~ f hemolizada hemolyzed blood; ~ f heparinizada heparinized blood; ~ f humana citrada citrated whole human blood, CWHB; ~ f íntegra whole blood; ~ f total whole blood; ~ f venosa venous blood, deoxygenated blood
sangría f phlebotomy, bloodletting
sangriento adj bloody
sanguijuela f leech; ~ f artificial artificial leech; ~ f medicinal medicinal leech
sanidad f health, wellness, being well
sano adj able-bodied, healthy, physically fit, having a sound, strong body
saponinas f pl saponins
saprofito m saprophyte

sarampión m measles, rubeola; ~ m alemán rubella, German measles; ~ m de los tres días rubella, German measles; ~ m negro black measles
sarcoide m de Boeck benign lymphogranulomatosis, Boeck's sarcoid, lupus pernio, sarcoidosis
sarcoidosis f sarcoidosis, Besnier-Boeck disease, lupus pernio, benign lymphogranulomatosis; ~ f pulmonar pulmonary sarcoidosis
sarcolema m sarcolemma, plasma membrane of a striated muscle fiber
sarcoma m sarcoma; ~ m de Ewing Ewing's sarcoma; ~ m de Kaposi Kaposi sarcoma, Kaposi syndrome, Kaposi's sarcoma; ~ m dérmico dermal sarcoma; ~ m gigantocelular giant cell sarcoma; ~ m óseo osteosarcoma; ~ m osteógeno osteogenic sarcoma, osteosarcoma; ~ m retroperitoneal retroperitoneal sarcoma; ~ m testicular sarcoma of the testicle
sarcoptes m scabiei acarus scabiei, mange mite, itch mite, sarcoptes scabiei
sarcosina f sarcosine
sarna f scabies
sarnoso adj mangy, scabbed
sarpullido m eruption, break out
sarro m tartar, plaque, fur; ~ m dental dental calculus, tartar, dental plaque
saturación f saturation; ~ f del sangre arterial con oxígeno arterial oxygen saturation; ~ f de oxígeno oxygen saturation; ~ f oxihemoglobinada arterial oxygen saturation
sebo m grease, fat, tallow; ~ m cutáneo sebaceous matter, sebaceous secretion
seborrea f seborrhea, oily skin
secante m siccative, desiccant
secarse v to dry out, to dessicate
secas f pl buboes, swollen lymph nodes
sección f section; ~ f cesárea cesarian section
seco adj dry
secreción f secretion, discharge, excretion; ~ f cervical cervical smear; ~ f de leche lactation, milk production; ~ f del páncreas secretion of the pancreas; ~ f endocrina endocrine secretion; ~ f holocrina holocrine

S

secretion; ~ f **lacrimal** lacrimal fluid;
~ f **nasal** nasal secretion; ~ f **sebácea
cutánea** sebaceous matter, sebaceous
secretion; ~ f **vaginal** vaginal secretion

secretina f secretin

secretor m secretory

secuela f sequel, sequelae, complication

secuencia f sequence; ~ f **cognada** cognate
sequence; ~ f **de consenso** consensus
sequence; ~ f **de control** enhancer element;
~ f **de corte** cutting sequence; ~ f **de
replicación autónoma** autonomus replicating
sequence; ~ f **flanqueadora** flanking
sequence; ~ f **guía** leader sequence;
~ f **nucleotídica** nucleotide sequencing;
~ f **remolque** trailer sequence; ~ f **repetitiva
de ADN** DNA sequence, redundant DNA

secuenciación f sequencing; ~ f **de
nucleótidos** nucleotide sequencing; ~ f **del
ADN** DNA sequencing; ~ f **del genoma
humano** sequencing of human genome

secuenciador m **rápido de ADN** DNA
sequencing system

secuestro m sequestra, sequestrum, pieces of
bone

secundario adj secondary

secundinas f pl placenta, afterbirth

sed f thirst

sedación f sedation

sedante m sedative, tranquilizer

sedativo m sedative, tranquilizer

sedentario adj sedentary, sitting

sedimentación f sedimentation; ~ f **sanguínea**
sedimentation of the blood; ~ f **de la sangre**
blood sedimentation

sedimento m sediment, pellet; ~ m **urinario**
urinary sediment, urine sediment;
~ m **curativo** medicinal mud, healing
mudpack, fangotherapy, mud pack

segmentación f cleaving, cleavage

segmento m segment

segregación f segregation, prevention,
protection

seguimiento m monitoring; ~ m **génico** gene
tracking; ~ m **médico** medical exam, physical
exam, medical examination

seguir v to stay

según las necesidades p.r.n., pro re nata

segundo adj second; ~ adj **parto** afterbirth,
placenta

seguridad f safety; ~ f **instrumental**
instrumental dependability; ~ f **profesional**
occupational safety

seguro m insurance, lock, safety catch;
~ m **colectivo de asistencia médica** group
hospitalization insurance; ~ m **de accidentes
del trabajo** workers'compensation insurance,
workmen's compensation; ~ m **de
enfermedad** Medicaid - government medical
assistance to the poor & elderly; ~ m **de
incapacidad** disability insurance, invalidity
insurance; ~ m **de salud del gobierno**
Medicare, health insurance; ~ m **médico**
insurance (medical)

seis adj six

selectina-P f P-selectin

selectivo adj selective

selenio m selenium

sello m cachet

semana f week; ~ f **pasada** last week

semejante like

semejanza f affinity, attraction

semen m semen, seminal fluid; ~ m **fresco** fresh
semen

semiconductor m **iónico** ionic semiconductor

semicuantitativo adj semiquantitative

seminario m workshop

semiología f semeiology

semisintético adj semisynthetic

semivida f half-life; ~ f **biológica** biological
half-life

señal f signal

senilidad f senility, old age

seno m breast; ~ m **cavernoso** cavernous sinus;
~ m **costodiafragmático** diaphragmatic sinus;
~ m **de Aschoff–Rockitansky** Rokitansky
sinus; ~ m **frontal** frontal sinus; ~ m **maxilar**
maxillary sinus; ~ m **nasal** nasal sinus, cavity
of the cranial bones; ~ m **periférico** peripheral
sinus

señor m man, gentleman, Mr.

señora f woman, lady, Mrs.

señorita f young lady, Miss

sensación f sensation; ~ f **de estrechez**
tightness; ~ f **de hormigueo** paraesthesia,
paresthesia; ~ f **de pánico** sense of panic,

sensation of panic; ~ **f de pinchazos**
paraesthesia, paresthesia; ~ **f de presión**
sensation of pressure
sensato *adj* sensible, wise
senscencia *f* aging, getting older, senescence
sensibilidad *f* sensitivity; ~ **f a la ampicillina**
sensitivity to ampicillin; ~ **f a la vibración**
sensitivity to vibrations; ~ **f de contraste**
contrast sensitivity; ~ **f diagnóstica** diagnostic
sensitivity; ~ **f metrológica** metrological
sensitivity; ~ **f nosográfica** nosographic
sensitivity; ~ **f nosológica** nosologic
sensitivity; ~ **f química multiple** multiple
chemical sensitivity
sensibilización *f* sensitization
sensible *adj* sensitive
sensitivo *adj* susceptible
sensor *m* sensor
sensorial *adj* sensory
sentarse *v* to sit down
sentido *m* sense; ~ *m* **del espacio** space sense;
~ *m* **del gusto** sense of taste, ability to taste,
gustation; ~ *m* **del tacto** sense of touch,
tactile sense, tactile perception;
~ *m* **gustativo** sense of taste, ability to taste;
~ *m* **olfativo** olfactory organ, sense of smell
sentimiento *m* affect, emotion
sentir *v* to feel; ~ *v* **hormigueo** to tingle, to
prickle; ~ *v* **picazón** to tingle, to prickle
sentirse *v* **desamparado** to feel helpless, to feel
abandoned, to feel forsaken; ~ *v*
desfalleciente to feel faint, to be woozy
separación *f* dissociation, separation, sorting,
classifying; ~ **f lateral** lateral separation
separador *m* separator
sepsis *f* sepsis, septicemia; ~ **f focal** focal
sepsis; ~ **f puerperal** puerperal sepsis,
puerperal infection, puerperal eclampsia,
puerperal abscess
septicemia *f* sepsis, septicemia, blood
poisoning; ~ **f melitocócica** brucella sepsis
séptico *adj* septic
septiembre *m* September
séptimo *adj* seventh
septostomía *f* septostomy; ~ **f de balón** balloon
atrial septostomy
septum *m* dividing wall, septum;
~ *m* **pellucidum** septum lucidum, septum

pellucidum
sequedad *f* dryness, dessication; ~ **f vaginal**
vaginal dryness
ser *v* to be
serenidad *f* sobriety
serie *f* series, run
serina *f* serine
serio *adj* serious
sermorelina *f* sermorelin
seroconversión *f* seroconversion, development
of resistance
serodiagnóstico *m* serodiagnosis, serologic tests
seroglobulinas *f pl* serum globulins
serología *f* serology; ~ **f anti-VIH** anti-HIV
serology; ~ **f forense** forensic serology
serológico *adj* serological, blood study-related
seropositivo *adj* HIV positive, HIV-infected;
~ *adj* **con VIH** HIV positive
serotipificación *f* serological typing
serotipo *m* serotype
serotonina *f* serotonin
serpiente *f* snake
servicio *m* service, bathroom, toilet;
~ *m* **ambulatorio** ambulatory care; ~ *m* **de
ambulancias** ambulance service; ~ *m* **de
referencias** referral service, information
service; ~ *m* **médico de urgencia** emergency
room, emergency unit, emergency service,
emergency medical services; ~ *m* **psiquiátrico**
psychiatric ward
servicios *m pl* **de salud comunitario**
community health center, community health
care, community health services; ~ *m pl* **de
salud mental** mental health services;
~ *m pl* **de terapia de convalescencia** after
care services, follow-up treatment;
~ *m pl* **sanitarios preventivos** preventive care
sesenta *adj* sixty
setenta *adj* seventy
seudoartrosis *f* pseudarthrosis
seudociesis *f* phantom pregnancy, false
pregnancy, pseudopregnancy
seudocilindro *m* pseudocast
seudoembarazo *m* phantom pregnancy, false
pregnancy, pseudopregnancy
seudohermafroditismo *m*
pseudohermaphroditism; ~ *m* **masculino**
androgyny, masculin pseudo-hermaphroditism

S

seudomembrana *m* pseudomembrane, false membrane

seudomembranoso *adj* pseudomembranous, like a pseudomembrane

seudotumor *m* pseudotumor, tumor-like growth

severo *adj* severe

sexo *m* sex, gender; ~ *m* **cromosómico** chromosomal sex; ~ *m* **nuclear** nuclear sex

sexología *f* sexology

sexto *adj* sixth

sexualidad *f* sexuality

Shigella *f* **dysenteriae** Shigella dysenteriae; ~ **flexneri** Shigella flexneri; ~ **sonnei** Shigella sonnei

shigellosis *f* shigellosis

shock *m* shock, fright; ~ *m* **afectivo** psychic shock, mental shock, emotional shock; ~ *m* **anafiláctico** anaphylactic shock, anaphylaxis, acute hypersensitivity shock; ~ *m* **cardiogénico** cardiogenic shock, cardiac shock; ~ *m* **hipoglicémico** hypoglycemic shock, hypoglycemic attack; ~ *m* **hipovolémico** hypovolemic shock, volume deficiency collapse; ~ *m* **retardado** delayed shock

shunt *m* shunt

si if, yes

sialorrea *m* excessive salivation, ptyalism, sialorrhoea

sicología *f* psychology

sicológico *adj* psychological

sicosis *f* **de la barba** sycosis of the beard, barber's itch, tinea barbae

sicotecnia *f* psychotechnics, psychotechnology

SIDA *m* acquired immunodeficiency syndrome, AIDS

siderosis *f* siderosis, welder's lung

siembra *f* scatter

sien *f* temple

sieso *m* anal orifice, anus

siete *adj* seven

sievert *m* sievert

sifilítico luetic, syphilitis-related, pertaining to syphilis

sigma *f* **iliaca** sigmoid colon

sigmoide *adj* sigmoid, S-shaped

significativo *adj* significant

signo *m* symptom, sign, phenomenon; ~ *m* **de**

Babinski Babinski's sign, paradoxical extensor reflex; ~ *m* **de Gowers** Gowers contraction; ~ *m* **del pistón** mobility of head of femur

signos *m pl* **vitales** vital signs

siguiente *adj* secondary

silbar *v* to whistle; ~ *v* **el pecho** to wheeze

silencio *m* silence; ~ *m* **electroencefálico** electro- cerebral inactivity

sílice *f* **gelatinosa** silica gel

silicio *m* silicon, a nonmetalic element analogous to carbon, silicium

silicosis *f* silicosis

silicotuberculosis *f* silicotuberculosis, infective silicosis

silla *f* seat, chair; ~ *f* **de ruedas** wheelchair; ~ *f* **de ruedas eléctrica** electric wheelchair; ~ *f* **plegable** folding chair; ~ *f* **turca** sella turcica

silueta *f* silhouette; ~ *f* **cardíaca** cardiac shadow

simétrico *adj* symmetric

simpático *adj* sympathetic, nice

simpático *m* sympathetic; ~ *m* **lumbar** lumbar sympathetic; ~ *m* **torácico** thoracic sympathetic

simpaticomimético *m* sympathomimetic

simpatolítico *m pl* sympatholytic agent, sympathetic blocking agent

simple vista with the naked eye

simposio *m* conference

simulación *f* simulation

simulador *m* simulator

simultáneo *adj* simultaneous

sin *prep* without; ~ **aliento** out of breath, puffing & panting; ~ **dormir** sleepless, insomniac; ~ **fuerzas** exhausted, worn out, run-down; ~ **lupa** *f* with the naked eye; ~ **resuello** *m* out of breath, puffing & panting; ~ **resultado** *m* negative; ~ **retorno** *m* irreversible; ~ **trabajo** *m* out of work

sinapismo *m* poultice, sinapism, mustard plaster; ~ *m* poultice, sinapism, mustard plaster

sinapsis *f* nerve synapse; ~ *f* **nervio-músculo** neuromuscular synapse, nerve-nerve synapse

sináptico *adj* synaptic

sincitio *m* syncytium, coenocyte

síncope *m* syncope, fainting, fainting spell;
~ *m* **cardiaco** cardiac syncope;
~ *m* **postoperatorio** post-operative shock,
surgical shock; ~ *m* **provocado por la tos**
tussive syncope, fainting from a severe
coughing spell; ~ *m* **sinocarotídeo** carotid
syncope

síndrome *m* syndrome; ~ *m* **adrenogenital**
adrenogenital syndrome, congenital adrenal
hyperplasia; ~ *m* **agudo de las radiaciones**
radiation sickness; ~ *m* **cerebeloso** cerebellar
syndrome; ~ *m* **clínico** clinical syndrome,
clinical symptomatology; ~ *m* **cubital** cubital
syndrome; ~ *m* **de Albright** Albright-McCune-
Sternberg syndrome; ~ *m* **de asfixia
traumática** traumatic syndrome of asphyxia;
~ *m* **de colon irritable** irritable bowel
syndrome; ~ *m* **de compresión de la cava
inferior** vena cava compression syndrome;
~ *m* **de compresión del nervio ulnar** ulnar
nerve compression syndrome, cubital tunnel
syndrome, ulnar nerve entrapment; ~ *m* **de
compresión nerviosa** nerve entrapment,
compression neuropathy; ~ *m* **de Corvisart**
Corvisart syndrome, Fallot disease, Fallot's
tetralogy; ~ *m* **de Cushing** Cushing syndrome;
~ *m* **de declive** failure to thrive syndrome;
~ *m* **de desgaste personal** burnout,
exhaustion, inability to cope, weariness;
~ *m* **de Down** Down syndrome, translocation
mongolism, trisomy 21; ~ *m* **de Dressler**
Dressler's syndrome; ~ *m* **de Erasmus** Erasmus'
syndrome; ~ *m* **de exfoliación** capsular
glaucoma, exfoliation syndrome; ~ *m* **de
fatiga crónica** chronic fatigue syndrome,
myalgic encephalomyelitis, postviral fatigue
syndrome; ~ *m* **de Fisher** Fisher syndrome;
~ *m* **de Gilles de la Tourette** Gilles de la
Tourette syndrome; ~ *m* **de Goodpasture**
pulmonary-renal syndrome, vascular collagen
disease, Goodpasture's syndrom; ~ *m* **de
Gowers** Gowers disease, Gowers syndrome,
vasovagal syncope; ~ *m* **de Gradenigo**
Gradenigo's syndrome; ~ *m* **de Hamman**
Hamman mediastinal emphysema, Hamman
disease; ~ *m* **de HELLP** HELLP syndrome,
acronym for hemolysis, elevated liver enzymes

& low platelet count; ~ *m* **de hipercalcemia**
hypercalcemia syndrome; ~ *m* **de
inmunodeficiencia adquirida** acquired
immunodeficiency syndrome, AIDS; ~ *m* **de
insuficiencia respiratoria del adulto** adult
respiratory distress syndrome, ARDS, shock
lung; ~ *m* **de la apnea del sueño** sleep apnea
syndrome; ~ *m* **de la cápsula interna** capsular
hemiplegia, capsular paralysis; ~ *m* **de
malabsorción** malabsorption syndrom; ~ *m* **de
Melkersson-Rosenthal** factor XI deficiency,
Rosenthal's syndrome, plasma thromboplastin,
antecedent deficiency, PTA deficiency; ~ *m* **de
Menière** Ménière's disease, auditory vertigo,
Ménière's syndrome, labyrinthine vertigo;
~ *m* **de Moebius** ophthalmoplegic migraine,
Möbius disease, Möbius syndrome, relapsing
periodic oculomotor paralysis; ~ *m* **de
Münchausen** Munchausen syndrome by proxy,
facticious disorder by proxy; ~ *m* **de muerte
infantil súbita (SIMS)** sudden infant death
syndrome (SIDS), crib death; ~ *m* **de Noonan**
Noonan's syndrome; ~ *m* **de Pancoast**
Pancoast's syndrome; ~ *m* **de Pierre Robin**
Pierre Robin syndrome; ~ *m* **de Reye** Reye's
syndrome; ~ *m* **de salida capilar** capillary leak
syndrome; ~ *m* **de Senear-Usher** pemphigus
erythematosus, Senear-Usher disease; ~ *m* **de
Sjoegren** Sjögren's syndrome, sicca-
syndrome; ~ *m* **de Smith** Smith syndrome,
acute infectious lymphocytosis; ~ *m* **de
Turner** Turner's syndrome, gonadal dysgenesis
XO, monosomy X; ~ *m* **de Wolff-Parkinson-
White** Wolff-Parkinson-White syndrome;
~ *m* **del alcoholismo fetal** fetal alcohol
syndrome; ~ *m* **de la uña-patella** nail-patella
syndrome, hereditary osteo-onychoplasia
syndrome; ~ *m* **del canal de Guyon** Guyon's
canal syndrome; ~ *m* **del cayado aórtico**
aortic arch syndrome; ~ *m* **del edificio
enfermo** sick building syndrome; ~ *m* **del
miembro fantasma** phantom pain, phantom
limb syndrome, phantom sensation; ~ *m* **del
tunel carpiano** carpal tunnel syndrome, CTS;
~ *m* **hemolítico-uremico** hemolytic-uremic
syndrome; ~ *m* **medular** medullary syndrome;
~ *m* **mucocutáneo adenopático** Kawasaki
syndrome, mucocutaneous lymph node

syndrome, Kawasaki disease; ~ **m nefrótico de Epstein** Epstein nephrosis, Epstein's syndrome; ~ **m neuropático de Jamaica** Jamaica neuropathic syndrome; ~ **m de nevo displásico** dysplastic naevus-cell-naevus syndrome; ~ **m de Werner** Werner's syndrome; ~ **m pos-poliomielitis** post-poliomyelitis syndrome, Postpoliomyelitis Muscular Atrophy; ~ **m postinfarto de miocardio** Dressler's syndrome; ~ **m sideropénico** iron deficiency syndrome

sinergético adj synergistic, combined

sinergia f synergism, synergy

sinérgico adj synergetic

sínfisis f **pericárdica** pericardial concretion

singulto m singultus, hiccup; ~ **espasmódico** spasmodic hiccup, spasmolygmus

siniestrado m victim of a disaster, victim of an accident, casualty

siniestral adj left-handed

sino m but

sinovial adj synovial

sinovitis f synovitis, inflammation of a joint-lubricating membrane

sintasa f synthetase, ligase

síntesis f synthesis; ~ **f de las enzimas** enzymic synthesis, enzymic biosynthesis

sintetizador m synthesizer; ~ **m de ADN** DNA synthesizer, oligonucleotide synthesizer

síntoma m symptom; ~ **m facultativo** facultative symptom

síntomas m pl **carenciales de vitaminas** vitamin deficiency symptoms, vitamin deficiency disease

sintomático adj symptomatic

sintomatología f symptomatology

sinus m sinus; ~ **m aórtico** aortic sinus

sinusal adj sinusal

sinusitis f sinusitis

sinvastatina f simvastatin

siquiatra m/f psychiatrist

siquiatría f psychiatry

siquiátrico adj psychiatric

siriasis f heat stroke, siriasis

sismoterapia f sismotherapy, vibratory massage, vibrational therapy

sisomicina f sisomicin, an antibiotic related to gentamicin

sistema m system; ~ **m anaeróbico de incubación** anaerobic incubation system; ~ **m analítico** analytical system; ~ **m cromafínico** chromaffin system; ~ **m de activación metabólica** metabolic activation system; ~ **m de administración de medicamentos** drug delivery system; ~ **m de hemovigilancia** hemovigilance system; ~ **m de HLA de histocompatibilidad** HLA histocompatibility system; ~ **m de identificación** identification system; ~ **m de informática hospitalaria** Hospital Information System; ~ **m de medición** system of measurement; ~ **m de medida** measuring system; ~ **m de retención** restraint system; ~ **m de secuenciación de proteínas** protein sequencing system; ~ **m de sujeción** restraint system; ~ **m endocrino** endocrine system; ~ **m extrínseco de coagulación** extrinsic coagulation system, extrinsic coagulation pathway, thromboplastin system; ~ **m hematopoyético** hematopoietic system; ~ **m HLA de histocompatibilidad** HLA histocompatibility system; ~ **m inmunitario** immune system; ~ **m intrínseco de coagulación** intrinsic coagulation pathway, intrinsic coagulation cascade; ~ **m límbico** limbic system, group of subcortical structures; ~ **m linfático** lymphatic system; ~ **m nervioso** nervous system; ~ **m nervioso autónomo** autonomic nervous system; ~ **m nervioso central** central nervous system; ~ **m nervioso periférico** peripheral nervous system; ~ **m nervioso simpático** sympathetic nervous system; ~ **m olfativo** olfactory system; ~ **m parasimpático nervioso** parasympathetic nervous system; ~ **m porta** portal system; ~ **m radiomédico** radio medical system, medical consulting by radio; ~ **m respiratorio** respiratory system, airways; ~ **m TNM de estadiaje** TMN staging system; ~ **m vascular** vascular system

sistemático adj systematic

sistémico adj systemic, pertaining to the whole body

sistólico adj systolic (pressure)

sitio m place; ~ **m activo** active site; ~ **m antigénico** antigenic site; ~ **m de**

iniciación de la transcripción transcription initiation site

situación f status, state; ~ f **jurídica del hijo concebido** legal status of the child conceived

situado adj situated, placed; ~ **detrás** posterior

sobaco m armpit

sobadora f medical practitioner in Mexico

sobaqueras f pl crutches

sobaquina f body odor, B.O., underarm odor, smell of sweat

sobar v to massage

sobre on, about, above; ~ **todo** especially, particularly

sobredosis f overdose, overdosing, overdosage

sobreestimar v to overestimate

sobreexcitación f stimulation, excitation

sobrefatigarse v to overexert oneself

sobreparto m in childbed

sobrepeso adj overweight, fat, chubby, pudgy, portly, stout

sobresaliente adj relevant

sobresalir v to bulge, to protrude

sobresalto m startle reaction, startle response, jumping when startled

sobreviviente adj surviving

sobreviviente m/f survivor; ~ m pl **a largo plazo** long-term survivor

sobrina f niece

sobrino m nephew

socioterapeuta m social therapist

sodio m sodium

sofocar v to suffocate, to choke, to asphyxiate

sofocos m pl hot flashes

sol m sun

solamente only

solanera f heat stroke, siriasis

solitaria f tapeworm, cestode

sólo only

soltarse v to break loose

soltero m single

solución f solution, fluid; ~ f **amortiguadora de fosfatos** phosphate buffered saline solution; ~ f **de carga** loading solution, buffered solution; ~ f **de compromiso** compromise, trade-off; ~ f **de Lugol** Lugol's solution; ~ f **de perfusión** perfusion solution, infusion solvents; ~ f **de Ringer** Ringer's solution; ~ f **fisiológica** physiological salt, physiological

saline solution, normal saline solution; ~ f **isotónica** isotonic solution; ~ f **para perfusión** perfusion solution, infusion solvents; ~ f **salina isotónica** isotonic saline solution; ~ f **tampón de fosfatos** phosphate buffered saline solution; ~ f **tamponada** loading solution, buffered solution

solvatación f solvatation

solvente m solvent, dissolvent

somático adj somatic, physical

somatización f somatization

somatoliberina f growth hormone-releasing factor, somatoliberin, GH-RF, somatotropin-releasing factor

somatología f somatology, physical anthropology

somatomedina f somatomedin

somatorelina f somatorelin

somatostatina f somatostatin, growth-hormone-release-inhibiting hormone

somatotropina f GH, growth hormone, somatotrophin

somnolencia f sleepiness, somnolence

sonambulismo m somnambulism, sleep-walking

soñar v to dream; ~ v **despierto** to daydream

sonarse v **las narices** to blow one's nose

sonda f probe, catheter; ~ f **de ácidos nucleicos** nucleic acid probe, DNA probe, molecular probe; ~ f **de Fogarty** Fogarty balloon catheter; ~ f **intestinal** intestinal probe, intestinal catheter; ~ **a permanencia** f indwelling catheter

sonido m sound; ~ m **asmático** wheezing, whistling

sonograma m ultrasonogram, sonogram, echogram

soñoliento adj sleepy, drowsy

sopa f soup

soplo m puff, souffle; ~ m **cardíaco** heart murmur; ~ m **cardíaco sistólico** systolic murmur, ejection murmur; ~ m **de expulsión** vasodilatation murmur, ejection click; ~ m **del corazón** heart murmur; ~ m **protodiastólico** protodiastolic murmur; ~ m **sistólico** systolic murmur, ejection murmur

soponcio m fainting, swoon, collapse

soporífico adj soporific, sleep-inducing

soporte m support, bracket; ~ m **para la caja**

S

toracica fracture appliance for ribs;
~ m **pélvico** pelvic support

sorbitol m sorbitol

sordera f hearing impairment, impaired hearing, deafness, surdity; ~ f **accidental** acquired deafness, adventitious deafness; ~ f **adquirida** acquired deafness, adventitious deafness; ~ f **de percepción** labyrinthine hearing loss, inner-ear deafness, nerve deafness, sensorineural hearing loss; ~ f **neurosensorial** labyrinthine hearing loss, inner-ear deafness, nerve deafness, sensorineural hearing loss; ~ f **parcial** hearing disorder, defective hearing, auditory disorder, partial hearing loss; ~ f **por trauma acústico** deafness due to acoustic trauma, noise-induced hearing loss; ~ f **profesional** occupational hearing loss, deafness due to occupational noise, noise induced hearing loss; ~ f **sensorineural** labyrinthine hearing loss, inner-ear deafness, nerve deafness, sensorineural hearing loss

sordo adj deaf, dull; ~ adj **de nacimiento** born deaf, congenitally hearing impaired

sordo m hearing-impaired person

soroche m mountain sickness, altitude sickness

sosa f soda; ~ f **cáustica** caustic soda; ~ f **líquida** lye, caustic soda, sodium hydroxide

sostén m support, woman's bra, brassiere

spondylotherapy f spondylotherapy, spinal manipulation

spotting (inglés) spotting

spray m spray

stent m stent; ~ m **coronario** intraluminal coronary artery stent

stockinette f stockinet, tubular gauze

streptococcus m streptococcus

streptomicina f streptomycin, a broad-spectrum antibiotic

su, sus your, her, his

suave adj soft

suavizar v to soften

subagudo adj subacute, somewhat acute

subalimentación f inanition, starvation, malnutrition

subaracnoideo adj subarachnoid

subastragalina f subtalar

subcapsular adj subcapsular, beneath a tough outer covering

subclínico adj mild; ~ adj subclinical, mild, asymptomatic

subcondral adj subchondral, situated beneath cartilage

subconjuntival adj subconjunctival, situated beneath the conjunctiva

subconjunto m subset, subsystem

subcutáneo adj subcutaneous, below the skin

subdivisión f breakdown, decomposition

subespecie f subspecies

subgrupo m subset, subsystem

subir v to lift, to raise, to pull up; ~ v **una escalera** climbing stairs

súbito adj suddenly adj

subjetivo adj subjective

sublingual adj sublingual, under the tongue

subluxación f subluxation, an incomplete dislocation; ~ f **unilateral** subluxation, dislocation

substitutivo m substitute; ~ m **del plasma** plasma substitute

substituto m substitute; ~ m **sanguíneo** blood substitute, substitute blood product

substitutos m pl **de grasa** fat substitutes, artificial fats

substrato m substrate; ~ m **tampón** buffer substrate, buffer solution

subtilisina f subtilisin

succión f suction, aspiration

sucesión f succession; ~ f **ecológica** ecological succession

sucio adj dirty, soiled, grubby

sudación f perspiration, sweating; ~ f **exagerada** hyperhidrosis, excessive sweating

sudar v to sweat

sudor m sweat, perspiration, sweating; ~ m **frío** cold sweat; ~ m **nocturno** night sweats

sudoración f perspiration, sweating

suegra f mother-in-law

suegro m father-in-law

suelo pélvico m pelvic floor, floor of the pelvis

sueño adj sleepy, drowsy

sueño m sleep; ~ m **paradójico** paradoxical sleep; ~ m **profundo** sound sleep, deep sleep; ~ m **REM** REM sleep, paradoxical sleep

suero m serum; ~ m **antialérgico** serum against

allergic diseases; ~ m **antiestreptocócico** streptococcic serum; ~ m **antigangrenoso** serum against gangrene; ~ m **antiglobulinas humanas** anti-human globulin immune serum, Coombs' reagent, Coombs serum; ~ m **antilinfocítico** antilymphocyte serum; ~ m **Coombs** anti-human globulin immune serum, Coombs' reagent, Coombs serum; ~ m **inorgánico** inorganic serum; ~ m **sanguíneo** blood serum

sufocar v to suffocate, to choke, to asphyxiate

sufrimiento m distress, suffering; ~ m **fetal** fetal distress

sufrir v to suffer; ~ v **una recaída** to have a relapse, to get sick again; ~ v **una reincidencia** to have a relapse, to get sick again; ~ v **un tirón** to pull a muscle

suicida m/f suicide

suicidarse v to commit suicide

suicidio m suicide; ~ m **deliberado** deliberate suicide

sujeción f restraint, retention, immobilization, uptake, absorbing, retention; ~ f **de precisión** precision grip, precision grasp; ~ f **de una pelota** span grip, course grip

sujetalengua f tongue depressor

sulbactam m sulbactam

sulfadiacina f sulfadiazine; ~ f **de plata** silver sulfadiazine, an antibacterial used topically in burn therapy.

sulfadimidina f sulfamethazine

sulfhemoglobina f sulph hemoglobin, sulfhemoglobin

sulfamethoxazol m sulfamethoxazole, an antibacterial agent that interferes with folic acid synthesis in susceptible bacteria

sulfanilamida f sulfonilamide, sulfa drug

sulfato m sodium sulfate; ~ m **de amonio** ammonium sulphate; ~ m **de bario** barium sulfate; ~ m **de cinc** zinc sulphate; ~ m **de condroitina** chondroitin sulfate; ~ m **de magnesio** magnesium sulphate; ~ m **de protamina** protamine sulfate; ~ m **de quinina** quinine sulphate; ~ m **magnésico** magnesium sulphate

sulfonamidas f pl sulfonamides

sulindac m sulindac

sulphite lye m sulphite lye, sulfite lye

superenrollamiento m **del ADN** DNA supercoiling

superficie f surface; ~ f **gástrica del hígado** gastric surface of the liver

supergén m supergene

superhélice f superhelix, supercoil

superinfección f superinfection, secondary infection

supersticioso adj superstitious

supervisión f supervision

supervivencia f survival; ~ f **sin enfermedad** disease-free survival, event-free survival

supinación f supination

supino adj supine

suplemental adj additional

suplemento m supplement

suposición f hypothesis, theory

supositorio m suppository

suprarrenal adj adrenal

suprarrenales f pl suprarenal glands

supraventricular adj supraventricular, above the heart chambers

supresión f suppressing, suppressive, withdrawal

suprimir v to suppress

supuración f suppuration, discharging pus

surco m line, wrinkle, track, fissure, groove, sulcus; ~ m **dental primitivo** night guard, mouth guard, biteguard, occlusal splint, peridontal splint, dental prosthesis

sus their

susceptible adj irritable, cranky, touchy, short-tempered, in a bad mood

suspender v to hang, to hang up, to suspend, to stop; ~ v **la respiration** to hold the breath

suspensión f suspension; ~ f **bacteriana** bacterial suspension; ~ f **de virus** virus suspension, viral suspension

sustancia f substance, agent, essence, matter; ~ f **activa** active principle, active ingredient, active agent; ~ f **añadida** additive, add-on; ~ f **básica** substrate, substance on which an enzyme acts; ~ f **blanca** white matter, substantia alba; ~ f **blanca del cerebro** white matter of the cerebellum; ~ f **mimética** mimetic substance; ~ f **probiótica** probiotic substance; ~ f **psicotropa** psychotropic substance; ~ f **reguladora** modulator

sustitución f substitution; ~ f **alélica** allele

displacement, allele replacement; ~ f de tejidos tissue replacement

sustituto m substitute; ~ m de la sangre blood substitute, substitute blood product

susto m shock, fright

sustrato m substrate

sutura f wound suture; ~ f ligadura de Blalock Blalock suture ligature; ~ f patelar patellar suture, prepatellar suture, cerclage of the patella

suturar v to suture; ~ v una herida to stitch up a wound, to suture it

T

tabaco m tobacco; ~ m sin humo smokeless tobacco, chewing tobacco

tabaquera f anatómica anatomist's snuff-box

tabaquismo m tobacco smoking, tabacco use; ~ m involuntario passive smoking, second-hand smoke; ~ m pasivo passive smoking, second-hand smoke

tabes m dorsal tabes dorsalis, spinal paralysis

tabique m thin wall; ~ m de separación dividing wall

tabiques m pl placentarios placental septa, incomplete partitions between placental cotyledons

tabla f plank, board, panel; ~ f oftálmica vision chart, eye chart; ~ f periodica de los elementos periodic table of the elements

tablilla f night guard, mouth guard, biteguard, occlusal splint, peridontal splint, dental prosthesis; ~ f digital finger splint

tacto m touch

tálamo m thalamus

tal vez maybe

talasemia f thalassemia, Mediterranean anemia

talidomina f thalidomide

taller m workshop; ~ m de protesis dental prosthetic dentistry laboratory

tallo m height

talón m heel of the foot

tambalear v to stagger, to weave, to be unsteady on one's feet

tambaleos m pl en la marcha unsteady gait,

staggering gait

tamizaje m screening, detection, preventive medical checkup; ~ m genético presymptomatic genetic testing

tamoxifén m tamoxifen, antioestrogen drug

tampón m buffer, ink pad; ~ m de fosfato phosphate buffer; ~ m higiénico tampon

tanatología f thanatology

tántalo m tantalum

tapado adj hidden, occult, concealed

tapón m cap, top, plug, cork; ~ m de oidos earplug

taponamiento m cardiac tamponade; ~ m cardíaco cardiac tamponade

taquiarritmia f tachyarrhythmia, rapid irregular heartbeat

taquicardia f tachycardia, racing heart beat; ~ f sinusal sinus tachycardia

taquifilaxia f tachyphylaxis, loss of effectivity

tara f tare, defect, disability; ~ f física physical disability, physical deterioration; ~ f mental physical & mental disability, physical & mental deterioration

tarde f afternoon

tardio adj tardive, late

tarjeta f card; ~ f de crédito credit card

tarsos m pl tarsals

tartamudear v to stutter, to stammer

tartamudez f stutter, stuttering, stammering

tartrato m tartrate; ~ m de antimonio y potasio antimony-potassium tartrate

tasa f rate; ~ f absoluta de curación absolute healing index; ~ f de dosis dose-rate; ~ f de fertilidad fertility rate; ~ f de infección infection rate; ~ f de metabolismo basal fasting metabolism, basal metabolic rate, basal metabolism; ~ f de morbilidad morbidity rate; ~ f de mortalidad death rate; ~ f de mortalidad infantil infant mortality; ~ f de reincidencias relapse rate; ~ f de supervivencia global overall survival rate

tasicinesia f acathisia, cathisophobia

tatuaje m tattoo

taxonomía f taxonomy; ~ f numérica numerical taxonomy

TC f (tomografia computada) CT scanning (computed tomography); ~ f cerebral CT scan of the brain

té *m* tea; **~ con leche** tea with milk

tebaína *f* dimethylmorphine, thebaine, paramorphine

técnica *f* technique, procedure; **~ f de fenolftaleina** phenolphthalein test, PST; **~ f de ventana pericárdica** pericardiostomy, pericardial window technique; **~ f médica** medical engineering, medical technique, medical technology

técnicas *f pl* **para inmunoenzimas** immunoenzyme techniques, enzyme immunoassay, enzyme-labeled antibody technique

técnico *m* technician, expert, specialist; **~ m de radiología** radiology technician, radiological technologist

tecnología *f* technology; **~ f celular** cell technology

tecoma *m* thecoma, theca cell tumor

teicoplanina *f* teicoplanin

tejido *m* tissue; **~ m adiposo** fatty tissue, adipose tissue; **~ m blando** soft tissue; **~ m blando rodeando** surrounding soft tissue; **~ m calloso** callosity, calloules; **~ m canceroso** cancerous tissue; **~ m celular subcutáneo** subcutaneous cellular tissue; **~ m ciatrizal** scar tissue; **~ m conjuntivo** fatty lymphoid tissue, connective tissue; **~ m conjuntivo embrionario** embryonal connective tissue, mesenchyme; **~ m conjuntivo hialino** hyaline connective tissue; **~ m conjuntivo retroperitoneal** retroperitoneal connective tissue; **~ m conjuntivo subepitelial** subepithelial connective tissue; **~ m de granulación** granulation tissue; **~ m embrionario** germinal tissue; **~ m epitelial** epithelial tissue, epithelial layer of cells; **~ m grasoso** fatty tissue, adipose tissue; **~ m hematopoyético** hematopoietic tissue, blood-forming tissue; **~ m indiferente** formative tissue (botany); **~ m óseo** bone tissue, osseous tissue; **~ m osteoide** osteoid tissue, osseous tissue prior to calcification

tela *f* cloth, fabric, sheet; **~ f hospital** hospital sheet

telangiectasia *f* telangiectasia, permanent dilation of existing blood vessels

teléfono *m* telephone

telemedicina *f* telemedicine

telemetría *f* telemetry; **~ f médica** biotelemetry, medical telemetry

temblar *v* to shiver, to tremble, to shake

temblor *m* tremor; **~ m cerebeloso** cerebellar tremor; **~ m de la enfermedad de Parkinson** Parkinson's tremor; **~ m de las manos** tremor of hands, unsteady hands, trembling of hands; **~ m intencional** intention tremor, shakiness

temperatura *f* temperature; **~ f ambiente** room temperature; **~ f Celsius** Celsius temperature; **~ f corporal** body temperature; **~ f cutánea** skin temperature; **~ f de la piel** skin temperature; **~ f termodinámica** thermodynamic temperature

templo *m* temple

temporada *f* season, period; **~ f de cría** child bearing period

tenacillas *f pl* forceps, tweezers

tendencia *f* tendency, predisposition, trend, addiction

tendencias *f pl* **suicidas** suicidal tendencies

tendinitis *f* tendinitis, inflamed tendons; **~ f bicipital** bicipital tendonitis; **~ f del hombro** shoulder tendon inflammation

tendinopatía *f* **del hombro** rotator cuff tendinitis, shoulder tendon inflammation

tendón *m* tendon; **~ m de Aquiles** Achilles tendon, tendo calcaneaus, tendo calcaneus; **~ m desgarrado** pulled tendon, desmectasia, strained tendon

tendovaginitis *f* tendosynovitis, tendovaginitis

tener *v* to get, to have; **~ v ansias** to be anxious; **~ v dolor de cabeza** to have a headache; **~ v el hipo** to have the hiccups; **~ v escalofríos** feel queasy, to, feel out of sorts, to, feel shivery, to, be unwell, to, be quivering, to, be under the weather, to; **~ v estreñimiento** to be constipated; **~ v frío** to be cold, to, freeze; **~ v la menstruación** to be menstruating, to have one's period; **~ v náuseas** to be nauseated, to throw up, to vomit; **~ v relaciones sexuales** to have intercourse, to have sex, to copulate, to make love

tenesmo *m* urge to evacuate rectum or bladder, tenesmus, the runs

tenia *f* tapeworm, cestode

tenosinovitis f tenosynovitis, inflammation of a tendon sheath; ~ f de De Quervain tenosynovitis

tensioactivo adj tensioactive, affecting surface tension

tensión f tension, tone; ~ f aumentada hypertension, high blood pressure, hypertonia; ~ f muscular muscle tone, tension; ~ f premenstrual premenstrual dystonia, premenstrual syndrome, PMS; ~ f superficial surface tension

teofilina f theophylline

teorema m theorem; ~ m de Bayes Bayes' theorem

teoría f theory; ~ f delta delta theory

teórico adj theoretical

TEP f (tomografía por emisión de positrones) PET, positron-emission tomography

terapeuta m therapist; ~ m de reeducación occupational therapist; ~ m ocupacional occupational therapist

terapéutica f therapeutics, treatment; ~ f respiratoria respiratory therapy, the therapeutic treatment of respiratory diseases

terapéutico adj therapeutic

terapia f therapy, treatment; ~ f antibiótica antibiotic therapy; ~ f anti-hongo anti-fungal therapy; ~ f antineoplásica antineoplastic therapy; ~ f biológica biological therapy; ~ f citorreductora debulking (of a tumor), cytoreductive therapy, cytoreductive resection; ~ f cognitiva cognitive therapy, cognitive behavior therapy; ~ f concomitante concomitant therapy; ~ f de afirmación assertiveness training; ~ f de la voz voice therapy, rehabilitation of the voice; ~ f de ozono ozone therapy; ~ f de radiación radiation therapy, radiotherapy; ~ f de rehidratación oral oral rehydration therapy; ~ f de relajación relaxation therapy; ~ f de sustitución hormonal hormone replacement therapy; ~ f fotodinámica PDT, photodynamic therapy, phototherapy; ~ f genética genetic therapy; ~ f germinal gene therapy; ~ f herbaria phytotherapy, herbal treatment, herbal medicine; ~ f neurovegetativa electroneural therapy; ~ f ocupacional occupational therapy, ergotherapy; ~ f por ultrasonido ultrasonic therapy; ~ f tisular tissue therapy

teratogenicidad f teratogenicity

teratogénico adj teratogenic producing a fetal abnormality

teratógeno adj teratogen, teratogenic, tending to produce anomalies of formation or teratism

teratológico adj teratological

teratoma m teratoma, made up of a heterogeneous mixture of tissues; ~ m testicular testicular teratoma

terbinafina f terbinafine

terbutaline f terbutaline

tercero adj third; ~ adj trimestre del embarazo third trimester of pregnancy

tercio m third (part)

terementina f turpentine

térmico adj thermal, heat related

terminador m terminator

terminal adj terminal

término m term, end, conclusion; ~ m del embarazo term of pregnancy

términos m pl médicos medical terms

termocauterio m thermocautery

termocoagulación f thermocoagulation

termografía f thermography

termolisina f thermolysin

termómetro m thermometer; ~ m de hipotermia hypothermic thermometer; ~ m registrador recording thermometer

termorregulación f thermoregulation, heat regulation

tesaurismosis f cálcica calcium thesaurismosis

test m test, exam; ~ m de Apgar Apgar index, Apgar-score; ~ m de Coombs Coombs' test, Coombs reaction; ~ m de mutagenicidad mutagenicity test; ~ m de toxicidad toxicity test; ~ m epicutáneo skin testing, patch test, epicutaneous test

testicular adj testicular

testículo m testicle, testis, male gonad; ~ m endurecido hardened testicle; ~ m no descendido undescended testicle, cryptorchism

testosterona f testosterone

testuz m forehead

tetania f tetany, muscle spasm; ~ f gravídica gestation tetany

tetanígeno adj tetanus-prone
tétano(s) m tetanus
tetilla f nipple
tetina f nipple of baby bottle
tetraciclina f tetracycline
tetracloruro m **de carbono** carbon tetrachloride
tetralogía f tetralogy; ~ f **de Fallot** Corvisart syndrome, Fallot disease, Fallot's tetralogy; ~ f **del pequeño mal** petit mal quartet
tez f complexion; ~ f **blanca** fair-skinned, fair complected
THC (tetrahidrocannabinol) THC, tetrahydrocannabinol
tía f aunt
tiabendazol m thiabendazole, an anthelmintic
tiamazol m methimazole
tiamfenicol m thiamphenicol
tiamina f thiamine, vitamin B1, aneurin
tiaminasa f thiaminase
tibia f tibia
tibio adj lukewarm, tepid
tic m tic; ~ m **doloroso** trigeminal neuralgia, tic douloureux, an intense paroxysmal neuralgia of the trigeminal nerve, prosopalgia
ticarcilina f ticarcillin
tiempo m time, geather; ~ m **de coagulación** clotting time; ~ m **de entrega** turnaround time; ~ m **de protrombina** prothrombin time; ~ m **de recuperación** recovery time, recovery period; ~ m **de retracción del coágulo** clot-retraction time; ~ m **de sangría** bleeding time; ~ m **de trombina** thrombin time; ~ m **de tromboplastina parcial** partial thromboplastin time; ~ m **libre** spare time, leisure time, time off; ~ m **medio** mean time
tiesa f erect, stiff, rigid
tiesura f rigidity, stiffness
tifo m typhus
tifoidea f typhoid
tifus m typhus; ~ m **abdominal** typhoid fever; ~ m **exantemático endémico** murine typhus, endemic typhus
tijeras f pl scissors
tilacoide m thylakoid
timbre m call bell
timerosal m thimerosal, a crystalline organic mercurial antiseptic with antifungal and bacteriostatic properties
timidina f thymidine, deoxythymidine; ~ ~ **cinasa** f thymidine kinase
timina f thymin
tímpano m eardrum, tympanic membrane
timpanograma m tympanogram
tina f bathtub
tiña f ringworm, tinea; ~ f **de la barba** tinea barbae, barber's itch, sycosis of the beard, impetigo sycosiformis; ~ f **podal** tinea pedis, foot infection; ~ f **tonsurante** ringworm of the scalp, herpes tonsurans capillitii, barbae, corporis, vesiculosus
tinción f stain, coloring; ~ f **de ácidorresistencia** acid-fast stain; ~ f **de Giemsa** Giemsa stain; ~ f **de Gram** Gram stain; ~ f **de Papanicolaou** Papanicolaou stain; ~ f **de Wright** Wright stain; ~ f **de Ziehl-Neelsen** Ziehl-Neelsen stain; ~ f **flagelar** flagellar stain; ~ f **fluorescente** fluorescent stain
tinidazol f tinidazole
tinitus m tinnitus
tinoso adj mangy, scabbed
tinte m dyeing, stain; ~ m **amarillento** yellowish complexion; ~ m **ictérico** yellowish complexion
tintineo m tinnitus, ringing in the ears
tintura f tincture; ~ f **de yodo** tincture of iodine
tío m uncle
tioflavina f thioflavine
tioglucosidasa f thioglucosidase
típico adj classic
tipificación f typing; ~ f **con colicina** colicin typing; ~ f **con fagos** phage typing; ~ f **de HLA** HLA typing, human lymphocyte antigen typing; ~ f **del ADN** DNA profiling; ~ f **serológica** serotyping, serological typing
tipo m type, kind, sort; ~ m **de magnitud** kind-of-quantity; ~ m **de propiedad** kind-of-property
tira f strip, strap; ~ f **reactiva** dipstick, reagent strip, testing strip
tirantes m pl braces, suspenders
tirantez f tightness, tension, strain
tirar v to pull; ~ v **al retrete** to flush (a toilet)
tiritar v to quiver, to shiver, to tremble, to shake

tiriton *m* shivering attack, uncontrollable trembling

tiro *m* gunshot

tirocalcitonina *f* thyrocalcitonin

tiroglobina *f* thyroglobin

tiroides *m* thyroid, thyroid gland

tiroidismo *m* disease of the thyroid

tiroiditis *f* thyroiditis; ~ *f* **autoinmune** autoimmune thyroiditis; ~ *f* **de Hashimoto** Hashimoto thyroiditis

tiroliberina *f* thyroliberin, thyrotropin-releasing factor, TRF

tirón *m* pulled tendon, desmectasia, strained tendon; ~ *m* **muscular** muscle twitch

tirones *m pl* wrenching pain

tiropexina *f* thyropexin

tirosina *f* tyrosine; ~ *f* **descarboxilasa** decarboxylase; ~ *f* **quinasa** tyrosine kinase

tirostático *m* thyrostatic, antithyroid product

tirotoxicosis *f* thyrotoxicosis, excess of thyroid hormone

tirotropina *f* thyroid-stimulating hormone, thyrotrophin, TSH

tiroxina *f* thyroxine, T4, thyroid hormone; ~ **desiodinasa** *f* thyroxine 5-deiodinase

tísico *adj* tubercular

tisis *f* pulmonary tuberculosis

titubear *v* to stagger, to weave, to be unsteady on one's feet

título *m* titre, concentration of a substance in solution

tlacotillo *m* perianal abscess

toalla *f* towel; ~ *f* **sanitaria** sanitary napkin

tobillo *m* ankle

tobramicina *f* tobramycin

tocino *m* bacon

tocoferol *m* tocopherol, vitamin E

todavía *adv* still

todo all, entire

tofo *m* tophus

tolbutamida *f* tolbutamide

tolerabilidad *f* tolerability

tolerancia *f* tolerance; ~ *f* **a la glucosa** glucose tolerance; ~ *f* **al estrés** tolerance to stress; ~ *f* **al tetrazolio** tetrazolium tolerance; ~ *f* **del dolor** threshold of pain; ~ *f* **gastrointestinal** gastro-intestinal tolerance

tolnaftato *m* tolnaftate, a synthetic antifungal agent

tolondro *m* lump

toma *f* ingestion, swallowing; ~ *f* **cervicovaginal** cervical-vaginal swab; ~ *f* **de decisones médica objetiva** objective medical decision making

tomaína *f* ptomaine

tomar *v* to take; ~ *v* **asiento** to sit down; ~ *v* **el pulso** to take your pulse; ~ *v* **frío** to catch a cold; ~ *v* **una píldora** to take a pill

tomografía *f* tomography; ~ *f* **computada** computer tomography, diagnostic imaging, CT scanning; ~ *f* **en decúbito horizontal** horizontal tomography; ~ *f* **por emisión de positrones** PET scan, positron-emission tomography

tomógrafo *m* laminagraph, planigraph, stratigraph

tónico *adj* tonic

tono *m* tension, tone; ~ *m* **muscular** muscle tone, tension

tonometría *f* corneal tonometry, a procedure to measure the intraocular pressure

tonsila *f* tonsil

tonsilitis *f* tonsillitis

tópico *adj* local, topical, regional, applied to the surface

torácico *adj* thoracic, chest-related

toracocentesis *f* thoracentesis, thoracocentesis

toracolumbar *adj* thoracolumbar

toracotomía *f* thoracotomy, a surgical procedure opening the chest cavity; ~ *f* **doble** double thoracotomy

tórax *m* chest, thorax; ~ *m* **hidatádico** hydatid thorax

torcedura *f* sprain, dislocation, torsion, twist, twisting

torcido *adj* crooked

torniquete *m* tourniquet, Esmarch bandage

toronjil *m* lemon balm, citronnelle

torrente *m* torrent, stream, rush; ~ *m* **sanguíneo** bloodstream, flow of blood

torsade de pointes torsade de pointes

torsión *f* sprain, dislocation, torsion, twist, twisting; ~ *f* **del pedículo de un hidátide** hydatid torsion; ~ *f* **testicular** inverted testicle, torsion of the testicle

torta *f* cake

tortícolis f torticollis, twisting of head and neck

torunda f swab

tos f cough; ~ f **crupal** croupous cough;
~ f **espasmódica** convulsive cough, spastic cough; ~ f **faríngea** pharyngeal cough;
~ f **ferina** whooping cough, pertussis;
~ f **pleural** pleural cough

toser v to cough

tosferina f pertussis, whooping cough

total m total, whole; ~ m **de la población** the whole of the population

toxemia f blood poisoning, toxemia; ~ f **de la sangre** blood toxemia

toxicidad f poisonousness, toxicity; ~ f **aguda** acute toxicity; ~ f **para los riñones** nephrotoxicity

tóxico adj toxic, m poison; ~**-farmacológico** adj pharmatoxicological;
~ m **protoplasmático** protoplasmatic poison

toxicología f toxicology; ~ f **clínica** clinical toxicology; ~ f **genética** genetic toxicology;
~ f **inhalatoria** respiratory toxicology, inhalation toxicology; ~ f **respiratoria** respiratory toxicology, inhalation toxicology

toxicológico adj toxicologic, toxicological

toxicomanía f toxicomania; ~ f **múltiple** multiple addiction, multiple drug abuse

toxina f toxin, poison; ~ f **botulínica** botulinum toxin; ~ f **de staphylococus aureus** staphylococcus aureus toxin; ~ f **del cólera** cholera toxin, enterotoxin from Vibrio cholerae; ~ f **diftérica** diphtheria toxin;
~ f **estafilocócica** staphylotoxin

toxoide m anatoxin, toxoid; ~ m **tetánico** tetanus toxoid

toxoplasma f toxoplasma

toxoplasmosis f toxoplasmosis; ~ f **cerebral** cerebral toxoplasmosis

trabajador m worker; ~ m **en una fábrica** factory worker; ~ m **lastimado** injured worker

trabajar v to work

trabajo m labor, work; ~ m **de parto inducido** induced labor; ~ m **del corazón** heart action, cardiac work

trabécula f trabecula

trabecular adj trabecular

tracción f traction, extension treatment

tracoma m pink-eye, trachoma

tracto m bundle, tract, sheaf of fibers;
~ m **alimentario** digestive tract, alimentary channel, gastrointestinal tract, digestive system; ~ m **intestinal** digestive tract, gastrointestinal tract; ~ m **respiratorio superior** respiratory tract; ~ m **ureteral** ureteral tract

traducción f translation

traductor m translator

tragadero m esophagus, gullet, throat

tragante m esophagus, gullet

tragar v to swallow

traje m **protector** protective clothing

trama f **pulmonar** pulmonary trama;
~ f **pulmonar esclerótica con estrías** striated pulmonary trama

tranquilizante m sedative, tranquilizer;
~ m **mayor** neuroleptic, antipsychotic

tranquilo adj still

transaminasa f transaminasa

transbordación f **de cromosomas** translocation of chromosomes

transcetolasa f transketolase

transcripción f transcription; ~ f **genética** genetic transcription, gene transcription;
~ f **inversa** reverse transcription

transcriptasa f **inversa** reverse transcriptase, RNA-dependent DNA polymerase

transcrito m transcript

transcutáneo adj transcutaneous

transdérmico adj transdermal

transducción f **restringida** restricted transduction

transductor m transducer

transferasa f transferase

transferencia f transfer; ~ f **de embriones** embryo transfer; ~ f **de gametos en las trompa** gamete intrafallopian transfer, GIFT;
~ f **genética** genetic transfer; ~ f **intratubaria de gametos** gamete intrafallopian transfer, GIFT; ~ f **intratubaria de zigotos** zygote intrafallopian transfer, ZIFT;
~ f **transplacentaria de gammaglobulina** gamma globulin transfer

transferibilidad f transferability

transferrina f transferrin

transformación f transformation

transformado m transformant

transfusión f transfusion; ~ f **de sangre** blood transfusion; ~ f **de sangre intrauterina** intrauterine blood transfusion

transgenética f transgenetics

transgénico, -ica adj transgenic

tránsito m intestinal intestinal transit

transitorio adj transitory, temporary, brief

translectura f readthrough

translocación f translocation; ~ f **bacteriana** bacterial translocation; ~ f **centrómero-telómero** centromere-telomere translocation; ~ f **de un gen** gene translocation, translocation of a gene; ~ f **de X-autosomas** X-autosome translocation

translucidez f transparency, translucence

transmisible adj communicable, contagious

transmisión f transmission, conduction; ~ f **aérea** airborne transmission; ~ f **de infección** transmission of infection; ~ f **del impulso nervioso** conduction of nerve impulses; ~ f **maternofilial** vertical transmission, mother-to-child transmission; ~ f **perinatal** transmission, vertical transmission, mother-to-child transmission; ~ f **sináptica de excitación** synaptic transmission of excitation; ~ f **vertical** transmission, vertical transmission, mother-to-child transmission

transmitancia f transmittance

transparencia f transparency, translucence

transparente adj transparent

transpeptidasa f transpeptidase

transpiración f perspiration, sweating

transplacentario adj transplacental, diaplacental

transplante m transplant; ~ m **alogénico** allograft, allogenic graft, allogenic transplant, homologous graft; ~ m **cardíaco** heart transplant, heart transplantation; ~ m **cardíaco-pulmonar** heart-lung transplant; ~ m **de médula ósea** bone marrow transplant; ~ m **hepático** liver transplant; ~ m **heterólogo** heterograft, heteroplasty; ~ m **homoplástico** homoioplastic transplant, homograft

transponible adj transponible

transportador m vehicle, base; ~ m **de dopamina** dopamine reuptake transporter

transporte m transport; ~ m **de pacientes** patient transport; ~ m **discreto** discrete transport

transposición f transposition immunity

transposón m transposon; ~ m **compuesto** composite transposon

transtiretina f transtyretin

transuretral adj transurethral, through the urine tube

tráquea f trachea, windpipe

traqueítis f tracheitis

traquelectomía f trachelectomy, cervicectomy

traqueomalacia f tracheomalacia

traqueotomía f tracheotomy, tracheostomy

traslación f **de mellas** nick translation

trasladar v to transfer

trasplantación f transplant; ~ f **de células de sangre periférico** peripheral blood stem cell transplant, PBSCT; ~ f **de la córnea** cornea transplant, corneal transplant

trasplante m transplantation, grafting; ~ m **autólogo** autologous transplantation; ~ m **de riñón** kidney transplant; ~ m **de un órgano** organ transplanation

trastorno m disturbance, disorder, derangement; ~ m **afectivo** affective disorder, mood disorder; ~ m **afectivo estacional** seasonal affective disorder, winter blues; ~ m **afectivo mayor** affective psychosis; ~ m **alimentar** eating disorder; ~ m **amnesico alcohólico** m alcohol amnesic disorder, cerebropathia psychica toxemica, Korsakoff's disease; ~ m **bipolar** bipolar disorder; ~ m **cervicobraquial laboral** cervicobrachial disorder, machinist's disease; ~ m **circulatorio** circulation problems, circulatory disorder; ~ m **cognitivo** cognitive dysfunction, cognitive disorder; ~ m **congénito del metabolismo** inborn metabolic disease; ~ m **de adaptación** reactive depression, adjustment disorder; ~ m **de déficit de atención** attention deficit disorder, attention deficit hyperactivity disorder, ADHD; ~ m **de humores** affective disorder, mood disorder; ~ m **de la audición** hearing disorder, defective hearing, auditory disorder, partial hearing loss; ~ m **de la memoria** memory disturbance, memory disorder, trouble remembering; ~ m **de la**

nutrición nutritional disturbance, dietary deficiency, nutritional disorder; ~ m **de la personalidad esquizotípica** borderline psychosis; ~ m **de los cromosomas** chromosome disorder, chromosomal abnormality; ~ m **del cerebro** brain damage brain dysfunction, intracranial disorder; ~ m **del desarrollo** developmental disorder, developmental disturbance; ~ m **del lenguaje** speech disorder, speech defect; ~ m **del metabolismo** metabolism misadaptive; ~ m **del sueño** sleep disorder, somnipathy, sleep disturbance; ~ m **mental** thought disorder, thinking disorder, mental retardation, mental disorder, feeblemindedness, dementia; ~ m **metabólico** metabolic disturbance; ~ m **muscular atrofico** atrophic muscular disorder, disuse atrophy; ~ m **neurológico** neurological disorder; ~ m **nutricional** nutritional disturbance, dietary deficiency, nutritional disorder; ~ m **obsesivo-compulsivo** obsessive-compulsive disorder, obsessive-compulsive psychoneurosis; ~ m **psicofisiológico** psychosomatic illness; ~ m **psicótico afectivo** affective psychosis; ~ m **visual** visual disturbance, defective vision

trasudado m transudate

tratamiento m treatment; ~ m **ambulatorio** outpatient clinic, ambulatory care, outpatient treatment, outpatient care; ~ m **antibiótico** antibiotic therapy; ~ m **antirretroviral** antiretroviral therapy; ~ m **de desinfección** disinfection treatment; ~ m **digitálico** digitalis therapy; ~ m **esclerosante de las varices** varicosclerosation; ~ m **intensivo** intensive therapy, intensive treatment; ~ m **médico** medical treatment; ~ m **obligatorio** compulsory treatment; ~ m **ortofónico** speech therapy, speech training; ~ m **paliativo** palliative therapy, palliative treatment, palliative care; ~ m **permanente de diabético** long-term treatment of diabetes; ~ m **por extensión** traction, extension treatment; ~ m **por oscilaciones de relajamiento** treatment by relaxation oscillations; ~ m **por perfusión** m infusion therapy; ~ m **postoperatorio** postoperative care,

postoperative treatment; ~ m **preventivo** preventive measures; ~ m **zootécnico** zootechnical treatment

tratar v to treat

trauma m physical trauma; ~ m **acústico** acoustic trauma, trauma from acoustic overload

traumático adj traumatic

traumatismo m lesion, injury, trauma, wound, affected area; ~ m **abdominal** abdominal trauma; ~ m **agudo** acute trauma; ~ m **cerebral** brain injury; ~ m **craneoencefálico** craniocerebral trauma; ~ m **del nacimiento** birth injury, birth trauma; ~ m **por esfuerzo** strain trauma

traumatología f traumatology

trazabilidad f traceability

trazador m tracer

trece adj thirteen

trecientos adj three hundred

treinta adj thirty

treonina f threonine

tres adj three; ~ **veces al día** t.i.d. (ter in die)

tretinoina f vitamin A acid

triacilglicerol-lipasa f triglyceride lipase

triazina f triazine

tricíclico adj tricyclic

triclorometano m chloroform, trichloromethane

tricomoniasis f trichomoniasis

triflupromazina f triflupromazine, a phenothiazine used as an antipsychotic agent or as an antiemetic

trifosfato m **de adenosina** adenosine triphosphate

triglicérido m triglyceride

trigo m wheat

trígono m **cerebral** fornix cerebri

triiodotironina f triiodothyronine, T3; ~ f **inversa** reverse triiodothyronine

trimepracina f trimeprazine, a phenothiazine derivative used as an antipruritic

trimetoprima f trimethoprim

tripanosoma m trypanosome, a protozoan blood parasite that causes African sleeping sickness and leishmaniasis

tripanosomiasis f trypanosomiasis, sleeping sickness, African sleeping sickness

tripsina f trypsin

tripsinógeno m trypsinogen, the inactive proenzyme of trypsin secreted by the pancreas

triptófano m tryptophan

triquina f trichinella spiralis, an intestinal roundworm

triquinosis f trichinosis

trismo f trismus, lockjaw, tetanus, gnathospasm

trisómico m trisomic, a person with Down syndrome

trivalente adj trivalent

tRNA m atransfer RNA; ~ m daptador adaptor RNA; ~ m cargado charged tRNA; ~ m cognado cognate tRNA

trocánter mayor greater trochanter

trocar m de Cushing Cushing trocar

trófico adj trophic, nutrition-related

trofismo m trophism

trofoblasto m trophoblast, outer layer of the blastocyst

trofozoíto m trophozoite

trolamina f triethanolamine

trombastenia f thrombasthenia, defective platelet aggregation

trombectomia f thrombectomy

trombidiosis f scrub itch, trombidiasis; ~ f fibrinogenase, thrombin

trombo m thrombus, blood clot, coagulum, ~ m esferico ball thrombus; ~ m oclusivo occlusive thrombus, obstructive thrombus

tromboangitis f thromboangiitis; ~ f obliterante thromboangiitis obliterans

trombocinasa f thrombokinase, factor xa, thromboplastin, prothrombinase

trombocitemia f hemorrágica esencial essential hemorrhagic thrombocythemia

trombocito m thrombocyte

trombocitopenia f thrombocytopaenia, low blood platelet count

trombocitosis f thrombocytosis, increased platelets in the blood

tromboembolismo m thromboembolism, blood clotting

tromboflebitis f thrombophlebitis, inflammation of a vein

trombólisis f thrombolysis, reabsorption of blood clots into bloodstream

trombolítico adj thrombolytic

tromboplastina f thrombokinase, factor xa, thromboplastin, prothrombinase; ~ f tisular tissue thromboplastin

trombosis f thrombosis; ~ f capilar capillary thrombosis; ~ f cerebral cerebral thrombosis; ~ f coronaria coronary thrombosis; ~ f del seno cavernoso cavernous sinus thrombosis; ~ f venosa profunda deep vein thrombosis, DVT

tromboxano m thromboxane; ~ ‑sintasa f thromboxane synthase

trompa f tube, conduct, mouth; ~ f de falopio fallopian tube

tronar v to crack, to pop

tronco encefálico brainstem, brain stem; ~ m simpático sympathetic trunk

troponina fT troponin T

trueno m popping, clicking; ~ m de una articulatión clicking of a joint

tu you, your

tus your

tubercular adj tubercular, nodular

tuberculina f tuberculin

tuberculización f de rutina tuberculin testing

tubérculo m tubercle

tuberculosis f tuberculosis; ~ f de los anexos adnexal tuberculosis; ~ f ganglionar lymph node tuberculosis; ~ f por deglución deglutition tuberculosis; ~ f pulmonar pulmonary tuberculosis

tuberculostático adj tuberculostatic, anti-TB medication

tuberosidad f tuberosity

tubo m tube, catheter; ~ m auditivo Eustachian tube; ~ m de ensayo test tube; ~ m de Eustaquio Eustachian tube; ~ m digestivo gastrointestinal tract, intestinal tract, alimentary canal; ~ m urinario urinary catheter

tubular adj tubular

tubulina f tubulin, an abundant cytoplasmic protein

túbulo m renal renal tubule

túbulos m pl uriniferos uriniferous tubules

tularemia f tularemia, rabbit fever, deer fly fever

tumefacción f extumescence, swelling,

tumefaction; ~ f acuosa hydroncus; ~ f del disco óptico papilledema, papilloedema, swollen optical disk; ~ f infecciosa swelling due to infection

tumescencia f pilosa hair bulge

tumor m tumor, neoplasm; ~ m benigno non-malignant tumor, benign tumor, neoplasm; ~ m carcinoide carcinoid tumor; ~ m cerebral brain tumor; ~ m coloide colloid tumor, myxoma, mucous tumor, collonema, gelatinous polyp, gelatinous tumor; ~ m de Burkitt Burkitt's lymphoma, non-Hodgkin's lymphoma caused by the Epstein-Barr virus; ~ m de Calabar calabar swelling; ~ m de células gigantes giant cell tumor; ~ m de los anejos adnexal tumor, adnexal mass; ~ m de Pancoast tumor of pulmonary sulcus, Pancoast's tumor; ~ m de transición transition tumor; ~ m del cerebro brain tumor; ~ m del mediastino mediastinal cancer, mediastinal neoplasm; ~ m en el sobaco tumor in the armpit; ~ m falso phantom tumor, pseudotumor, false tumor; ~ m fantasma phantom tumor, pseudotumor, false tumor; ~ m férreo Riedel's thyroiditis, iron-hard tumor, a rare fibrous induration of the thyroid gland; ~ m gelatinoso colloid tumor, myxoma, mucous tumor, collonema, gelatinous polyp, gelatinous tumor; ~ m mixto de glándulas salivares mixed tumor of salivary glands; ~ m mucoso colloid tumor, myxoma, mucous tumor, collonema, gelatinous polyp, gelatinous tumor; ~ m nocivo carcinoma, cancer; ~ m pigmentario pigmentary tumor, colored tumescence; ~ m testicular tumor of the testicle

tumoración f growths

tumorectomia f lumpectomy, tylectomy

tumorigénico adj tumorigenic, oncogenic, carcinogenic

tumoroso adj tumorous

túnel m carpiano carpal tunnel

tunelización f tunneling

túnica f tunica; ~ f adventicia tunica adventitia, tunica externa; ~ f intima tunica intima, the thin inner lining of blood vessels, consisting of endothelial cells

turbidimetría f turbidimetry, nephelometry

turgente adj distended, rounded swollen, bloated

turnover (inglés) turnove, renewal

U

ubiquitina f ubiquitin

úlcera f ulcer; ~ f anastomótica ulceration of anastomosis; ~ f crural ulcus cruris, foot ulcer; ~ f de estómago peptic ulcer, stomach ulcer; ~ f de la córnea corneal ulcer; ~ f duodenal duodenal ulcer; ~ f en la boca canker sore, aphthous ulcer; ~ f gástrica gastric ulcer; ~ f péptica peptic ulcer, stomach ulcer; ~ f por decúbito bedsore, decubitus ulcer, pressure sore; ~ f sifilítica syphilitic abscess, gummatous abscess

ulceración f ulceration; ~ f del tabique nasal ulceration of the nasal septum; ~ f chromique tanner's disease

ulcerógeno adj ulcerogenic, leading to the production of ulcers

ulcus (latín) ulcer

última f vez last time

último adj terminal

ultracentrifugación f ultracentrifugation

ultracentrifugadora f ultracentrifuge

ultraestructura f ultrastructure

ultrafiltración f ultrafiltration

ultrasonido m ultrasound; ~ m cardiaco cardiac ultrasound; ~ m transrectal transrectal ultrasound; ~ m transvaginal trans-vaginal ultrasound

ultrasonografía f ultrasound scanning, ultrasonography; ~ f Doppler Doppler ultrasonography

umbral m threshold; ~ m de consciencia threshold of consciousness; ~ m del dolor threshold of pain; ~ m discriminante discrimination threshold

un m, **una** f a, an; ~ **cuarto** quarter; ~ **poco a little**; ~ **tercio** m third (part)

uña f fingernail, toenail, unguis, nail; ~ f del pie encarnado ingrown toenail

una vez once

uñas f pl claws (animal term)

uncartrosis f uncarthrosis

undécimo eleventh

uñero m panarition, inflammation around the fingernail

ungüento m ointment; ~ m **para heridas** salve for wounds, ointment for wounds

único adj exclusive

unidad f unit; ~ f **de cuidado intensivo** intensive care unit, ICU; ~ f **de día** halfway house; ~ f **de digital** digitalis unit; ~ f **de ictus** stroke center; ~ f **de insulina** unit of insulin; ~ f **de masa atómica** atomic mass unit; ~ f **de medida** unit of measurement; ~ f **de prematuros** premature baby unit; ~ f **derivada** derived unit; ~ f **genética** genetic unit; ~ f **internacional** international unit, IU

uniforme adj homogeneous, uniform

unilateral adj unilateral, one-sided

unión f association; ~ f **a proteínas** protein binding; ~ f **cruzada** cross link, cross linking; ~ f **iónica** ionic bond, adsorption immobilization; ~ f **neuromuscular** neuromuscular junction, myoneural junction

uno adj one

unos, algún, algunos some

uracilo m uracil, the pyrimidine base from which uridine is derived

urato m urate

urato-oxidasa f urate oxidase

úrea f urea

ureasa f urease

uremia f uremia

uréter m ureter

uretra f urethra

uretritis f urethritis

urgencia f emergency

uricosúrico m uricosuric, drug to promote uric acid excretion

uridina f uridine, ribonucleoside formed when ribose & uracil combine

urinario m urinary

urobilinógeno m urobilinogen

urogenital adj urogenital, urinary and genital apparatus-related

urografía f excretion pyelography, urinary tract x-ray, pielography, ureteropyelography; ~ f **intravenosa** intravenous urography, excretory urography, intravenous pyelography

urología f urology

urólogo m urologist

uroporfirina f uroporphyrin

uroporfirinógeno-III-sintasa f uroporphyrinogen-III synthase

uropoyesis f uropoiesis, secretion of urine

uroquinasa f urokinase, an enzyme produced in the kidney that activates plasminogen, and that is used to dissolve blood clots

urticaria f hives, urticaria; ~ f **alérgica** allergic urticaria; ~ f **papular** strophulus, lichen urticatus, papular urticaria; ~ f **por esfuerzo** effort urticaria; ~ f **a frigore** congelation urticaria

urusiol m urushiol, an oily toxic irritant present in poison ivy

usar v to use

uso m use; ~ m **de tabaco** tobacco use

usted / Vd. (s, formal), ustedes / Vds. (p, formal) you

usualmente usually

útero m uterus, womb

utilizar v to use

utrículo m utricle (of the inner ear)

uva f grape

úvea f **del ojo** uvea

uveítis f uveitis, inflammation of the uvea

úvula f uvula

V

vaccinia f vaccinia

vacuna f vaccine, inoculation, shot; ~ f **antigripal** influenza vaccine, flu vaccine, antiinfluenza vaccine; ~ f **anti-paratífico** paratyphus vaccine; ~ f **anti-peste** swine fever vaccine; ~ f **antitetánica** tetanus vaccine, tetanus shot; ~ f **atenuada** attenuated vaccine, attenuated-virus vaccine; ~ f **BCG** BCG vaccination; ~ f **con células diploides humanas** human diploid cell vaccine; ~ f **conjugada** conjugated vaccine; ~ f **contra la polio** polio vaccine, poliomyelitis

vaccine; ~ f **contra la tuberculosis**
tuberculosis vaccine; ~ f **contra la varicela**
chickenpox vaccine, varicella vaccine;
~ f **contra las paperas** mumps vaccine; ~ f **de
viruela** smallpox vaccine; ~ f **oral** oral
vaccine; ~ f **recombinante** recombinant
vaccine; ~ f **viva recombinante** recombinant
live vaccine

vacunación f vaccination, immunization; ~ f **de
emergencia** emergency vaccination, ring
vaccination; ~ f **de urgencia** emergency
vaccination, ring vaccination; ~ f **preventiva**
prophylactic inoculation; ~ f **sistemática**
routine vaccination

vacunar v to inoculate, to vaccinate

vacunas f pl shots

vacuola f vacuole; ~ f **contráctil** contractile
vacuole

vacuolación f vacuolation

vagal adj vagal, pertaining to the vagus nerve

vagina f vagina

vaginal adj vaginal

vaginismo m vaginal spasm, vaginismus

vaginitis f vaginitis, colpitis, inflammation of
the vaginal mucosa; ~ f **adhesiva** adhesive
colpitis, adhesive vaginitis; ~ f **micótica**
colpitis mycotica, vaginal yeast infection;
~ f **senil** adhesive colpitis, adhesive vaginitis

vaginosis f vaginosis; ~ f **bacteriana** bacterial
vaginosis

vagolítico adj vagolytic

vagotomía f vagotomy, surgical division of the
vagus nerve

vagotonía f vagotonia, hyperexcitability of the
vagus nerve

vahído m vertigo, dizziness

vahidos m pl heart palpitation, cardiac
palpitation, heart throb

vaina f sheathing, involucrum; ~ f **de mielina**
myeline sheath; ~ f **del recto** rectal sheath

vainas f pl **protectoras del folículo** epithelial
hair sheaths

valentón m bully

valeriana m valerian

validez f validity

valina f valine

Valium m Valium

valor m value; ~ m **aberrante** outlier value;
~ m **asignado** assigned value, target value;
~ m **biológico límite** biological limit value;
~ m **certificado** certificate value;
~ m **consensual** consensus value; ~ m **de
captación estándar** standard uptake value,
suv; ~ m **de referencia** reference value;
~ m **definitivo** definitive value; ~ m **del
blanco** blank value; ~ m **discriminante** cut-
off point; ~ m **globular** blood count quotient;
~ m **numérico** numerical value;
~ m **predictivo** predictive value;
~ m **predictivo de un resultado negativo**
negative predictive value; ~ m **predictivo de
un resultado positivo** positive predictive
value; ~ m **semiológico** semeiologic value;
~ m **verdadero** true value

valoración f titration; ~ f **ética** ethical
evaluation

valores m pl **de referencia** normal values

valorización f assessment, evaluation

valva f **pulmonaria** pulmonic valve, pulmonary
valve, pulmonary semilunar valve

válvula f valvule, small valve; ~ f **cardiaca** heart
valve; ~ f **cardiaca de origen animal**
bioprosthetic heart valve; ~ f **pulmonar**
pulmonic valve, pulmonary valve, pulmonary
semilunar valve; ~ f **tricúspide** tricuspid valve
(between right atrium & right ventricle of
heart)

valvuloplastia f pulmonary valvuloplasty,
pulmonic valvuloplasty; ~ f **cardíaca** cardiac
valvuloplasty, surgery on a heart valve

vancomicina f vancomycin

vanguardia f cutting edge, on the forefront,
avant-garde

variabilidad f variability; ~ f **biológica**
biological variability; ~ f **genética** genetic
variability; ~ f **metrológica** metrological
variability

variable f variable; ~ f **experimental**
experimental variable, observable variable

variación f variation; ~ f **biológica** biological
variation; ~ f **fisiológica** physiological
variation

variado adj multiple

variancia f variance

várice f varicose vein

varicela f chickenpox (varicella), varicela

várices f pl varix, varicose veins;
~ f esofagicas esophageal varices

varicosidad f varicosity, varicose condition

varix m varix, varicose veins

varón adj masculine, male

varonil adj virile, manly

vascular adj vascular, pertaining to the blood vessels

vascularización f vascularization

vasculitis f vasculitis, blood vessel inflammation (small vessels)

vasectomía f vasectomy

vaselina f vaseline; ~ f en bruto crude petroleum jelly, petrolatum; ~ f purificada refined petroleum jelly, vaseline

vaso m glass; ~ m capilar sanguíneo blood capillary; ~ m sanguíneo ocluido occluded blood vessel

vasoactivo adj vasoactive, affecting the blood vessels

vasoconstricción f vasoconstriction, narrowing of the small arteries; ~ f arterial arterial vasoconstriction

vasoconstrictores m pl vasoconstrictive agents, vasoconstrictors

vasodilatación f vasodilatation, widening of the blood vessels

vasodilatador m vasodilator; ~ m directo direct vasodilator

vasomotor m vasomotor, pertaining to blood blood flow

vasoparálisis f vasoparalysis

vasoplegia f vasoparalysis

vasopresina f vasopressin, adiuretin

vasopresor m vasopressor, substance affecting blood flow

vaso m vessel

vasos m pl sanguíneos blood vessels

vávula f mitral mitral valve

vecino m neighbor

vectocardiograma m vectorcardiogram

vector m vector; ~ m adenoviral adenoviral vector, adenoviral construct; ~ m de enfermedad disease vector, carrier of infection; ~ m genético genetic carrier, gene vector; ~ m por sustitución replacement

vector; ~ m recuperador retriever vector;
~ m transportador shuttle vector

vegetativo adj vegetative, without consciousness

vehículo m carrier, vehicle of infection transmission, excipient; ~ m de transmisión de la infección carrier, vehicle of infection transmission

veinte adj twenty

vejamen m annoyance

vejez f senility, old age

vejiga f blister, bulla, bleb, pomphus, bladder, vesicle; ~ f aneurismal aneurysmal bladder;
~ f aneurismática aneurysmal bladder;
~ f urinaria urinary bladder

vello m body hair; ~ m pubiano pubic hair, pubic hairs

vellosidades f pl coriónicas chorionic villi, chorial villosities

velocidad f speed, velocity; ~ f de filtración glomerular glomerular filtration rate; ~ f de procesamiento input rate; ~ f de reacción rate of reaction; ~ f de transformación rate of conversion

vena f vein; ~ f cefálica cephalic vein;
~ f safena saphenous vein; ~ f trabecular trabecular vein; ~ f yugular jugular vein

venas f pl varicosas

venda f bandage, surgical dressing;
~ f adhesiva adhesive bandage, sterile strip, adhesive dressing, finger dressing; ~ f de gasa para apósito gauze strip for bandages;
~ f elástica elastic bandage, Ace bandage

vendaje m dressing; ~ m abdominal abdominal bandage, abdominal belt, binder;
~ m adhesivo adhesive bandage, sterile strip, adhesive dressing, finger dressing;
~ m enyesado plaster cast (on a limb);
~ m para la hernia hernial truss, hernia bandage; ~ m tubular stockinet, tubular gauze

veneno m toxin, poison; ~ m de serpiente snake venom

venenoso adj toxic; ~ adj para el feto toxic to the fetus

venéreo adj venereal, sexually transmitted

venir v come, to

venombina f venombin, a thrombin-like enzyme from the venom of snakes of the viper/

rattlesnake group

venoso adj venous, pertaining to the veins

ventaja f advantage

ventana f window; ~ f **aórtica** aortic window;
~ f **mediastínica** mediastinal window;
~ f **pulmonar** pulmonary window, aortic septal defect, aortopulmonary window

ventanilla f nostril, nostrils

ventilación f ventilation, breathing; ~ f **máxima voluntaria** maximum voluntary ventilation, MVV, maximum breathing capacity, MBC;
~ f **pulmonar** pulmonary ventilation

ventral adj ventral, pertaining to the belly

ventricular adj ventricular, pertaining to a small cavity

ventrículo m ventricle; ~ m **cardiaco** ventricle of heart; ~ m **lateral** lateral ventricle, a cavity in each cerebral hemisphere

ventriculografía f ventriculogram, ventriculography; ~ f **cerebral** cerebral ventriculography

ver v to see; ~ v **puntos luminosos** flickering of the visual image

veracidad f trueness

verano m summer

verde adj green

verdolaga f purslane

verdugo m welt (on the skin), wea

verdugón m welt (on the skin), weal

verduras f pl vegetables

vergencia f **fusional** fusional vergence, fusional movement

vergüenza f shame

vergüenzas f pl private parts, genitalia, genitals

verijas f pl pubic region, groin

verosimilitud f plausibility, credibility, probability; ~ f **biológica** biological plausibility

verruga f wart; ~ f **común** common wart, verruca vulgaris; ~ f **plantar** plantar wart

verrugas f pl **genitales** genital warts, fig wart, condyloma acuminatum

vértebra f vertebra; ~ f **cervical** cervical vertebra; ~ f **lumbar transicional** transitional lombosacral vertebra

vertebral adj vertebral

vértebras f pl vertebrae; ~ f pl **cervicales** cervical vertebrae; ~ f pl **dorsales** thoracic vertebrae; ~ f pl **lumbares** lumbar vertebrae

vértigo m dizziness, vertigo, altitude sickness; ~ m **ocular** ocular vertigo

vesical adj vesical

vesícula f blister, bulla, bleb, pomphus, vesicle; ~ f **biliar** gall bladder; ~ f **de sangre** blood blister, blood bleb; ~ f **seminal** seminal vesicle

vesicular adj vesicular

vesículas f pl **de eccema** eczema vesicles

vestibular adj vestibular, pertaining to the space or cavity at the entrance to a canal

vestigial adj vestigial, greatly reduced from the original ancestral form and no longer functional

vestigio m **embrionario** embryonic vestige

vestimenta f **para quirófano** surgeon's gown, operating room gown

vestirse v to dress

vetas f pl linea albicante, stretch marks, striae atrophicae, striae cutis distensae

veteaduras f pl linea albicante, stretch marks, striae atrophicae, striae cutis distensae

veterinario m veterinarian, vet

vetusto adj decrepit, to be worn out, feeble, infirm, sickly, doddering

vía tract, via, channel, passage, conduit;
~ f **alternativa** alternative pathway; ~ f **biliar** bile duct, biliary duct; ~ f **catabólica** catabolic pathway; ~ f **clásica** classical pathway; ~ f **de la síntesis metabólica de lípidos** metabolic lipid synthesis pathway

vial m cartridge, vial, small bottle

vías f pl ways; ~ f pl **aerodigestivas** upper airways; ~ f pl **eferentes** efferent path;
~ f pl **respiratorias** respiratory system, airways; ~ f pl **urinarias** urinary tract

víbora f viper

vibraciones f pl **bronquiales** bronchial fremitus; ~ f pl **vocales** vocal fremitus

vibrador m vibro-massage machine, vibrator, vibratory-massage devic

vicio m bad habit, addiction, craving

víctima f **de un accidente de trabajo** victim of an accident at work

vida f life; ~ f **afectiva** emotional life;
~ f **media** half-life, mean life

video-cirugía f video surgery, videosurgery

viejo adj old

viento *m* fart, wind, expelled gas, flatus

vientre *m* abdomen, gut, stomach;
~ **hinchado** swollen abdomen, swollen belly

viernes *m* Friday

vigilancia *f* vigilance, surveillance, observation;
~ *f* **de guardia** sentinel health event, sentinel surveillance; ~ *f* **de la glucosa sanguínea** blood glucose monitoring, blood glucose measuring; ~ *f* **nutricional** nutritional surveillance

vigilar *v* to monitor, to observe

vigilia *f* vigilance; ~ *f* **anormal** insomnia, sleeplessness

VIH *m* HIV

vinagre *m* vinegar

vinculación *f* **afectiva** emotional bonding, affective rapport

vínculo *m* **ser humano-animal** human-pet bonding, emotional attachment of humans and pets

vino *m* wine

vinorelbina *f* vinorelbine

vinorelbina *f* nevirapine, Viramune

viola *f* viola

violación *f* rape, violation; ~ *f* **conyugal** marital rape; ~ *f* **de menores** statutory rape

violencia *f* violence; ~ *f* **doméstica** domestic violence, family violence; ~ *f* **sexual** sexual assault, sexual violence

virago *f* virago, masculine woman

viral *adj* viral

Viramune *f* nevirapine, Viramune

viremia *f* viremia

virgen *f* virgin

viril *adj* virile, manly

virilismo *m* virilism, masculinity

virilización *f* virilization, masculinization

virión *m* viral particle, virion

viroide *m* viroid

viruela *f* cowpox, vaccinia, smallpox; ~ *f* **loca** chicken pox

virulencia *f* virulence, ability of a pathogenic organism to cause disease

virus *m* virus; ~ *m* **cancerígeno** carcinogenic virus; ~ *m* **circulante** circulating virus;
~ *m* **Coxsackie** Coxsackie virus; ~ *m* **de Epstein-Barr** Epstein-Barr virus; ~ *m* **de la fiebre Dengue** dengue fever virus, dengue virus; ~ *m* **de la hepatitis A** hepatitis A virus;
~ *m* **de la hepatitis D** hepatitis D virus,

hepatitis delta virus; ~ *m* **de la inmunodeficiencia humana** immunodeficiency virus, HIV; ~ *m* **de la parainfluenza humana** human parainfluenza virus, ~ *m* **de la parotiditis** mumps virus;
~ *m* **de la rabia** rabies virus; ~ *m* **de la varicela** varicella-zoster virus; chickenpox virus; ~ *m* **de las paperas** mumps virus;
~ *m* **defectuoso** defective virus; ~ *m* **del molusco contagioso** molluscum contagiosum virus; ~ *m* **del sarampión** measles virus;
~ *m* **ébola** Ebola virus; ~ *m* **Hantaan** hantavirus, Hantaan virus; ~ *m* **Lassa** Lassa virus, a member of Arenaviridae;
~ *m* **oncogénico** oncogenic virus, tumor virus, oncovirus; ~ *m* **papova humano** human papiloma virus; ~ *m* **respiratorio sincitial** respiratory syncytial virus, chimpanzee coryza agent; ~ *m* **varicella-zóster** varicella-zoster virus; chickenpox virus

visceral *adj* visceral

visceroptosis *f* visceroptosis

viscosidad *f* viscosity, thickness of a liquid;
~ *f* **de la sangre** blood viscosity viscosity, thickening of blood

visible *adj* manifest, visible, evident

visión *f* vision; ~ *f* **amarillenta** xanthopsia, yellow vision; ~ *f* **bizcada** amblyopia, lazy eye syndrome; ~ *f* **borrosa** blurred vision, blurry vision; ~ *f* **doble** diplopia, double vision;
~ *f* **negra** blackout, seeing black, fainting, losing consciousness; ~ *f* **reducida** amblyopia, lazy eye syndrome

visita *f* **médica preventiva** screening, preventive medical checkup, prophylactic medical examination

vista *f* sight, ability to see; ~ *f* **corta** myopia, near-sightedness, short-sighted;
~ *f* **empañada** blurred vision, blurry vision

visual *adj* visual

visualizar *v* to display, to show

vitalidad *f* vitality

vitamina *f* vitamin; ~ *f* **B1** thiamine, vitamin B1, aneurin; ~ *f* **B9** folic acid, pteroyl glutamic acid, folacin, vitamin B9; ~ *f* **B12** cobalamin, vitamin B12, cyanocobalamin, anti-pernicious

factor, animal protein factor, APF; ~ f **C** f
vitamin C, ascorbic acid; ~ f **D** f **(calciferol)**
vitamin D (calciferol); ~ f **D3** vitamine D3;
~ f **H** biotin, vitamine H
vitiligo m vitiligo, skin disorder with blotchy
skin due to a loss of pigmentation
vitrectomía f vitrectomy, removal of all or part
of the vitreous body
vítreo adj vitreous, glassy
viuda f, **viudo** m widow / widower
viudo adj widowed
vivo adj alive
volátil adj volatile
volt m volt
volumen m volume; ~ m **de gaz intratorácico**
thoracic gas volume; ~ m **de reserva**
espiratoria expiratory reserve volume; ~ m **de**
ventilación pulmonar tidal volume,
respiratory volume; ~ m **diastólico** diastolic
volume, diastolic filling; ~ m **eritrocítico**
medio average erythrocyte volume;
~ m **específico** specific volume;
~ m **expiratorio forzado** expiratory volume (in
one second); ~ m **minuto del corazón** cardiac
output, cardiac pressure output, cardiac
minute ouput; ~ m **molar** molar volume;
~ m **sanguíneo** vascular volume, blood
volume; ~ m **sistólico** systolic volume, stroke
volume
volumetría f volumetry
volúmico, -ica adj-ica volumic
voluntario adj voluntary
voluntario,-a m/f volunteer
volver v to return; ~ v **en sí conocimiento** to
regain consciousness, to come to
consciousness
vólvulo m ileocecal twisted intestine
vomitar v to be nauseated, to throw up, to
vomit
vómito m emesis, vomiting, vomitus;
~ m **acetonémico** acetonemic vomiting, cyclic
vomiting; ~ m **de sangre** hematemesis,
vomiting blood; ~ m **negro** black vomit
vórtice m vortex
vosotros m pl, **-as** f pl **(fam)** you
voz f voice
vuelta f **superhelicoidal** superhelical turn
vuestro m, **-a** f, **vuestros** m pl, **-as** fp your

vulva f vulva
vulvar adj vulval
vulvitis f vulvitis
vulvovaginitis f vulvovaginitis, vaginal
inflammation; ~ f **por Candida** vulvovaginal
candidiasis

W

warfarina f warfarin
watt m watt

X

xantina f xanthin; ~ **–oxidasa** f xanthine
oxidase
xantoma m xanthoma, fatty skin tumour
xantomatosis f xanthomatosis; ~ f **de la**
córnea xanthomatosis corneae, dystrophia
adiposa corneae, steatosis corneae
xantopsia f xanthopsia, yellow vision
xenobiótico m xenobiotic
xenodiagnóstico m xenodiagnosis
xenogénico m xenogenic, heterologous
xenotrasplante m xenograft, heterologous
transplant, xenotransplant
xeroderma f xeroderma
xeroftalmía f xerophthalmia, dry eyes
xerostomía f xerostomia, dry mouth
xilometazolina f xylometazoline, a
sympathomimetic agent used as a nasal
decongestant
xilosa f xylose
xister m xyster, raspatory, rugine

Y

y and
yatrogénico iatrogenic, due to the activity of a
physician or therapy
yema f **del dedo** fingertip
Yersinia f **pestis** Yersinia pestis
yeso m cast, plaster of Paris
yeyuno m jejunum, part of the small intestine

yeyunoileostomía f jejunoileostomy
yodato m **de calcio** calcium iodate
yodo m iodine
yoduración f iodization, iodine disinfection
yoduro m iodide; ~ m **de plata** silver iodide;
  ~ m **de sodio** sodium iodide; ~ m **potásico**
  potassium iodide; ~ m **radiactivo** radioiodine,
  radioactive iodine
yogur m yogurt

Z

zalenquear v to limp, to hobble
zalzitabina f zalcitabine, dideoxycitidine
zanahoria f carrot
zanamivir m Relenza, Zanamivir
zapato m shoe; ~ m **ortopédico** orthopedic
  shoe
zarpa f paw, foot (animal term)
zeaxantina f zeaxanthin, E161h, a carotinoid
zidovudina f zidovudine
zigótico adj zygotic
zigoto m zygote, fertilized ovum
zimógeno m proenzyme, zymogen
zimógenos m pl zymogenic bacteria
zimótico adj zymotic, pertaining to
  fermentation
zinc m zinc
zona f domain; ~ f **cardiaca** cardiac region,
  cardiac zone; ~ f **de excitabilidad
  aumentada** trigger zone; ~ f **postal** zip code,
  postal code; ~ f **tropical** tropical area
zoonosis f zoonosis, diseases communicable
  from vertebrate animals to humans, epizootic
zooterapia f zootherapy, pet therapy; ~ f **de
  oído** tinnitus, buzzing, ringing in the ears
zumbidos m pl buzzing, ringing in the ears,
  tinnitus
zurdo adj left, left-handed

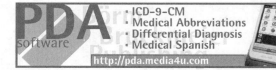

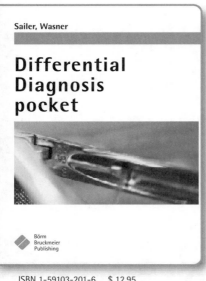

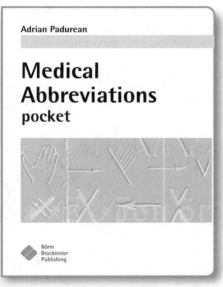

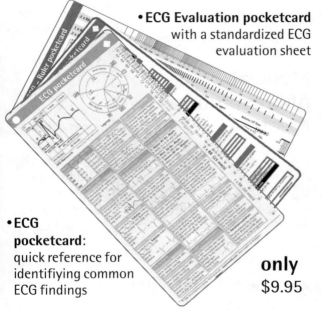

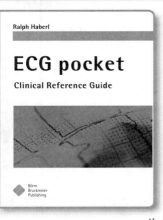
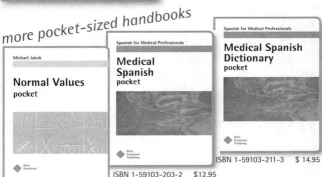

Börm Bruckmeier pockets

Additional Titles in this series:
Differential Diagnosis pocket
Drug pocket 2003
Drug Therapy pocket
ECG pocket
Homeopathy pocket
Medical Abbreviations pocket
Medical Spanish pocket
Medical Spanish pocket plus
Normal Values pocket

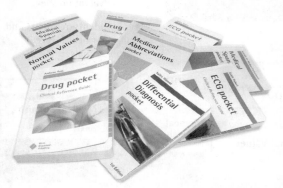

For students, residents and all other health care professionals